D0025723

DISEASES

of the

HUMAN BODY

6TH EDITION

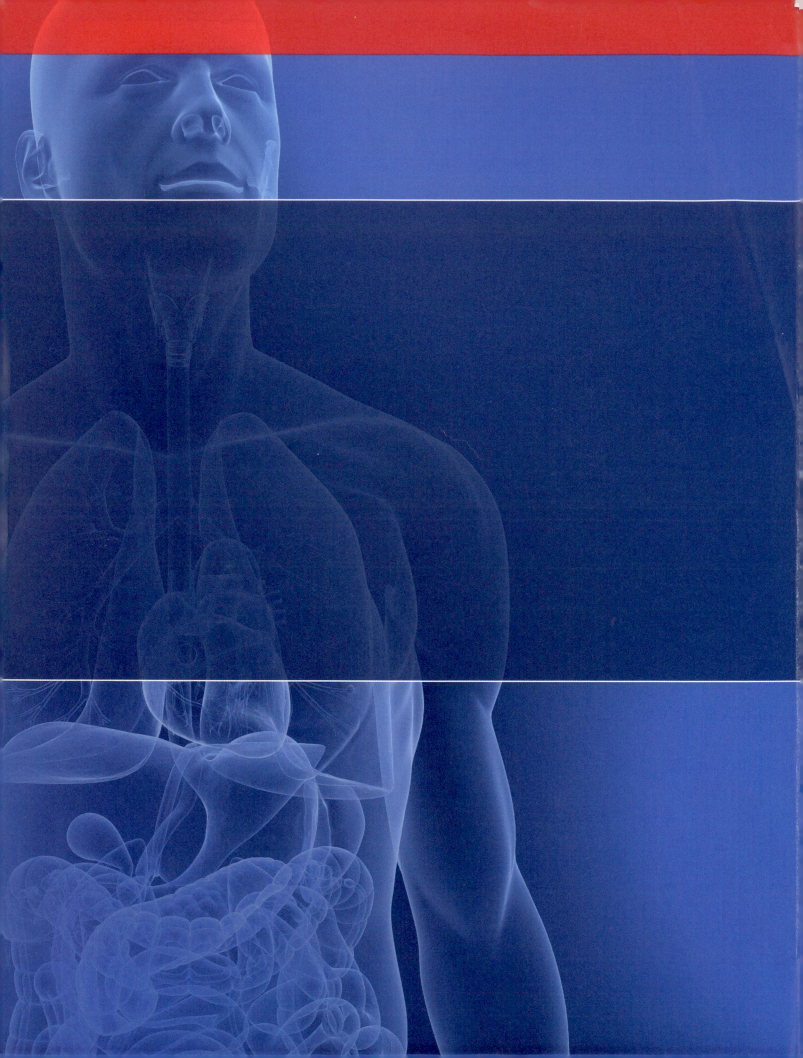

DISEASES
of the
HUMAN
BODY

6TH EDITION

CAROL D. TAMPARO, PhD, CMA-A (AAMA)
Formerly Dean of Business and Allied Health
Lake Washington Institute of Technology
Kirkland, Washington
Coordinator, Medical Assistant Program
Highline Community College
Des Moines, Washington

F.A. Davis Company • Philadelphia

F.A. Davis Company
1915 Arch Street
Philadelphia, PA 19103
www.fadavis.com

Copyright © 2016 by F.A. Davis Company

Copyright © 2016 by F.A. Davis Company. All rights reserved. This product is protected by copyright. No part of it may be reproduced, stored in a retrieval system, or transmitted in any form or by any means, electronic, mechanical, photocopying, recording, or otherwise, without written permission from the publisher.

Printed in the United States of America

Last digit indicates print number: 10 9 8 7 6 5 4 3 2 1

Senior Acquisitions Editor: Andy McPhee
Developmental Editor: Donna Morrissey
Director of Content Development: George Lang
Art and Design Manager: Carolyn O'Brien

As new scientific information becomes available through basic and clinical research, recommended treatments and drug therapies undergo changes. The author(s) and publisher have done everything possible to make this book accurate, up to date, and in accord with accepted standards at the time of publication. The author(s), editors, and publisher are not responsible for errors or omissions or for consequences from application of the book, and make no warranty, expressed or implied, in regard to the contents of the book. Any practice described in this book should be applied by the reader in accordance with professional standards of care used in regard to the unique circumstances that may apply in each situation. The reader is advised always to check product information (package inserts) for changes and new information regarding dose and contraindications before administering any drug. Caution is especially urged when using new or infrequently ordered drugs.

Library of Congress Cataloging-in-Publication Data

Names: Tamparo, Carol D., 1940- author.
Title: Diseases of the human body / Carol D. Tamparo.
Description: Sixth edition. | Philadelphia, PA : F.A. Davis Company, [2016] |
  Includes bibliographical references and index.
Identifiers: LCCN 2015048556 | ISBN 9780803644519
Subjects: | MESH: Disease | Internal Medicine | Handbooks
Classification: LCC RC46 | NLM WB 39 | DDC 616—dc23 LC record available at
http://lccn.loc.gov/2015048556

Authorization to photocopy items for internal or personal use, or the internal or personal use of specific clients, is granted by F.A. Davis Company for users registered with the Copyright Clearance Center (CCC) Transactional Reporting Service, provided that the fee of $.25 per copy is paid directly to CCC, 222 Rosewood Drive, Danvers, MA 01923. For those organizations that have been granted a photocopy license by CCC, a separate system of payment has been arranged. The fee code for users of the Transactional Reporting Service is: 978-0-8036-4451-9/16 0 + $.25.

DEDICATION

There are so many individuals and so many experiences that bring me to this edition. I wish to express my gratitude and give recognition to those who had such a powerful influence on my life and have brought me to this place as an author.

There was the Alliance High School teacher in Northwestern Nebraska who triggered my passion for writing and editing the school newspaper. In the same school, the English teacher taught me the value of good grammar, which was stressed even more by shorthand classes in both high school and at the University of Wyoming where I earned a BS in Secretarial Science/Business Administration.

Blue Mountain Community College in Pendleton, Oregon, gave me my first teaching position—the first quarter teaching all levels of typewriting on about five different manual typewriters. (Oh how the world has changed.) In Des Moines, Washington, the Highline Community College Dean of Occupational Education gave me the opportunity to build the Medical Assistant program, furnish the classroom and clinic environment, and support the program through its first and many subsequent national accreditations through Commission on Accreditation of Allied Health Education Programs CAAHEP) and the American Association of Medical Assisting (AAMA).

Teaching classes in the Medical Assistant program at that time required writing much of my own material. That led to a lasting friendship with Marti Lewis, another instructor in the field, dealing with similar issues. Thus, the first edition of the *Law and Ethics in the Medical Office* was created. Later we wrote *Diseases of the Human Body* so medical assisting students would better understand the diseases process. Here you have the 6th edition of that text. Together Marti and I taught and mentored hundreds of students, struggled through our doctoral programs, shared meals with our families at home and on the Oregon coast, and along the way became closer than most sisters. I still miss her.

From early years, my parents stressed that I could do about anything I set my mind to. I am so grateful to their encouragement. I am forever indebted to those who believed I could teach, to those who believed I could write, to F.A. Davis and Robert Martone who saw potential in that first book and a future in medical assisting for their company, and to Andy McPhee, Senior Acquisitions Editor at F.A. Davis who is a champion for health-care textbooks, and has also become a good friend.

I am so blessed to share it all with my husband and my daughters and to have had such a cherished friend as a co-author.

What I am today is because of all of you. I am eternally thankful. I dedicate this edition to you!

—CAROL D. TAMPARO, PhD, CMA (AAMA)
ctamparo@comcast.net

PREFACE

This totally new and completely updated text provides clear, succinct, and basic information about common medical conditions. *Diseases of the Human Body,* 6th edition, is carefully designed to meet the unique educational and professional needs of health-care personnel. The book focuses on human diseases and disorders that are frequently first diagnosed or treated in ambulatory health care. Each entry considers what the disease or disorder is, how it might be diagnosed and treated, and the likely consequences of the disease or disorder for the person experiencing it.

Chapters 1 through 7 provide a solid foundation for subsequent chapters and include:

- The Disease Process
- Integrative Medicine and Complementary Therapies
- Pain and Its Management
- Infectious and Communicable Diseases
- Cancer
- Congenital Diseases and Disorders
- Mental Health Diseases and Disorders

The remaining 10 chapters cover major conditions organized by body system. This pattern of organization is easily integrated with medical terminology or anatomy and physiology courses that health-care professional students often take concurrently with the study of human disease. Within each system chapter, there is an anatomy and physiology review of that system for further assistance. Each disease condition is highlighted by means of a logical, nine-part format consisting of:

- Description
- Etiology
- Signs and Symptoms
- Diagnostic Procedures
- Treatment
- Complementary Therapy
- Client Communication
- Prognosis
- Prevention

The balance of information in each of these subsections varies according to the relative frequency and severity of the condition. In every case, the information selected is chosen to reflect the need for thorough yet concise information about the condition.

Research for this edition indicates that alternative and complementary therapies are now more often viewed as "integrative medicine," providing the best of both traditional and complementary therapies for treating clients. Viable complementary or alternative therapy was included when documentation was found regarding effectiveness and lack of harm.

The organization of the text is thoroughly contemporary and designed to help you retain and understand basic concepts within the context of your chosen profession. Color in the interior further enhances its appeal. Features include clear chapter outlines, chapter learning outcomes that can be easily matched to questions in the electronic test bank, pronunciation of key terms, review questions, and case studies to encourage critical thinking. Client Communication sections will remind you to think about teaching opportunities for your clients. You will also find reference to the most common "reportable diseases" as required by state and/or federal government. This feature prompts you to recall your reporting responsibility.

The "Chapter Episode" feature makes a particular disease or disorder very personal and asks you to respond to related questions at the end of each episode. The episode appears at the beginning of the chapter and is further explained throughout the chapter, becoming more complex each time. There also is a Reality Episode in each chapter as well as accompanying questions. Answers to the episode questions, review questions, and case studies are found in the Instructor's Guide to this textbook. Throughout the text, carefully chosen illustrations help you visualize body structures and conditions.

The sixth edition provides the International Classification of Diseases, 10th revision, Clinical Modification (ICD-10-CM) codes for each disease. This valuable tool reinforces the importance of proper coding for reimbursement and research. See the note at the end of this preface regarding this update on coding.

The comprehensive glossary appears at the end of the text, using *Taber's Cyclopedic Medical Dictionary,* 22nd edition, as the main reference. The appendices include succinct descriptions of most of the diagnostic procedures mentioned in the text and a comprehensive list of over 200 commonly used abbreviations, along with a reference list that includes Internet sites. These features help make *Diseases of the Human Body*, 6th edition, a valuable classroom text and a useful reference after you begin your professional career. Finally, in addition to a general subject index, a specialized index of diseases covered in this text directs the reader to the nine-part presentation of each disease covered.

Herman cartoons, a special favorite of the author, provide a little levity to what can be "worrisome" topics of disease. Jim Unger, their creator, has a unique understanding of human nature, of life, and of all its travails. We hope you will giggle and even laugh out loud. Such "internal jogging" is good for the soul.

The study of human disease is never easy. Every effort has been made to make it clear and accessible by presenting information to benefit both students and health-care professionals. Students will be able to access many online ancillary pieces to enhance their study and learning process. There are numerous interactive exercises that include case studies, and 17 podcasts can be downloaded for listening and review. New to this edition is the inclusion of nine videos that illustrate one or more applications of the chapter content. These resources are available at http://davisplus.fadavis.com (keyword *Tamparo*). Twice yearly, updated information on diseases and disorders is provided on Davis*Plus* by F.A. Davis. To assist instructors, there is an Instructor's Guide, an electronic test bank, and PowerPoint presentations, which are available to adopters.

—Carol D. Tamparo

ICD-10-CM

The implementation of ICD-10-CM occurred October 1, 2015. After many extensions granted by the U.S. Department of Health and Human Services (HHS), the transition from ICD-9-CM to the new ICD-10-CM code set became a reality.

The implementation of ICD-10-CM coding expanded the ICD-9-CM codes from approximately 17,000 codes to approximately 69,000 in the ICD-10-CM. The increase is due to the greater level of specificity in the coding process. More extensive and accurate documentation is necessary to be able to code to the highest level of specificity. ICD-10-CM is an alphanumeric classification system that has been expanded from five to seven characters. ICD-10-CM uses the letter "X" as a placeholder to allow for expansions in the future. This placeholder is used in the fifth, sixth, and seventh character positions. ICD-10-CM has been used in other countries for many years. Once the United States adopted ICD-10-CM coding, we are now able to compare health data and statistics worldwide. Proponents of ICD-10-CM state that areas such as public health, research, and reimbursement will greatly benefit from using the new codes.

The health-care industry has taken many steps in preparation for the conversion to ICD-10-CM. System updates needed to be installed to be compatible with the new format. Changes were necessary on any forms that previously utilized ICD-9-CM. Internal and external testing was conducted to ensure payers are able to receive data with ICD-10-CM codes. Training on the new coding system was offered in various formats. Online courses, seminars, and boot camps were just some of the options in becoming proficient in ICD-10-CM. Several studies predict a shortage of coders in the next several years. This is a great opportunity for anyone interested in a career as a certified coding professional.

I would like to take this opportunity to thank my mentor, Richard K. Brown, for his willingness to share his skills, knowledge, and expertise.

—Donna Firn, CPC, CMA (AAMA), CRCS-I
Masters of Arts in Counseling Psychology
Kitsap Mental Health Services
Bremerton, Washington

CONTRIBUTORS

JENNIFER T. DAVIS, BSN, RN, CBC
Medical Assisting Program Director
Harcum College
Bryn Mawr, Pennsylvania
NICU RN and ECMO Specialist
St. Christopher's Hospital for Children
Philadelphia, Pennsylvania
Jennifertdavisrn@verizon.net

DONNA M. FIRN, CPC, CMA (AAMA), CRCS-I
Medical Assisting Clinical Coordinator
Harcum College
Bryn Mawr, Pennsylvania

MARTIANN C. LEWIS, MA, LMHC
Lewis and Clark College
Portland, Oregon

REVIEWERS

LISA MICHELLE BAKER, BS, CMA
Medical Office Administration
Forsyth Tech Community College
Winston-Salem, North Carolina

TRICIA BERRY, PhD, MATL, OTR/L
Medical Assisting
Kaplan University
Chicago, Illinois

DARLENE BOSCHERT, RHIA, CPC, COC, CPC-I
Medical Programs
Bayside Medical Consultants
Holiday, Florida

JENNIFER BOYER, CMA (AAMA), AAT
Medical Assisting
Lanier Technical College
Oakwood, Georgia

SONYA M. BURNS, BBA, RHIA, CMA (AAMA)
Allied Health Sciences and Nursing
Augusta Technical College
Augusta, Georgia

WILLIAM TRAVIS BUTLER, MHA
Health Science
ECPI University
Raleigh, North Carolina

SCOTT CRAWFORD, MS, ATC, CSCS
Athletics/College of Health and Human Services
Concordia University
Portland, Oregon

BRIAN DICKENS, RMA, MBA, CHI
Dean of Academic Affairs of Southeastern College
Lakeland, Florida

SANDRA M. ERLEWINE, CMA (AAMA), CPC
Allied Health Technology Department
Yakima Valley Community College
Yakima, Washington

DONNA FIRN, CMA (AAMA), CPC, CRCS-I
Allied Health Science
Harcum College
Bryn Mawr, Pennsylvania

DEBORAH R FLOWERS, MS
Medical Assisting
Guilford Technical Community College
Jamestown, North Carolina

TRACIE FUQUA, BS, CMA (AAMA)
Medical Assisting
Wallace State Community College
Hanceville, Alabama

CAROLYN JEAN GAARDER, MLA RHIA
Health
MN State Community and Technical College
Moorhead, Minnesota

DOLLY HORTON, CMA, EdD
Allied Health
Asheville Buncombe Technical Community
College
Asheville, North Carolina

SUSAN W. KINNEY, RN, BSN, CNOR, RMA
Health Science
Piedmont Technical College
Greenwood, South Carolina

JUDITH KIMELMAN KLINE, NCRMA
Health Science
Miami Lakes Educational Center & Technical
College
Miami Gardens, Florida

GREG KLINGLER, MPAS, DHSc, PA-C
Health, Recreation, Human Performance
Brigham Young University
Rexburg, Idaho

JENNIFER LAME, MPH, RHIT
Health & Human Services
Southwest Wisconsin Technical College
Fennimore, Wisconsin

EBONY S. LAWRENCE, BS, MHA, DrPH (ABD)
Medical Assisting/Medical Administration
ECPI University—Medical Careers Institute
Charlotte, North Carolina

DEB LeHEW, CMA
Medical Assisting
Anoka Technical College
Anoka, Minnesota

BARBARA MARCHELLETTA, BS, CMA (AAMA), RHIT,
CPC, CPT, AHI
Allied Health
Beal College
Bangor, Maine

NIKKI A. MARHEFKA, EdM, MT (ASCP), CMA (AAMA)
School of Health Sciences
Central Penn College
Summerdale, Pennsylvania

MARY M. MARKS, FNP, RMA (AMT)
Nursing, Public Service, and Allied Health
Mitchell Community College
Mooresville, North Carolina

JUDY MARTIN, MEd
Continuing Education
Trident Technical College
Charleston, South Carolina

TATYANA PASHNYAK, CHIS-TR, COI
Health Sciences & Professional Studies
Bainbridge State College
Bainbridge, Georgia

VICTOR SCHUELLER, DC
General Education
Lakeshore Technical College
Cleveland, Wisconsin

ROBIN SNIDER-FLOHR, EdD, RN, CMA (AAMA)
Health & Public Services
Eastern Gateway Community College
Steubenville, Ohio

LORI STARNES, CMA (AAMA)
Allied Health—Medical Assisting
South Piedmont Community College
Monroe, North Carolina

SUSAN D. STOCKMASTER, MHS
Patient Care Services
Trident Technical College
Charleston, South Carolina

HOLLY A. TUMBARELLO, RN, BSN
Certified Allied Health Instructor
Allied Health
Clatsop Community College
Astoria, Oregon

PAM VENTGEN, CMA (AAMA), CCS-P, CPC, CPC-I
Medical Assisting
University of Alaska Anchorage
Anchorage, Alaska

KARON G. WALTON, BS, AAS, CMA
Medical Assisting
Augusta Technical College
Augusta, Georgia

KARI WILLIAMS, BS, DC
Medical Office Technology
Front Range Community College
Longmont, Colorado

STACEY F. WILSON, MT/PBT (ASCP), AHI, CMA
(AAMA), MHA
General Education
Cabarrus College of Health Sciences
Concord, North Carolina

BARBARA D.S. WORLEY, BS, DPM, RMA (AMT)
Medical Assisting
King's College
Charlotte, North Carolina

SANDRA WRIGHT, PhD
Administration
Atlanta Medical Academy
Palmetto, Georgia

ACKNOWLEDGMENTS

There is the saying, "It takes a village to raise a child." The same can be said for the creation of a book. So many individuals, working in concert with just the proper instrumentation at the correct time, are essential to the process. It began with a time of development, strategy planning, and decision making in the F.A. Davis conference room with two days of discussion. We discovered we would be the first team to work through a new process where all the ancillary pieces would be completed at the time each chapter was submitted. While it appeared cumbersome in the beginning, it soon became fun to visualize the entire picture for each chapter. The result was a more cohesive and comprehensive package to be delivered to students.

Jennifer Davis, BSN, RN, CBC, is the primary author of Chapters 8, 16, and 17. Martiann Lewis, MA, LMHC, is the primary author of Chapter 7. Jennifer and Martiann were a part of the team lending their dedication, wisdom, and support for their particular chapters and the entire book. Their unique knowledge and expertise was essential to the finished product. Donna Morrissey, developmental editor, provided valuable editing along the way and assisted in the incorporation of Blooms taxonomy into our learning outcomes and test questions. Donna Firn, CMA (AAMA), CPC, CRCS-I, provided all the ICD-10-CM codes for each chapter in a timely and efficient manner. The ICD-10-CM coding is much more complex and detailed than the ICD-9-CM and required a great deal of deliberation on her part in order to determine the specificity of each code for the purposes of the book.

All the staff at F.A. Davis make delivery of the 6th edition most pleasurable. Andy McPhee, Senior Acquisitions Editor, is not only visionary in his thinking, but he is also gracious, lends delightful humor to the project, and hosts a wonderful meal gathering. The time and talent of the reviewers who made helpful suggestions is invaluable to the caliber of the finished product.

I acknowledge all the authors of the many reference resources used in this edition. The content of this text cannot be entirely new because it is based on the work of a community of researchers, clinicians, and authors; it is hoped, however, that it has been presented in a manner that is unique and in a style that is useful to all readers.

Finally, without my husband and my family, this book would never have been finished. Tom knew just when to say, "It looks like nothing has been started for dinner; how about I take you out to eat." His loving support and encouragement were vital to my well-being and stamina. Interestingly enough, some grandchildren are now beginning to refer to this text for use in their classes at three different universities in Washington State. I am honored to be able to make that small contribution to them.

—CAROL D. TAMPARO, CMA (AAMA) PhD
ctamparo@comcast.net

My love for the medical world paired with my desire to take my knowledge and teach beyond the bedside and classroom have come true. I am truly thankful to Carol Tamparo, Donna Morrissey, Andy McPhee, F.A. Davis, and the entire team that offered and helped guide me through this wonderful opportunity.

Special thanks to Troy, my wonderful husband, who is my rock; MacKenzie and Aiden, my awesome children who inspire me to be a better person every day; Jill Tillman, my mom, nurse, mentor, and amazing friend; Craig Tillman, my dad, #1 fan, and supporter; and the many friends and family who have provided constant love and support.

If it weren't for others believing in me when I didn't, I wouldn't be where I am today. Remember, life is full of opportunities to learn, so take it in, always look for opportunities to learn, and share that knowledge with the world.

—JENNIFER DAVIS, BSN, RN, CBC
jennifertdavisrn@verizon.net

CONTENTS

chapter 14
Digestive System Diseases and Disorders, 343

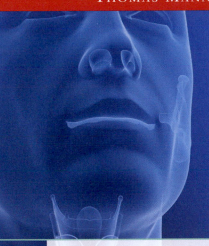

All interest in disease and death is only another expression of interest in life.
—THOMAS MANN

1

The Disease Process

● *chapter outline*

● *key words*

Amino acid (ă•mē'nō ă'sĭd)
Analgesic (ăn"ăl•jē'sĭk)
Anaphylaxis (ăn"ă•fĭ•lăk'sĭs)

Antibody (ăn'tĭ•bŏd"ē)
Antiemetic (ăn"tĭ•ē•mĕt'ĭk)
Antigen (ăn'tĭ•jĕn)

Chromosome (krō'mō•sōm)
Diuretic (dī"ū•rĕt'yk)
Dyspnea (dĭsp•nē'ă)
(key words continues)

1

(key words continued)

Edema (ĕ•dē'mă)
Erythema (ĕr''ĭ•the'mă)
Genotype (jĕn'ō•tīp)
Heterozygous
  (hĕt''er•ō•zī'gŭs)
Homeostasis
  (ho''mē•ō•stā'sĭs)
Homozygous (hōm''ō•zī'gŭs)
Hypovolemic shock
  (hī''pō•vō•lē'mĭk shŏk)
Hypoxemia (hī''pŏks•ē'mē•ă)

Incontinence (ĭn•kŏn'tĭ•nĕns)
Lymphadenopathy
  (lĭm•făd''ĕ•nŏp'ă•thē)
Macrophage (măk'rō•fāj)
Metastasis (mĕ•tăs'tă•sĭs)
Nosocomial (nŏs''ō•kō'mē•ăl)
Osteomalacia
  (ŏs''tē•ō•măl•ā'shē•ă)
Pathogenic (păth''ō•jĕn'ĭk)
Phagocytosis (făg''ō•sī•tō'sĭs)
Phenotype (fē'nō•tīp)

**Polymorphonuclear
  leukocyte**
  (pŏl''ē•mōr''fō•nū'klē•ăr
  loo'kō•sīt)
Pruritus (proo•rī'tŭs)
Sequela (sē•kwē'lă)
Stridor (strī'dōr)
Syncope (sĭn'kō•pē)
Syndrome (sĭn'drōm)
Tachycardia (tăk''ē•kăr'dē•ă)
Urticaria (ŭr''tĭ•kā'rē•ă)

● *learning outcomes*

On successful completion of this chapter, you will be able to:

- Interpret key terms.
- Explain three ways the body is protected from disease.
- Contrast illness and disease.
- Restate the predisposing factors of disease.
- Identify the three classifications of hereditary diseases.
- Describe the genetic activity of DNA.
- Distinguish between genotype and phenotype.
- Categorize the common types of monogenic disorders, giving an example of each.
- Explain chromosomal disorders and give at least one example.
- Summarize multifactorial disorders and give at least one example.
- Restate the process of inflammation.
- Describe how infections are transmitted.
- Compare the five main groups of microorganisms.
- Recall trauma statistics and major trauma injuries.
- Compare/contrast concussion, traumatic brain injury, and contusion.

- Restate the physical and chemical agents that may cause disease.
- Compare "Rule of Nines" and "Lund and Browder's" burn charts.
- Compare neoplasm to cancer.
- Contrast benign and malignant tumors.
- Differentiate between:
  - Natural and acquired immunity
  - Humoral and cell-mediated immunity
  - B-cell and T-cell immunity
  - Active and passive immunity
- Describe three malfunctions of the immune response and recognize an example of each.
- Recognize allergic reactions.
- Explain how anaphylactic shock can occur in any of the allergic reactions.
- Recognize the main examples of nutritional imbalance.
- Calculate your personal body mass index.
- Differentiate between idiopathic and iatrogenic causes of disease.

CHAPTER EPISODE—PART I

Ian Sumner was a rough-and-tumble kid. He was a daredevil. He played junior peewee football when he was only 8 years old. On many occasions, he hurt his head in play and practice but never experienced any problems as a result. When he discovered soccer, he quit football because he did not like having to wear all the heavy protective gear. He was a good player, good enough to play in college. He butted the ball with his head too many times to keep track. One time, he got hit exceptionally hard and afterward was confused and disorientated. Another time he was involved in an automobile crash, which threw him into the windshield. He was unconscious when the medics arrived but did not seem to suffer any serious injury.

- Should Ian be concerned about his personal and medical history?
- Justify your response.

INTRODUCTION

Despite a rapid increase in the number of medical research discoveries and the phenomenal development in technology, accompanied by society's increased awareness of wellness and health, we have not been able to eradicate disease. An ideally designed body would be free from disease, and a careful study of body chemistry and cellular function does reveal a blueprint for maintaining a disease-free state. The body is protected in three ways: (1) Normal body structures function to block the entry of germs through the use of tears, mucous membranes, intact skin, cilia, and body pH; (2) the inflammatory response rushes leukocytes to a site of infection, where the invading organisms are engulfed and destroyed in a process called **phagocytosis;** (3) specific immune responses of the body react to foreign antigens to protect and defend against disease.

Disease is a pathological condition of the body that occurs in response to an alteration in the normal body harmony. Disease is usually tangible or measurable. It may be the direct result of trauma, physical agents, and poisons, or it may be the indirect result of genetic anomalies and metabolic and nutritional disturbances.

There is a difference between illness and disease. *Illness* describes the condition of a person who is experiencing a disease. It encompasses the way in which individuals perceive themselves as suffering from a disease. Illness is highly individual and personal. A *disease*, on the other hand, is known by its medical classification and distinguishing features. For most health-care providers, a disease is easier to treat than an illness. Proper and effective medical management, however, attends to both the disease and the illness.

Fear, anxiety, embarrassment, and concern about the cost of treatment or about possible incapacity or disfigurement may be some of the troubling emotions persons feel when faced with an illness. Some people desire to know everything about their particular disease; others choose complete ignorance. The medical community is generally expected to have a "cure," but not many individuals understand the importance of their participation in the "getting well" process.

This chapter provides a brief synopsis of the causes of disease and disorders. When considering the disharmony that occurs in the body in the form of disease, remember the harmony that exists most of the time.

PREDISPOSING FACTORS

A *predisposing factor* is a condition or situation that may make a person more at risk or susceptible to disease. Some predisposing factors include heredity, age, gender, environment, and lifestyle.

Heredity is a predisposing factor when a trait inherited from a parent puts an individual at risk for certain diseases. Heredity is not easily controlled, changed, or altered. Cystic fibrosis (ICD-10: E84.9), sickle cell anemia (ICD-10: D57.1), and trisomy 21 or Down **syndrome** (ICD-10: Q90.9) are examples of hereditary diseases related to genetic abnormalities.

Age is a risk factor related to the life cycle. For example, adenoid hyperplasia (ICD-10: J35.2), acute tonsillitis (ICD-10: J03.90), and otitis media (ICD-10: H66.90) are more common among children than adults. Older adults are at greater risk than younger adults for degenerative arthritis (ICD-10: M15.9 or M19.90) and senile dementia (ICD-10: F03.9). Older adults have unique problems that arise from the aging process itself. Physiological changes occur in the body systems, and some of these changes can cause functional impairment. Older persons generally experience problems with temperature extremes, have lowered resistance to disease as the result of decreased immunity, and have less physical activity tolerance.

Gender is a predisposing factor when the disease is physiologically based. For example, prostate cancer (ICD-10: C61, C79.82, D07.5) occurs only in men; ovarian cancer (ICD-10: C56.9, C79.60, D09.10, or D09.19) occurs only in women. Men are more likely to develop gout (ICD-10 M10.00), whereas osteoporosis (ICD-10: M81.0) is more common in women. However, lung cancer (ICD-10: C34.90, C78.00, D02.20) is as prevalent in women as in men. Also, women experience heart disease as often as men do.

The *external environment* can be a risk factor. Exposure to air, noise, and other environmental pollutants may predispose individuals to disease. For example, drinking water became contaminated with methane during drilling at some fracking sites because of faulty well construction. With a warming climate and increased logging in our forests, new fungal growths are now identified where they previously did not exist. Some geographical locations have a higher incidence of insect bites and exposure to venom. Living in rural areas where fertilizers and pesticides are commonly used can predispose individuals to disease. Even office employees may be affected by environmental or occupational health problems, as seen with carpal tunnel syndrome (ICD-10: G56.00) and eye strain, which can result from heavy computer use.

Lifestyle choice may predispose some diseases. Lifestyle is the consistent, integrated way of life of an individual, as typified by mannerisms, attitudes, and possessions. From the time a person is born, lifestyle is influenced by (1) modeling of family members and peers, (2) education and knowledge, (3) personal attitudes, (4) degree of self-confidence, (5) individual responsibilities, and (6) life's opportunities. Lifestyle choices have great influence, whether positive or negative, on personal health and the health of others.

An increasing number of individuals suffer from such diseases as diabetes, heart disease, and some cancers that are preventable or delayed when lifestyle factors are appropriately addressed. Numerous medical studies identify highly effective preventive measures and lifestyle choices that include following a healthy diet, exercising regularly, maintaining an ideal weight, managing stress, and quitting smoking.

HEREDITARY DISEASES

The problem with the gene pool is there is no lifeguard. — David Gerrold

Hereditary diseases are the result of a person's genetic makeup. It is uncertain to what extent environmental factors influence the course of a hereditary disease, but the two do interact. Hereditary diseases do not always appear at birth. Mild hemophilia (ICD-10: D66) and muscular dystrophy (ICD-10: G71.0) may go undetected until adolescence or adulthood.

Thousands of genetic diseases are identified in humans—some are fatal. All genetic information is contained in DNA, a complex molecular structure found in the nucleus of cells. The DNA is incorporated into structures called **chromosomes.** The normal number of chromosomes in humans is 46 (23 pairs). In the formation of the ovum and sperm cells (sex cells, or gametes), this number is reduced by half, with each gamete having 23 chromosomes. When the two sex cells unite at the time of fertilization, the 23 chromosomes from the ovum combine at random with the 23 chromosomes from the sperm,

producing a cell with a full complement of 46 chromosomes. Two of these chromosomes determine sex.

A gene is the basic unit of heredity. Each gene consists of a fixed segment of the DNA on a specific chromosome. Physical traits are the result of the expression of gene pairs. Gene pairs are **homozygous** when they possess identical genes from each parent for a particular trait and when they are both dominant (one parent contributes) or both recessive (both parents contribute) in their expression of a trait. Gene pairs are **heterozygous** when they possess different genes from each parent for a particular trait and if one gene is dominant and one is recessive. Recessive genes are expressed only when the gene pair is homozygous, whereas dominant genes are expressed whether the gene pair is homozygous or heterozygous.

To determine a person's genetic makeup, a family history is taken to ascertain their **genotype,** which is a description of the combination of a person's genes with respect to either a single trait or a larger set of traits. Genotype includes all of the genes that are inherited from one's parents. The **phenotype** consists of the observable physical characteristics, determined by the combined influences of a person's genetic makeup and the effects of environmental factors. Phenotype is revealed in a person's appearance—the color and texture of the hair, shape of the nose, height, and so on.

An X- or sex-linked hereditary disease can occur when one parent contributes a defective gene from the sex chromosome. In color blindness (ICD-10: H53.50), the inability to distinguish reds from greens is the result of a recessive gene located on the X chromosome. The trait shows up when there is no dominant gene for normal color vision to override the recessive gene.

Changes in the structure of genes, called *mutations,* may cause disturbances in body functions. Mutations occur when the normal sequence of DNA units is disrupted. How such a disruption is manifested depends on whether the affected gene is dominant or recessive and whether it is homozygous or heterozygous. The causes of mutations are largely unknown, but they could be the result of environmental factors, such as exposure to certain chemicals or radiation.

Classification of Hereditary Diseases

Genetic diseases are the result of monogenic (Mendelian) alterations, chromosome aberrations, and multifactorial errors and are classified similarly.

Monogenic (Mendelian) Disorders

Monogenic disorders are those caused by mutation in a single gene. The way in which the disorder is passed on to succeeding generations (the pattern of inheritance) is determined by whether the gene is dominant, recessive, or sex-linked. (A sex-linked gene is carried on the X chromosome. Because males have only one X chromosome, a sex-linked gene will be expressed in males whether it is dominant or recessive.) Figure 1.1 illustrates the three most common patterns of inheritance of monogenic disorders. Monogenic disorders are classified as autosomal dominant, autosomal recessive, X- or sex-linked, chromosomal, and multifactorial. They are described below.

Autosomal Dominant

Only one abnormal gene from a parent is needed for an autosomal-dominant gene disease to be inherited. One parent often has the disease. When one parent has the faulty gene, there is a 50% chance the offspring will have the defect. Examples of autosomal-dominant diseases include:

- Huntington disease (ICD-10: G10): Also called *Huntington chorea*, this disease is caused by a genetic defect on chromosome 4 that results in the degeneration of neurons in certain areas of the brain. Individuals show signs of uncontrolled movements, emotional disturbances, and mental deterioration. Symptoms often do not develop until the affected person is in their 30s or 40s. Beta blockers are often given to minimize abnormal movements and behavior. The medications tetrabenazine (Xenazine) and amantadine (Symmetrel) can reduce the jerky, involuntary movements of the

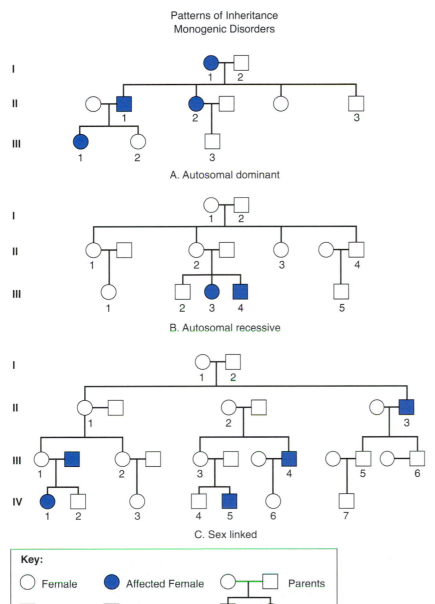

Figure 1.1 Patterns of inheritance monogenic disorders.
A. Pedigree displaying autosomal-dominant inheritance. Autosomal-dominant traits can be inherited by either gender. The female individual I-1 is heterozygous autosomal dominant. If she were homozygous for the mutant trait, then all progeny in generation II would show the trait.
B. Pedigree displaying autosomal-recessive inheritance. Autosomal recessive traits can be inherited by either gender. A recessive allele needs to be inherited from both the mother and the father for the trait to be seen. Recessive traits may not be seen for several generations, as shown by the progenies III-3 and III-4, who received both alleles.
C. Pedigree showing sex-linked inheritance. Males are most often affected by sex-linked disorders due to a mutation on the X chromosome. The II-3 male is affected, so his mother, individual I-1, must have been a carrier. The female individuals II-2 and III-3 each had a son with the trait, so both are carriers. Notice that the female individual III-1 had progeny with a male that carries the mutant trait. The female progeny IV-1 shows the trait because she inherited two mutant X chromosomes, so III-1 must also be a carrier.

disease by increasing the amount of dopamine available in the brain.

- Retinoblastoma (ICD-10: C69.20): A rare type of eye cancer that develops in the retina, retinoblastoma appears in early childhood and tends to occur in only one eye. The cancer often can be cured if diagnosed early, but it can spread to other areas of the body and become life-threatening. Treatment is varied and partially dependent on the spread of the disease.

Autosomal Recessive

There must be two copies (both parents) of the abnormal gene in order for an autosomal-recessive disease or trait to develop. Some examples include:

- Cystic fibrosis: This is a chronic, generalized disease that affects the cells that produce mucus, sweat, and digestive juices. The defective gene makes the secretions thick and sticky, causing tubes, ducts, and passageways to become clogged. The glands primarily affected are the pancreas, respiratory system, and sweat glands (see Chapter 6).
- Tay-Sachs disease (ICD-10: E75.02): This disease is a rare lipid abnormality in which harmful amounts of fatty substances build up in the nerve cells of the brain and spinal cord. It is distinguished by progressive neurological deterioration and a cherry-red spot with a gray border on both retinas. It chiefly affects infants of Eastern European Jewish (Ashkenazi) ancestry. It is also seen in certain French Canadian areas of Quebec, the Old Order Amish community in Pennsylvania, and the Cajun population of Louisiana. The progressing disease can result in deafness, blindness, and paralysis. Recurrent bronchopneumonia is a problem after age 2. Death usually occurs by age 5.
- Phenylketonuria (PKU): PKU is a rare inherited disease caused by an inability to metabolize phenylalanine, an essential **amino acid.** Amino acids are organic compounds that constitute the primary building blocks of proteins. Mental disability results unless a special diet begins within the first few weeks of life (see Chapter 6).
- Sickle cell anemia: A disease affecting mostly black populations around the world, it is one of the most common single-gene disorders. It occurs because the body produces a defective form of hemoglobin that causes red blood cells to roughen and become sickle shaped when deoxygenated. These cells clump together, making it difficult for them to pass through blood vessels (see Chapter 6).

X- or Sex-Linked

Dominant X-linked diseases occur when a single abnormal gene on the X chromosome can cause a disease;

this abnormal gene dominates the gene pair. There are only a few known dominant X-linked diseases, including:

- Vitamin D–resistant rickets (ICD-10: E83.39, E83.31, E83.30, E83.32): This disease is defined as such because it is resistant to the vitamin D treatment usually given for rickets and is evidenced by deficient amounts of mineral in the cartilage growth plates and by **osteomalacia,** or softening of the bones.
- Rett syndrome (ICD-10: F84.2): This is a severe disorder affecting the way the brain develops. It occurs most frequently in girls, producing symptoms similar to autism. Children with Rett syndrome have problems with motor functions that affect their ability to speak, walk, chew, use their hands, and even breathe. They may need a feeding tube in order to get sufficient dietary nutrients.

Recessive X-linked diseases occur when both of the genes in a pair are abnormal. If only one gene in the pair is abnormal, the disorder is quite mild or does not show at all. The two identified here are hemophilia and Duchenne muscular dystrophy:

- Hemophilia: This rare bleeding disorder is caused by a deficiency of specific types of serum proteins called *clotting factors*. A person with hemophilia bleeds longer following any kind of injury because the blood does not clot normally. Hemophilia can be mild, moderate, or severe, depending on how much clotting factor is in the blood. It is more common in males.
- Duchenne muscular dystrophy: This disorder manifests as a progressive bilateral wasting of skeletal muscles in males. Symptoms appear between ages 2 and 5 and include difficulty walking. The child has a stumbling gait and falls easily (see Chapter 6).

Chromosomal Disorders

Chromosomal disorders are caused by abnormalities in the number of chromosomes or by changes in chromosomal structure, such as *additions* (more than necessary), *deletions* (missing genes), or *translocations* (genes shifted from one chromosome to another or to a different location on the same chromosome). Diseases caused by chromosomal alterations include:

- Klinefelter syndrome (ICD-10: Q98.4): This condition occurs when there is an additional X chromosome in males. The male body shape is elongated, the testes are small, the mammary glands are abnormally large, and men with this syndrome do not produce sperm.
- Turner syndrome (ICD-10: Q96.9): This condition is caused by the loss of or an incomplete

X chromosome in either the ovum or the sperm. It affects only females and is often characterized by shortened stature; swollen hands and feet; and coarse, enlarged, prominent ears. Most females affected are infertile.

- Trisomy 21 or Down syndrome: This is a condition in which an individual has three copies of chromosome 21 instead of two; it is more likely to occur in children born to parents aged 35 to 50. Infants with this condition typically have a sloping forehead and folds of skin over the inner corners of their eyes, and they may have heart defects. They generally show evidence of moderate to severe mental disability. This condition is one of the most common birth defects (see Chapter 6).

Multifactorial Disorders

Multifactorial disorders result from the interaction of many factors, both hereditary (mutations in multiple genes) and environmental. Among the multifactorial diseases are:

- Diabetes mellitus: This disorder of carbohydrate, fat, and protein metabolism is due primarily to insufficient insulin production by the pancreas (see Chapter 11).
- Congenital heart anomalies: This category includes six major anatomic defects that change the blood flow through the heart, causing circulatory problems (see Chapter 6).

INFLAMMATION AND INFECTION

Inflammation is the body's immunologic response to tissue damage caused by the invasion of foreign bodies, microorganisms, or harmful chemicals. This invasion may result from trauma; physical agents (e.g., temperature extremes, radiation) or chemical agents (e.g., poisons, venoms); allergens; and disease-producing, or **pathogenic,** organisms (e.g., bacteria, viruses, fungi). Inflammation occurs when microorganisms gain entry into the body, most likely through a break in the skin. How well the body responds to inflammation depends on (1) an individual's general health, nutritional state, and age; (2) tissue factors; and (3) type of physical irritant.

Inflammation may be acute or chronic. In its acute phase, there is redness, swelling, pain, heat, and maybe even loss of function. At a site of injury, there are a large number of **polymorphonuclear leukocytes,** which are white blood cells (WBCs) that possess a nucleus composed of 200 or more lobes or parts. Examples of acute inflammation include insect bites, mild burns, and minor abrasions and cuts. The inflammation may persist, spread to adjacent or distant tissue, and become chronic. In chronic inflammation, there is an increase in the number of lymphocytes, monocytes, and plasma cells.

When microorganisms gain entry into the body, they release a toxin that causes the capillaries of the host to become permeable and allow access to WBCs—hence, the redness, swelling, heat, and pain. Factors that help in abating the inflammatory response include topical applications of ice packs, adequate hydration and nutrition, rest, and good blood supply. NSAIDs such as ibuprofen (e.g., Aleve, Advil) are useful in managing inflammation.

Inflammation is a beneficial biological response in most instances; however, if it becomes chronic, inflammation can be debilitating, as is the case in rheumatoid arthritis. Whatever the cause of inflammation, it is the body's protective response.

Infection is the invasion and multiplication of pathogenic or disease-producing microorganisms in the body. Most microorganisms in the body are nonpathogenic and are often necessary to maintain **homeostasis,** a state of stability that the body tries to maintain even though it is exposed to continually changing outside forces. When one or more of the requisite factors in the infectious process are present, a microorganism can become a potential pathogen.

People as well as animals serve as hosts for organisms. A host does not necessarily have to be "diseased" or "sick" but simply serves as a reservoir for the microorganisms. Transmission can be through exposure to a host's coughing or sneezing, through touching something contaminated by the infected host, or through direct contact with the microorganism. If the receiving host is not susceptible, then the microorganism has little chance of becoming a pathogen. The susceptible host, however, may have low resistance or provide the microorganism with an unusual means of entry, such as an open wound.

Whenever a pathogenic microorganism finds a suitable environment for growth in an appropriate host, disease may result. Growth factors for microorganisms vary and include the presence or absence of oxygen, a ready source of food, an optimal temperature, moisture, and darkness.

The most common microorganisms that cause disease can be classified as fungi, protozoa, viruses, bacteria, and parasites.

Fungi

This group includes yeasts and molds that may be present in the soil, air, and water. Only a few species cause disease (Fig. 1.2). Fungal diseases, called *mycoses,* usually develop slowly, are resistant to treatment, and are rarely fatal. The more common mycoses include histoplasmosis, coccidioidomycosis, and thrush (see Chapter 13); tinea corporis, or ringworm; and tinea pedis, or athlete's foot (see Chapter 8).

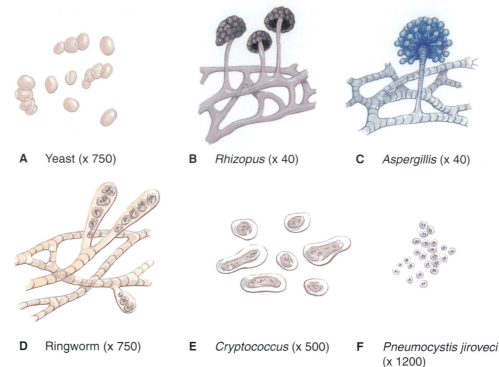

Figure 1.2 Fungi. *(From Scanlon, VC, and Sanders, T: Essentials of Anatomy and Physiology, ed. 5. FA Davis, Philadelphia, 2007, p 513, with permission.)*

A   Yeast (x 750)   **B**   *Rhizopus* (x 40)   **C**   *Aspergillis* (x 40)

D   Ringworm (x 750)   **E**   *Cryptococcus* (x 500)   **F**   *Pneumocystis jiroveci* (x 1200)

Protozoa

These single-celled organisms have animal-like characteristics (Fig. 1.3). Malaria (ICD-10: B50.9 or B50.8), amebic dysentery (ICD-10: A06.0), and African sleeping sickness (ICD-10: B56.9) are examples of protozoan diseases. *Trichomonas vaginalis* is a protozoon that causes trichomoniasis or vaginitis, a disease fairly common among women.

Viruses

These are the smallest microorganisms, visible only through the use of electron microscopy. Figure 1.4 illustrates common viruses and compares the size of the three viruses with that of the *Escherichia coli* bacillus. Viruses are independent of host cells, they are difficult to isolate, and few respond to drug therapy. Viruses may remain dormant in a host for long periods before

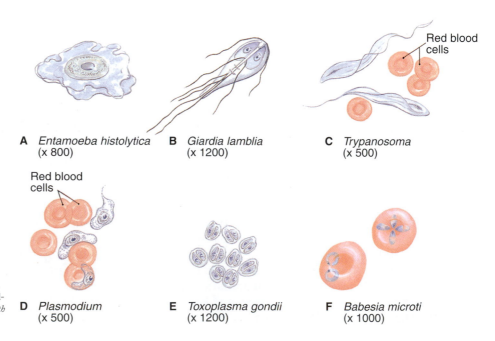

Red blood cells

A   *Entamoeba histolytica* (x 800)   **B**   *Giardia lamblia* (x 1200)   **C**   *Trypanosoma* (x 500)

Red blood cells

Figure 1.3 Protozoa. *(From Scanlon, VC, and Sanders, T: Essentials of Anatomy and Physiology, ed. 5. FA Davis, Philadelphia, 2007, p 514, with permission.)*

D   *Plasmodium* (x 500)   **E**   *Toxoplasma gondii* (x 1200)   **F**   *Babesia microti* (x 1000)

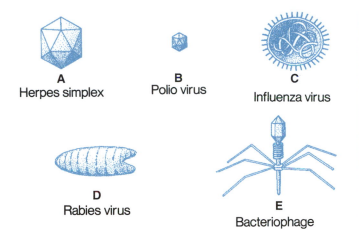

Relative sizes
(× 25,000)

E. coli

Rabies

Influenza

Polio

Figure 1.4 Viruses: representative shapes and relative sizes. *(From Scanlon, VC, and Sanders, T: Essentials of Anatomy and Physiology, ed. 5. FA Davis, Philadelphia, 2007, p 511, with permission.)*

becoming active. Viral infections include the common cold, West Nile virus, measles, mumps, rabies (ICD-10: A82.9), chickenpox, herpesviruses, poliomyelitis, hepatitis, influenza, and certain types of pneumonia and encephalitis.

Bacteria

There are many varieties of these single-celled organisms. Most are nonpathogenic and useful. Bacteria, including those that cause disease, are classified according to their shape (Fig. 1.5).

- Bacilli are rod-shaped bacteria. Diseases caused by bacilli include tuberculosis, whooping cough, tetanus, typhoid fever, and diphtheria.
- Spirilla are spiral-shaped bacteria. Diseases caused by spirilla include syphilis and cholera (ICD-10: A00.0).
- Cocci are dot-shaped bacteria. Diseases caused by cocci include gonorrhea, meningitis, tonsillitis (ICD-10: J03.90), bacterial pneumonia, boils (ICD-10: L02), scarlet fever (ICD-10: A38.9), sore throats (ICD-10: J02.9), and certain skin and urinary infections.

Parasites

This is a group of host-requiring organisms that includes external and internal parasites. External parasites include lice and mites (insects) and are discussed in Chapter 8. Helminths (ICD-10: B83.9) are wormlike internal parasites that are typically transmitted from person to person via fecal contamination of food, water, or soil. Three classes of helminths may infect humans (Fig. 1.6):

- Pinworms (ICD-10: B80) are the most common worm infection in the United States. They look like small threads about the size of a staple and often live in the human colon and rectum. During an individual's sleep, female pinworms leave the intestine via the anus to deposit their eggs on the surrounding skin tissue, causing itching and restlessness.
- Tapeworms (ICD-10: B68) are long and narrow, as their name indicates, and they depend on two hosts, one human and one animal, from the development of the egg to the larva to the adult. The easiest way to remember their names is by the name of the animal that acts as the second host: beef tapeworm (ICD-10: B68.1), pork tapeworm (ICD-10: B68.0), fish tapeworm (ICD-10: B70.0), and dog tapeworm (ICD-10: B71.8 or B71.1). Intestinal infection occurs when raw or contaminated meat or fish is eaten.
- Flukes (ICD-10: B66.0) are small, leaf-shaped, flat, nonsegmented worms. Fluke infection occurs from eating uncooked fish, plants, or animals from water infested with flukes.

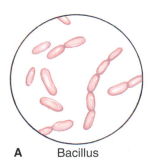

A Bacillus

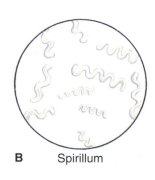

B Spirillum

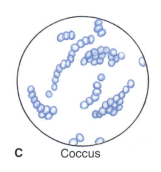

C Coccus

Figure 1.5 Bacteria (magnification x2000). *(From Scanlon, VC, and Sanders, T: Essentials of Anatomy and Physiology, ed. 5. FA Davis, Philadelphia, 2007, p 509, with permission.)*

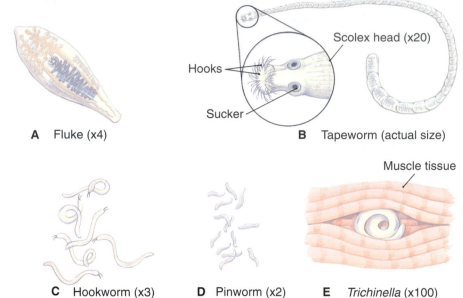

Figure 1.6 Helminths. *(From Scanlon, VC, and Sanders, T: Essentials of Anatomy and Physiology, ed. 5. FA Davis, Philadelphia, 2007, p 515, with permission.)*

TRAUMA

The Centers for Disease Control and Prevention (CDC) reports that the leading cause of death in the United States for persons younger than 35 is physical trauma, an injury or a wound caused by external force or violence, which occurs in one person every 3 minutes. According to the National Center for Health Statistics (NCHS), trauma is the fifth leading cause of death in the United States, following cardiovascular disease, cancer, chronic respiratory diseases, and stroke.

CHAPTER EPISODE—PART II

After college, Ian entered the military. During his second term in Iraq, the Humvee he was driving was hit by an improvised explosive device. The buddy next to him died, but Ian survived. He spent many weeks in rehabilitation and was later discharged from service because of injuries to his brain. The physician explained to his spouse that brain injuries can change the way a person thinks, acts, feels, and moves the body. The physician also noted that while he believed Ian's traumatic brain injury (TBI) was permanent, Ian could learn to cope.

• Where might Ian and his spouse turn for help?
• What special needs might Ian have?

Head Trauma

Injuries to the head include concussion; traumatic brain injury; cerebral contusion; skull, nose, and jaw fractures; and perforated eardrum.

Concussions cause temporary neural dysfunction but are not severe enough to cause a contusion. A concussion results from a closed-head type of injury and does not include injuries in which there is bleeding under the skull or into the brain. This kind of trauma is normally the result of a fall, a severe blow to the head area, or a motor vehicle accident. A mild concussion may involve no loss of consciousness, may leave a person feeling "dazed," or may result in a very brief loss of consciousness. A severe concussion may cause prolonged loss of consciousness and a delayed return to normal.

Traumatic brain injury occurs when the brain collides with the inside of the skull, bruising the brain and tearing nerve fibers. It is often the result of an external force so strong that temporary or permanent impairment of cognitive, physical, and psychosocial functions may occur. Many returning veterans suffer from TBIs.

Cerebral contusions, a form of TBI, are more serious than concussions because they bruise the brain tissue and disrupt normal nerve function. Damage to a major blood vessel within the head can cause a hematoma or heavy bleeding into or around the brain when a contusion occurs. The main causes of cerebral contusions are motor vehicle accidents, sports activities, and assaults. Falls are a common cause for individuals over age 65. Contusions may cause loss of consciousness, hemorrhage, and even death.

If unconsciousness, convulsions, forceful and persistent vomiting, blurred vision, staggering walk, or hemorrhage occurs after a blow to the head, the person should be immediately taken to a hospital where the seriousness of the event can be assessed and proper treatment given. (See further discussion in Chapter 10.)

Skull fractures often are accompanied by scalp wounds and profuse bleeding. The concern in the individual with a skull fracture is possible damage to the brain. Fractures generally are accompanied by pain, tenderness, and swelling of the affected areas. Surgery may be required to remove foreign bodies or bone fragments. The person is closely monitored in a hospital.

Perforated eardrums normally result from the insertion of sharp objects into the ear canal or from a severe blow to the side of the head. Sudden and excessive changes in air pressure can cause perforation. Children who have acute otitis media (earache) may experience a perforated eardrum as a complication of this disease.

Chest Trauma

Penetrating chest injuries are often caused by knife and gunshot wounds. These wounds typically produce a sucking sound as air enters the chest cavity through the chest wall opening. The person may be in severe pain. **Tachycardia,** or an abnormally rapid heartbeat, is apt to occur. There may be a weak pulse, blood loss, and possible **hypovolemic shock** (ICD-10: E86.1), a condition of severe physiological distress. Hypovolemic shock is caused by a decrease in the circulating blood volume so great that the body's metabolic needs cannot be met. It is important to control blood loss in penetration wounds.

Nonpenetrating chest injuries such as rib fractures usually result from motor vehicle crashes in which the driver is thrown against the steering wheel. There is a sensation of tenderness and worsening pain with deep breathing or exertion. A potential complication of rib fractures is the penetration of a rib into the pleura, lung tissue, or myocardium. Immediate assessment and medical attention are paramount. Surgical repair is often necessary.

Abdominopelvic Trauma

Injuries to the abdominopelvic region may cause hemorrhages within the liver, spleen, pancreas, and kidneys and/or rupture of the stomach, intestine, gallbladder, and urinary bladder. Rupture of the organs results in the spilling of the contents of the organs (including bacteria) into the abdominopelvic cavity. This spillage is a major cause of infection. Blood loss (ICD-10: R58) and hypovolemic shock are also concerns. Emergency attention is necessary to determine the extent of the damage and the necessary treatment. Most abdominal injuries require surgical repair. The prognosis depends on the extent of the injury, but prompt attention generally improves the outcome.

Neck and Spine Trauma

Neck and spine injuries include fractures, dislocations, contusions, and compressions of the vertebral column. The greatest concern with this type of trauma is damage to the spinal cord and paralysis. Spinal cord injuries are discussed in connection with the nervous system (see Chapter 10).

Extremities Trauma

The various types of sprains, strains, and fractures to the arms and legs are common. They are discussed in Chapter 9.

EFFECTS OF PHYSICAL AND CHEMICAL AGENTS

Physical and chemical agents can adversely affect the body, and the severity of the effects depends on many factors. If exposure to the irritant is short in duration and frequency, is fairly localized, and the person is healthy, the damage may be unnoticed or reversible. However, if the person is debilitated, diseased, very young or elderly, has lowered resistance, or is on certain medications, the irritant may cause irreversible systemic damage.

Some of the more common physical and chemical agents include extreme heat and cold; ionizing radiation; extremes of atmospheric pressure; electric shock; poisoning; near drowning; bites of insects, spiders, and snakes; asphyxiation; and burns.

Extreme Heat and Cold

Extreme heat (ICD-10: T67.0XXA) may result in **syncope** (a transient loss of consciousness [ICD-10: T67.1XXA]), heat exhaustion (ICD-10: T67.5XXA), or heatstroke (ICD-10: T67.0XXA). Causes of these disorders include overexertion in heat, prolonged heat exposure, salt depletion, dehydration, failure of the body's heat-regulating mechanisms, or a combination of these causes.

Heat exhaustion, sometimes resulting in syncope, is caused by overexposure to heat and insufficient water and salt intake (ICD-10: T67.4XXA). The person is usually pale and the skin is clammy. There is a rapid, weak pulse and shallow breathing. Individuals treated at this stage generally respond promptly to rest, cooling, and weak salty liquids administered orally. Heat cramps in the legs and abdomen result from heavy salt loss.

If the person does not respond or heat exhaustion is not treated, heatstroke may result when the body's temperature-control mechanism malfunctions. **Heatstroke is a medical emergency.** Sweating ceases and the body temperature rises. The skin becomes hot, dry, and flushed. Heatstroke may require hospitalization with IV therapy, cooling therapy, increased fluid intake, temperature monitoring, and muscle massaging. Hypersensitivity to heat may remain for some time. Any of the heat disorders mentioned can be fatal.

Extreme cold may cause such disorders as chilblain (ICD-10: T69.1XXA), frostbite (ICD-10: T33–T34), and hypothermia (ICD-10: T68.XXA). Causes include overexposure to cold air, wind, or water. Chilblain, a mild frostbite, produces red, itching skin lesions, usually on the extremities, whereas frostbite, the freezing of exposed areas, causes tingling and redness followed by paleness and numbness of the affected areas. Untreated, either condition can lead to gangrene and may necessitate amputation. Hypothermia is a systemic reaction when more heat escapes from the body than the body can produce, which can be fatal. Treatment of any of the cold disorders includes gradually warming the person, monitoring body temperature, protecting the affected part, preventing infection, and administering pain relievers, or **analgesics,** as necessary.

Ionizing Radiation

Depending on the duration and intensity of exposure and the form of the irradiating agent, the effects of ionizing radiation (ICD-10: T66.XXXA) range from mild skin burns (ICD-10: L58.9) to fatal tissue destruction. The exposure to radiation may be via ingestion, inhalation, or direct contact. Causes include (1) occupational or accidental exposure and (2) the misuse of radiation for diagnostic or treatment purposes. Persons at risk include those with cancer who are receiving radiation therapy and employees in nuclear power plants. The harmful effects of radiation may be immediate or delayed and acute or chronic. Treatment is symptomatic and supportive and may include **antiemetics** (drugs used to prevent or stop vomiting), simple and palatable foods, blood transfusions, and emotional support.

Extremes of Atmospheric Pressure

Extremes of atmospheric pressure result from a rapid change from a high-pressure to a low-pressure environment or from a low-pressure to a high-pressure environment. Decompression sickness (ICD-10: T70.3XXA) is an occupational hazard for deep-sea divers and airplane pilots who descend or ascend too quickly and for hospital personnel who work in hyperbaric chambers. Systemic damage occurs following rapid decompression when gases dissolved in the blood and other tissues escape faster than they can be diffused through respiration. Nitrogen gas bubbles form in the blood and tissue, causing respiratory problems and pain. Treatment consists of emergency oxygen until the person can be transported to a hyperbaric chamber, where recompression is followed by slow decompression. Supportive measures are also important.

Electric Shock

Electric shock (ICD-10: T75.4XXA) can occur anywhere there is electricity—home, work, or school. The causes of electric shock can be natural (as from lightning [ICD-10: T75]) or contrived (because of carelessness or ignorance or from faulty equipment). The victim must be freed from the source of electric current without the rescuer contacting the current, and treatment must begin immediately. There may be very little external evidence of injury or severe and obvious burns. Other injuries may occur if the victim was thrown clear of the electrical source by forceful muscular contraction. In this case, possible spinal injuries should be considered. Cardiopulmonary resuscitation (CPR) may be necessary. If the damage is severe, hospitalization may be required to observe the individual, treat any burns, and prevent infection.

Poisoning

Poisoning is a common occurrence, especially among curious children. In addition, society has become increasingly aware of poisonous chemicals that have been dumped or buried. Such chemicals cause soil and water contamination that result in ecological and personal damage.

Poisons may be accidentally ingested, inhaled, injected, or absorbed through the skin, but poisoning can also be the result of occupational exposure when working with toxic chemicals; improper cooking, storage, and canning of food; and drug overdoses or abuse. Treatment consists of administering first aid, identifying and providing the correct antidote if one exists, and instituting supportive measures. The local poison control center offers valuable help. Prompt, correct treatment can save a life.

Near Drowning

Near drowning (ICD-10: T75.1XXA) is more common during the warm summer months and can be prevented in many cases by following water safety precautions. In near drowning, the person generally aspirates fluid or may have an obstructed airway caused by a spasm of the larynx when gasping underwater, resulting in **hypoxemia** (ICD-10: R09.02) (insufficient oxygenation of the arterial blood). Later, within minutes or possibly days of near drowning, the person may experience respiratory distress. Emergency treatment is critical. Hospitalization may be required for oxygenation, airway maintenance, observation of the cardiovascular status, and prevention of further complications.

Bites of Insects, Spiders, and Snakes

Insect, spider, and snake bites occur most often during the warm summer months. Bee, yellow jacket, wasp, and hornet stings may cause localized pain, but they usually require little more than symptomatic treatment. Allergic reactions and multiple stings or bites, however, are a more serious matter and are treated as medical emergencies. There are only two poisonous spiders in the United States—the black widow and the brown recluse. Their bites are rarely fatal but do cause redness,

REALITY EPISODE

Fred and Dot were fishing about 150 yards from the lakeshore in their small motorboat. It was a beautiful day: The water was calm, and the fish were biting. They were having fun and laughing when Fred caught a big one. He rose up in the boat to lean over to grab his catch in the net and suddenly felt dizzy. Before he could say anything to Dot, he fainted and fell into the lake. As he began to sink underwater, Dot was able to get a good hold on his jacket and keep his head out of water. However, Fred was a big man. Dot knew she could not hold on for too long. She began to yell and scream as loud as she could. A man working in his flower bed on the shore heard her shouts for help and he could see the boat. He jumped into his own motorboat and raced to the scene. He managed to pull Fred into his boat and turn him on his side; Fred was beginning to cough and choke.

What might be the outcome of this situation? What could have prevented Fred from sinking into the water?

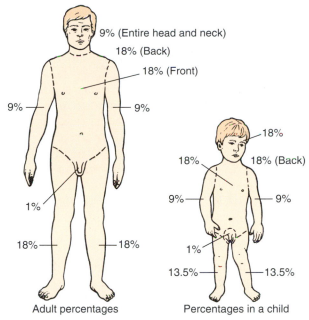

Figure 1.7 Rule of nines and burn classification. *(From Venes, D [ed]: Taber's Cyclopedic Medical Dictionary, ed. 22. FA Davis, Philadelphia, 2013, p 2069, with permission.)*

irritation, and discomfort. Venomous snake bites require quick emergency measures to prevent venom absorption and life-threatening symptoms from occurring. The victim should be immobilized, with the affected area kept below the heart, and transported immediately to a hospital, where the specific antidote can be administered. Whether the bite is considered serious or mild, close observation of the victim is essential.

Asphyxiation

Asphyxiation (ICD-10: R09.01), which is the lack of oxygen coupled with accumulating carbon dioxide in the blood, may result from carbon monoxide poisoning, near drowning, hypoventilation, airway obstruction, or inhalation of toxic fumes. Emergency treatment is generally required, and it may involve removal of any obstruction, CPR, oxygenation, and intubation. Hospitalization may be necessary to stabilize the victim's vital signs. Obviously, any breathing difficulty is frightening to the victim, so reassurance and encouragement are needed.

Burns

Burns are classified by extent, depth, person's age, and associated illness and injury. Two commonly used measures to assess the extent of burns are discussed here. The Wallace rule of nines, a formula for estimating medium to large burns in adults, determines the percentage of a body surface burned by using multiples of nine. It is generally believed not to be accurate when used with children (Fig. 1.7). The Lund and Browder chart is more accurate in that it considers the body's shape and size, thus making it more appropriate for use in both children and adults (Fig. 1.8). Burns are classified according to depth and how severely they penetrate the skin's surface. **Erythema,** or redness of the skin, is generally not considered because it may be hours before the redness begins to fade.

- First-degree or superficial burns affect only the epidermis or outer layer of skin. A mild sunburn is an example. The skin is red, painful, and dry, but there are no blisters.
- Second-degree or partial-thickness burns involve the epidermis and part of the dermis. The skin appears red and blistered and it may be swollen. Second-degree burns that injure deeper skin layers are known as *deep partial-thickness burns.*
- Third-degree or full-thickness burns destroy the epidermis and dermis skin layers. The skin most likely appears white, pearly, or leathery.
- Fourth-degree burns extend into underlying bones, muscles, tendons, nerves, and blood vessels. The skin appears white or charred; sensation is lost because nerve endings are destroyed.

Second-, third-, and fourth-degree burns require immediate medical attention. Emergency measures may be necessary to maintain the burn victim's airway, cool the wound, and prevent serious loss of body fluids. After hospitalization, frequently in a special burn center, the focus is on maintaining fluid balance and preventing infection. Severe burns can be

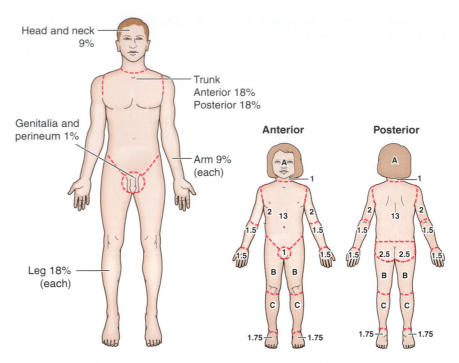

Body Part	Age				
	0 yr	1 yr	5 yr	10 yr	15 yr
A = ½ of head	9 ½	8 ½	6 ½	5 ½	4 ½
B = ½ of 1 thigh	2 ¾	3 ¼	4	4 ¼	4 ½
C = ½ of 1 lower leg	2 ½	2 ½	2 ¾	3	3 ¼

Relative percentage of body surface area (% BSA) affected by growth

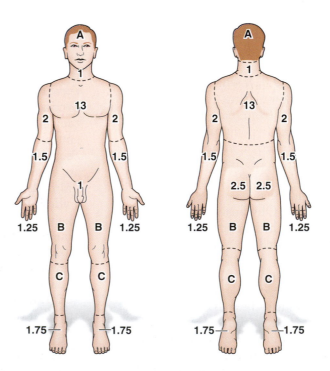

Figure 1.8 Lund and Browder chart to assess burns in adults and children. *(From Roy, S: The Rehabilitation Specialist's Handbook, ed. 4. FA Davis, Philadelphia, pp 552–553, with permission.)*

extremely painful and require a lengthy rehabilitation period, including possible skin grafting and plastic surgery. Emotional support is essential.

NEOPLASIA AND CANCER

Neoplasia means "new formation" or "new growth." A *neoplasm* is a new and abnormal formation of tissue. The abnormal tissue may form a *tumor;* in leukemia, however, the abnormal tissue is found in the blood cells without evidence of a tumor. The actual cause of neoplasms is not known, but an alteration in genes does occur, allowing independent and uncontrollable growth. As was discussed earlier under "Hereditary Diseases," an alteration in a gene on a chromosome is a mutation. The mutant cell differs from the normal cell in that the abnormal cell is no longer subject to normal control mechanisms. Apparently, mutations such as this occur relatively frequently, but the body usually is able to destroy the resulting mutant cells as soon as they appear. Therefore, a neoplasm may represent a failure on the part of the body's immune system. The harmful effects of the neoplastic growth may be from the growth itself or from the destruction of surrounding tissue.

Tumors are further classified as benign or malignant, depending on their growth pattern. A *benign* tumor is one that remains circumscribed, although it may vary in size from small to large. A *malignant* tumor, or cancer, is one that spreads to other cells, tissues, and parts of the body through the bloodstream or lymphatic system. The spreading process is called **metastasis.**

Cancer is a general term for approximately 100 diseases, all of which are characterized by the uncontrollable growth of abnormal or malignant cells. The diagnosis, treatment, prognosis, and prevention of cancer are discussed in Chapter 5.

IMMUNE-RELATED FACTORS IN DISEASE

The Immune Response

Immunity is the security against a particular disease or the state of being nonsusceptible to pathogenic effects of disease-causing organisms. The body's immune system is both natural and acquired. Natural immunity is a genetic feature specific to race, sex, and the individual's ability to respond. This form of immunity is also called *genetic immunity.* The term *acquired immunity* indicates that the body has developed the ability to defend itself against a specific agent. Acquired immunity is called *active immunity* when protection occurs as a result of prior exposure to an infectious agent or its antigens. Acquired immunity is *passive* when a person is given antibodies to a disease rather than producing them. Therefore, active acquired immunity can occur after having a disease, and passive acquired immunity occurs after receiving immunization against a disease. Although the human body does not begin developing antibodies (protein substances produced by the body's immune system in response to and interacting with specific antigens) until 3 to 6 weeks of age, an infant has passive and temporary immunity because it receives antibodies produced by its mother's immune system in utero. Some medical personnel refer to this as *maternal immunity.*

There are two types of acquired immunity:

1. *Humoral immunity* is the body's major defense against bacteria. Here the body produces antibodies or immunoglobulins that combine with and eliminate the **antigen** or foreign substance. An antigen is any substance that, when introduced into the body, causes the immune system to produce a specific **antibody.** These antibodies are formed by WBCs called *B-cell lymphocytes.* The humoral response is rapid, beginning immediately or within 48 hours of antigen contact. Humoral immunity, in the presence of an antigen, causes an antibody to be released, which in turn reacts exclusively with that antigen. This binding of antibody to antigen encourages phagocytosis of the antigen and activates the complement system. The complement system is responsible for enzyme development, which helps remove the antigen from the body.

2. *Cell-mediated immunity* is action by another group of WBCs, called *T-cell lymphocytes.* These lymphocytes provide the main protection against viruses, fungi, parasites, some bacteria, and neoplasms. T cells mature in the thymus and are stored in the lymphatic system and spleen. Cell-mediated immunity is initiated when a T lymphocyte becomes sensitized by contact with a specific antigen. In response to additional contacts with the antigen, the T lymphocyte releases sensitized lymphocytes, which migrate to the inflammation site. These lymphocytes help to transform local cells within the body tissues, enabling the cells to engulf particular substances and microorganisms, or **macrophages,** and activate them into "killer" T lymphocytes that are highly phagocytic. The migration of antigens also is prohibited. Some normal tissue can be destroyed during this very intense process.

The ability to generate an immune response is controlled by genetics. Immune response genes regulate B-cell and T-cell proliferation; therefore, they influence resistance to infection and neoplasms. The immune response normally recognizes its own body cells, thereby preventing damage to tissue.

Although this complex system is designed to protect the body and keep it disease-free, the immune response can malfunction. Immunologic malfunctions are classified as (1) *allergy,* when the immune response is inappropriate; (2) *autoimmunity,* when the immune response is misdirected; and (3) *immunodeficiency,* when the immune response is inadequate.

Allergy

Allergic reactions that reflect malfunctioning immunity are often caused by certain foods (especially milk, nuts, eggs, and wheat), seasonal pollen, dust mites, mold, pets, insect bites, certain fabrics, inhalants, and cosmetics. Familial history, stress, and general physical condition may predispose a person to allergies.

Another allergic reaction results from transfusion of the wrong type of blood or blood components, which become toxic to the body's cells. Transfusion reactions (ICD-10: T80.89XA) may be mild or severe, depending on the amount of transfused fluid and the person's condition. Symptoms of transfusion reaction range from chills and fever, pain, nausea, and vomiting to a sudden, unusually severe, and possibly life-threatening allergic reaction, or **anaphylaxis** (ICD-10: T80.89XA), and congestive heart failure. Blood and laboratory tests have to be performed to confirm the type and severity of reaction. Medical attention is necessary to prevent complications.

Allergy is also seen in hypersensitivity reactions to drugs (ICD-10: T50.995A). In some people, certain drugs can act as antigens, stimulating the formation of sensitizing antibodies. Although any drug can be the offender, common ones include penicillin, sulfa drugs, and anticonvulsants. The degree of hypersensitivity depends on the extent and duration of exposure to the drug; the person's genetic background, age, and sex; and the presence of underlying disease. Symptoms range from a local rash, **urticaria, pruritus** (ICD-10: L29.9) or severe itching, flulike symptoms, and erythema (diffuse redness of the skin) to such severe conditions as swelling of the lip, tongue, or face and anaphylaxis.

Anaphylactic shock (ICD-10: T78.2XXA) is considered by some authorities to be an allergic reaction. This reaction is acute and potentially life threatening. It may be caused by drug hypersensitivity, foods (the most common offenders are nuts, legumes, berries, and seafood), and insect stings (honeybees, wasps, yellow jackets, mosquitoes, ants, and certain spiders). Anaphylaxis may occur after a single exposure to an antigen or after repeated exposures. For this reason, it is important to be alert for an allergic reaction in any person at any time. In some cases, the reaction may occur within seconds, but it is usually no later than 40 to 50 minutes after contact with the allergen.

Cardiovascular symptoms can include hypotension, shock, and cardiac irregularities. Respiratory symptoms can include nasal congestion, profuse watery rhinorrhea, itching, and sudden sneezing. **Edema** (ICD-10: R60.1, R60.9 or R60.0), or excessive accumulation of fluid in bodily tissues, of the nose or throat can cause a high-pitched sound during respiration; **stridor,** which is labored and difficult breathing; or **dyspnea,** which is acute respiratory failure (ICD-10: J96.90 or J96.00). Gastrointestinal (GI) and genitourinary symptoms include stomach cramping (ICD-10: R10.9), nausea (ICD-10: R11.0), diarrhea (ICD-10: R19.7), urinary urgency (ICD-10: R39.15), and the inability to control the passage of urine, or **incontinence** (ICD-10: R32). Anaphylactic shock is a medical emergency. It requires immediate countermeasures, which may include injection of epinephrine. It is important to maintain the individual's airway and to administer CPR in the event of cardiac arrest.

Autoimmunity

In autoimmune disease, self-antigens, or abnormal immune cells, develop and incite the immune response into abnormal or excessive activity of T cells or B cells that attack their own tissues and organs. What causes an autoimmune response is largely unknown; however, there is an inherited predisposition in some cases. There currently is no cure for autoimmune diseases. The goal of treatment is to relieve symptoms and lessen tissue and organ damage. Temporary remission of symptoms also may occur. In this text, most of the autoimmune diseases are discussed in conjunction with the specific organ systems affected; however, a brief summary of five types follows:

- Gastrointestinal: primary biliary cirrhosis, ulcerative colitis, and atrophic gastritis (see Chapter 14)
- Cardiovascular: pernicious anemia, hemolytic anemia, idiopathic thrombocytopenia, and leukopenia (see Chapter 12)
- Endocrine: insulin-dependent diabetes, thyrotoxicosis, and Hashimoto thyroiditis (see Chapter 11)
- Musculoskeletal: mixed connective-tissue diseases, rheumatoid arthritis, systemic lupus erythematosus, and myasthenia gravis (see Chapter 9)
- Dermatologic: dermatomyositis and scleroderma (see Chapter 8)

Immunodeficiency

Immunodeficiency diseases are a result of B-cell, T-cell deficiency, or both or some unknown immunodeficient factor. Most immunodeficient diseases are diagnosed by immunologic analyses, because many persons are asymptomatic except for recurrent infections. Most immunodeficient persons have impaired resistance to infections, and these infectious conditions may cause death.

AIDS (see Chapter 4) is a severe form of acquired immunodeficiency. Another immunodeficiency disease is Hodgkin lymphoma, a neoplastic malignancy of the lymph system. The immunodeficiency is thought to be due to impaired T-cell function, which leaves the person more susceptible to infections. Once a fatal disease, it is now potentially curable, even in advanced stages. Hodgkin lymphoma is discussed in detail in Chapter 5.

Malignant lymphomas, also known as *non-Hodgkin lymphomas* and sometimes lymphosarcomas, are malignant neoplasms of the lymphoreticular system. Persons with genetic, or acquired, immunodeficiency disorders clearly are predisposed to these malignant neoplasms. A symptom is swelling of the lymph glands. Diagnosis is made chiefly by lymph node biopsy to differentiate lymphoma from Hodgkin disease and other causes of **lymphadenopathy** or diseases of the lymph nodes. Identification of the disease is necessary for proper treatment, and chemotherapy and radiation are used with some success. Non-Hodgkin lymphomas cause more deaths than Hodgkin disease.

NUTRITIONAL IMBALANCE

Nutritional imbalance can cause growth problems, specific diseases, and even death. Nutritional imbalances, deficiencies, and excesses are becoming more apparent as causes of health problems worldwide. Nutritional deficiencies can cause grave intellectual and physical impairments as well as affect an individual's overall well-being. Causes of nutritional imbalances include malnourishment, vitamin and mineral deficiencies and excesses, obesity, and starvation.

Malnourishment

Malnourishment (ICD-10: E44.0) may be due to:

- Improper intake of foodstuffs in both quality and quantity, as seen in people with alcoholism (ICD-10:F10.229), anorexia nervosa, and bulimia or in those who engage in diet faddism
- Improper intake of foodstuffs because of GI problems, as exhibited in individuals who have no sense of taste or smell and little tolerance for food, those with postoperative anorexia, those being treated with chemotherapy, or those who have a lesion in the throat
- Malabsorption or poor utilization of foodstuffs, as seen when an individual is unable to absorb nutrients properly
- Increased need for food or certain nutrients, as seen in marathon runners, people in a febrile state, and those with cancer
- Impaired metabolism of foodstuffs, as in both hereditary and acquired biochemical disorders

- Food and drug interactions, as seen in those taking corticosteroid medications, which are known to deplete muscle protein, lower glucose tolerance, and induce osteoporosis

Vitamin Deficiencies and Excesses

Early signs of vitamin deficiency (ICD-10: E56.9) are generally vague and nonspecific. Vitamin deficiency diseases include scurvy (ICD-10: E54), which is caused by a lack of vitamin C and is characterized by abnormal bone formation and hemorrhages of mucous membranes, as well as rickets and some cancers and infectious diseases that are due to a lack of vitamin D (ICD-10: E55.0) and a prolonged lack of vitamin B_{12} (ICD-10: E53.8), causing neurological damage. Vitamin D deficiency is increasingly common among all age-groups. Treatment typically consists of a diet high in protein and the required vitamin. Vitamin excess (ICD-10: E669) may occur when people take vitamins in an attempt to cover missed or inadequate meals, when they hope to prevent some disease, or when they self-treat a condition. Large doses of a number of vitamins can accumulate in the body and become toxic. They may cause illness, especially when taken over a long period of time.

Mineral Deficiencies and Excesses

Minerals are a vital component of a balanced diet. Mineral deficiencies (ICD-10: E50-E64) of chloride, potassium, sodium, calcium, and magnesium are the most common deficiencies. Causes include dietary deficiencies and metabolic disorders. Treatment may involve increasing the intake of a deficient mineral through foodstuffs or medication or addressing any underlying metabolic disorder. Mineral excess also may be caused by diet, medication, or a metabolic error. Treatment consists of locating the cause and correcting the problem.

Obesity

Obesity (ICD-10: E66.9) is when body weight is 10% to 20% above the ideal. Of course, "ideal" is difficult to determine, and such factors as family history and body build must be considered. One measure of obesity is a calculation known as the *body mass index,* or BMI. This index expresses the relationship between height and weight. Another measure, often used in conjunction with the BMI, is a body shape index, or ABSI. ABSI accounts for height and is more sensitive to the relationship between abdominal fat and muscle mass and bone structure. The Internet provides formulas for personal use for both the BMI and the ABSI.

The cause of obesity may be too many calories, too little activity, or, less frequently, an endocrine and metabolic problem. In addition, fluid retention may cause an increase in weight. Treatment may include lowering caloric intake, increasing physical activity, or correcting metabolic disorders. If fluid retention is a problem, drugs that promote the secretion of urine, or **diuretics** may be prescribed, and any underlying cause of the retention should be detected and treated.

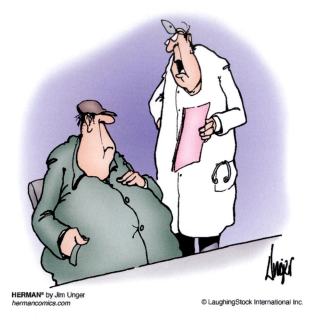

HERMAN® by Jim Unger
hermancomics.com   © LaughingStock International Inc.

"In some parts of the world, whole villages could live on your food intake."

(HERMAN© is reprinted with permission from LaughingStock Licensing, Inc., Ottawa, Canada. All rights reserved.)

The prognosis for obesity is not good. Although a small percentage of obese individuals are able to lose weight, an even smaller percentage are able to maintain permanent weight reduction. Obesity poses a serious risk for the development of hypertension and stroke, diabetes mellitus, gallbladder disease, and heart disease.

Gary Whitlock, a member of a research group at the University of Oxford in the United Kingdom, reported the following data gathered from nearly 900,000 men and women from Western Europe and North America who participated in 57 studies related to obesity*:

- A BMI over 25 translates to a 40% increase in the risk of heart disease and stroke and a 60% increase in the risk of diabetes.
- A BMI over 30 reduces a person's life span by 2 to 4 years; a BMI over 40 reduces life span by 8 to 10 years.

Much media attention regarding obesity has translated into healthier choices available at school cafeterias and restaurants and a greater awareness of food choices.

Also, a number of obese individuals opt for gastric bypass or lap band surgery in search of a more permanent solution to obesity.

Starvation

Causes of starvation (ICD-10: T73.0XXA) include lack of food or an unbalanced diet over a long period of time, causing metabolic and physiological body changes. A starved person generally does not have adequate food, whereas someone who is malnourished generally has enough food available but it is of inadequate nutritive value. Starvation can be the result of illness, poverty, and poor dietary planning. It is seen at any age; however, infants and children aged 1 to 3 suffer more severely than adults. Pregnant women and elderly people are also vulnerable.

OTHER CAUSES OF DISEASE

Some diseases, having no known cause, are described as *idiopathic*. When the cause is unknown, the disease can only be treated symptomatically.

Some diseases are *iatrogenic*—that is, they are caused by medical treatment and its effects. For example, the chemotherapy drugs used to treat some cancers can cause severe anemia, or hepatitis can develop as a result of a contaminated blood transfusion. A term closely related to iatrogenic is **nosocomial.** It refers to a hospital-acquired or health-care-associated infection. A nosocomial infection appears 48 hours or more after hospital admission or within 30 days after discharge. Another term often associated with disease is **sequela.** Sequela is a pathological condition that results from a prior disease, injury, or attack. For example, a sequela to polio is paralysis.

CHAPTER EPISODE—PART III

Ian has difficulty in his thinking process. He is often overwhelmed when too much information comes to him. In the beginning of his recovery, it was much worse. In time, however, he was able to manage better. Occupational therapists were helpful in identifying how Ian could be more productive in some kind of vocation.

- Search the Internet to determine how many individuals have a TBI each year. Visit other sites that show how individuals cope with TBI.
- Might there be any long-term adverse outcomes to Ian's injuries?

*These data are still referred to today. For Gary Whitlock's Mortality Trends website, see http://www.mortality-trends.org/.

SUMMARY

The disease process is varied, complex, and sometimes unknown. When the body is out of harmony, there is a need for care and treatment. Only when the disease process is understood are the best care and treatment possible. The body's disharmony affects each individual differently and for many different reasons. Health-care professionals must remain aware of the *person* with the illness who is affected by the disease or disorder.

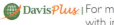 | For more resources and to sharpen your skills with interactive exercises, visit DavisPlus at http://davisplus.fadavis.com. Keyword *Tamparo*.

ONLINE RESOURCES

Body mass index calculator, sponsored by the National Heart Lung and Blood Institute, National Institutes of Health
http://www.nhlbi.nih.gov/health/educational/lose_wt/BMI/bmicalc

Burns
http://www.ncbi.nlm.nih.gov/pmc/articles/PMC449823/

Huntington Disease
U.S. National Library of Medicine
http://www.ncbi.nlm.nih.gov/pubmedhealth/PMH0001775/

Immunodeficiency Disorders
http://www.nlm.nih.gov/medlineplus/ency/article/000818.htm

Spider Bites
http://www.medicinenet.com/spider_bites_black_widow_and_brown_recluse/article.htm

CASE STUDIES

Case Study 1

Just off the Oregon coast, a fishing boat filled with eager tourists pulled out of the harbor on a beautiful, sunny, cool day. The tide was unusually low as the boat was crossing the bar. This was the third boat to go out that morning, and the first two encountered no problems. This boat, however, was hit broadside by a wave and capsized. About half of the passengers were wearing life jackets. Some of the passengers were trapped below deck in the overturned boat and attempted to break through the glass barriers to swim to the surface. Hypothermia set in within minutes, and 10 of the 17 passengers drowned. Two persons were not recovered.

Case Study Questions
1. Describe the physiological effects of hypothermia.
2. What preventative measures could the tourists have taken?
3. What preventative measures could the captain of the boat have taken?

Case Study 2

Jayne and Brandon have three active children, aged 7, 9, and 11. Tonight they have to take the two boys, Jason and Kyle, to a baseball game and their daughter, Miranda, to karate practice. Both Jayne and Brandon leave work a bit early to allow time to take the family to the local fast-food drive-through. Everyone orders "supersize." Jayne drops the boys and Brandon off at the baseball game and drives the van to karate practice with Miranda. Jayne and Miranda return to the baseball game as the coach is giving his winning players candy bars, soda, and chips. The family leaves for home, and on the way, Miranda asks the boys to share their candy and chips. Mom ponders the nutritional value of the evening's meal, activities, and snacks.

Case Study Questions
1. Identify the nutritional implications of the meal.
2. What are the negative and positive effects of tonight's activities and the family's habits?

REVIEW QUESTIONS

Matching
Match each of the following definitions with its correct term:

1. Genes inherited from parents
2. Describes condition of a sick person
3. Disrupted DNA sequence
4. Smallest microorganism
5. Not in harmony
6. Contains all genetic information
7. Worms
8. Process of engulfing invading organisms at the site of infection
9. Caused by treatment
10. Helps assess extent of burns

a. Disease
b. Illness
c. Genotype
d. DNA
e. Mutation
f. Virus
g. Helminths
h. "Rule of nines"
i. Phagocytosis
j. Iatrogenic
k. Homeostasis
l. Phenotype

Short Answer

1. Can you explain the three ways that the body is protected from disease?
   a. _____
   b. _____
   c. _____

2. What is the leading cause of death in the United States for those younger than 35?
   _____

3. What are the common predisposing factors for disease?
   a. _____
   b. _____
   c. _____
   d. _____
   e. _____

4. Briefly describe the three types of monogenic hereditary disorders.
   a. _____
   b. _____
   c. _____

5. Identify five groups of microorganisms, and give an example of a disease caused by each.
   a. _____
   b. _____
   c. _____
   d. _____
   e. _____

Multiple Choice
Place a check next to the correct answer:

1. Which of the following best describes trisomy 21, or Down syndrome?
   _____ a. Is caused by a missing gene
   _____ b. Is an uncommon birth defect
   _____ c. Is indicated by three copies of chromosome 21
   _____ d. Is caused by an additional X chromosome in males

2. How are B-cell lymphocytes likely characterized?
   _____ a. Provide cell-mediated immunity
   _____ b. Are responsible for acquired humoral immunity
   _____ c. Are the slowest and least aggressive responses of antigen contact
   _____ d. Are processed in the thymus

3. What is an important key to recall about anaphylactic shock?
   _____ a. May occur after single or repeated exposures to an antigen
   _____ b. Most often presents mild symptoms of distress
   _____ c. Is an example of both B-cell and T-cell deficiency
   _____ d. Is not an allergic reaction

4. Malignant tumors are best described how?
   _____ a. Are circumscribed
   _____ b. Are not cancerous
   _____ c. Do not spread through the lymphatic system
   _____ d. Are characterized by uncontrollable growth cells

5. At what point does the risk of diabetes in obesity increase by 60%?

    _____ a. When the BMI is under 25

    _____ b. If there is an additional metabolic disorder

    _____ c. When the BMI is over 25

    _____ d. The result of mineral deficiencies in the blood

Discussion Questions/Personal Reflection

1. Compare and contrast the two situations that follow. What potential causes of disease do you think either or both persons might have?
   Nathan Zimmer lives in an area of northeastern Pennsylvania where hydraulic fracturing for natural gas has elevated methane gas levels in his drinking water. Sandi Smith lives in rural western Nebraska working outdoors much of the time managing her wheat farm.

   _____

   _____

   _____

   _____

   _____

   _____

   _____

   _____

   _____

   _____

2. Discuss malnourishment and vitamin/mineral deficiencies and the influence of poverty.

   _____

   _____

   _____

   _____

   _____

   _____

   _____

   _____

   _____

   _____

> *Some patients, though conscious that their condition is perilous, recover their health simply through contentment with the goodness of the physician.*
> — HIPPOCRATES, 460–400 BC

2

Integrative Medicine and Complementary Therapies

● *key words*

Endorphin (ĕn•dŏr′fĭn)   **Enkephalin** (ĕn•kĕf′a•lĭn)

● *learning outcomes*

Upon successful completion of this chapter, you will be able to:

- Define key terms.
- Define other terms for *alternative medicine*.
- Identify the growth of complementary and alternative forms of medical treatment.
- Recall the history and philosophy of conventional medicine.
- Restate the history and philosophy of alternative medicine.
- Examine at least five hurdles to clear as society moves toward integrative health care.
- Apply the points in separating fact from fallacy to selecting an alternative medical treatment.
- Assess the role of the National Center for Complementary and Integrative Health (NCCIH).
- Describe the treatment model of at least five alternative health-care providers licensed to practice.
- Assess the validity of nonlicensed alternative therapies.
- Support the connection of mind and body in relation to the disease process.

- Recognize the effects of unexpressed negative emotions on the body.
- Discuss the importance of laughter and play in health.
- Explain the importance of personal responsibility in relation to health.
- List at least four influences of personal lifestyle on health.
- Assess the influence of *stress* and *distress* on health.
- Identify at least three dietary goals for the population of the United States.
- Evaluate Dr. Andrew Weil's philosophy on the importance of accepting one's circumstances in chronic illness.
- Compare and contrast conditional and unconditional love.
- Discuss the effects of spirituality on a healthy lifestyle.

CHAPTER EPISODE—PART I

Jesse Mach, a 56-year-old man, was coming home from work each day more tired than ever. Sleep and rest did not seem to increase his energy. Because he was a 7-year survivor of chronic lymphocytic leukemia, he was alert to symptoms that might signal a return of the disease. He and his wife, Lexi, were preparing for the first vacation they had taken in quite some time—a trip to France and Spain. Jesse wisely made an appointment with his primary care provider, who ordered blood tests. The tests confirmed their suspicions. The disease had returned. This time, it was also accompanied by hairy cell leukemia. After much discussion and

agreement with the doctor, Jesse and Lexi decided to take their trip. An appointment was made with the oncologist for the week of their return. During the vacation, Jesse and Lexi were able to discuss treatment and what they hoped to do differently for this round of treatment.

- Do a little research to determine if/how either type of leukemia is life-threatening. How do these leukemias attack the body? Are they fast- or slow-growing?
- What might the discussion about treatment during vacation include?

THE CHANGING CLIMATE FOR COMPLEMENTARY AND ALTERNATIVE THERAPIES

In 2008, $33.9 billion was spent by individuals for alternative health care in the United States. Most of this amount was out-of-pocket expense. Statistics released in December 2008 from the National Center for Complementary and Integrative Health (NCCIH) (established in 1998 by the U.S. Congress) and the National Center for Health Statistics (part of the Centers for Disease Control and Prevention) indicate that over 38% of adults and 12% of children in the United States are using some form of complementary and alternative medicine. That number has continued to grow. Furthermore, Alan Mozes noted in a "Health Day" article in 2011 that health-care workers (doctors, nurses, their assistants, health technicians, and health-care administrators) are more apt to seek some form of complementary medicine and/or treatment than the average population. The most common complementary medical options sought were massage, yoga, acupuncture, Pilates, and herbal medicines.

DEFINITION OF TERMS

Many terms are used to refer to alternative medicine: *integrative*, *complementary*, and *alternative* are increasingly popular. Practitioners in the field are not totally satisfied with the terms *complementary* or *alternative* that are often referred to in the NCCIH. *Alternative* can imply that one medical treatment is to be used instead of another. *Complementary* medicine can imply that it is being used alongside traditional medicine, but the term is often misspelled and *complimentary* is used instead—there is no desire among any practitioners for this form of treatment to be seen as something "nice." The term *integrative*, introduced by Andrew Weil, MD, promotes the blending of the best of both conventional and nonconventional therapies and is reflected in the tittle.

The authors use *integrative* to refer to this model of care and *complementary* to refer to the therapies themselves. It should be noted that, increasingly, integrative medicine and alternative therapies actually do complement the more traditional form of health care.

HISTORY OF CONVENTIONAL MEDICINE

Conventional medicine can be traced back to René Descartes (1596–1650), a scientist and philosopher characterized by his rationalistic and dualistic worldview. Whether or not intended, his philosophy eventually led to the separation of the "mind" from the "body." Today's specialization of various branches of medicine and treatment by body systems is partly a result of this separation. During the mid-19th century, the discovery of disease-producing microbes and Louis Pasteur's (1822–1895) theory that germs caused illness opposed the earlier theory and approach to medicine that such microbes became infectious only if conditions inside the body were out of balance. Modern medicine went on to expand its role in the treatment of illness.

The development of microscopy, bacterial cultures, radiography, vaccines, and antibiotics led medical science more into the germ theory of disease and away from the idea that an individual had an important role to play in his or her own health. Medical schools organized into various departments, forcing students to focus their studies on one organ at a time, independent of all other organs. Even today, diseases are identified by a specific organ or system—gallbladder disease (ICD-10: K81.0), colitis (ICD-10:K50.10; inflammation of the large intestine), prostatitis (ICD-10: N41.9; inflammation of the prostate gland). Even cancers are named by the organ they affect. This terminology diverts attention away from the interrelatedness of all parts of the body as one whole person. This system-based approach to medicine was coined *allopathic medicine* by the German physician and chemist Samuel Hahnemann (1755–1843), who questioned the inherent limitations of this form of treatment.

HISTORY OF ALTERNATIVE MEDICINE

As early as 5000 BC, healing traditions from Chinese medicine and ayurvedic medicine, which is practiced in India, were based on the belief that health represented a balance and harmony that included body, mind, and spirit. Health was linked to harmony, whereas disease was linked to disharmony or imbalance. Even Hippocrates (477–360 BC), the father of Western medicine, recognized and taught that health depended on living in harmony with life forces.

Although conventional medicine is unsurpassed in its treatment of acute life-threatening illness and injuries, alternative medicine practitioners recognized that the most effective form of health care treats a person's entire being and educates and empowers individuals to take personal responsibility for their health.

INTEGRATION OF BOTH WORLDS

The most sensible form of health care for individuals seeking treatment would be a form of integrated medicine where practitioners in both worlds accepted conventional and complementary methods of treatment. There are a number of health-care issues to address, however, as society advances toward such integration:

1. Controlling spiraling health-care costs resulting from the need for and the use of increased technology.
2. Spending "little" to treat the cause of chronic disease but spending "much" when major illness results.
3. Spending huge sums on heroic measures, especially at both ends of life.
4. Ignoring lifestyle causes of diseases and disorders.
5. Integrating preventive medicine with rescue medicine.
6. Learning not to rely on only drug-based therapies to bring relief.
7. Seeking answers that address the root causes of health problems.
8. Obtaining increased insurance coverage for complementary therapies.

While progress has been made in a number of these areas, there still is a long way to go. Changing the paradigm is not easily accomplished when the issues are so very personal or force recognition of the fact that the current mode of medical care often lacks in progress.

SEPARATING FACT FROM FALLACY

Moving more toward integrative medicine has been slow, due in part to the skepticism of many traditional providers. An individual seeking to embrace a particular alternative or complementary method of care has to determine who the legitimate providers are and separate those who would do no harm from those whose particular treatment protocol has little or no value. The Mayo Clinic has gathered and summarized recommendations on how to evaluate the success of any alternative medicine treatment. Consider the following main points when evaluating any kind of health-care information:

- Seek information from the most recent date.
- Search major medical centers, universities, government agencies for data.
- Be wary of commercial sites on the Web or those loaded with advertisements.
- Watch for such red flag words such as *miracle cure, purify,* and *detoxify.*
- Look for clinical studies and randomized, controlled trials.
- Seek providers who work collaboratively with conventional practitioners.
- Get information about licensure, certification, and appropriate credentials.

- Remember that "natural" does not always mean "safe."
- Discuss any alternative treatment with the primary care provider.
- Be very careful of drug interactions when using any dietary supplements.

Another method of evaluation considers the licensure of alternative practitioners. Although their number has greatly increased, not all are licensed or regulated in their practice by the states in which they work. Osteopaths, chiropractors, and acupuncturists are licensed in every state. Naturopaths are licensed in Alaska, Arizona, California, Connecticut, Hawaii, Idaho, Kansas, Maine, Minnesota, Montana, New Hampshire, Oregon, Utah, Vermont, and Washington. Five Canadian provinces, the District of Columbia, and the U.S. territories of Puerto Rico and the U.S. Virgin Islands also license naturopaths. Homeopaths are licensed only in Arizona, Connecticut, and Nevada. Midwives and massage therapists are licensed in all states. Many licensed practitioners incorporate one or more of the alternative methods of treatment identified in their practices. NCCIH, one of the 27 institutes and centers that make up the National Institutes of Health, was charged with studying the various forms of alternative therapies to separate fact from fallacy and to present their findings to the public. Four main categories are identified here.

Alternative Systems of Medical Practice

There are a number of alternative medical systems to consider. Two of these alternative forms are also classified as ancient healing systems—Ayurveda and traditional Chinese medicine.

Ayurveda is based on a 5,000-year-old system from India. It identifies three fundamental energies important to the mind and body: Vata (wind), Pitta (fire), and Kapha (earth). Each person holds a unique proportion of these three, usually with one being dominant. The goal is to keep the forces in balance. This system stresses mind–body practices such as yoga and meditation. Proper nutrition, herbal medicines, and massage are also involved.

Traditional Chinese medicine (TCM) is as ancient as Ayurveda. TCM is based on the five elements of fire, earth, metal, water, and wood. The feminine aspect of life, or *yin,* and the male element of life, or *yang,* are included. Some authorities refer to this system as "ancient medicines" and include Asian, Pacific Islander, American Indian, and Tibetan practices. TCM considers qi (pronounced "chee") to be the life force or energy that flows in channels or meridians to all parts of the body to nourish, protect, and heal.

Acupuncture is a common component of TCM, as is acupressure and moxibustion, massage, herbal medicine, meditation, and exercise (often in the form of tai chi). Acupuncture is placement of very thin, sterile, flexible needles into one of the 365 points along 12 meridians of the body to transmit qi (Fig. 2.1). Moxibustion practiced today uses various substances to apply heat to a broad area of skin. The direct heat source helps to relax muscles and relieve aching and mild pain without making skin blisters, as was often the case in the ancient moxibustion technique.

Homeopathy is a system of healing developed and published by Samuel Hahnemann in 1796. He believed that low doses of certain substances, prescribed in miniscule amounts, could bring about a cure. The idea is that highly diluted substances leave an "energy imprint" in the body and stimulate the immune system, thereby helping to cure an illness. This system is generally accepted in England, parts of Europe, and India. Homeopathy is increasingly known in the United States, but there is much controversy surrounding it.

Naturopathy is a system of medicine that stresses prevention and the use of nontoxic, natural therapies. Naturopathy treats the whole person and stresses a positive mental attitude and a healthy lifestyle that includes exercise, sleep, and a healthy diet. Nutritional supplements, vitamins and minerals, and physical modifications in breathing and posture may be emphasized.

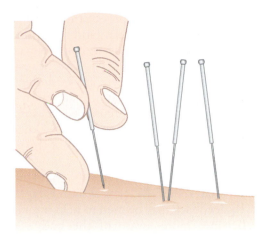

Figure 2.1 Acupuncture needles used in traditional Chinese medicine.

Additional Therapies Referred to as Alternative

Bioelectromagnetic or *bioenergetic therapies* concentrate on modifying the disease processes by directing energy (electrical or magnetic) within or through the body. Drugs and surgery are not used. Healing touch and therapeutic touch are also included. Bioelectromagnetic therapy encourages the individual to be aware of the body's own signals or energy field and strives to help create a more healthy or positive energy force.

Diet and nutrition therapies emphasize general dietary goals, in particular ensuring sufficient amounts of essential fatty acids, amino acids and enzymes, and minerals and vitamins. Most conventional practitioners stress diet and nutrition as well.

Herbal medicine therapies use any number of herbs to assist in the healing process. The practice of herbal medicine is considered mainstream in many cultures. Much of modern traditional medications are based on the use of herbs. Although herbal medicines do not go through the rigor of approval by the U.S. Food and Drug Administration (FDA), the World Health Organization has indicated that the historical use of herbal preparations is evidence of safety unless there is scientific evidence to the contrary. Attention to FDA rulings is beneficial, however. For example, dietary supplements that contain synthetic ephedrine (used mostly for weight loss) are not permitted for distribution.

Manual healing methods include osteopathic medicine, chiropractic, and massage therapy. Osteopathy was founded in 1874 by Dr. Andrew Taylor Still, who believed the musculoskeletal system played a more significant role than is usually believed in allopathic medicine. Osteopathic manipulation is often used to deal with the body's dysfunction. Many osteopaths also practice conventional medicine. Chiropractic officially began in 1895. Much like osteopathy, chiropractic

---

CHAPTER EPISODE—PART II

After vacation, Jesse keeps his appointment with the oncologist. They discuss treatment and the number of ways it has been improved since he was last treated. He is reminded, however, that recovery is still difficult but that remission is a very strong possibility. Jesse tells the oncologist that he would like to add some alternative therapy to his treatment—namely acupuncture and the part of mind–body medicine he believes is known as *psychoneuroimmunology*. The physician is a little surprised by Jesse's wish but understands when he is told that Jesse's oldest daughter is a nurse practitioner and has discussed with him how these avenues of treatment might enhance his more traditional therapy.

- Was it helpful that Jesse shared his ideas with his oncologist? Why or why not?
- What might the oncologist wish to do?
- What can Jesse do to see that his treatment plan is integrated with both the traditional and the alternative forms of care?

principles involve spinal biomechanics and musculoskeletal, neurological, vascular, and nutritional relationships. Massage therapy is well known and has been increasingly popular in the past decade, especially in sports medicine arenas. There are a number of different techniques, but all apply therapy with gliding strokes, kneading, rubbing, percussion, and sometimes vibration. Thai massage uses the elbows, knees, and feet as well as the hands in application of the massage to provide therapeutic relief.

Mind–body medicine integrates the mind and body and teaches that, medically, each system is equally significant. Biofeedback may be used to help train individuals to become more aware of the body's signals. Psychoneuroimmunology is another concept used in mind–body medicine; it is derived from -*logy* ("study of"), *psych-* ("mind"), *neuro-* ("brain"), and *immuno-* ("immune system"). This system promotes a strong interrelatedness among emotions, stress, and the body's reaction through the immune system. Participants are taught how to use relaxation and visualization to reduce stress in their lives. Deep breathing from the diaphragm, meditation, repetitive exercise and/or prayer, progressive muscle relaxation, yoga or tai chi, and imagery may be used as part of this therapy. Hypnotherapy may be suggested. The use of humor and laughter, journaling exercises, music, dance, and art also may be used as therapy.

NCCIH has a comprehensive website that disseminates up-to-date information on which complementary and alternative modalities work and why. One of the goals of the NCCIH is to promote the integration of scientifically proven complementary and alternative modalities into conventional medicine. Fact sheets are available that cover general information about complementary and alternative medicine on specific topics and treatments.

Whether only traditional medicine is embraced, only alternative medicine is embraced, or the two are integrated, there are several general themes that run through all three possibilities. Those themes are identified here.

THE MIND'S CONNECTION WITH HEALTH AND DISEASE

It is difficult to identify or even define the mind. The writer Candace Pert, PhD, has described the mind as "an enlivening energy in the information realm throughout the brain and body that enables the cells to talk to each other, and the outside to talk to the whole organism." The mind has everything to do with health. Moods and attitudes embodied in a person's emotions are part of the mind's physical expression. Emotions affect all of the organs and tissues. Negative emotions have a negative effect on health, especially over a long period of time; positive emotions have a positive effect on health.

It appears that sustained negative emotions over a long period of time can seriously hinder the body's immune system and keep it from functioning at an optimal level. Such links between the psychological state and the body's biological processes call on the medical community and each individual to pay closer attention to emotions and levels of stress.

Managing Negative Emotions

Humans are emotional creatures. Feelings of joy, sorrow, anger, jealousy, love, resentment, fear, and hate are part of existence. How those emotions are dealt with has much to do with physical health.

Emotions may be categorized as positive or negative. Fear is a negative emotion if, for instance, it prevents functioning as normal human beings; it is a positive emotion if it cautions safety. Anger or resentment may cause the fist to clench, breathing to accelerate, the heart to pound, the head to ache, and muscles to tighten. Feelings of despair, panic, depression, fear, and frustration cause the healing resources of the human brain to be underutilized.

It can be helpful to realize that negative emotions that are not dealt with in a wholesome manner probably express themselves physically in the body. Some individuals may be sensitive to and recognize the physical signals given by the body. All too often, however, these negative emotions are "buried" somewhere in their inner consciousness and later may exhibit themselves during an illness. Even then, illness may not be attributed to repressed negative emotion. The kind of disease that results from unexpressed negative emotion is called *psychosomatic illness*. The symptoms of the disease are very real but are likely the result of one or more unexpressed negative emotions. Individuals must learn how to express negative feelings without destroying themselves or others if they wish to live a healthy life.

Table 2.1	Some Positive Ways to Work Out Negative Emotions

Weed the garden
Scrub and wax a floor
Run a mile—or several
Ride a bike
Beat a pillow
Relax in a tub
See a counselor
Wash the car
Play with a puppy or kitten
Lift weights
Cry, weep
Accept yourself
Read a funny book or go to a funny movie. Laugh!
Roll up the car windows; scream a little or a lot
Make certain there is someone who loves you unconditionally.

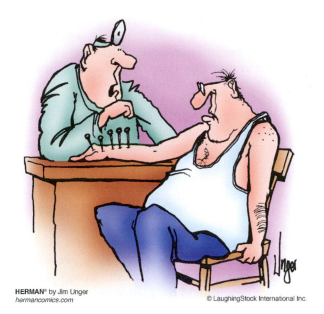

HERMAN® by Jim Unger
hermancomics.com

© LaughingStock International Inc.

**"I'll work my way up your arm and you
tell me when you feel anything."**

HERMAN© is reprinted with permission from LaughingStock Licensing Inc., Ottawa, Canada. All rights reserved.

Teach clients to check their bodies to see which part is most affected the next time anger or other emotions have a negative effect. If they can feel a headache coming on, can feel the fire in the gut, or feel the heart pounding, it is important to remember that there may be the need of an emotional release.

Enhancing Positive Emotions

When individuals have a great will to live and expect the best in life, their brains have a greater ability to produce chemicals, such as **endorphins** and **enkephalins,** that have a very positive effect on the body. For example, a sense of joy may warm the body, cleanse the spirit, relax muscles, lighten air passages, and generally make people feel good all over. Laughter, one sign of positive emotion, has often been described as "internal jogging." Despair and joy cannot be experienced at the same time. Therefore, it is important for individuals to allow, even plan for, laughter and play in their lives.

There are several examples of the use of laughter and play in today's health care. The late Dr. O. Carl Simonton, a noted radiation oncologist, told of his work with teaching cancer patients how to juggle. On his first visit, he gave individuals a set of juggling bags and some simple instructions. He juggled for them and told them to practice every day and that they would do some juggling together each time they met. Simonton reported that this activity (1) enabled

 REALITY EPISODE

Marcia was in the middle of a devastating divorce. She was trying hard to maintain control and move forward. To assist in that process, she sought counseling and learned about grieving. At one point, the counselor challenged Marcia: "When are you going to get angry?" That question made Marcia instantly angry, and she retorted, "I already did that." The counselor explained what happens when anger is repressed, where and how it often surfaces physiologically, and how to realistically express the anger in order to release it. The counselor gave Marcia several possibilities of how she might release her anger. The one that was of most interest to Marcia was putting old bottles and jars into a heavy-duty plastic bag and smashing them with a hammer, all the while allowing the surfaced thoughts to be expressed verbally.

Although Marcia felt a little silly, the next time she was really angry, she rushed to the garage, grabbed a big bag, and headed for the jars. She stopped short, however, when she spotted the cast-off pottery her husband (a novice potter) had abandoned when he left. She became excited. She threw a bunch of the pottery pieces into the bag, closed it, and gave the first big smash with the hammer. Then she hit the bag again. The shouting followed as she continued to smash the pottery. Afterward, she did not recall what she had said, but she was on the floor of the garage, crying, laughing, and feeling so good. Marcia also realized for the first time the rage she had been feeling and how much lighter she felt now.

Describe what is good about this activity. What might have happened had Marcia not discovered a way to release her anger?

him and his clients to develop a relationship outside of "doctor-client," (2) encouraged a lot of laughing together, and (3) gave the client something other than an illness to think about. Simonton also promoted the healing aspects of music, specifically the psychoneuroimmunological effects of active drumming. Dr. Simonton popularized the mind–body connection in fighting cancer and helped push the once-controversial notion into mainstream medicine. Simonton died at the age of 66 from an unfortunate accident, but many carry on his work at the Simonton Cancer Center.

They say laughter is the best medicine, and it appears there may be some truth to the statement. The art of laughter yoga was developed in 1995 by Dr. Madan Kataria, a physician practicing medicine in India. Intrigued by the claimed health benefits of laughter, he started a laughter club with people just telling jokes. Today, there are over 6,000 laughter clubs in 60 different countries. Usually the sessions start with a warm-up, which includes stretching and some body movement to help establish a feeling of playfulness. This is followed by exercises of deep breathing from the diaphragm. Then the laughter begins. With names like "the milkshake laugh" and "the lion laugh," it comes as no surprise that these exercises are quite childlike. Children can be our models, because children are great laughers, and they laugh even without jokes.

The well-known story reported by Norman Cousins in *Anatomy of an Illness* tells how laughter helped in healing his illness. He watched old Marx Brothers movies several times a day, laughing to near tears. Following this time of laughter, he was always able to function without pain medication for a greater period of time.

PERSONAL RESPONSIBILITY

Because the body is not indestructible, individuals need to be taught self-care and responsibility from birth. Often, however, it is not until individuals see someone become disabled or die that they gain a proper appreciation for their own bodies. From the moment of birth, the road to death begins. And during the period of life, individuals make choices about their body's well-being. Early in life, individuals are taught and learn by observation of those close to them either to respect or to ignore their bodies.

If individuals accept themselves, feel self-worth, and are taught well, they are able to listen to their body's signals and seek necessary attention. There is little or nothing a medical practitioner can do when the body breaks down if one does not want help or is unwilling to ask for it.

Andrew Weil, MD, says that the most common correlation between mind and healing in people with chronic illness is total acceptance of the circumstances of a person's life, including illness. This acceptance seems to allow and encourage a profound internal relaxation that enhances a person's spirit and immune system.

INFLUENCE OF LIFESTYLE

Lifestyle is an individual's consistent, integrated way of life, as typified by mannerisms, attitudes, and possessions. From the time a person is born, choices are made that influence lifestyle. These influences come from the following: modeling of family members and peers, education and knowledge, personal attitudes, degree of self-confidence, individual responsibilities, where the individual is in life, and life's opportunities. From this list, it is clear that individuals have a great deal of control over their own lifestyles. Lifestyle choices have great influence, whether positive or negative, on personal health and the health of others. Parents who provide a model of healthful living influence their children toward a healthy lifestyle.

Personal responsibility requires a person to act safely in a potentially dangerous situation. Conversely, being responsible for oneself requires that the individual avoid potentially harmful behaviors and attitudes, such as smoking, failing to exercise, driving without a seat belt, or disregarding treatments prescribed by health-care providers. It requires individuals to listen to their bodies. Living a healthy lifestyle can lessen one's chances of developing heart disease, diabetes, hypertension, and other chronic diseases. It is unfortunate, however, that disease can still ravage the body even when an individual exercises regularly, eats healthy foods, maintains a proper weight, sleeps well, manages distress appropriately, never smokes or uses recreational drugs, and rarely drinks. As you learned in Chapter 1, there are still many predispositions to disease not managed by one's choices.

If individuals seek an integrative approach to health care, they must remember that they have a personal responsibility to share *all* of their treatment methods with their primary care provider. The traditional or allopathic practitioner should be a part of an individual's decision to seek complementary or alternative therapies. Likewise, an alternative practitioner must be aware of any treatment the individual is receiving from the allopathic practitioner.

Value of Good Nutrition

Gluttony is not a secret vice.—Orson Wells

Improper nutrition may result in disorders or diseases. Bowel cancer is more common among groups of people who consume high amounts of animal fat and little fiber. There also is evidence that breast cancer may be linked to a high-fat, low-fiber diet and that where there is high meat consumption, cancer mortality rates are correspondingly high.

The *Dietary Goals for Americans*, adapted from the U.S. Department of Agriculture, includes the ABCs with the following suggestions:

A. *Aim for Fitness*
   • Aim for healthy weight.
   • Be physically active each day.
B. *Build a Healthy Base*
   • Let the Food Pyramid guide choices.
   • Choose a variety of whole grains daily.
   • Choose a variety of fruits and vegetables daily.
   • Keep food safe for eating.

C. Choose Sensibly
- Choose a diet low in saturated fat and cholesterol and moderate in total fat.
- Choose beverages and foods to moderate intake of sugars.
- Choose and prepare foods with less salt.
- Drink alcoholic beverages only in moderation, if at all.

It is important to realize that individuals have the power to improve their lifestyle by eating properly each and every day. Good nutrition can make a difference—if not in prolonging life, at least in enabling individuals to face life's stresses with greater ease.

Stress and Distress

It is generally believed that biological organisms require a certain amount of stress in order to maintain their well-being. Stress is always present. "Good" stress enables the body to meet the challenges of everyday activity. For example, stress keeps individuals alert when driving in heavy traffic or helps them respond to needs of family members in crises. Without a correct balance of stress, people would be unable to respond to any stimuli.

Distress, however, tends to be a negative influence. When distress occurs in quantities that the system cannot handle, it may produce pathological changes. These stressors can be either a person or a condition; some examples of stressors are children, spouses, bosses, unemployment, weather, traffic, noise, money, school, environment, retirement, divorce, death, disease—any change that occurs in life. The amount of distress experienced depends a great deal on how individuals respond to these stressors.

The recognition of stressors in life and their subsequent management constitute one of the keys to a healthy lifestyle. It has been shown that good nutrition, proper exercise, and a quality support system can help alleviate distress.

LOVE, FRIENDSHIP, AND SPIRITUALITY

We learn in most psychology classes that we must love ourselves before we can love another. But what is love? In his book *Love,* Leo Buscaglia defined love as "a learned, emotional reaction. If we wish to know love, we must live love, in action." Love is spontaneous. If someone is loved, share that love now. Love must be given unconditionally. (Striking evidence of the positive effects of unconditional love comes from the successful use of

pets in various kinds of therapy.) To expect something in return for love is an error. We love because we feel it and want to share it. And we never "run out of" love.

Friendship is one part of love. Everyone needs at least one friend or mentor with whom he or she can share anything at any time. The friend must love unconditionally and not expect anything in return. Friendship may be short-lived or lifelong. Whatever the duration, friendships enable growth and development and are to be encouraged.

Not every person embraces religion or senses a strong spiritual influence in life, but all have witnessed its influence in the life of someone some time. Some call it worship. Others call it prayer. For many, it may be meditation. Yoga has been very helpful to some; for others, it is a mental discipline. The experience is a devotion, a setting aside, an adoration, a refreshing, or an enlightening. It may include service, witnessing, sharing, and a sense of community and belonging. Whatever it is, it is a very personal experience.

Practitioners of integrative health recognize the worth of such experiences in a person's life. A faith in something or someone greater and more powerful than oneself can make coping with the most desolate of times a little less difficult.

CHAPTER EPISODE—PART III

The outcome of Jesse's diagnosis is not known at this point, but can you talk a little about what difference, if any, complementary therapies might make in his treatment?

- What mind–body therapies might he have chosen?
- What would you choose in the same circumstances?

SUMMARY

Complementary therapies and integrative medicine play an important role in the treatment of diseases and disorders in today's climate. The greatest success in treatment will be seen in clients cared for by health-care practitioners who are able to integrate the traditional and alternative modalities, who are effective in encouraging their clients to be open and honest about their choices, and who are unafraid to take a bold step forward in uncharted waters.

DavisPlus | For more resources and to sharpen your skills with interactive exercises, visit DavisPlus at http://davisplus.fadavis.com. Keyword *Tamparo*.

ONLINE RESOURCES

Complementary and Alternative Medicine: Evaluate Treatment Claims

http://www.mayoclinic.org/healthy-living/consumer-health/in-depth/alternative-medicine/art-20046087

http://www.fda.gov

National Center for Complementary and Integrative Health

http://nccih.nih.gov/

The Healing Art of Laughter

http://www.mondaymag.com/news/146909085.html

http://www.laughteryoga.org/english

CASE STUDIES

Case Study 1

Joyce Garcia, a 64-year-old surgical nurse, is diagnosed with breast cancer. After consulting with her primary care provider, undergoing mammography and ultrasonography, and seeing a specialist, a treatment protocol is determined. Joyce undergoes a lumpectomy. The lymph nodes are found to be clear of the cancer. Radiation treatment follows. Joyce notifies her closest friends and the women in her Bible study group. She asks for prayer and support. She uses visualization in her healing. She visualizes the cancer as a black, nasty-looking glob being removed in its entirety from her breast. Joyce's recovery is uneventful, and she regularly returns to her primary care provider for evaluation. She is so grateful that breast self-examination helped her find the lump.

Case Study Questions

1. Identify the conventional and traditional methods of treatment that Joyce sought.
2. Are there any other complementary therapies that might have helped in Joyce's recovery?

Case Study 2

Robert Busabarger, MD, is the only physician in a small rural East Coast village. He is all things to all people—physician, counselor, surgeon, obstetrician, pediatrician, and psychiatrist. He works 10-hour days and is rarely away from his practice unless on the ocean in his fishing vessel. He is frustrated that there is never enough time to meet all the needs of his clients as fully as he would like.

Case Study Questions

1. How might Dr. Busabarger use complementary therapies with his clients and decrease his workload?
2. Discuss how clients in this kind of setting might be able to help Dr. Busabarger and each other obtain medical treatment that treats the "whole" person.

REVIEW QUESTIONS

Matching

Match each of the following definitions with its correct term:

_____ 1. Father of Western medicine

_____ 2. NCCIH

_____ 3. Licensed in every state

_____ 4. Philosopher of conventional medicine

_____ 5. Medicine from India

a. René Descartes

b. Ayurvedic medicine

c. Hippocrates

d. Osteopaths, chiropractors, and acupuncturists

e. National Center for Complementary and Integrative Health

f. Naturopaths and homeopaths

Short Answer

1. What are four of the health-care issues most important to you that society must address in advancing toward integrative care?

   a. _____

   b. _____

   c. _____

   d. _____

2. When evaluating any alternative form of medicine, what are four main points you might consider?

   a. _____

   b. _____

   c. _____

   d. _____

3. Traditional Chinese medicine (TCM) can be identified by three main philosophies. Can you name them?

   a. _____

   b. _____

   c. _____

4. Create a day's eating plan to allow for four servings of fruits and vegetables.

   _____

   _____

   _____

5. What are four constructive outlets for expressing negative feelings that might be beneficial to an individual?

   a. _____

   b. _____

   c. _____

   d. _____

Multiple Choice

Place a checkmark next to the correct answer.

1. What term does Andrew Weil, MD, use for nontraditional medicine?

   _____ a. Complementary

   _____ b. Holistic

   _____ c. Alternative

   _____ d. Integrative

2. Which of the following statements is true concerning conventional medicine?

   _____ a. It is often referred to as allopathic or traditional medicine.

   _____ b. It was strongly influenced by Chinese and Ayurvedic medicine.

   _____ c. It treats a person's entire being and empowers an individual to take personal responsibility.

   _____ d. It does not include specialization as various branches of medicine.

3. Which of the following group of alternative practitioners are licensed in only a few states?

   _____ a. Naturopaths

   _____ b. Homeopaths

   _____ c. Midwives

   _____ d. Acupuncturists

4. Acupuncture, often a component of TCM, likely includes what other practices?

   _____ a. The use of nutritional supplements, vitamins, and minerals

   _____ b. Especially encourages laughter yoga

   _____ c. Moxibustion and tai chi

   _____ d. Using highly diluted substances to leave an imprint on the body

5. When clients are taught how to use relaxation, visualization, deep breathing, and progressive muscle relaxation, they are embracing what form of medical practice?

_____ a. Manual healing methods

_____ b. Mind–body medicine

_____ c. Bioenergic therapies

_____ d. Herbal medicine therapy

Discussion Questions/Personal Reflection

1. Identify a negative emotion you have difficulty expressing. Discuss with a friend what may be the consequences of such repression.

_____

_____

_____

_____

_____

_____

_____

_____

_____

_____

_____

_____

_____

2. Share a cartoon, joke, or funny story with a classmate. Describe how you felt after sharing a laugh.

_____

_____

_____

_____

_____

_____

_____

_____

_____

_____

_____

_____

_____

_____

Hold on, hold on to yourself, for this is gonna hurt like hell.
—SARAH MCLACHLAN

Pain and Its Management

● *key words*

Adjuvant analgesics
  (ăd'jū•vănt ăn"ăl•jē'sĭks)
Cordotomy (kŏr•dŏt'ŏ•mē)
Endorphin (ĕn•dŏr'fĭn)
Enkephalin (ĕn•kĕf'ă•lĭn)
Hypophysectomy
  (hī•pŏf'ĭ•sĕk'tō•mē)
Intrathecal (ĭn"tră•thē'kăl)

Neuromodulator
  (nū"rō•mŏd'ū•lā•tŏr)
Neuropathic pain
  (nū"rō•pă'thĭk pān)
Neurotomy (nū•rŏt'ŏ•mē)
Neurotransmitter
  (nū"rō•trăns'mĭt•ĕr)

Nociceptive pain
  (nō"sĭ•sĕp'tĭv pān)
Nonopioids (nŏn•ō'pē•oyds)
Opioids (ō'pē•oyds)
Prostaglandins
  (prŏs"tă•glăn'dĭns)

● *learning outcomes*

Upon successful completion of this chapter, you will be able to:

- Define key terms.
- Summarize three types of pain clinics.
- Discuss the major barriers to pain management.
- Describe *pain*.
- Discuss the purpose of pain.
- Compare and contrast acute and chronic pain.
- Explain nociceptive pain and neuropathic pain and give examples of each.
- State five factors that influence how pain is experienced.
- Explain the gate control theory of pain.

- Critique the two most common pain assessment tools.
- List and describe the types of OTC medication therapies for treating pain.
- List and describe the types of prescription medication therapies for treating pain.
- List and describe the types of complementary therapies for treating pain.
- Discuss the role of placebos in pain management.

CHAPTER EPISODE—PART I

Allan is 76 years old. He is retired and goes regularly to the neighborhood gym. He has been physically active all his life. Most of his friends are from the gym. Recently, Allan has been having some pain issues in his lower back and down his legs. He changed his stretching routine and that helped some. He would take a couple of Tylenol before going to the gym, which helped for a while. This morning when he awoke, he had trouble walking because the pain was so bad.

- Is Allan's workout routine the source of his discomfort? Explain your answer.
- What might be the next step for Allan?

PAIN AND ITS TREATMENT MODELS

Pain affects everyone at one time or another. It can be acute or chronic. Many diseases and disorders of the human body are accompanied by pain. It is feared by many people, as much as or more than the diseases themselves. Pain is one of the most common complaints of those seeking medical attention. Pain can be debilitating, interfering with sleep and daily activities. What is pain? What purpose, if any, does it serve? What happens in the body when a person feels pain? How is pain assessed? What are the different types of pain? Can pain be treated? If so, how?

Pain is an expanding science, and an increasing number of specialty clinics are emerging. The International Association for the Study of Pain (IASP) identifies the following models for pain treatment:

Pain clinic: Usually outpatient, these clinics focus mainly on diagnosis and management of individuals with chronic pain. The focus most likely is on specific pain issues, such as back pain or headache, but these clinics can also provide treatment for general pain conditions.

Multidisciplinary pain clinic: These clinics may be inpatient or outpatient and include specific treatment. They provide services from different health-care professionals, who can assess and manage physical restoration or rehabilitation and medical needs and can provide educational and psychological services.

Multidisciplinary pain center: This is usually found in a medical school or teaching hospital. The pain center provides the most complex model for managing and treating pain. Pain centers also engage in research. Two of the earliest multidisciplinary pain centers were the University of Washington in Seattle and the City of Hope Medical Center in Duarte, California.

EFFECTIVE PAIN MANAGEMENT

According to the Agency for Healthcare Research and Quality (AHRQ), a federal agency established in 1989, there are three major barriers to effective pain management: (1) the health-care system, (2) health-care professionals, and (3) clients. The health-care system is often slow to hold itself accountable for assessing and relieving pain. Many professionals suggest that assessment of pain be included when measuring vital signs, such as temperature, pulse, respiration, and blood pressure. Pain assessment would be the fifth vital sign. It is helpful to remember that heart rate and blood pressure may increase with acute pain but not necessarily with chronic pain. The belief is that routinely assessing and relieving pain can prove more cost-effective than ignoring the issue. Health professionals are not always educated about the meaning of and assessment of pain management and may be concerned about the use of **opioids** (narcotics), mainly due to possible addiction. Clients and their families also have concerns about opioid use and potential addiction. They may believe that chronic pain cannot be effectively treated. Health-care professionals can be frustrated in their attempt to treat individuals who experience pain, especially when its cause is not readily identifiable. Clients in pain may be frustrated and confused, too, especially if the pain is unbearable. In all situations, education is a key element for health-care professionals and for clients and their families.

WHAT IS PAIN?

Definition of Pain

In dictionaries, *pain* (ICD-10: R52 or G89.X) is defined as a sensation of hurting or of strong discomfort in some part of the body, caused by an injury, a disease, or a functional disorder and transmitted through the nervous system. A nurse, Margo McCaffery of Los Angeles, worked for years with clients in pain and conducted extensive research in the field of pain. She defines pain as "whatever the experiencing person says it is, existing when he or she says it does." This definition is perhaps the most useful because it acknowledges the client's complaint, recognizes the subjective nature of pain, and implicitly suggests that diverse measures may be undertaken to relieve pain.

The IASP and the American Pain Society define pain as an unpleasant sensory and emotional experience arising from actual or potential tissue damage or described in terms of such damage. Again, this definition further confirms the multiple components of pain in a person's psychological and physiological existence. Pain is the most common complaint of persons seeking medical attention.

Acute Pain

Acute pain (ICD-10: R52 or G89.1X*) is a helpful warning that something is wrong in normal body functioning. It warns of inflammation, tissue damage, infection, injury, trauma, or surgery somewhere in the body. Acute pain is often accompanied by anxiety. It is usually sudden and can last for hours or days, perhaps even longer. Such pain may manifest as an increase in heart rate, blood pressure, and muscle tension and a decrease in salivary flow and gut motility. The primary goal of treatment is to diagnose the source of pain and remove it. Acute pain disappears once the underlying cause of the pain is treated.

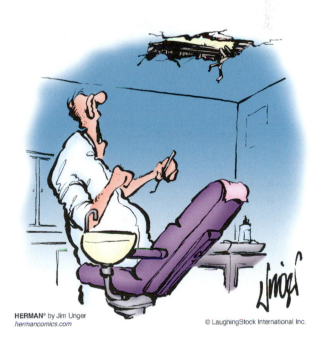

HERMAN® by Jim Unger
hermancomics.com

© LaughingStock International Inc.

**"OK, that's enough for one day.
I'll see you next Tuesday."**

HERMAN© is reprinted with permission from LaughingStock Licensing Inc., Ottawa, Canada. All rights reserved.

Chronic Pain

Approximately 100 million adults in the United States suffer from chronic pain (ICD-10: G89.2x or G89.4). This type of pain often starts as acute pain but continues beyond the normal expected time for resolution.

*The X represents the fourth digit that is often required and supplied once more detailed information about the disease or disorder is made known to the provider.

Chronic pain is no longer useful or beneficial. It may be described as a pain that recurs. It can be debilitating, exhausting an individual's physical and emotional resources. It is often difficult to manage, can aggravate other health conditions, and may lead to depression and anxiety. Complete relief of chronic pain does not always occur. In 2011, the Institute of Medicine reported that "the annual cost of chronic pain in the U.S. is estimated to be $560-$635 billion, including health care expenses and lost productivity." In light of this information, the treatment goal of chronic pain is to minimize the pain and maximize a person's functioning. The intent is to decrease the level of pain so that everyday activities can be performed. Because of this goal, a multidisciplinary approach to treatment is often necessary. This approach blends physical, emotional, intellectual, and social skills.

Chronic pain can further be described as:

1. **Nociceptive pain**
2. **Neuropathic pain**

Nociceptive pain is sometimes called *tissue pain*. It is derived from damage to tissues rather than nerves and is experienced mostly in the back, legs, and arms. The nerve cells (called *nociceptors*) carry the pain sensation to the spinal cord, where it is then relayed to the brain. This pain is well localized, often has an aching or throbbing quality, and is constant. The pain is called *somatic* if it is the result of damage or injury to muscles, tendons, and ligaments, usually in the back and thighs. Somatic pain may be further classified as *cutaneous* if the pain comes from the skin, or *deep* if the pain comes from deeper musculoskeletal tissues.

Neuropathic pain comes from a nervous system lesion. It may be further identified as *neural pain* if the lesion is in the brain or spinal cord. It is referred to as *peripheral neuropathic pain* if the lesion is along the cranial or spinal nerves (see Chapter 10). Neuropathic pain is often described as severe, sharp, stabbing, burning, cold, numbing, tingling, or weakening. Some individuals feel the pain move along the nerve path from the spine to the extremities. This type of pain does not usually respond to routine analgesics.

It is quite possible for individuals to experience nociceptive and neuropathic pain at the same time in certain conditions. Specialists in pain management define additional types of pain. The most common are listed here:

- Angina pain (ICD-10: R07.2) occurs when the blood supply to the heart muscle is disrupted. It is often described as crushing or tightness and burning pain in the chest.
- Breakthrough pain (ICD-10:R52) results from the reoccurrence of chronic pain that earlier responded to pain management.

- Malignant (cancer) pain (ICD-10: G89.3) comes from cancer (tumor, abnormal growth) or the treatment for cancer (surgery, radiation, chemotherapy).
- Phantom limb pain (ICD-10: M79.2) is the pain felt from an amputated body part. Military personnel who suffered the loss of a limb often describe this pain as squeezing or burning. The brain mistakenly interprets the nerve signals as coming from the missing limb.
- Psychogenic pain (ICD-10: F45.41) is often experienced by individuals with psychological disorders. They have very real pain but without a physical cause.

The Experience of Pain

How pain is experienced is based, in part, on several variables:

1. *Early experiences of pain.* Did management of pain in the past have a positive or negative impact? Generally, a person's fear of pain increases with each pain experience.
2. *Cultural backgrounds.* Research shows that culture generally does not influence how a person perceives pain but does influence how a person responds to pain. Early in life, children learn from those around them. For example, children may learn that a sports injury does not hurt as much as trauma from an automobile crash. Further, they learn what behaviors are acceptable or unacceptable. These behaviors vary among cultures. Rarely are these expectations changed; in fact, these perceptions are believed to be normal and acceptable.
3. *Anxiety and depression.* Does anxiety increase or decrease pain? Is depression the cause or result of pain? Some believe there is a relationship between anxiety and depression and pain. The longer the duration of pain, the greater is the occurrence of depression. It is important to address anxiety and depression when treating individuals in pain.
4. *Age.* Pain perception does not change significantly with age, yet the way an elderly person responds to pain treatment may differ from that of a younger person. For example, as a person ages, a slower metabolism and greater ratio of body fat to muscle mass dictates that a smaller dosage of analgesics may be required.
5. *Sex.* Recent research suggests that females and males experience pain differently. In fact, females demonstrate a greater frequency of pain-related symptoms in more bodily areas than do males. In addition, when pain-free individuals were exposed to a variety of painful stimulus, females exhibited greater sensitivity to the experimentally induced pain than did males. It was also evident that women attach an emotional aspect to the pain they experience, while men concentrate only on the physical sensations they experience. This sensory focus for

men allowed them to endure more pain and suffer less than the women.

GATE CONTROL THEORY OF PAIN

What occurs at the cellular level when pain is experienced? The gate control theory of pain, created by P. D. Wall and Ronald Melzack, offers a useful model of the physiological process of pain. Gate control is recognized as a major pain theory.

According to the gate control theory, pain is a balance between information traveling into the spinal cord through large nerve fibers and information traveling into the spinal cord through small nerve fibers (Fig. 3.1). Without any stimulation, both the large and small nerve fibers are quiet, and the substantia gelatinosa (SG) blocks the signal to the transmission cell (T cell) connected to the brain. The "gate is closed," and there is no pain. With pain stimulation, small nerve fibers are active. They activate the T-cell neurons but block the SG neuron, making it impossible for the SG to block the T-cell transmission to the brain. The "gate is open" and there is pain. In other words, pain is experienced whenever the substances that tend to propagate a pain impulse across each "gate" in a nerve pathway overpower the substances that tend to block such an impulse.

Studies of coping factors support a wider version of the gate control theory. These factors are to be considered before determining treatment for pain, and they raise several questions:

1. How well is the client experiencing life?
2. Does the client have pain, and if so, does he or she think that it is under control?
3. Does the client feel adequately informed about the painful condition?
4. Is the client occupied? How does the individual fill his or her time?
5. Is the client coping with other problems?
6. Does the client feel dissatisfied with his or her past life, or does he or she have any substantial regrets?
7. Are there any reasons why the client may not be coping?

Answers to these questions may help determine the best treatment protocol for pain, but they are not always easily related by clients to health-care professionals.

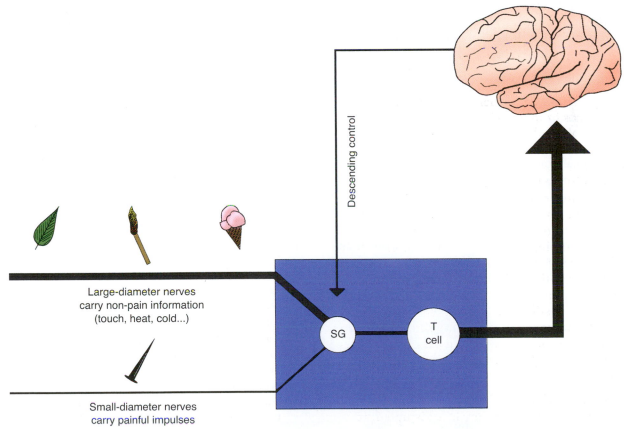

Figure 3.1 The gate control theory of pain transmission. The substantia gelatinosa (SG) accepts input both from large-diameter (nonpain) and small-diameter (pain) nerves. Based on the rate of input, the SG allows either the pain or nonpain stimulus to be passed on to the transmission cell (T cell) and up to the brain. Because nonpain impulses travel faster than pain impulses, stimulation of nonpain fibers can override the transmission of pain. In addition, the brain has an inhibiting influence both on the SG and the spinal cord that can work to limit the perception and reaction to pain. *(From Starkey, C.* Therapeutic Modalities for Athletic Trainers. *Philadelphia: FA Davis, 1993, p 28, with permission.)*

ASSESSMENT OF PAIN

Pain gives the body warning and often is accompanied by anxiety and the need to relieve the pain. Pain is both sensation and emotion. As noted earlier, it can be acute or chronic. Health-care professionals may find the following mnemonic tool useful for assessing a client in pain:

P = place (client points with one finger to the location of the pain)

A = amount (client rates pain on a scale from 0 [no pain] to 10 [worst pain possible])

I = interactions (client describes what worsens the pain)

N = neutralizers (client describes what lessens the pain)

The scale of 0 to 10, as described in the mnemonic, is a useful method of assessing pain. Further pain assessment skills include observing the client's appearance and activity. Monitoring the client's vital signs may be of value in assessing acute pain but not necessarily chronic pain.

To assess the pain of children or those with some cognitive dysfunction or dementia, a "smiley face" model often proves beneficial (Fig. 3.2). The first smiley face shows a content or happy face with no pain or hurt, whereas the last face shows pain that "hurts worst." Individuals are asked to point to the face that describes his or her smile. Note the faces are on a numeric scale.

TREATMENT OF PAIN

The objective of pain treatment is to remove or correct the cause of pain or to lessen its severity; however, there can be a lag in time between identifying the cause of the pain and providing relief. Treatment is diverse and can be difficult. Pain relief is not a "one-size fits all" proposition. A multidisciplinary approach to chronic pain management is often most successful but is not always available to everyone. This team approach involves both medical and nonmedical personnel and may include any number of approaches. There are several integrative/complementary pain control protocols that may be effective. Treatment of pain depends on the type of pain. Medications, too, are different in their pain control management.

Medications

Medications tend to be the main treatment of choice for many clients experiencing pain. Analgesics, anesthetics, and anti-inflammatory agents may be prescribed to decrease or eliminate pain, although they do not eliminate the cause of pain. Analgesics can be **opioid** (formerly referred to as *narcotic*) or **nonopioid** (formerly referred to as *non-narcotic*) or prescription or over-the-counter (OTC) and can be of varying strengths. Opioid analgesics may include morphine-like drugs, whereas nonopioid drugs include acetaminophen and NSAIDs. A third category of drugs called **adjuvant analgesics** include those whose primary purpose is not generally used or prescribed for pain. For example, drugs used for depression may be prescribed to effectively treat pain. Other adjuvant medications include those used for seizure control and corticosteroids. Medication may be administered orally, intravenously, nasally, by injection, or from a skin patch. Additionally, medications may be used alone or in conjunction with other treatment modalities.

Nonprescription Drug Therapy

OTC medications may be useful in relieving milder forms of pain. These medications include acetaminophen (Tylenol) or such NSAIDs as aspirin, naproxen, or ibuprofen. Both acetaminophen and NSAIDs can relieve pain due to muscle aches, but NSAIDs are able to reduce inflammation as well. There are many creams and salves on the market that can reduce pain. These topical analgesics give a "warm" sensation when applied to the area. Capzasin is known to give a "hot" feeling to the skin. Salicylates that have the pain-relieving substance found in aspirin, such as Aspercreme and Bengay, can provide pain relief from arthritic pain.

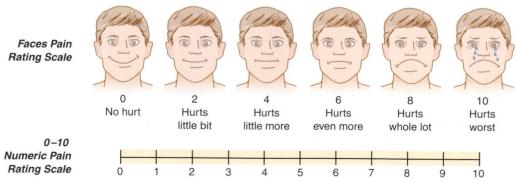

Figure 3.2 Pain assessment scales for adults and children.

REALITY EPISODE

Leslie Suianoa suffers from serious chronic pain that is difficult to relieve. She is 78 years old and is surprised when her primary care provider cautions her about preventing falls and suggests she use a walker or a cane. She comments, "I thought you were just increasing my pain medication; I can walk just fine."

What is the concern of the primary care provider? Of the client?

Nonprescription medications are taken so readily and freely by consumers that warning labels are often ignored. Those warnings, however, are quite important. Gastroenterologists advise all their clients that acetaminophen and NSAIDs can have an adverse effect on the digestive system. For example, the second major cause of ulcers is the overuse of NSAIDs. Long-term use of these medications should be monitored by a primary care provider who can help weigh the benefits of the drug treatment against possible side effects.

Prescription Drug Therapy

Prescription drug therapy may include muscle relaxants, antianxiety medications, antidepressants, prescription NSAIDs, steroids, and opioids.

Muscle relaxants have an overall sedative effect on the body and act on the brain rather than the muscles to create a total-body relaxant. They can be beneficial for muscle spasms and early treatment of low-back pain and can aid in sleep when pain keeps individuals awake. Side effects should be carefully considered. They can be habit-forming and may create changes in sleep cycles.

Antianxiety and antidepressant medications help to reduce depression and anxiety, but some can also reduce pain in muscles and joints. They can be particularly helpful for migraine headaches and neuropathic pain. These medications are powerful central nervous system depressants that may be used alone or in conjunction with other analgesic medications.

Prescription NSAIDs reduce inflammation and pain when they block enzymes and **prostaglandins** (proteins) made by the body. Prostaglandins cause pain when they irritate nerve endings, but they also help to protect the stomach lining, so blocking this enzyme may produce an adverse effect. These drugs do not alter a person's cognitive functioning, cause respiratory depression, or cause nausea. A common NSAID is Celebrex, which carries the additional warning of risk for heart attack and stroke.

Steroids are very potent anti-inflammatory drugs that also reduce pain. They work directly on the brain's chemistry to elevate mood and reduce pain. Unfortunately, steroids can suppress the body's immune function, cause fluid retention and weight gain, worsen diabetes, and reduce bone density when used for long periods of time.

Epidural steroid injections are very useful in alleviating pain that radiates from the lower back into the leg (as seen in spinal stenosis [ICD-10: M48.00]) or neck pain that radiates into the arm. The physician uses x-ray fluoroscopy to guide the needle directly into the neural foramen or the point where the affected nerve root exits the spinal canal to bathe the inflamed nerve root, thus reducing irritation and pain. These injections do not have the side effects attributed to oral steroids.

Opioids are strong and potentially addictive; therefore, they are to be carefully monitored by the provider giving the prescription. While opioids do not actually rid a person of pain, they work to separate or distance individuals from the feeling of pain. Common opioids are codeine, hydrocodone, oxycodone, and morphine. They are effective pain relievers for all types of pain. There are, however, side effects such as impairment of mental function, constipation, and interaction with acetaminophen.

Research indicates that health-care professionals and family members tend to undermedicate for pain because of incorrect assumptions, prevailing attitudes, the complexity of pain assessment, and unfounded fears, mainly those of addiction (psychological dependence). However, no medical research testifies to such an addiction. In fact, the use of opioids is indicated in many cases of pain management, and evidence is overwhelming that such fears are greatly exaggerated. Untreated pain adversely affects pulmonary, gastrointestinal, and circulatory systems and can cause insomnia, depression, and irritability if the pain becomes chronic. Pain must be reduced for healing to occur.

Patient-Controlled Analgesia Pump

A common treatment of some pain is the patient-controlled analgesia (PCA) pump. The pump allows clients to administer their own pain medication, offering some sense of control of the pain, which is an important psychological benefit. In PCA, the amount of drug dispensed by the pump is determined by the primary care provider. The device is designed to not release more than the prescribed amount within a set period of time, thus guarding against overmedication. Clients who should not use a PCA are those with hypersensitivity to the medication used, those with physical impairments that make it difficult to activate the pump, and those with any emotional or cognitive disability.

Intrathecal Drug Delivery

This method to control pain is similar to the PCA pump except that a surgeon places a medicine pump in a small pocket under the skin that delivers medicine from the pump to the **intrathecal** space around the spinal cord. This system can provide significant pain control with far fewer drugs than required with pills.

Surgery

Surgery for the treatment of pain is not normally considered until after all other treatments have failed. While surgery may reduce pain, it also can permanently damage the ability to feel other sensations. When necessary to block the transmission of pain or to remove the cause of pain, surgery may include such procedures as **neurotomy,** the dissection or division of a nerve; **cordotomy,** the surgical division of one or more of the lateral nerve pathways emerging from the spinal cord; and the removal of any causative factor.

Placebos

An interesting phenomenon is the use of placebos in pain management. A placebo is defined as a medication that produces an effect in a client because of its intent rather than because of its specific physical or chemical properties. In the placebo effect, the treatment works because the person believes it to be effective. When such placebos are used, studies show that 20% to 40% of those with objective stimuli report pain relief, at least for a short time. This is a powerful example of the mind–body connection. The placebo effect results from the natural production of **endorphins** and **enkephalins** in the descending control system. The more cues the client receives about the placebo's effectiveness, the more likely it will be effective in relieving pain.

Mobile Technology to Manage Chronic Pain

While not an actual treatment for pain, the use of a mobile electronic device may be used to help manage pain. Smartphones can be equipped with applications to monitor pain levels, connect to peer-support programs, or connect with the primary care provider. They can also collect data and track changes in pain, mood, and medication use. Many clients using this technology reported that they felt like they had greater control over their pain.

CHAPTER EPISODE—PART II

Allan is not happy about taking medications in order to feel comfortable. When the pain made it hard to walk, however, he knew something was wrong. He called his primary care provider (PCP). After a thorough examination, including x-rays and blood work, an oral steroid was prescribed. When the PCP called 3 days later to report his findings on the x-rays and blood workup, he asked about the pain level. Allan reported that in a day, his pain was gone. All the blood work was normal. However, the x-rays showed some moderate to severe degenerative changes at the L4-L5 level, as well as possible spinal stenosis. Anterolisthesis also was revealed. Conservative treatment was discussed, including a steroidal injection, and a physical therapy appointment was made.

- Using your medical dictionary, summarize the x-ray findings.
- Because Allan does not like to take medications, what would you say to him about both the oral and the injectable steroid? Identify the classification of these medications.

COMPLEMENTARY THERAPIES

The following pain treatments have proved effective in the treatment and management of pain, and they illustrate the blending of traditional and complementary medicine. Many, if not all, are used in conjunction with more traditional pain control, creating an integrative approach.

Physical Therapy

Physical therapy is a common adjunct to other pain therapies. By improving movement and body function that has been impaired by injury or disability, pain is reduced. Various stretching and movement exercises are shown to be pain relieving. Physical therapists may also use ultrasound for pain treatment. Using sound waves, ultrasound generates heat within a body part and stimulates blood flow circulation. Physical therapy sometimes includes warm water therapy pools in which clients exercise. Regular exercise and movement will also improve muscle tone, strength, and flexibility—all of which help to lower pain levels.

Biofeedback

Biofeedback is aimed at helping an individual gain voluntary control over normally involuntary physiological functions. Various forms of electronic feedback produced by monitoring physiological events may promote blood flow and reduce muscle tension, which in turn may reduce the concentration of neurotransmitters at the site of pain. The client has sensors attached to the skin with a device to measure the temperature of the skin site, which registers the tension in sore muscles. As the client relaxes, the blood flow increases with the temperature rise. After 10 to 12 sessions, the biofeedback procedure becomes so ingrained that the client is able to call on it whenever pain relief is needed.

The Association for Applied Psychophysiology and Biofeedback recommends the use of biofeedback for controlling pain for migraine headaches (ICD-10: G43.9x), tension headaches (ICD-10: G44.20X), and certain types of chronic pain.

Relaxation

Relaxation therapy can be used to modify muscle tension that is believed to cause or exacerbate pain. The individual is taught a series of techniques for relaxation to be used any time pain occurs. This includes both visual imagery and body awareness to move a person into a deep state of relaxation. Relaxation therapy is especially successful when used in conjunction with biofeedback and imagery. Almost all people experiencing pain benefit from some form of relaxation. It also helps combat fatigue (ICD-10: R53.x) and muscle tension.

Imagery/Visualization

Imagery is used to produce relaxation and increase the production of endorphins and enkephalins. It may consist of slow, rhythmic breathing with a mental image of comfort and relaxation. The person imagines and concentrates on a pleasant scene or experience and is taught to relax. To be effective, imagery necessitates a positive relationship to the image scene; otherwise, the imagery may only exacerbate the pain. To be effective, the guided imagery should be done for at least 5 minutes, three times a day.

Hypnosis

Hypnosis is a method of achieving a state that resembles sleep but is induced by a hypnotist, who makes readily accepted suggestions to the client. Autohypnosis, or self-induced hypnosis, is most effective when a person is motivated—and pain is a strong motivating force. Autohypnosis can be learned in a few hours. The mechanism whereby hypnosis works is thought to be mediated by the endorphin system. It is especially useful in clients with burns. The period of pain relief from hypnosis is from 4 to 6 hours, and the time of relief is extended with repeated hypnotic reinforcement. Hypnosis is also helpful in the management of psychogenic pain.

Transcutaneous Electrical Nerve Stimulation

Transcutaneous electrical nerve stimulation (TENS) is a therapeutic procedure that uses TENS pads to induce an electrical impulse in the large nerve fibers that carry nonpain information to block or reduce the transmission of painful impulses. The electrodes are connected by lead wires to a stimulator called a TENS unit, and the frequency and intensity of the electric current can be varied. The current produces a tingling, vibrating, or buzzing sensation in the area of pain. It is used by physical therapists for both acute and chronic pain. For example, it may be used on a surgical client to stimulate the nonpain or noxious receptors. This is consistent with the gate control theory and explains the effectiveness of cutaneous stimulation when applied to the same area as the injury.

Massage

Massage consists of manipulation, methodical pressure, friction, and kneading of the body. Oils or creams may be used to increase stimulation. Massage may be performed over or around an area of pain or at trigger points. This type of treatment stimulates blood flow, induces relaxation, and increases the production of endorphins and enkephalins. Massage also promotes comfort because it promotes muscle relaxation. The adjustment of joints in the spine and neck given by a chiropractor or an osteopath can be used in conjunction with massage therapy. Otherwise, massage is generally provided by massage therapists or physical therapists.

Humor, Laughter, and Play

Norman Cousins, former editor of the *Saturday Review*, popularized the concept of making laughter and humor an antidote for pain. While quite ill in the hospital, he discovered he could go much longer without his pain medication when he had been doing a great deal of laughing. He watched comedy films and read humorous books. Humor and laughter control pain in four ways: (1) by distracting attention, (2) by reducing tension, (3) by changing expectations, and (4) by increasing production of endorphins and enkephalins—the body's natural painkillers. Dr. Franz Ingelfinger, former editor of the *New England Journal of Medicine*, stated that "building a positive focus in your life—which includes a regular dose of laughter—can play a key role in supporting the body's ability to heal itself."

Play is another activity that is helpful in reducing pain, even for the severely debilitated person. Play can be childlike or quite adult. Consider the following: Two toddlers, riding tricycles, approach the charge nurse on the floor of the burn unit in a major city hospital. The burns of both are obvious, but their "race" through the corridors has become part of their treatment. One child is quite concerned over the loss of his baseball hat—a gift to all the children from a Major League team. The reason for the concern? All the children were leaving shortly to play ball with one of the therapists. Who can play ball without a cap? The tricycle race and the game afterward focus the child's attention on play—not on pain.

Music

Many health-care providers and dentists have discovered that music helps to alleviate pain. Dentists know that some clients are receptive enough to music to have their teeth extracted without anesthesia. Some hospitals allow music to be piped into their surgical rooms because it puts both clients and practitioners in a more relaxed state.

John Diamond, MD, practices preventive medicine and psychiatry in Valley Cottage, New York, and spent more than 25 years researching music and its therapeutic value and life-enhancing quality. His books *The Life Energy in Music*, volumes 1, 2, and 3, are particularly interesting to any person seeking more knowledge about music therapy and its healing powers.

A recent study conducted on 60 individuals who had experienced pain for an average of 6.5 years were able to reduce both their pain level and the depression related to the pain by about 20% when they listened to music for 1 hour per day for 7 days. Music is a safe and inexpensive way to help clients reduce their pain level and give them a measure of power over their symptoms.

Acupuncture

Acupuncture, which originated in China more than 5,000 years ago, began to receive attention in Western culture in the 1970s and was approved by the U.S. Food and Drug Administration in 1997. Acupuncture is a technique for treating certain painful conditions and for producing regional anesthesia via the passage of long, very thin needles through the skin to specific points. The free ends of the needles are twirled or, in some cases, used to conduct a weak electric current. Most acupuncturists use only 10 to 12 needles per treatment, and the person feels only a slight pricking sensation when the sterile, disposable needles are inserted. The treatment is painless and can take anywhere from a few seconds to 45 minutes.

Acupuncture appears to stimulate release of the body's natural painkillers, endorphins and enkephalins. It has been suggested that acupuncture influences the production and distribution of **neurotransmitters** and **neuromodulators,** which in turn modifies the person's perception of pain. Acupuncture, used as treatment for pain, is most effective in the treatment of postoperative pain (ICD-10: G89.18), dental pain following surgery, neck pain (ICD-10: M54.2), myofascial pain syndrome (ICD-10: M79.1 or M60.9), muscle tension headaches (ICD-10: G44.20X), and migraines (ICD-10: G43.XX)

Aromatherapy

Aromatherapy is the use of essential oils found in plants and herbs to relieve pain. This therapy is used extensively in Europe. Some believe the effects of the oils come from their pharmacological properties and their small molecular size, making them easier to penetrate the body tissues. Health-care professionals may use essential oils in massage to relieve pain and induce sleep. Oil baths, hot and cold compresses, or a simple topical application can also help alleviate pain. A very warm compress of eucalyptus oil on the forehead can help relieve stress and reduce headache pain.

Therapeutic Touch and Reiki

Therapeutic touch is a technique that has been taught to thousands of practitioners. The practitioner begins the therapeutic touch session with a client assessment wherein the practitioner places his or her hands 2 to 6 inches above the client's body and makes slow, rhythmic hand motions to find blockages in the client's energy field. The practitioner's hand motions then replenish the client's energy field. The session lasts about 20 to 25 minutes. In therapeutic touch, there usually is no physical touching of the client. Sometimes, however, touching may be necessary, especially in pain associated with fractures or physical trauma. Proper use of therapeutic touch has been shown to reduce pain and ease problems associated with the autonomic nervous system.

Reiki is similar. It is a Japanese technique that promotes stress reduction and healing. It is based on a "laying on of hands" that enables a "life force energy" to flow from one individual to another. The idea is that when one person's life energy is low, illness and stress may follow. When life energy is high, a person is healthy and happy. Reiki technique is used to enhance the energy in an individual. To be most effective, the technique requires that the receiver accept responsibility for his or her role in the healing experience.

Yoga/Tai Chi

Yoga, which means "union," is a system of beliefs and practices whose goal is to teach mind and body unity. In the Western world, yoga generally is associated with physical postures, relaxation, and regulation of breathing. These yoga poses and exercises are often used in the treatment of pain to promote relaxation, aid circulation, reduce fatigue, lower blood pressure, regulate heart rate, stimulate particular body areas, strengthen muscles, and develop flexibility. Tai chi, a common Chinese practice, consists of gentle, graceful, movements found to be a safe way to relieve arthritis pain and gain balance, strength, and flexibility. Tai chi is used to promote the movement of energy through the body. For the best results, yoga and tai chi should be practiced regularly. Both have become very popular in the United States in the past decade, with most health and fitness clubs offering classes for participants.

CHAPTER EPISODE—PART III

Between Allan's appointment with the physical therapist (PT) and his actual visit, the pain returned. He quit going to the gym for several days. The pain was a little more tolerable, but he was very unhappy about not being able to work out. The PT was quite helpful in identifying the types of exercises Allan could do without causing more harm. It meant changing his routine a little, but Allan thought it might work. He was also more accepting of a steroid injection if necessary.

- What is the client's main concern here? The PCP's concern? The PT's concerns?
- If the steroid injection is recommended, will it correct Allan's problem? What are the limitations of these injections?
- If neither an adjusted exercise regimen nor steroid injections lessen Allan's pain, what other options are there?

SUMMARY

Despite its multitude of forms and sometimes highly subjective qualities, pain is real. Pain is to be understood and accepted in the terms of the person experiencing it, because each person experiences pain differently. Pain should be managed as aggressively as its cause. The health-care professional and the person in pain benefit most when both are willing to investigate many forms of pain management to determine what best suits the individual's needs.

Finally, a useful attitude toward pain management is captured in the following statement by David Black in *The Laughter Prescription*: "Pain is an energy monster, we give it the power to hurt us. And we take that power away—depending on how we choose to view ourselves. All pain is real, but you can change your reality."

 DavisPlus | For more resources and to sharpen your skills with interactive exercises, visit Davis*Plus* at http://davisplus.fadavis.com. Keyword *Tamparo*.

ONLINE RESOURCES

American Pain Society
http://www.ampainsoc.org

Association for Applied Psychophysiology and Biofeedback
http://www.aapb.org

International Association for the Study of Pain
http://www.**ia**sp-pain.org

The Institute of Medicine. *Relieving Pain in America. A Blueprint to Transforming Prevention, Care, Education, and Research.* Washington, DC: The National Academies Press; 2011.

CASE STUDIES

Case Study 1

Brenda, a 56-year-old carpenter, injured her back years ago, had major surgery, and felt "normal" within 6 months. She returned to work and for 3 years was accident free. Then she reinjured her back four times within a 3-year period. Physical therapy and analgesia were unsatisfactory. She was referred to a multidisciplinary pain center when nothing seemed to control the pain, and she began missing too much work and could not pay her bills. At the pain center, she saw a medical doctor, a psychologist, a social worker, an occupational therapist, and a pharmacist. Her husband was involved in the pain assessment as well and was interviewed separately by team members. At the end of the daylong session, Brenda and her husband met with the team, who discussed their findings and detailed their treatment plan.

Case Study Questions
1. What do you think the team advised Brenda to do?
2. Why do you think the team involved her husband?
3. What else would you advise?

Case Study 2

John, a 35-year-old stockbroker, is near death. His treatment for pancreatic cancer has been discontinued. He rates his pain as a 9 on a scale of 1 to 10. He is not receiving the maximum dosage of opioids that he could receive. When you, as a health professional, talk with him about his pain, John responds, "My wife says I'm strong enough to take it." John's wife is his main caregiver.

Case Study Questions
1. Discuss the assessment of John's pain. Can further pain assessments be done?
2. What strategies might be used in working with John? And with his wife?

Case Study 3

Ten-year-old Madison was riding the brand-new scooter she received from her parents as a birthday gift. Going down a rather steep hill, Madison lost control of the scooter around the curve at the base of the hill and sideswiped a tree. Her parents rushed her to the emergency department, where she was treated and sent home with instructions for her care, including a medication for pain. Her parents gave her the acetaminophen every 3 to 4 hours, but it was not adequately addressing her pain. The physician from the emergency department did not want the parents to administer any other medication because it could mask further symptoms.

Case Study Question

1. Discuss what complementary therapies could be used to relieve Madison's pain.

REVIEW QUESTIONS

Matching

Match the following by placing the correct letter in the column:

_____ 1. Finds and replenishes a person's energy field with rhythmic hand movements

_____ 2. Electric impulses block transmission of painful impulses

_____ 3. Characterized by manipulation, pressure, friction, and body kneading

_____ 4. Slow, rhythmic breathing accompanied by a mental picture of relaxation

_____ 5. Long, hair-thin needles placed into the skin produce regional anesthesia

_____ 6. Achieves a state similar to sleep

_____ 7. Uses essential oils and plants

_____ 8. Gentle movements to move energy through the body

_____ 9. Blocks enzymes and prostaglandins

_____ 10. Sometimes called issue pain

a. TENS
b. Acupuncture
c. Massage
d. Therapeutic touch
e. Tai chi
f. Imagery
g. Physical therapy
h. Hypnosis
i. Relaxation
j. Biofeedback
k. Aromatherapy
l. Reiki
m. NSAIDs
n. Nociceptive pain

Short Answer

1. What is the 1 to 10 scale tool used for?

_____

2. What are three major barriers to effective pain management according to the AHRQ?

   a. _____

   b. _____

   c. _____

3. What is the term for morphine-like drugs used to control pain? _____

4. Clients with cancer experience what type of pain?

_____

5. Pain that comes from a nervous system lesion is called what? _____

Multiple Choice

Place a checkmark next to the correct answer:

1. Acute pain is pain that:

   _____ a. Is no longer useful

   _____ b. Starts slowly but lasts a long time

   _____ c. Provides a warning that something is wrong

   _____ d. Is difficult to manage

2. Biofeedback is a complementary therapy used in treating pain for:

   _____ a. Epilepsy

   _____ b. Low blood sugar

   _____ c. Migraine headaches

   _____ d. Psychogenic pain

3. Which of the following is/are a variable(s) considered in the experience of pain?

   _____ a. Cultural background

   _____ b. Height and weight

   _____ c. Pulse and blood pressure

   _____ d. Gate control theory

4. What might nonprescription drug therapy include?

   _____ a. Muscle relaxants

   _____ b. Antidepressants and antianxiety medications

   _____ c. Steroids

   _____ d. Topical analgesics

5. An Iraq war veteran who lost a leg might feel what kind of pain?

   _____ a. Psychogenic pain

   _____ b. Phantom limb pain

   _____ c. Peripheral neuropathic pain

   _____ d. Angina pain

Discussion Questions/Personal Reflection

1. Identify the two definitions of pain given in the text. Explain what pain means to you.

_____

_____

_____

_____

_____

_____

_____

_____

_____

_____

_____

2. Of the pain therapies outlined in the text, which have you tried? What works best for you? Which would you like to try the next time you have pain? Which therapy would you never try, and why?

_____

_____

_____

_____

_____

_____

_____

_____

_____

_____

_____

_____

_____

What is to give light must endure burning.
—VIKTOR E. FRANKL

4

Infectious and Communicable Diseases

● *chapter outline*

key words

Anorexia (ăn•ō•rĕk'sē•ă)
Antipruritic (ăn"tĭ•proo•rĭt'ĭk)
Antipyretic (ăn"tĭ•pī•rĕt'ĭk)
Arthralgia (ăr•thrăl'jē•ă)
Bacteremia (bak-tə -'rē-mē-ə)

Enanthems (ĕn•ăn'thĕms)
Exanthems (ĕg•zăn'thĕms)
Leukopenia (loo"kō•pē'nē•ă)
Myalgia (mī•ăl'jē•ă)
Nosocomial (näsə´kōmēəl)

Orchitis (ər•kī'tĭs)
Rhinitis (rī•nī'tĭs)
Scotomata (skō•tō'mă•tă)
Sepsis ('sep-səs)
Spirochete (spī'rō-kēt)

learning outcomes

Upon successful completion of this chapter, you will be able to:

- Define key terms.
- Compare and contrast infectious and communicable diseases.
- Recall at least five reasons for the surge in new infectious and communicable diseases.
- Identify and define emerging and reemerging infectious diseases.
- Explain the health crisis from antimicrobial resistance.
- Identify the peculiar nature of the H1N1 virus.
- Discuss the route of food-borne infection caused by *Escherichia coli* O157:H7.
- Summarize the prognosis of *E. coli* O157:H7.
- Identify the etiology and three stages of Lyme disease.
- Discuss the infectious characteristics of severe acute respiratory syndrome (SARS).
- Assess the current threat of Middle East respiratory syndrome (MERS).
- Describe the six infectious diseases that could be used as possible weapons.
- Explain the four characteristics of Category A diseases as potential weapons.
- Compare/contrast the three forms of anthrax.
- Recall how botulism has been used in warfare.
- List the signs/symptoms of pneumonic plague.
- Discuss the pros and cons of keeping the smallpox virus.
- Explain the treatment protocol for tularemia.
- Identify the four main groups of viral hemorrhagic fevers.
- Summarize the treatment for hemorrhagic fevers.
- Restate the preventative methods for West Nile virus.
- Recall the etiology of malaria and the threat to travelers.
- Discuss alternative therapies for the treatment of colds and influenza.
- Recall the treatment of influenza.
- Summarize the possible prognosis of MRSA.
- List two major criteria used to diagnose chronic fatigue syndrome.
- Discuss the etiology of HIV/AIDS.
- Recall the number of persons living with HIV/AIDS in the world.
- Compare/contrast the common infectious and communicable diseases of childhood and adolescence.
- Identify the etiology of infectious diarrheal diseases.
- Recall the etiology and incubation period of rubeola.
- Distinguish rubeola and rubella.
- Define the classic symptoms of mumps.
- Describe the treatment of varicella.
- Describe the infectious period of erythema infectiosum (fifth disease).
- Discuss the two stages of pertussis.
- Explain measures to prevent diphtheria.
- Outline preventive strategies for tetanus.
- Discuss inoculation schedules for children and adults.

CHAPTER EPISODE—PART I

Rodney is a single father, widowed when his wife died of cancer shortly after their son, Jed, was born. He brings Jed to the pediatrician for his 3-month well-baby examination. Rodney is concerned about vaccinations for Jed. He is reluctant to give permission for the vaccinations because he believes they may cause other problems, especially autism. The pediatrician explains to Rodney that Jed is due for a series of vaccinations that include the following: hepatitis B (not given at birth), rotavirus, DTaP, Hib, PCV, and IPV. Rodney reacts by saying, "That is too much for my little guy!"

- What might be happening with Rodney and his son?
- Are Rodney's fears related to autism founded? Justify your response.

ETIOLOGY OF INFECTIOUS AND COMMUNICABLE DISEASES

As we learned in Chapter 1, infection is a major cause of disease. An *infectious disease* is caused by a microorganism that can transfer to new individuals. It may or may not be easy to catch and is thus not a great threat to others. A *communicable* (or *contagious*) *disease* is an infectious disease that is readily transmitted from one individual to another, either directly or indirectly. Table 4.1 lists several communicable diseases, their methods of transmission, and incubation periods. The Centers for Disease Control and Prevention (CDC), the World Health Organization (WHO), and the National Foundation for Infectious Diseases supply a great deal of detail related to infectious and communicable diseases. Their websites are particularly informative.

Table 4.1 Transmission and Incubation Period for Some Communicable Diseases

DISEASE	HOW ORGANISM IS TRANSMITTED	INCUBATION PERIOD
AIDS	Intimate sexual contact, semen, blood, blood products, contaminated needles, placental transmission, breast milk	Uncertain; antibodies appear within 1–3 months of infection
Anthrax	Break in skin; inhaled from air; consumed from contaminated meat	Varies depending on strength and amount of exposure; 1–43 days
Botulism	Eating contaminated food; wound or break in the skin	6 hours–10 days from exposure
Common cold (coryza)	Airborne respiratory droplets; hand-to-hand contact; contact with contaminated items	2–5 days from exposure
Diphtheria	Intimate contact with discharges from nose, throat, eye, and skin lesions	2–5 days from exposure
E. coli O157:H7	Eating/drinking contaminated food/water; swimming in sewage-contaminated water	Between 1 and 8 days
Erythema infectiosum (fifth disease)	Respiratory secretions; direct contact	Generally 4–14 days
H1N1 influenza	Respiratory secretions; hand-to-hand contact	1–7 days from exposure
Infectious diarrheal diseases	Oral-fecal route of transmission; possibly respiratory	48 hours
Influenza	Respiratory secretions; hand-to-hand contact; contact with contaminated items	1–3 days
Methicillin-resistant *Staphylococcus aureus* (MRSA) infection	Close contact with infected persons; indirect contact with towels, wound dressings; sports equipment	Very unpredictable; usually 1–10 days after MRSA enters the bloodstream
Mumps	Droplets of saliva; airborne route	18 days
Pertussis (whooping cough)	Droplets of respiratory secretions; contact with contaminated items	7–10 days
Plague (pneumonic)	Close contact with infected individuals; respiratory droplets	1–6 days
Rubeola (hard measles)	Respiratory droplets from nose and throat	8–13 days from exposure; 14 days until rash appears
Rubella (3-day measles)	Respiratory droplets from nose and throat	Ranges from 14–23 days; commonly 16–18 days
Smallpox	Respiratory droplets; infected dried scales from lesions; contact with contaminated items	10–14 days after exposure
Varicella (chickenpox)	Respiratory secretions and direct contact	Usually between 13 and 17 days
Viral hemorrhagic fevers	Airborne transmission; contact with infected hosts (animals, flies, mosquitoes)	2–21 days

Source: Adapted from Thomas, CL (ed): Taber's Cyclopedia Medical Dictionary, ed. 22. Philadelphia: FA Davis, 2013, pp 702–703, with permission.

Modern sanitation methods, immunizations, and potent antibiotics have not eradicated infectious and communicable diseases. Persons can refuse immunizations, and some infections are now resistant to antibiotics; hence, they flourish. Over the past two decades, 26 new human pathogens have been identified; many are recognized as either emerging or reemerging. The Institute of Medicine, a research arm of the U.S. government, has identified 13 factors for the surge in new infectious and communicable diseases:

1. Microbial adaptation and change
2. Human susceptibility to infection
3. Climate and weather
4. Changing ecosystems
5. Human demographics and behavior
6. Economic development and land use
7. International travel and commerce
8. Technology and industry
9. Breakdown of public health measures
10. Poverty and social inequality
11. War and famine
12. Lack of political will and/or clout
13. Biological warfare

Regardless of the precautions taken, microbes continue to be virulent, can appear in unsuspecting places, and can cause infection leading to a serious illness.

It is helpful to know the infectious period for a communicable disease, so anyone who has been exposed can be alerted. In some cases, isolation may be necessary to prevent further exposure and transmission.

Medical personnel and hospital staff members are required to notify county and state health departments of confirmed cases of certain communicable diseases. This reporting helps to monitor epidemics and alerts the medical community to special problems. Known reportable communicable diseases are identified throughout this text. The occurrence and incidence of reportable diseases are made to local or county health departments. Some diseases should be reported immediately, others are reported within 24 hours, and the remainder are reported within 72 hours. Reporting requirements vary a little by state but are usually made via telephone or fax.

EMERGING AND REEMERGING INFECTIOUS DISEASES

The National Institute of Allergy and Infectious Diseases, an arm of the National Institutes of Health, publishes a list of emerging and reemerging infectious diseases when the incidence in humans has increased within the past two decades or threatens to increase in the near future. The list changes fairly regularly. One new infection called "antimicrobial resistance" (see the "Antimicrobial Resistance" box) is particularly important because of its unique circumstances. Six of the infections included on this list also carry the greatest threat if used as weapons. Many infectious diseases are featured in this chapter; others are included in their appropriate body system chapters.

Antimicrobial Resistance

Many infections are increasingly difficult to treat because of their resistance to antibiotics. They may include staphylococcal infections, tuberculosis, influenza, gonorrhea, candida infection, and malaria. Also, several are **nosocomial,** or hospital-acquired infections. It is estimated that close to 10% of hospital patients develop an infection, and nearly 90,000 die as a result of their infection. In 2011, the CDC reported that antibiotic resistance in the United States costs nearly $20 billion a year and more than 8 million additional days in the hospital.

In 2013, microorganisms with a threat level of serious were identified. Many of the microorganisms cause **sepsis** or **bacteremia.** Sepsis occurs when microorganisms released into the bloodstream from infection trigger inflammation throughout the body. This inflammation can damage multiple organ systems, sometimes causing them to fail. Some of these microorganisms cause watery or bloody diarrhea; others cause respiratory tract infections, urinary tract infections, pneumonia, and skin infections. *Bacteremia* literally means "bacteria in the blood."

Drug resistance is a target area for the CDC in its plan for preventing infectious diseases. Its report Emerging Infectious Diseases: A Strategy for the 21st Century recommends that primary care providers educate clients regarding why antibiotics should not be given for most colds, coughs, sore throats, and runny noses. The CDC is encouraging providers not to write prescriptions for treating viral illnesses when the use of antibiotics is inappropriate.

Unfortunately, however, the public frequently demands antibiotics and providers continue to prescribe them, often when the specific microorganism has not yet been isolated and identified. Thus, bacteria and other microorganisms have developed resistance to antimicrobial drugs both inside and outside of the hospital settings. Antibiotics are no longer the "miracle drugs" they once were. In fact, antimicrobial resistance already affects virtually all pathogens previously considered to be easily treatable.

According to the CDC, the most common organisms to develop resistance are methicillin-resistant *Staphylococcus aureus* (MRSA); vancomycin-resistant enterococci (VRE);

Antimicrobial Resistance—cont'd

extended-spectrum beta-lactamase, which is resistant to cephalosporins and monobactams; and penicillin-resistant *Streptococcus pneumoniae* (PRSP). MRSA and VRE are more common in nonhospital health-care settings, such as hemodialysis centers, long-term care facilities, and in-home care. PRSP is more common in outpatient clinics of primary care providers, especially in pediatric settings. Staphylococci are one of the most common causes of skin infections in the United States and have, over the years,

become resistant to various antibiotics. *Streptococcus pneumoniae* (ICD-10: J18.1or J13) is the leading microorganism in most cases of pneumonia (ICD-10: J18.9), otitis media (ICD-10: H66.4X), and meningitis (ICD-10: G00.X–G03.X). These specific diseases are detailed in Chapter 10 (meningitis); Chapter 13 (pneumonia); and Chapter 17 (otitis media). For more information, go to http://www.cdc.gov/drugresistance/threat-report-2013/pdf/ar-threats-2013-508.pdf.

When there is illness from an emerging or reemerging infectious disease, immediate medical attention from a primary care provider (PCP) is essential. Little information is available on complementary therapies for emerging infectious diseases and disorders. However, complementary therapies and integrative medicine that encourage client comfort with proper nutrition, fluid balance, and symptomatic treatment are noted.

Pandemics

Outbreaks of the influenza virus (ICD-10: J10.XX*), causing upper respiratory discomfort, occur each year. While vaccines are readily available in the United States, influenza virus is particularly threatening to elderly people and young children. Influenza pandemics occur when the virus spreads quickly into many countries, becoming almost unstoppable. The 1918 flu pandemic caused 50 million deaths, and the 1957 flu pandemic caused 2 million deaths. The WHO predicts that a pandemic flu event today could cause as many as 2 to 7 million deaths throughout the world, and tens of millions more would require health care. Any new influenza virus identified is closely monitored, such as with H1N1. The CDC's early predictions were that the H1N1 flu pandemic might possibly infect 2 billion individuals worldwide. Fortunately, it was not so serious.

H1N1 FLU

✔ REPORTABLE DISEASE

ICD-10: J09.XX

Description

Infection with the H1N1 flu virus was first reported in April 2009. This virus is caused by a never-before-seen mixture of viruses typical among pigs, birds, and humans. The H1N1 virus contains DNA found in avian,

swine, and human viruses, including elements from Europe and Asian swine viruses. H1NI was raised to the pandemic level by the WHO in June 2009. Just over 30,000 cases were reported in 2013 by the CDC.

Etiology

Normally, a flu virus from animals does not infect humans; however, it is believed that genetic changes in the swine flu that normally infects pigs has allowed it to more easily pass to humans.

Signs and Symptoms

The symptoms are the same as for seasonal flu. They include fever, cough, sore throat, nasal congestion, body aches, fatigue, and headaches. Some experience diarrhea and vomiting.

Diagnostic Procedures

A severe upper respiratory infection plus confirmation by one of the following tests is necessary for diagnosis: (1) real-time polymerase chain reaction, (2) viral culture to measure the amount of virus in the blood, and (3) a fourfold increase in the H1N1-specific neutralizing antibodies. Additionally, in 2010, the U.S. Food and Drug Administration (FDA) approved tests to detect the H1N1 in just 4 hours.

Treatment

Antiviral medications Zanamivir (Relenza) and Oseltamivir (Tamiflu) have been beneficial in treatment when caught early.

Complementary Therapy

Rest, sufficient hydration, hot chamomile tea, hot chicken soup, nasal saline, and vitamin C supplements can complement antiviral medications.

➡ CLIENT COMMUNICATION

Remind clients of methods to protect themselves from H1N1, and encourage them to be vaccinated.

*The X represents the fourth digit that is often required and supplied once more detailed information about the disease or disorder is made known to the provider.

Prognosis

Presently, the prognosis is much like any other influenza infection, with symptom relief in 7 to 10 days. Most schools, colleges, and communities have contingency plans for closing public meeting places should the H1N1 flu virus or any other infection become epidemic in their area.

Prevention

Avoiding contact with infected individuals is highly recommended. It is important to practice regular hand washing, cover the mouth when sneezing or coughing, and stay home if flu infection is suspected. It is believed that individuals may be contagious from 1 day before symptoms develop to up to 7 days after they are ill. The H1N1 vaccination is available for everyone either by injection or nasal spray and is the best prevention.

ESCHERICHIA COLI O157:H7

✔ **REPORTABLE DISEASE**

ICD-10: B96.29 or B96.20

Description

E. coli O157:H7 is only one of hundreds of strains of the bacterium *E. coli* (ICD-10:B96.21). Most strains are harmless and live in the intestinal tract of healthy humans and animals, but the O157:H7 strain produces a powerful toxin and can cause serious illness. *E. coli* O157:H7 is an emerging cause of food-borne illness, with an estimated 20,000 cases of infection in the United States each year. This number has decreased due to increased awareness of prevention. This infection is associated with eating undercooked, contaminated ground beef; consuming contaminated lettuce or spinach; or drinking unpasteurized milk and fruit juices. The website http://www.cdc.gov/ecoli provides the latest information on outbreaks.

Etiology

The organism, which can be found on some cattle ranches, lives in the intestines of healthy cattle. Meat may become contaminated during slaughter. Organisms can be thoroughly mixed into beef when it is ground. Bacteria present on the cow's udders or on equipment may get into raw milk. Swimming in sewage-contaminated water also can cause infection. Bacteria in the diarrheal stools of infected persons can be passed from one person to another if hand washing and personal hygiene are inadequate.

Signs and Symptoms

The infection causes bloody diarrhea, nausea and vomiting, and abdominal cramps, although in some cases, the person is asymptomatic. Usually, no fever is present and the illness will resolve in 5 to 10 days. In elderly persons and children, the infection can cause a complication called *hemolytic uremic syndrome* (ICD-10: D59.3). In this condition, the red blood cells are destroyed, creating low platelet counts that can lead to acute kidney failure. Complications of the syndrome include end-stage renal disease (ICD-10: N18.6), hypertension (ICD-10: I10), seizures (ICD-10: R56.9), blindness (ICD-10: H54.XX), and paralysis (ICD-10: G83.X). These complications are associated with death and long-term difficulties in a small percentage of individuals.

Diagnostic Procedures

The infection from *E. coli* O157:H7 is diagnosed by detecting the bacteria in the stool. Some laboratories in the United States do not routinely test for these bacteria. Therefore, it may be necessary to request that the stool specimen be tested specifically for the organism in all individuals who suddenly have bloody diarrhea.

Treatment

Persons with only diarrhea usually recover without specific treatment in 5 to 10 days. However, hospitalization may be necessary for those with hemolytic uremic syndrome, which is life-threatening and is treated aggressively. Blood transfusions and kidney dialysis are usually required.

Complementary Therapy

Complementary therapy is supportive only and designed to make clients more comfortable. Rest, eating a balanced diet, and drinking ample fluids is recommended.

⊕ **CLIENT COMMUNICATION**

The disease process can linger with complications or may be acute; hence, educate clients on how to specifically follow the treatment plan.

Prognosis

Persons with only diarrhea usually recover completely with a good prognosis. The prognosis is guarded if hemolytic uremic syndrome develops. About one-third of people with the syndrome either develop abnormal kidney function or require long-term dialysis.

Prevention

Consumers can prevent illness by cooking all ground beef thoroughly to an internal temperature of at least 160°F, by consuming only pasteurized milk and fruit juices, and by making certain that all persons, especially children, regularly wash their hands carefully with soap and water. Washing counters, utensils, and surfaces where raw meat has been prepared or handled will help prevent cross-contamination. Washing fruit and vegetables thoroughly is important as well. Do not swallow water when swimming anywhere, but especially in lakes and ponds. Meat processing plants are more regulated as a result of *E. coli* O157:H7.

LYME DISEASE

✔ *REPORTABLE DISEASE*

ICD-10: A69.20

Description

Lyme disease is caused by *Borrelia burgdorferi*, a tiny tick-transmitted **spirochete,** or bacterium, that has a slender spiral shape. The disease occurs in stages. Each stage has different clinical manifestations, and between stages there may be remissions and exacerbations. Lyme disease was named for Lyme, Connecticut, a town in which it was first recognized in 1975. The incidence has increased, and although the disease has spread west, most cases have occurred in the northeastern United States.

Etiology

B. burgdorferi is carried by blacklegged ticks found on the white-tailed deer, the white-footed mouse, and even raccoons, rabbits, dogs, horses, cattle, and migrating birds. The tick injects its saliva into the host's bloodstream, or it deposits fecal material on the skin (Fig. 4.1).

Signs and Symptoms

Stage 1 signs include a rash called *erythema chronicum migrans* (ECM), which appears at the site of the bite and may resemble a bull's eye. ECM is very distinct, with a dark-red rim and faded center. ECM does not occur in all cases. Other signs of stage 1 include such flulike symptoms as fatigue, headache, fever, chills, stiff

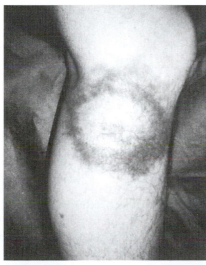

Figure 4.1 **Lyme disease rash.** *(From Thomas, CL [ed]: Taber's Cyclopedia Medical Dictionary, ed. 21. Philadelphia: FA Davis, 2009, p 1373, with permission.)*

neck, and joint and muscle pain, which can last from several weeks to several months. Stage 2 symptoms affect the central nervous system, causing such diverse problems as meningitis, nerve damage, and facial palsy. Stage 3 symptoms include chronic arthritis and continuing neurological problems. Stage 1 usually lasts for several weeks, stage 2 occurs during the following several months, and stage 3 occurs months to years after the onset of the initial infection. Except for fatigue and lethargy, which are often constant, the early signs of the disease are typically intermittent and changing.

Diagnostic Procedures

The easiest diagnosis is likely determined in stage 1 by the appearance of the ECM and a history of possible exposure to infected ticks. Blood tests are used to assist in diagnosis; however, it can take more than 6 weeks for the antibodies to appear in the blood, making diagnosis by this method alone inconclusive. The most common laboratory abnormalities are a high erythrocyte sedimentation rate (ESR), an elevated total serum immunoglobulin (IgM) level, or an increased aspartate aminotransferase level. The enzyme-linked immunosorbent assay (ELISA) test detects antibodies to *B. burgdorferi*. The Western blot will confirm the diagnosis.

Treatment

The treatment of choice in all three stages is the use of antibiotics, such as doxycycline or amoxicillin.

Complementary Therapy

Along with the antibiotic therapy, complementary medicine practitioners suggest avoidance of alcohol and sugar, because the bacteria feed on them. Proper nutrition can help bolster immune function. Practice stress-reduction techniques and encourage ample rest. The following therapies are not helpful, or may even be harmful, and are to be avoided in the treatment of Lyme disease: malariotherapy, intracellular hyperthermia therapy, hyperbaric oxygen therapy, colloidal silver, dietary supplements, and herbs. For more information see: http://www.quackwatch.com/01QuackeryRelated Topics/lyme.html.

➲ CLIENT COMMUNICATION

Because the disease occurs in stages and may have exacerbations and remissions, clients need different support systems during the course of the disease. Encourage clients to follow the treatment plan, especially taking the medication as directed. Eating a balanced diet and drinking plenty of fluids are recommended. Education about exacerbations and remissions is warranted, while helping clients understand that having Lyme disease once does not protect them from getting it again.

Prognosis

Although minor recurrences of headaches, musculoskeletal pain, or lethargy are consistent with the disease, eventually, complete recovery occurs with proper treatment.

Prevention

The best prevention is to cover as much of the body as possible when in the woods. Watch for tiny pinpoint specks that may be ticks on the body and clothing. If a tick is found on the body, remove it with tweezers, making sure to get the head. Use an insect repellent as directed on clothes and exposed areas of arms and hands. Make certain pets that go outside have protection against fleas and ticks and inspect them after outings.

CORONAVIRUSES: SEVERE ACUTE RESPIRATORY SYNDROME AND MIDDLE EAST RESPIRATORY SYNDROME

✔ *REPORTABLE DISEASES*

Description

Severe acute respiratory syndrome (SARS) is a respiratory illness that may present in varying degrees of severity. SARS was first reported in Asia in 2003. During the next few months, the illness spread rapidly through North America and Europe before it was contained. Middle East respiratory syndrome (MERS) was first reported in 2012 in Saudi Arabia. On May 2, 2014, a traveler to the United States was diagnosed with the first case of MERS reported in this country.

Etiology

SARS is caused by a virus known as SARS-associated coronavirus (ICD-10: B97.21). Studies showed the virus survived for at least 24 hours on a plastic surface at room temperature and that the microbe remained viable for as long as 4 days in human waste. Consequently, potential ways to contract SARS include touching the skin of other people or objects that are contaminated with infectious droplets and then touching the eyes, mouth, or nose. Most cases of SARS in the United States occurred among travelers returning to the country from other parts of the world where SARS was diagnosed.

MERS (ICD-10-CM J12.81) is caused by a coronavirus known as MERS-CoV. It is not known where the virus comes from but is thought to be an animal source—perhaps camels or bats. To date, all reported cases have been linked to the Arabian Peninsula.

Signs and Symptoms

Individuals with SARS may be asymptomatic or may experience a mild respiratory illness. The moderate form of SARS begins with a temperature greater than 100.4°F. Additionally, some symptoms may include headache, an overall feeling of discomfort, and body aches. With the more severe forms of SARS, people develop a dry cough, have trouble breathing, and may show evidence of pneumonia or respiratory distress syndrome (severe impairment of respiratory function). The onset of symptoms in the moderate and severe forms is generally 2 to 7 days after exposure. Most people who have been confirmed to have MERS-CoV developed severe acute respiratory illness. They had fever, cough, and shortness of breath. About 30% of these people died.

Diagnostic Procedures

Testing should include chest x-ray, pulse oximetry, blood and sputum cultures, and testing for viral respiratory pathogens. The CDC has developed diagnostic tests to allow scientists to detect antibodies to the MERS virus. The tests will tell whether a person is, or has been, infected. Much is still being learned about MERS; where it came from, the best way to treat it, and how to prevent it are still under investigation.

Treatment

The CDC recommends that persons infected receive the same treatment used for anyone with a community-acquired atypical pneumonia. Otherwise, treatment choices generally are symptomatic and may be influenced by the severity of the illness. For example, oxygen therapy and bed rest may be required. The death rate of MERS is presently at about 30%.

Complementary Therapy

Complementary therapy includes additional fluids, proper nutrition with some additional supplements, and supportive measures to keep clients comfortable.

➤ **CLIENT COMMUNICATION**

Remind clients to return for a follow-up visit with their primary care provider and to have all family members practice frequent hand washing.

Prognosis

The WHO reported that 8,098 persons became ill with SARS in the 2003 outbreak. A total of 774 individuals died of it. Containment of SARS was reported at the end of 2003. However, reappearance of SARS could occur at any time. At this writing, 463 cases of MERS were reported in Saudi Arabia, with a total of 126 deaths. A total of 184 cases of MERS, including 33 deaths have been reported in the Republic of Korea.

Prevention

Prevention includes good hygiene, especially if a family member has or is suspected of having SARS. Limit interactions with those suspected of having SARS. Disposable gloves and eye protection should be worn. Careful washing of shared eating utensils, towels, and bedding is good prevention as well. MERS-CoV spreads between individuals in close contact. When the case of MERS was diagnosed in May 2014 in the United States, quarantine was established and the route of travel and exposure to others was investigated.

Infectious Disease as Potential Weapons

While they are rarely seen in the United States, a number of emerging and reemerging diseases that could be used as weapons have been identified by the U.S. public health system. These diseases are listed in three categories (A, B, and C). Category A includes the highest-priority diseases for these reasons: (1) They can be easily disseminated or transmitted from person to person, (2) they result in high mortality rates and present a potential major public health threat, (3) they might cause public panic and social disruption, and (4) they require special action for public health preparedness. Category A diseases include anthrax, botulism, plague, smallpox, tularemia, and viral hemorrhagic fevers. They are the only ones discussed in this chapter. Visit the "Emergency Preparedness" section of http://www.cdc.gov, then click on "Bioterrorism" for podcasts on the various bioterrorism agents.

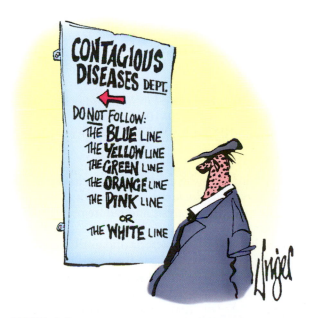

HERMAN by Jim Unger
hermancomics.com

© LaughingStock International Inc.

HERMAN© is reprinted with permission from LaughingStock Licensing Inc., Ottawa, Canada. All rights reserved.

ANTHRAX

✔ *REPORTABLE DISEASE*

ICD-10: A22.X

Description

Anthrax is an acute infection that can occur in three forms: (1) cutaneous or skin (ICD10: A22.0), (2) inhalation (ICD-10: A22.1), and (3) intestinal (ICD-10: A22.2). Farmers and ranchers have been aware of anthrax for many years because of possible exposure to infected cattle and sheep; the cutaneous form of the disease is most common.

Etiology

Humans develop anthrax after exposure to infected animals or tissue from infected animals and by direct exposure to *Bacillus anthracis*. Cutaneous anthrax infection occurs when the bacterium enters a cut or abrasion on the skin. Contact with infected tissue likely occurs during postmortem examination, slaughter, or handling of infected meat or hides. The first case of cutaneous anthrax in the United States was reported in 1992. Inhalation anthrax received high publicity in 2001 when it was found in mail that was distributed to members of the U.S. Senate and to national news media personnel. Intestinal anthrax is acquired by consuming contaminated meat, but there have been no confirmed cases in the United States.

Signs and Symptoms

The cutaneous form causes a raised itchy bump that resembles an insect bite but quickly develops into a vesicle—a painless ulcer that develops within 1 to 2 days. Symptoms of inhalation anthrax resemble those of a cold, with sore throat, mild fever, muscle aches, and malaise. Severe breathing problems and shock can occur. Intestinal anthrax is characterized by acute inflammation of the intestinal tract, causing nausea, vomiting, and severe diarrhea.

Diagnostic Procedures

Laboratory diagnosis consists of isolation and confirmation of *B. anthracis* from a clinical specimen collected from an affected tissue site. The bacteria can be cultured from blood, a skin lesion, and respiratory secretions. Other laboratory tests include evidence of the *B. anthracis* DNA by polymerase chain reaction and immunohistochemical staining.

Treatment

Individuals with cutaneous anthrax are treated with penicillin or doxycycline antibiotic therapy, regardless of their vaccination status. Broad-spectrum antimicrobial agents are beneficial in the treatment of inhalation anthrax, and antitoxin should be added to the combination antimicrobial treatment for intestinal anthrax. All treatments should be under the strict supervision of a healthcare provider, especially because prolonged treatment is necessary.

Complementary Therapy

No significant complementary therapy is indicated other than supportive measures to keep individuals comfortable. Rest, ample hydration, and strict adherence to prescribed medications are important. Reduction of the anxiety felt by those with the disease is beneficial.

 CLIENT COMMUNICATION

The near-panic a client senses when exposed to inhalation anthrax is real and must be considered in treatment. Help educate clients and family members that taking the full course of antibiotics is essential and that treatment may last for some time.

Prognosis

Early treatment of cutaneous anthrax is usually curative; the fatality rate without antibiotics is about 20%. Even with appropriate antimicrobial agents to treat inhalation anthrax, the mortality rate can be as high as 75%. Intestinal anthrax causes death in as many as 60% of cases.

Prevention

There is a vaccination for the prevention of anthrax. The vaccine contains no dead or live bacteria and is advised for the following individuals:

- Laboratory personnel who work directly with the organism
- Those working with imported animal hides or furs from areas where standards are insufficient to prevent exposure
- Persons who handle potentially infected animal products in high-incidence areas (i.e., veterinarians who travel to work in other countries)
- Military personnel deployed to areas with high risk for exposure (i.e., as a biological warfare weapon).

BOTULISM

✔ *REPORTABLE DISEASE*

Description

Botulism is a serious disease that paralyzes muscles. There are three forms of the botulism toxin:

- Food-borne botulism (ICD-10: A05.1) is caused by eating foods contaminated with the botulism toxin. This form is especially dangerous because many people can be poisoned at one time. In the

United States, food-borne botulism accounts for approximately 15% of cases.
- Wound botulism (ICD-10: A48.52) accounts for 29% of cases and occurs when a wound is infected with the botulism toxin.
- Infant botulism (ICD-10: A48.51) occurs when the spores of the botulism toxin grow in the intestines, resulting in 55% of the cases.

Botulism has been used as a warfare agent since before World War II. Hand grenades have been injected with botulism; it has been loaded into bombs and is quite lethal when used in enclosed areas.

Etiology

Botulism is caused by the bacterium *Clostridium botulinum*. This rod-shaped bacterium is found in the soil, growing best in low-oxygen conditions. The bacteria form spores that remain dormant until exposed to conditions supporting growth. The seven types of botulism toxin are designated by letters A through G. Types A, B, E, and F cause illness in humans.

Signs and Symptoms

The symptoms usually occur within 12 to 36 hours of eating contaminated food and include blurred or double vision, slurred speech, drooping eyelids, difficulty swallowing, and muscle weakness. Symptoms can appear, however, as early as 6 hours and as late as 10 days from exposure. The muscle weakness moves through the body, paralyzing arms and legs. Death may occur when respiratory muscles become paralyzed.

Diagnostic Procedures

History and physical examination may suggest botulism, but the evidence of the botulism toxin in the person's stool or blood serum is necessary for diagnosis. These tests are performed by some state health departments and the CDC. Special tests may be necessary to rule out stroke (ICD-10: I63.50), Guillain-Barré syndrome (an inflammatory disease of peripheral nerves; ICD-10: G61.0), or myasthenia gravis (ICD-10:G70.00).

Treatment

Treatment includes the use of an antitoxin derived from healthy horses to block the action of the toxin in the blood. Respiratory paralysis and failure requires the use of a respirator. Wounds usually require surgical removal of the toxin-producing bacteria and antibiotic therapy. A human-derived antitoxin is used to treat infants infected with the toxin. After several weeks of intensive therapy and hospital care, the paralysis slowly decreases.

Complementary Therapy

Inducing vomiting and using enemas to clear the body of the botulism toxin can be beneficial.

CLIENT COMMUNICATION

An effective defense against botulism is client education. Anyone who does home canning is advised to follow all precautions very carefully. Many universities have services regarding home canning. One source from Penn State is available at http://foodsafety.psu.edu/preserve.html. There are a number of topics to choose from at this site.

Prognosis

When an infected person's respiration has been severely compromised, months of recuperation may be necessary. Fatigue and shortness of breath may continue for years following botulism poisoning.

Prevention

Food-borne botulism usually occurs when home-canned foods with a low acid content are improperly prepared. The most common foods are asparagus, green beans, beets, and corn. Outbreaks have been found from chile peppers, tomatoes, chopped garlic in oil, and improper handling of baked potatoes wrapped in foil. Proper canning of foods and strict hygienic measures must be followed. Garlic-infused

REALITY EPISODE

Friday night at the sorority house was always busy with activities. This particular Friday, everyone was excited about tonight's homecoming football game and the following dance. Merilou and Kari, sorority roommates, hurriedly ate their dinner, one of their favorites—Swiss steak. They left the sorority dining room to get ready for the game and the dance. The evening went well. The home team won the game. Merilou was back at the sorority house first; her date wasn't too exciting. Kari followed about an hour later. As they talked and rehashed the day's activities, they decided they were hungry. They raided the kitchen to make some soup. They ate the soup, devoured half a box of soda crackers, and drank a couple bottles of soda. Soon they went to bed. Within 3 hours, they were both up running to the bathroom. They had diarrhea and were vomiting. It was quickly evident that about half of their sorority sisters were ill also. Many were far more ill than Merilou and Kari. Two were taken to the emergency room. Late the next morning, it was determined that the gravy on the Swiss steak had caused the illness.

What might be the offending bacteria?
What caused Merilou and Kari to be less ill than many of the others?
How long did the symptoms last for those who became ill?

oils should be refrigerated. Botulism is destroyed by high temperatures. Honey can contain the spores of *C. botulinum*, has been a source of infection for infants, and should not be given to children younger than age 1. Wound botulism can be prevented by seeking medical care for infected wounds. Not using injectable street drugs can keep the toxin from infecting the injection sites. The CDC and state health departments have information available to primary care providers anywhere in the country.

PLAGUE (BUBONIC AND PNEUMONIC)

✔ *REPORTABLE DISEASE*

Description

Plague is a communicable disease identified in two forms: Bubonic plague (ICD-10: A20.0) is transmitted through the bite of an infected flea or exposure to infected material through a break in the skin. Pneumonic plague (ICD-10: A20.2) is spread through close contact with infected individuals and affects the lungs. It is transmitted when a person breathes the bacteria from the air; it is this form of plague that carries the threat of bioterrorism.

Etiology

Plague is caused by the *Yersinia pestis* bacterium found in the fleas of rodents. If the *Y. pestis* was released in an aerosol attack, many individuals would become infected within 1 to 6 days. Once people have the disease, it spreads to others in close contact with them when their coughs and sneezes spread respiratory droplets carrying *Y. pestis*.

Signs and Symptoms

Fever, weakness, shortness of breath, chest pain, cough, and pneumonia are evident. There may be bloody or watery sputum, nausea and vomiting, and abdominal pain.

Diagnostic Procedures

Signs and symptoms along with an increased incidence of the disease are indicators to health-care professionals to begin testing for pneumonic plague. A blood or sputum sample sent to the laboratory for testing is the definitive diagnosis. Preliminary results are known within a few hours; confirmation can take 24 to 48 hours.

Treatment

Prompt treatment with antibiotic therapy is important—best within 24 hours of the first symptoms. There are large supplies of antibiotics available in the United States in the event of a bioterrorism attack using pneumonic plague.

Complementary Therapy

Keep individuals with the disease comfortable, and have them use cool compresses to lower a fever. Drinking chamomile tea or inhaling the vapors from the flowering tops of chamomile may be helpful.

 CLIENT COMMUNICATION

> If an outbreak of pneumonic plague were to occur, reassuring clients will be necessary to reduce the panic level. Have all individuals exposed begin antibiotics immediately. Encourage the use of tight-fitting surgical masks to prevent further exposure.

Prognosis

Without prompt treatment and antibiotic therapy, pneumonic plague leads to respiratory failure, shock, and death.

Prevention

There is no vaccine currently available to prevent pneumonic plague. Beginning antibiotic therapy upon exposure to someone who is infected can reduce the chance of becoming ill. Wearing tight-fitting, disposable surgical masks is indicated in an outbreak.

SMALLPOX (VARIOLA)

✔ *REPORTABLE DISEASE*

ICD-10: B03

Authors' note: there are only two places on earth where live smallpox virus is known to exist—Russia and the United States. Discussion has gone on for many years about the desire to destroy these tiny vials. There are those that say, "If a country that is a current or future enemy has the virus, then we better have it too." There are others who say it is better and safer if no country has the virus. In May 2014, the WHO again debated on whether the last samples should be destroyed or preserved. The stalemate continued, however, due to lack of consensus, and the virus has not been destroyed.

Description

Smallpox is a serious, contagious, and sometimes fatal disease. It typically causes systemic disease with rash. The last naturally occurring case of smallpox occurred in Somalia in 1977; the last case in the United States was in 1949. The WHO declared smallpox eradicated in 1979. Smallpox used as a weapon in the hands of terrorists could devastate a population that was not

vaccinated, and that includes most everyone in the United States under age 30. To view images of smallpox, search *smallpox* on the Internet and click on "Images" at the top of the page.

Etiology

Smallpox is caused by the variola poxvirus. It is spread directly via infected respiratory droplets or dried scales of virus-containing lesions or indirectly through contact with contaminated linens and other objects. Classic smallpox is contagious from onset until the last scab is shed. It affects people of all ages.

Signs and Symptoms

Early signs and symptoms are easily confused with those of other diseases and include fever, abrupt onset of chills (10 to 14 days after exposure), headache, backache, severe malaise, and vomiting. Skin lesions that progress from macular to papular, vesicular, and pustular soon develop. The pustules rupture, eventually dry, and form scabs that leave permanent pitting scars. Two days from onset, symptoms become more severe; thereafter, the person begins to improve. Sore throat with cough ensues. Generally, after 14 days, the symptoms subside.

Diagnostic Procedures

A culture of the vesicles and pustules confirms the presence of the variola virus. Signs, symptoms, and an increased incidence of the disease are indicators to health-care professionals to begin testing for smallpox.

Treatment

Treatment goals are to reduce contagion, prevent bacterial complications, and introduce symptomatic and supportive measures for individuals. **Antipyretics** (drugs that reduce fever) and pain medications may be given during the pustular stage.

Complementary Therapy

No significant complementary therapy is indicated.

 CLIENT COMMUNICATION

> It is important to provide ample fluids, electrolytes, and calories because many of the symptoms make drinking and eating difficult.

Prognosis

According to the CDC, death may occur in about 30% of cases.

Prevention

Since December 2002, there has been a smallpox vaccine program to better protect Americans against the threat of smallpox attack by hostile groups or governments.

Vaccination of the general public is not recommended at this time, but the United States currently has sufficient quantities of the vaccine for every person if an emergency occurs.

CHAPTER EPISODE—PART II

The pediatrician sits down with Rodney and little Jed, who passed his examination with flying colors, to further discuss his concerns about the needed vaccinations. He carefully explains any possible side effects as well as the protection each vaccine gives to Jed.

- Search the CDC site on the Internet to determine the latest information regarding autism and vaccinations to determine what might be said to Rodney.
- Explain the protection provided by each vaccination. (You may need to add some research to the information in your text.)

TULAREMIA (TYPHOIDAL OR PNEUMONIC)

✔ REPORTABLE DISEASE

ICD-10: A21.X

Description

Tularemia is also referred to as *rabbit fever* or *deer fly fever*. It is an acute, fever-causing, pneumonia-like infection. The microbe has been found in over 100 species of animals. The disease occurs throughout North American and Eurasia. It is contracted when skin or mucous membranes come in contact with infected animals or when individuals are bitten by infected ticks, deer flies, or mosquitoes. Also, inhaling contaminated dusts or ingesting contaminated foods or water may cause the disease. Tularemia was developed as a weapon during the 1950s and 1960s and is thought to be available in many countries.

Etiology

Tularemia is caused by the small, rod-shaped, nonmotile bacterium *Francisella tularensis* that can remain infectious in water, soil, animal hides, and even frozen meat. There are six forms of the illness, but the typhoidal and pneumonic forms of tularemia are the ones most likely considered to be a bioterrorism threat.

Signs and Symptoms

Symptoms of tularemia usually develop within 3 to 4 days of exposure. It spreads through the lymphatic system, multiplying within the macrophages. Fever, cough, shortness of breath, chills, malaise, muscle aches, and fatigue are the most common symptoms.

Diagnostic Procedures

Diagnosis is largely based on the signs and symptoms of the client and often may be confused with other illnesses. Chest x-ray may reveal infiltrates in the lungs. Exposure is an important clue to diagnosis.

Treatment

Antibiotic therapy, with streptomycin or gentamicin, both by injection and by mouth, is the treatment of choice. The CDC reports that initial studies show that treatment of tularemia exposure with ciprofloxacin or doxycycline within the first 24 hours can protect against the disease.

Complementary Therapy

Comfort measures are beneficial. Strict adherence to antibiotic therapy is important. Encourage rest and adequate nutrition.

➜ CLIENT COMMUNICATION

Caution should always be used when in contact with any wild animals or exposure to any water that may be contaminated.

Prognosis

With proper diagnosis and prompt antibiotic treatment, the mortality rate is greatly decreased.

Prevention

There is no vaccine available to the public. Individuals who come in contact with wild animals are advised to take precautions to prevent infection.

VIRAL HEMORRHAGIC FEVERS

✔ REPORTABLE DISEASE

ICD-10: 98-A99

Description

Viral hemorrhagic fevers (VHFs) are a group of viral illnesses that affect multiple organ systems in the body. The body's vascular system is damaged, and the body is unable to regulate itself. These agents are highly infectious and very stable via the aerosol route, which makes them potential bioterrorism weapons. There are four main groups of the viruses:

1. Arenaviruses—Lassa and Argentine, Bolivian, Venezuelan VHFs
2. Filoviruses—*Hantavirus* genus, Congo-Crimean, Rift Valley, Ebola, and Marburg VHFs
3. Bunyaviruses—Ebola and Marburg VHFs
4. Flaviviruses—Dengue and yellow fever, tick-borne encephalitis, Omsk hemorrhagic and Kyasanur Forest VHFs

Etiology

The viruses are generally derived from certain animals (mice and rats) and insects (ticks and mosquitoes) and are mostly restricted to the geographical location where their host species live. Humans are infected when they come into contact with infected hosts.

Signs and Symptoms

Symptoms include high fever, fatigue, muscle aches, and dizziness. There may be bleeding under the skin and from the mouth, eyes, and ears. Severely ill individuals suffer kidney failure, shock, coma, or seizures.

Diagnostic Procedures

Appearance of the symptoms in a number of individuals in a specified geographical location is strong evidence of a breakout. Laboratory findings can be helpful if infectious virus and viral antigens can be detected and identified by a number of tests such as ELISA using fresh or frozen serum or plasma samples. Diagnosis from cultivated virus samples can take 3 to 10 days.

Treatment

Close supervision is required. Intensive care and isolation may be required. Treatment is largely supportive and is basically the same as is provided to any person with multisystem failure. If clients are able, encourage fluids and nutrition. Rest and medications to alleviate pain can be helpful. The antiviral drug ribavirin may be helpful in some cases, especially if begun in the first 7 days of onset.

Complementary Therapy

Provide comfort measures if tolerated and if they can be given without risk of infection to others. Some may find hot tea soothing; others may have difficulty eating. Music and/or aromatherapy may be beneficial to some.

 CLIENT COMMUNICATION

Protection from insects, mice, and rodents is always important but is especially critical when traveling to countries that do not control insects. In the event of a bioterrorism attack, remind clients to carefully adhere to all recommendations made by community health practitioners.

Prognosis

There is no cure. Supportive therapy can reduce the rate of deaths for most VHFs.

Prevention

The best prevention is to control rodent populations and to spray for mosquitoes. There should be safe cleanup of rodent nests and droppings. The use of insect repellant, bed nets, proper clothing, and window screens is beneficial. Protection of medical personnel includes such strict precautions as hand washing and wearing double gloves, gowns, shoe and leg coverings, and face shields. Airborne precautions require the use of a filter-equipped respirator, a battery-driven air-purifying respirator, or a positive-pressure–supplied air respirator that is worn when coming within 6 feet of a client infected with a VHF. When several clients are infected, they should be housed together in isolation.

Mosquito-Borne Diseases

WEST NILE VIRUS

✔ **REPORTABLE DISEASE**

ICD-10: A92.30

Description

West Nile virus (WNV), or West Nile encephalitis, is an infectious disease that occurs when the virus from an infected mosquito bite multiplies in a person's blood, crossing the blood-brain barrier and causing inflammation of the brain. WNV emerged in North America in 1999 with encephalitis reported in humans and horses. Its spread to the United States was rapid. There were 4,156 cases in 2002, but in 2008, improved mosquito prevention and control brought cases down to 1,356. In 2013, the number of cases had again risen to 2,374 cases. This increase is probably because the virus was earlier underestimated and routine immunoglobulin M testing in 2013 revealed more cases.

Etiology

WNV is transmitted to humans via the bite of an infected mosquito. Scientists believe that mosquitoes feeding on birds infected with WNV carried the disease to New York, New Jersey, and Connecticut; then it quickly spread to other states. The incubation period from infection to disease symptoms is 3 to 14 days.

Signs and Symptoms

Symptom severity ranges from mild to severe and are flulike. A mild infection includes fever, headache, body ache, skin rash, and swollen lymph glands. Severe infections include all of the mild symptoms plus stupor, disorientation, tremors, convulsions, coma, and paralysis. Nearly 80% of individuals infected with the virus show no symptoms.

Diagnostic Procedures

Preliminary diagnosis may be determined by an individual's clinical picture, including places and dates of travel. The WNV IgM ELISA is the test of choice, using a single serum sample that can give a diagnosis within a few hours. This new blood test detects antibodies to the virus that are detectable within the first few days of the infection's onset.

Treatment

There is no known therapy for West Nile virus and no known cure. Treatment is aimed at alleviating the symptoms. Analgesics can help to relieve pain and discomfort. Encourage fluids and rest. Scientists are investigating interferon therapy.

Complementary Therapy

Complementary treatment goals are similar to the treatment above. Additionally, they are designed to help individuals feel better while dealing with their symptoms. The mind–body therapies seem to offer the best results.

⊕ CLIENT COMMUNICATION

When there is no cure, clients often feel fear. Reassure them regarding the success of treatment and that they will be monitored closely by the primary care provider.

Prognosis

Mild symptoms last a few days; severe symptoms can last several weeks. The neurological effect may be permanent. Fortunately, only about 2 out of every 10 individuals who are infected experience any illness. Persons over age 50 are particularly susceptible to the severe form of the illness.

Prevention

The best prevention requires the following actions:

- Use an insect repellant that contains DEET (N,N-diethyl-3-methylbenzamide) when going outside at dawn or dusk. DEET can be used safely for several weeks. Adults may use repellents that contain 30% to 35% DEET; children should use a maximum of 10%, and infants and pregnant women should not use DEET at all.
- Wear light, long-sleeved shirts and long pants for protection from mosquito bites.
- Empty any standing water that can become a breeding ground for mosquitoes.
- Install window and door screens.

MALARIA

✔ REPORTABLE DISEASE

ICD-10: B54

Description

Malaria is a great masquerader and must be differentiated from other febrile illnesses. In the United States,

the disease is seen in persons who have traveled abroad. In 2011, the CDC reported 1,925 cases in the United States.

The WHO reported that in 2012 there were 207 million cases of malaria in the world and that nearly 650,000 people (mostly children) died from the infection. The greatest number of cases occurs in Africa south of the Sahara.

Etiology

Malaria is transmitted from infected mosquitoes to humans. It is a protozoan disease. Once a person is bitten by an infected mosquito, parasites travel to the liver, where they multiply and change into another form of parasite called *merozoites*. Merozoites are then released from the liver and enter the red blood cells (RBCs), where they again grow and multiply. This growth causes the RBCs to burst, thus freeing the parasites and their toxins to attack other RBCs.

Signs and Symptoms

Symptoms are fever and flulike illness, including shaking chills, headache, muscle aches, and malaise. Nausea, vomiting, and diarrhea may also occur. Malaria can cause anemia and jaundice because of the destruction of RBCs.

Diagnostic Procedures

Under a microscope, the presence of the malaria parasites in the RBCs on blood smears confirms the diagnosis. Rapid diagnostic tests (RDTs) that detect antigens derived from the malaria parasites have been developed and approved. The RDTs reduce the amount of time it takes for a diagnosis of malaria.

Treatment

Medications that are effective against malaria depend on the strain of malaria diagnosed, the age of the person infected, and the severity of the illness. Antimalarial prescription medications can cure the disease. The medication also depends on resistance of the parasite to the drug, because so many strains of malaria are becoming increasingly resistant to treatment.

Complementary Therapy

Herbal, Ayurvedic, and traditional Chinese medicine may support traditional treatment by boosting the immune system but should always be used under the guidance of a practitioner.

⊕ CLIENT COMMUNICATION

Discuss prophylactic treatment before foreign travel. Remind clients to notify their PCP immediately of any flulike symptoms upon return.

Prognosis

When the person is treated promptly and correctly, the prognosis is good. However, in many developing countries, malaria is still the leading cause of death. Diet and nutrition should be emphasized.

Prevention

The best way to prevent malaria is to eliminate the malaria parasite and to educate people about the spread of malaria. International funding for malaria control has greatly increased in the past few years. New drug combinations have been developed to treat malaria strains that became resistant to former medications. It is hoped that soon, every person in malaria-endemic Africa will have a life-saving, long-lasting, insecticide-treated bed net to keep mosquitoes from biting during the night. Prompt diagnosis and early treatment are essential. Persons planning to travel to countries with a malaria risk should see their primary care provider 4 to 6 weeks before travel. An antimalarial drug may be prescribed. Using insect repellent products that contain DEET and wearing long pants and long-sleeved shirts are essential to protect against mosquito bites.

Viral Infections

COMMON COLD

ICD-10: J00

Description

The *coryza* or *common cold* is an acute infection that causes inflammation of the upper respiratory tract. Colds occur more frequently in children (as often as 6 to 10 times a year) and are the leading cause of time lost from school. Adults may have as many as 2 to 4 colds per year. The highest incidence of colds is during the fall and winter months.

Etiology

Colds are caused by hundreds of different viruses, the most common being the highly contagious rhinovirus. These microorganisms are transmitted by airborne respiratory droplets but can also be picked up by hand-to-hand contact and through the sharing of towels, telephones, keyboards, cups, and similar personal items.

Signs and Symptoms

The onset of symptoms is gradual and may include nasal congestion, pharyngitis, headache, malaise, burning and watery eyes, and low-grade fever (in children). A cough, either productive or nonproductive, may be present. The symptoms commonly last from 2 to 4 days, but nasal congestion may persist for an indefinite period. Reinfection is common, but complications are rare. The cold is contagious for 2 to 3 days after onset.

Diagnostic Procedures

There is no specific diagnostic test for the common cold. The goal is to rule out disorders that produce similar symptoms.

Treatment

Treatment of the cold is symptomatic and includes mild analgesics, ample fluid intake, and rest. Decongestants, nasal sprays (not more than a few days and not for children), throat lozenges, and a cool-mist humidifier may be helpful. In a child with a fever, acetaminophen is the drug of choice but must be given within the guidelines identified. If secondary bacterial infections are suspected, antibiotics may be prescribed, but they are not recommended for the common cold.

Complementary Therapy

A person with a cold will find it helpful to get extra sleep and drink large amounts of water and herbal teas, vegetable juices, and broths. The additional fluids help rehydrate the body and increase immune function. Chicken soup can help speed the removal of mucus through the nose as well as act as an anti-inflammatory. Saline nasal sprays will keep nasal passages moist. Baths with eucalyptus, lavender, lemon, or peppermint can be soothing to someone with a cold. Andrographis, an Indian herb, is likely to lessen the severity and duration of the common cold but is not to be taken by women who are pregnant. Taking additional vitamin C may prove helpful. Some find taking the herb echinacea, in tablet form or as an herbal tea, helpful during a cold, but it should not be taken long-term. Zinc lozenges taken at the cold's first symptoms may reduce the cold's duration. Foods such as yogurt, cheese, miso, some juices and soy drinks that contain beneficial bacteria or probiotics can reduce the risk and severity of the common cold. Remember that stress can increase susceptibility to disease.

⊙→ CLIENT COMMUNICATION

Teach clients to minimize the transmission of their cold, especially by hand washing and proper disposal of tissues and coughing into their sleeve at the bend of the elbow when a tissue is not available. Educate clients on when to see a doctor.

When to Seek Medical Care

The Mayo Clinic provides the following guidelines on when to seek medical attention: Adults should seek medical care if they have (1) a fever of 102°F (39°C) or higher; (2) a high fever plus fatigue and aches; (3) a fever with sweating, chills, and productive cough with colored phlegm; (4) significantly swollen glands; and (5) severe sinus pain.

Children should see a doctor if they have (1) a fever of 103°F (39.5°C), chills, or sweating; (2) a fever that lasts more than 3 days; (3) vomiting or abdominal pain; (4) unusual sleepiness or severe headache; (5) difficulty breathing; (6) persistent crying; (7) ear pain or persistent cough.

Prognosis

The disease is self-limiting, but it can lead to secondary bacterial infection. Complications can include otitis media (especially in children), sinusitis, and wheezing in individuals with asthma.

Prevention

There is no known prevention. Frequent hand washing and avoiding crowds can lessen the likelihood of contracting a cold.

INFLUENZA

ICD-10: J10.1 or J11.1

Description

Influenza (flu) is an acute, contagious respiratory disease characterized by fever, chills, headache, and **myalgia** (muscle pain and tenderness). The disease may affect anyone, but school-age children and elderly persons are especially susceptible. Flu often occurs in epidemic outbreaks, particularly in the winter and spring. Refer to the earlier section of this chapter regarding pandemics.

Etiology

Flu is caused by viruses that are members of the *Orthomyxoviridae* family. For diagnostic and treatment purposes, the viruses are classified as type A, B, or C on the basis of their antigenic properties. The A and B viruses commonly cause seasonal epidemics most winters. The C virus causes a mild respiratory infection that is rarely epidemic. Influenza viruses frequently mutate, creating new strains that easily infect populations that had acquired immunity to previous strains of the virus. Transmission generally occurs via cough, sneeze, hand-to-hand contact, and other personal contact.

Signs and Symptoms

The onset generally is abrupt, with fever, chills, croup (in children), malaise, muscle aches, headache, nasal congestion, laryngitis, and a cough.

Diagnostic Procedures

Because the signs and symptoms of flu resemble those of so many other illnesses, it is frequently difficult to diagnose solely on the basis of symptoms unless there is an ongoing epidemic. A throat culture may be performed to isolate the virus or to rule out bacteria. Various immunofluorescence techniques may be performed to detect viral antigens.

Treatment

Treatment consists of bed rest, adequate fluid intake, analgesics, and antipyretics. Note that aspirin should not be used to treat fever and muscle pain in children and adolescents with flu because of its association with an increased incidence of Reye syndrome. Acetaminophen may be given to children.

Complementary Therapy

Complementary therapies noted for colds are appropriate for the treatment of influenza. The use of antibiotics is not indicated, and therefore they are to be avoided. Warm baths may relieve myalgia.

⊕ CLIENT COMMUNICATION

Instruct clients, especially elderly ones, to rest, drink ample fluids, and eat a balanced diet. It is important to handle all tissue, utensils, and bedding with the usual precautions to prevent the spread of the disease. Encourage elderly clients to continue as many of the activities of daily living as possible to avoid the need for later rehabilitation from physical inactivity. Children are best kept home until 24 hours after the fever has subsided.

Prognosis

The prognosis is good with proper care. Complications include sinusitis, otitis media, bronchitis, and pneumonia. A large number of deaths occur as the result of influenza each year.

Prevention

Influenza vaccines prepared from the most recent strains of A- and B-type viruses are useful in preventing these particular strains of influenza. The CDC recommends influenza vaccine for children and adults, especially those with certain risk factors, such as diabetes, cardiac disease, and asthma. Proper disposal of contaminated tissues and frequent hand washing is important. There are instances when vaccinated individuals may still get influenza, but the cases will be milder than if they had received no vaccination.

Penicillin History

In 1942, a woman was hospitalized for a month with a life-threatening streptococcal infection. One night she was delirious, and her temperature soared to almost 107°F. Various treatments had been tried; none worked to break the fever. As a last resort, her physicians administered a tiny amount of penicillin, an obscure experimental drug at the time. Her hospital records showed that she had a sharp drop in temperature the following morning. This woman was the first person to receive penicillin. She lived until 1999, dying at age 90.

Multidrug-Resistant Organisms

METHICILLIN-RESISTANT STAPHYLOCOCCUS AUREUS

Description

An individual may have *staphylococci* present in or on the body and yet not become ill. The presence of *staphylococci* is known as colonization. The CDC reports that approximately 25% to 30% of population is colonized in the nose with *staphylococci* at a given time. Infection occurs when the *staphylococci* causes disease. Spread of methicillin-resistant *Staphylococcus aureus* MRSA (ICD-10:B95.62) among clients in outpatient departments generally occurs through close or direct contact with infected individuals. MRSA is not spread through the air. Indirect contact may occur when contaminated objects such as infected towels, wound dressings, clothes, or sports equipment are touched. Infections can result from sharing contaminated items, having recurrent skin diseases, and living in crowded areas; in addition, players in close-contact sports and persons in intimate relationships can spread infection. Sometimes it is unknown how the person contacted the infection.

Risk factors include severity of the MRSA infection; previous exposure to antimicrobial agents; invasive procedures, including dialysis; repeated contact with the health-care system; and any underlying diseases or conditions. Children and the elderly have increased risk.

Signs and Symptoms

Signs and symptoms depend on where the infection causes disease. For example, if the infection occurs in a wound, the wound will be painful, reddened, swollen, and warm to the touch (Fig. 4.2). If the skin infection spreads to the lung, causing pneumonia, or to the bloodstream, then the symptoms will be more systemic. Also, any antibiotic therapy prescribed may have little or no effect on the particular illness. For additional photos, go to: http://www.medicinenet.com/mrsa_infection/article.htm and click on "pictures."

Diagnostic Procedures

In 2008, the FDA approved a rapid blood test (StaphSR assay) that can detect the presence of MRSA genetic material in a blood sample in as little as 2 hours. The test is also able to determine whether the genetic material is from MRSA or from less dangerous forms of staph bacteria. The test should not be used as the only basis for the diagnosis of a MRSA infection. Culture and sensitivity is the main diagnostic tool strictly following the National Committee for Clinical Laboratory Standards. It can be difficult, however, to detect the exact organism and its sensitivity.

Treatment

Sometimes, draining a skin sore may be all the treatment that is necessary. However, in most cases, the treatment of choice is still antibiotic therapy, with doctors and pharmacists working together to determine the best antibiotic to use. Intravenous vancomycin often is the drug of choice for treatment for MRSA; however, it is not effective against vancomycin-resistant enterococci (VRE). In 2013, new discoveries about the cell wall of the bacteria led researchers to try new drugs that may breach this protective area, causing the MRSA bacteria to be susceptible to certain antimicrobial drugs.

Complementary Therapy

No complementary therapy is indicated.

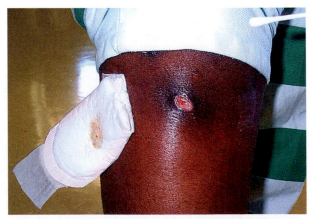

Figure 4.2 Infection caused by methicillin-resistant *Staphylococcus aureus* bacteria. *(Centers for Disease Control and Prevention. Bruno Coignard, MD; Jeff Hageman, MHS)*

⊙ CLIENT COMMUNICATION

Teach clients how infectious agents are spread and what preventive measures to take. Frequent hand washing cannot be overstressed. Individuals whose immune systems are compromised should avoid crowds and group settings.

Prognosis

MRSA can be difficult to treat and can progress to life-threatening blood or bone infections, lung infections, or skin/tissue infections. The prognosis may also depend on how quickly or aggressively the client is treated and on the client's general health. Individuals with suppressed immune systems or chronic illnesses may have a more difficult road to recovery.

Prevention

It is essential to use universal precautions at all times in medical clinics, outpatient departments, group homes, schools, group activities, and other settings. Hand washing is paramount. Some urgent care facilities and outpatient departments require staff and infected clients to wear masks while in the facility. Healthy people generally are at low risk of becoming infected through casual contact.

Immunosuppressant Diseases

CHRONIC FATIGUE SYNDROME

ICD-10: R53.82

Description

Chronic fatigue syndrome (CFS), although not fully understood, is aptly named. Individuals suffer from debilitating chronic fatigue that does not improve with rest and a host of other symptoms. Another name for the illness is *benign myalgic encephalomyelitis*. The symptoms are many and varied, and individuals may suffer for weeks or even years. It is twice as prevalent in women as it is in men, and generally it affects persons ages 25 to 45. Recent studies indicate that it may be an organic brain-based condition.

Etiology

There is no current agreement on the cause of CFS. It is most likely multifactorial. It was once thought to be attributed to the Epstein-Barr virus, but that hypothesis has been set aside. Viruses currently suspected include human herpesvirus 6, enteroviruses, or retroviruses. Other predisposing factors that may be partly responsible include the state of a person's immune system, genetic makeup, age, hormonal balance, sex, environment, and previous illness.

Signs and Symptoms

Two major criteria must be met for CFS to be diagnosed: persistent/relapsing fatigue (1) for at least 6 months that does not resolve with bed rest and (2) that is severe enough to reduce daily activity by at least 50%. In addition, at least four of the nine following minor criteria must be present:

- Fever or chills
- Sore throat; nonexudative pharyngitis
- Painful cervical or axillary lymph nodes
- Unexplained generalized muscle weakness
- Muscle discomfort and myalgia
- Migratory **arthralgia** or joint pain without joint swelling or redness
- Neuropsychological symptoms, including photophobia, forgetfulness, transient visual **scotomata** (an islandlike blind spot on the visual field of the eye), irritability, confusion, depression, inability to concentrate, difficulty thinking, brain fog
- Sleep disturbance
- Acute or subacute initial onset

Diagnostic Procedures

The challenge in diagnosis is that CFS remains a syndrome of symptoms and a diagnosis that comes from exclusion. A complete history and physical examination are essential for diagnosis. Laboratory testing—including complete blood cell count, ESR, electrolytes, thyroid-stimulating hormone, and a urinalysis—is used to rule out other possible causes.

Treatment

Treatment is supportive. The primary care provider will want to reassess the disease process frequently so that new symptoms can be treated. NSAIDs may be beneficial in the treatment of headache, pain, and fever. Medications to improve energy and emotional state may be used. At times, a psychiatric evaluation may be necessary if the person shows symptoms of depression. Lifestyle changes may be needed in the areas of sleeping and exercise. A holistic approach is essential.

Complementary Therapy

There are numerous therapy recommendations for CFS. Diet is crucial to reinforcing the immune system. Clients are advised to concentrate on high-nutrition, high-protein, and complex carbohydrate foods. A basic multivitamin/multimineral supplement with adequate amounts of trace minerals is beneficial. Acupuncture has shown promise in treatment. Herbal medications and Chinese medicine may be helpful but must always be discussed with the primary care provider prior to taking.

 CLIENT COMMUNICATION

Assure clients that although the disease may be chronic in nature, it is possible to make some lifestyle changes and live with it. Having a support system may prove helpful. Encourage clients to eat a balanced diet and drink ample fluids.

Prognosis

The disease is debilitating and lengthy in duration. Some individuals respond to a variety of treatment protocols based on symptoms. Research is under way to determine effective treatment.

Prevention

No prevention is known.

HIV INFECTION/AIDS

✔ **REPORTABLE DISEASE**

ICD-10: B20

Description

AIDS is a severe illness associated with HIV infection. Intimate contact resulting in the exchange of fluids such as semen, blood, blood products, or the use of shared needles is the route of transmission. In addition, infants born to HIV-infected women may become infected before or during birth via transplacental, parturition, or postpartum transmission. The virus also can be transmitted via breast milk.

Etiology

AIDS is caused by HIV, which is a retrovirus. HIV predominantly infects cells called T4 lymphocytes (T4-helper cells), which are critical to the operation of the body's immune system. The virus replicates by taking over the genetic machinery of the T cell it invades. The replication process continues until the host cell is destroyed. The newly produced HIV-infected cells can then infect other T4 lymphocytes, leaving the body open to opportunistic infections.

In 2013, AIDS.gov reported that there were more than 35 million individuals living with AIDS throughout the world—2.1 million of those are children. Two-thirds of the people living with AIDS are in sub-Saharan Africa.

Signs and Symptoms

After exposure to HIV, the majority of individuals experience no recognizable symptoms. Some persons, however, may develop a mononucleosis-like syndrome characterized by fever and flulike symptoms. The syndrome resolves spontaneously, with seroconversion usually occurring 8 to 10 weeks later. When symptoms of HIV later occur, the most common are generalized, persistent lymphadenopathy; weight loss; fever; fatigue; neurological symptoms; and malignancy.

The pulmonary, gastrointestinal, and neurological systems may be involved, and several forms of malignancy and chronic illnesses may result, presenting specific symptoms.

- Pulmonary symptoms include shortness of breath, dyspnea, coughing, chest pain, and fever, usually caused by a variety of opportunistic infections. The most common pulmonary infection is *Pneumocystis jiroveci* (formerly *P. carinii*) pneumonia, which has a high mortality rate. There also is an increased incidence of tuberculosis.
- Gastrointestinal symptoms may include loss of appetite, nausea, vomiting, oral and esophageal candidiasis, and chronic diarrhea or gastroenteritis. Diarrhea occurs in more than half of all clients with AIDS.
- Neurological symptoms may include memory loss, headache, depression, fever, confusion, and visual disturbances. Dementia and depression may also be seen.
- Malignancies commonly associated with AIDS include Kaposi sarcoma, a neoplasm evidenced by multiple vascular nodules in the skin and other organs. This malignant neoplasm is especially prevalent in the lymph nodes, the gastrointestinal tract, and the lungs. The purple lesions characterizing Kaposi sarcoma (ICD-10: C46.X) may appear on the skin and grow rapidly until wounds are produced, which increase the client's susceptibility to infections. Studies show that women infected with HIV experience a higher incidence of cervical cancer.
- Chronic illness results because persons with AIDS are often severely immunocompromised. Nearly all infected persons will eventually develop one or more chronic opportunistic infections during the course of the disease. Such illnesses may complicate treatment and produce debilitating symptoms.

Diagnostic Procedures

There are now four rapid HIV tests approved by the FDA that can return results the same day. They are OraQuick Advance Rapid HIV-1/2 Antibody Test, Reveal G2 Rapid HIV-1 Antibody Test, Uni-Gold Recombigen HIV Test, and Multispot HIV-1/HIV-2 Rapid Test. All four tests use oral fluid, fingerstick blood, or serum specimens collected by venipuncture. They can be interpreted visually and require no instrumentation. Another widely used screening test is the

ELISA, followed by the Western blot test for confirmation. These two tests can take several days for results, however.

The FDA has approved the OraQuick In-Home HIV Test, a rapid test kit that provides results in 20 to 40 minutes. The kit tests a sample of fluid from the mouth. It can be purchased in stores or online to anyone over age 17. A positive test result should be confirmed by follow-up laboratory testing.

A diagnosis of AIDS is made by a primary care provider using certain clinical and laboratory criteria. When HIV establishes itself in the body, the number of CD4 lymphocytes begins to decline. If the number falls below 300, individuals are at heightened risk for one or more opportunistic infections. If the CD4 cell number drops below 200, an individual is said to have AIDS.

Treatment

There is no cure for AIDS and no effective treatment to stop the HIV infection and the immunodeficiency it causes. Today, however, there are 31 antiretroviral drugs approved by the FDA to treat HIV infection. These medications can suppress the virus, even to undetectable levels, but they do not completely eliminate it from the body. HIV resistance to some antiviral agents prompts the need for highly active antiretroviral therapy (HAART) medications given daily. It is important to manage the opportunistic infections and malignancies as aggressively as possible. Chronic illnesses require symptomatic treatment for malnutrition, weakness, immobility, diarrhea, skin lesions, and altered mental state.

Complementary Therapy

Treatment focuses on the prevention of opportunistic infections and enhancing overall health. Vitamin supplementation with herbal medicines may be tried. Acupuncture has shown success in reducing fatigue, night sweats, and diarrhea. Mind–body therapies and spiritual practices have shown promise, because there is such an important relationship between an individual's emotional state and his or her immune system. Massage can improve circulation as well as reduce emotional and mental stress.

Garlic supplements can impede HIV medication, and St. John's wort can significantly compromise the effectiveness of antiviral drugs prescribed for the treatment of HIV.

⊖ CLIENT COMMUNICATION

Encourage clients to become part of a support system for persons with HIV/AIDS for education, support, and resource information that can prove valuable. Although the medication regimen can be daunting, teach clients the importance of following the regimen as closely as possible. Eating a balanced diet is important, as is an exercise program to fit the individual's needs. Because financial resources may be limited due to the cost of treatment and even the inability to work, a referral to a social worker may be helpful.

Prognosis

Recurrent bouts of opportunistic infections, with or without malignancies, usually cause the death of individuals with AIDS. Rapid testing for HIV, resulting in earlier treatment, and the use of HAART therapy have greatly increased the years a person may live following diagnosis.

Prevention

After years of research, there is still no effective vaccine against the infection. Education is the first defense against this epidemic. To avoid exposure to HIV, a person should practice safer sex. The use of latex condoms for any form of sexual intercourse is essential. Body fluids and items such as used hypodermic needles are considered potentially infective; therefore, universal precautions must be practiced when handling blood and body fluids. Eliminating risk factors for HIV-infected people can be as beneficial as treating the HIV infection. Eliminating malnutrition and needle sharing among those who abuse drugs is extremely important, and purifying blood-clotting factors for hemophiliacs has been very beneficial.

Infectious and Communicable Diseases of Childhood and Adolescence

CHAPTER EPISODE—PART III

Rodney seems to be more at ease following the discussion of the protection provided but is still a little hesitant. The pediatrician turns to his computer and pulls up a site that explains the risks and responsibilities of not having vaccinations. The information is available at http://www.cdc.gov/vaccines/hcp/patient-ed/conversations/downloads/not-vacc-risks-color-office.pdf and can be printed as a PDF. The pediatrician gives the information to Rodney and asks him to call tomorrow with his decision.

- For your own benefit, summarize the information in this file.

INFECTIOUS DIARRHEAL DISEASES

ICD-10: A09

Description

Infectious diarrheal disease usually affects children under age 5. The disease can be highly contagious and occurs frequently in day-care centers. In the United States, it is estimated that more than 20 million episodes of infectious diarrheal diseases occur in children under age 5.

Etiology

Diarrheal infections generally are transmitted via the oral-fecal route and possibly via airborne respiratory droplets. Individuals have natural defenses to combat pathogens taken in while eating, including normal flora, gastric acid, intestinal motility, and cellular immunity. However, when an individual ingests more than the host can combat, infection occurs. The incubation from ingestion to infection generally is 48 hours. The most common causative agents are rotaviruses and bacteria; the latter include *E. coli* O157:H7, *Salmonella*, *Shigella*, *Campylobacter*, and *Yersinia* species. Parasitic infections can also cause infectious diarrheal disease, generally from contaminated food and drink ingested by people who travel to high-risk areas in other countries of the world. Parasitic organisms include *Giardia* and *Cryptosporidium* species.

Signs and Symptoms

The most common symptom, diarrhea, may be bloody and may be preceded or accompanied by vomiting, nausea, and abdominal cramping. A low-grade fever may be present. In severe cases, dehydration, electrolyte imbalance, acidosis, and kidney failure may occur.

Diagnostic Procedures

History and physical examination with clinical presentation is important. Stool is examined for parasites, bacteria, and/or white blood cells. Repeat stool specimens may be required to confirm the infecting organism. Special laboratory tests may be needed, especially for *E. coli* O157:H7. A careful review of the child's diet for the previous 3 or 4 days may be helpful in determining the cause. The level of dehydration needs to be assessed.

Treatment

Rehydration is most important and must start immediately. If vomiting continues, it is better to rehydrate by offering small amounts of liquid frequently. If the infectious disease is caused by a virus, no medication generally is given; however, if the causative agent is bacterial, antibiotics may be administered. In parasitic infectious diarrheal disease, the drug chosen for treatment is determined by the specific parasite involved. Intake and output of fluids should be continually measured, and frequency of the stool should be noted. The infected child needs to maintain a high caloric intake and should avoid foods high in sugar; however, food may have to be offered slowly and in small amounts at first.

Complementary Therapy

Complementary therapy includes dietary limitations and appropriate nutritional therapy to replace fluid and electrolytes.

➔ CLIENT COMMUNICATION

Because the disease is highly contagious, it is paramount to teach all caregivers the proper care of clients during the contagious stage. Hand washing is essential, as is the proper handling of diapers and bedding. Encourage a balanced diet and ample fluids.

Prognosis

In the United States, the prognosis is good if detected early, if hydration is started immediately, and if antimicrobial treatment is begun. Unfortunately, if the infection is severe, a child can die within hours. Some children, especially those under age 2, may die from such complications as dehydration, shock, and bacteremia. In developing countries, there are an estimated 1.7 billion cases of infectious diarrhea per year that result in the death of 760,000 children under age 5.

Prevention

The importance of good hygiene cannot be overstressed, especially good hand washing when changing diapers or feeding children. Providing every child in the world with clean drinking water and food free from bacteria is a primary goal in prevention. Swimming should be avoided in ponds, lakes, or stagnant bodies of water.

RUBEOLA (MEASLES)

✔ REPORTABLE DISEASE

ICD-10: B05.X

Description

Rubeola (formerly known as *hard* or *red measles*) is a highly communicable respiratory infection. Its diagnostic signs are fever and the appearance of a characteristic rash. The disease is most common in school-age children, with outbreaks occurring in the winter and spring. In 2012, WHO reported 122,000 deaths from rubeola globally. The disease is less common in the United States, but from January to May 2014, 187 cases were reported in 15 outbreaks.

Etiology

Rubeola is caused by the *Morbillivirus rubeola* virus through direct contact with infectious droplets and occasionally through the air. The virus has an incubation period of 10 to 20 days.

Signs and Symptoms

The onset of symptoms is usually gradual. Initial symptoms may include **rhinitis** (inflammation of the nasal mucosa), cough, cold or coryza, drowsiness, **anorexia** (loss of appetite), and a slow but progressive rise in temperature to 101°F or 103°F by the second day. Small red spots with bluish white centers, called Koplik spots, appear on the oral mucosa by the second or third day. Photophobia and cough soon follow. By about the fourth day, the fever usually reaches its maximum (as high as 104°F to 106°F) and the characteristic rash appears. The rash first appears on the face as tiny maculopapular lesions that contain both discolored spots of skin called *macules* and red, raised areas of skin called *papules*. These rapidly enlarge and spread to other areas of the body. The lesions may be so densely clustered in certain areas that the skin surface appears generally swollen and red.

Diagnostic Procedures

The clinical picture of symptoms is usually a sufficient basis for a diagnosis of rubeola. Blood testing may reveal an abnormal decrease in the number of circulating white blood cells, or **leukopenia,** and antibody titers are used to detect the presence of measles antibody in both the acute and convalescent phases.

Treatment

Treatment for rubeola is essentially symptomatic. Bed rest is indicated, sometimes in a darkened room to alleviate the discomfort of photophobia. Antipyretics and liquids may be recommended. Keep infected children isolated until the rash disappears.

Complementary Therapy

No significant complementary therapy is indicated.

⊕ CLIENT COMMUNICATION

Educate caregivers about the incubation period, the spread of infection, and how to handle bedding, discarded tissues, and dishes. It is important to provide rest, ample fluids, and a balanced diet.

Prognosis

Rubeola is usually a benign disease, running its course in about 5 days after the rash appears. An attack of rubeola usually confers permanent immunity. Complications may arise, including croup, conjunctivitis, myocarditis, and opportunistic respiratory tract infections from staphylococci, streptococci, or *Haemophilus influenzae.*

Prevention

Active immunization can be produced by administration of a vaccine, preferably containing the live attenuated virus. The vaccine is normally a part of the measles/mumps/rubella immunizations (MMR) or measles/mumps/rubella/varicella (MMRV) vaccine given at 12 to 15 months of age and again at age 6. Prior to the vaccine, as many as 500,000 cases were reported yearly. The increase in incidence in the past few years is the result of children not receiving vaccinations as well as increased international travel, which is increasing the rate of exposure. Rubeola can be prevented within 5 days of exposure by administration of gamma globulin, a protein formed in blood that functions as an antibody to provide rapid, temporary immunity to the disease. Hand washing and discarding tissues contaminated with respiratory secretions may help prevent the spread of measles within a family.

RUBELLA (GERMAN MEASLES)

✔ *REPORTABLE DISEASE*

ICD-10: B06.X

Description

Rubella (German or 3-day measles) is an acute infectious disease characterized by fever and rash (Fig. 4.3). It closely resembles rubeola, but it differs in its short course, mild fever, and relative freedom from complications.

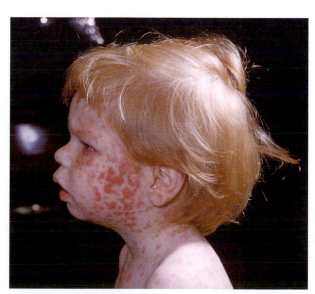

Figure 4.3 Rubella. *(Centers for Disease Control and Prevention.)*

Rubella is not as contagious as rubeola, and it occurs most frequently among teenagers and young adults.

Etiology

The disease is caused by the rubella virus. This virus has an incubation period of 14 to 21 days.

Signs and Symptoms

The onset of the disease is sometimes characterized by malaise, headache, slight fever, and sore throat. About 25% to 50% of cases are asymptomatic, especially among children. The rash typically appears the first or second day after onset. It may be composed of pale red, slightly elevated, discrete papules, or the rash may be highly diffuse and bright red. The rash begins on the face, spreads rapidly to other portions of the body, and usually fades so rapidly that the face may clear before the extremities are affected. Rash-covered portions of skin may itch or peel.

Diagnostic Procedures

Because rubella can be easily confused with other diseases, a definitive diagnosis can be reached with cultures of the throat, blood, and urine or with antibody titers. A culture of urine with antibody titers is generally done in the acute and convalescent phases.

Treatment

Symptoms are so mild that treatment usually is not necessary. Isolation from others (especially pregnant women) may be beneficial. Treatment is nonspecific and symptomatic. Bed rest is indicated. Topical **antipruritics** or warm water baths may be recommended to relieve itching. Antipyretics may be prescribed.

Complementary Therapy

No significant complementary therapy is indicated.

⊕ CLIENT COMMUNICATION

Because many clients are asymptomatic, teaching opportunities may be limited; however, it is a good idea to encourage clients to eat a balanced diet and drink ample fluids. Measures to reduce itching are helpful.

Prognosis

The prognosis for an individual with rubella is usually good. The disease is benign, seldom produces complications, and runs its course in 3 days. Rubella is dangerous, however, when it occurs in pregnant women, especially during the first trimester of pregnancy; the virus is capable of producing severe fetal malformation.

Prevention

Lasting immunization can be conferred through use of a live rubella vaccine. (See vaccine information in "Prevention" under "Rubeola [Measles].") This vaccine must not be administered to pregnant women or to those who may become pregnant within 3 months after immunization. Administration of gamma globulin shortly after exposure may prevent development of the disease, but it still may not prevent transfer of the virus to the fetus if exposure occurs during pregnancy. Prevention includes good hand washing and disposing of tissues contaminated with respiratory secretions.

MUMPS

✔ **REPORTABLE DISEASE**

ICD-10: B26.X

Description

Mumps is an acute contagious disease characterized by fever and inflammation of the parotid salivary glands. The disease is most common among children and young adults in late winter and spring. It is easily prevented by vaccination.

Etiology

The disease is caused by the mumps paramyxovirus, which has an incubation period of 18 days. The disease is transmitted via little droplets of saliva or the airborne route.

Signs and Symptoms

The classic symptoms of mumps are unilateral or bilateral swollen parotid glands. Headache, malaise, fever, and earache may occur, and other salivary glands may become swollen.

Diagnostic Procedures

The clinical picture of mumps and a history of recent exposure usually are sufficient for diagnosis. A nasopharyngeal culture is done. A blood test may be ordered.

Treatment

Analgesics, antipyretics, and adequate fluid intake are recommended. Isolation of the affected individual is important during the contagious period. Otherwise, there is no specific treatment for mumps.

Complementary Therapy

No significant complementary therapy is indicated.

 CLIENT COMMUNICATION

It is important to educate clients of the possible complications of mumps so that they can be prevented if at all possible. Encourage rest, increased fluids, and proper diet.

Prognosis

The prognosis for an individual with mumps is good. Complications can occur, however, and include **orchitis,** pancreatitis, and various central nervous system manifestations. Orchitis, which causes swelling of the testes in adult men, is extremely uncomfortable but rarely causes sterility, as is often feared.

Prevention

The best prevention is to receive the mumps vaccine (MMR or MMRV) and to avoid exposure to the disease during its communicable period. Good hand washing and proper disposal of contaminated tissues is essential for prevention.

VARICELLA (CHICKENPOX)

✔ *REPORTABLE DISEASE*

ICD-10: B01.X

Description

Varicella (chickenpox) is a highly contagious disease characterized by the appearance of a distinctive rash that passes through stages of macules, papules, small fluid-filled blisters or vesicles, and crusts (Fig. 4.4). The disease occurs most commonly among children and may occur in epidemic outbreaks.

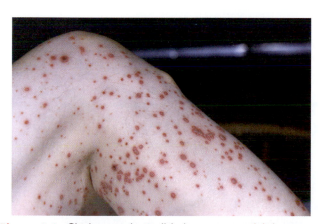

Figure 4.4 Chickenpox (varicella) shown on an adult knee. *(Centers for Disease Control and Prevention. Dr. Alexander D. Langmuir.)*

Etiology

The disease is caused by the varicella-zoster virus, which is a herpesvirus. Its incubation period is 2 to 3 weeks, usually between 13 and 17 days, and is spread via respiratory secretion and direct contact.

Signs and Symptoms

The sign of chickenpox is a pruritic rash, which begins as erythematous macules that produce papules and then clear vesicles. The rash usually contains a combination of papules, vesicles, and scabs in all stages. Anorexia, malaise, and fever may accompany the rash.

Diagnostic Procedures

The clinical signs are usually sufficient for the diagnosis. A history that indicates recent exposure helps confirm the diagnosis.

Treatment

Isolation is important during the infectious period—usually until all the scabs disappear. The only treatment necessary is to reduce the itching. Antihistamines may be given. Calamine lotion, cool bicarbonate of soda, or colloidal oatmeal baths can be very helpful. It is best not to scratch the lesions.

Complementary Therapy

No significant complementary therapy is indicated other than oatmeal baths, as suggested previously.

 CLIENT COMMUNICATION

Chickenpox requires strict adherence to proper hand washing, disposal of tissues, and proper cleaning of bedding and clothing. Teach clients or caregivers how to apply any lotions or medications to alleviate itching. Encourage bed rest and push fluids. Do not give children aspirin-containing products because of its link to Reye syndrome.

Prognosis

The prognosis for an individual with varicella is good. The disease runs its course in about 2 to 3 weeks. Complications may include secondary bacterial infections of the skin as a result of scratching open lesions, thrombocytopenia, arthritis, hepatitis, and Reye syndrome.

Anyone who has had chickenpox (or the chickenpox vaccine) is at risk for developing shingles (ICD-10; B02.X) later in life. After a varicella infection, the virus can remain inactive in nerve cells near the spinal cord and reactivate later as shingles. Shingles can cause tingling, itching, and pain followed by a rash of red bumps and blisters. Shingles is sometimes treated with antiviral drugs, steroids, and pain medications. In May 2006, the FDA approved a vaccine to prevent shingles in people over age 60. Anyone who has not had chickenpox can catch it from someone with shingles, but they cannot catch shingles.

Prevention

The best prevention is MMRV vaccination as a child. In certain situations, varicella-zoster immune globulin may be administered within 72 hours of exposure to stop the development of the disease. Good hygiene, including proper disposal of tissues contaminated with respiratory secretions, is important.

ERYTHEMA INFECTIOSUM (FIFTH DISEASE)

ICD-10: B08.3 or B09

Description

Erythema infectiosum is a common infection occurring predominantly in children, with flulike symptoms and diffuse redness of the skin, or erythema. It is called *fifth disease* because it was classified in the late 19th century as the fifth in a series of six childhood **exanthems**— rashes that occur on the skin as opposed to rashes that occur on the mucous membranes (or **enanthems**). It is a mild illness that exhibits a rash and develops quickly.

Etiology

Fifth disease is caused by the human parvovirus B19 (this not the same parvovirus pets may get) and is transmitted through respiratory secretions or direct contact. Parvovirus B19 can be transmitted during therapy with clotting factor concentrate. Its incubation period is generally 4 to 14 days but can be as long as 20 days. Unfortunately, the person is contagious before the onset of symptoms. It is most prevalent in elementary and junior high school children during winter and spring.

Signs and Symptoms

The child has a low-grade fever, coldlike symptoms, and a red facial rash that looks like a "slapped cheek." Later there is a circumoral pallor and symmetric lacy rash on the trunk and limbs (Fig. 4.5). The rash can recur for weeks with exposure to the sun, heat, stress, or exercise. Between 20% and 60% of the children in outbreaks are symptomatic, and many are asymptomatically infected.

Diagnostic Procedures

Diagnosis is generally made by clinical presentation. B19 can be detected in throat swabbings, respiratory tract secretions, and serum. The B19-specific antibodies can be detected with commercially available immunoassay kits.

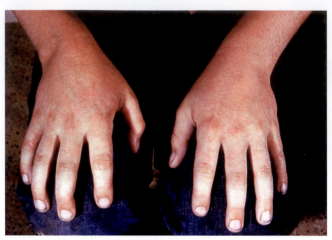

Figure 4.5 Hands of elementary school child showing symptoms of fifth disease. *(Centers for Disease Control and Prevention; http://phil. cdc.gov/phil/details.asp?pid=4511.)*

Treatment

Generally, no treatment is needed; however, it is important to manage any fever.

Complementary Therapy

No significant complementary therapy is indicated.

⊙ CLIENT COMMUNICATION

Inform caregivers that children are not contagious after the onset of a rash, so they can continue to attend school or work. Although the exact route of transmission is essentially unknown, it is important to discard any used tissues appropriately and to encourage clients to drink ample fluids and practice good hand washing.

Prognosis

Complications include arthralgia and arthritis.

Prevention

Good hygiene and proper disposal of tissues with contaminated respiratory secretions are necessary.

CHAPTER EPISODE—PART IV

Rodney calls the next day to say he is ready for Jed to have the vaccinations. You are to see them at 3:00 p.m.

- Is there anything you might say to Rodney to further ease his concerns?
- What information will you tell him about any reaction that might occur?

PERTUSSIS (WHOOPING COUGH)

✔ *REPORTABLE DISEASE*

ICD-10: A37.X

Description

Pertussis is an acute, highly infectious respiratory tract disease characterized by a repetitious, paroxysmal cough and a prolonged, harsh, or shrill sound during inspiration (the "whoop"). Pertussis affects infants and children more frequently and more severely than it does adults.

Etiology

Most cases of pertussis are caused by *Bordetella pertussis*. This bacterium has an incubation period of 7 to 10 days. It induces a mucopurulent secretion and hampers the natural ability of the respiratory tract to clear such secretions. Consequently, mucus accumulates in the airways and obstructs airflow. The route of transmission for the disease is direct contact with any discharge from the mucous membrane of an infected person.

Signs and Symptoms

The signs and symptoms of pertussis can be divided into three stages. The *catarrhal stage* is marked by the gradual onset of coldlike symptoms—mild fever, running nose, dry cough, irritability, and anorexia. This stage lasts from 1 to 2 weeks, during which the disease is highly communicable. The *paroxysmal stage* is marked by the onset of the classic cough, consisting of a series of several short, severe coughs in rapid succession followed by a slow, strained inspiration, during which a "whoop" (stridor) may be heard. The coughing occurs in periodic attacks. This stage, lasting 3 to 4 weeks, may be accompanied by weight loss, dehydration, vomiting, epistaxis, and hypoxia. After several weeks, a period of decline begins, marked by the gradual diminishment of coughing.

Diagnostic Procedures

A history of exposure to another infected individual and the presence of the classic cough may be sufficient to establish the diagnosis. A very high white blood cell count is another distinguishing feature of pertussis. A definitive diagnosis depends on a nasopharyngeal culture.

Treatment

Antibiotics administered during the catarrhal stage may check the development of the disease; if administration is delayed past this stage, antibiotics have little effect. The individual with pertussis requires meticulous care to ensure adequate nutrition, hydration, and clearance of mucous secretions.

Complementary Therapy

Fluids are encouraged. Light foods can be taken. The client should avoid all dairy products during the acute stage. Fruits, vegetables, brown rice, clear vegetable soups, potatoes, and whole grain toast may be tried. Aromatherapy with basil, chamomile, eucalyptus, peppermint, and lavender in a cool mist vaporizer may be useful. Osteopathic manipulation may be able to reduce the severity of the cough.

➤ CLIENT COMMUNICATION

Remind caregivers that the characteristic cough may sound worse than it is but that they need to be aware that mucus may accumulate and require attention if airways become clogged. Encourage proper fluid intake and a balanced diet. Educate clients about the necessity of following the treatment plan, including taking all of the prescribed medication.

Prognosis

The prognosis for an individual with pertussis varies from case to case. Uncomplicated pertussis may run its course in 12 weeks. Recovery may be considerably extended, however, particularly among infants. Complications can occur as a result of seizures, apnea, encephalopathy, and pneumonia. Young children can die. In 2014, 32,971 individuals were sickened by pertussis in the United States. Fifteen infants younger than 3 months died before they were old enough for the vaccination.

Prevention

A child can be rendered less susceptible to pertussis by receiving a series of immunizations with pertussis vaccine. The vaccine is part of the DTaP (diphtheria, tetanus, acellular pertussis) vaccine given around 3 months of age. Good hand washing and proper disposal of contaminated tissue from respiratory secretions are essential.

DIPHTHERIA

✔ *REPORTABLE DISEASE*

ICD-10: A36.X

Description

Diphtheria is an acute, life-threatening infectious disease. It is characterized by a gray to black membrane-like coating that forms over mucous membrane surfaces, particularly along the respiratory tract, which can block airways. It can cause a toxic reaction that primarily affects the heart and peripheral nerves. The disease may occasionally involve the skin. Most cases occur in children under age 10, but older children and adults also may be affected.

Etiology

Diphtheria is caused by *Corynebacterium diphtheriae*. The bacterium has an incubation period of 2 to 5 days. Most strains of *C. diphtheriae* also release a highly potent toxin capable of damaging the heart, kidneys, and peripheral nerves. Transmission is through contact with discharge from the nose, throat, eye, and skin lesions.

Signs and Symptoms

The specific symptoms vary with the site of infection. In typical cases, a slight headache, malaise, and a mild fever (100°F to 101°F) occur. There may be a strong, foul odor to the breath; bluish skin color; bloody, watery nasal drainage; and breathing problems. Some individuals infected with *C. diphtheriae* remain asymptomatic but become carriers of the disease.

Diagnostic Procedures

The appearance of the characteristic membrane may be sufficient to establish a diagnosis of diphtheria. A definitive diagnosis can be made only by identifying the bacterium in nose and throat cultures.

Treatment

The only specific treatment is administration of sufficient quantities of diphtheria antitoxin as early in the course of the disease as possible followed by antibiotic therapy. The affected individual must be isolated, and bed rest is required. A soft or liquid diet is recommended. Emergency measures may be required to maintain an airway or to control cardiac complications. Carriers of diphtheria are usually treated with antibiotics.

Complementary Therapy

No significant complementary therapy is indicated.

 CLIENT COMMUNICATION

Educate family members about diphtheria. Any nonimmunized members should receive diphtheria toxoid appropriate to age. Hospitalization of the infected child is often necessary for proper treatment and observation for complications.

Prognosis

The prognosis for an individual with diphtheria varies according to the severity of the disease. Mild cases resolve in 3 to 4 days or a week in moderate cases. Complications include myocarditis (the most common complication), thrombocytopenia, and vocal cord paralysis. Even with antitoxin therapy, death may result if complications are severe.

Prevention

Diphtheria is highly preventable. Inoculation with diphtheria toxoid at 3 months of age is routine. Booster doses should be administered at appropriate intervals during early childhood. Diphtheria toxoid is usually administered along with the vaccine for pertussis and the toxoid for tetanus (the DTaP vaccine), because higher levels of antibodies are produced when all three vaccines are administered simultaneously rather than individually. While today the incidence of diphtheria has greatly decreased, with only five cases reported in the United States in the last 10 years, it is a disease that must be recognized for its serious potential. Also, acknowledging the diseases prevented by the vaccination makes the public more aware of the consequences of refusing vaccinations.

TETANUS (LOCKJAW)

✔ **REPORTABLE DISEASE**

ICD-10: A35

Description

Tetanus is an acute, life-threatening infectious disease characterized by persistent, painful contractions of skeletal muscles. The disease may affect any person at any time—the elderly, migrant workers, children, and injection drug users. Puncture wounds are particularly prone to tetanus, but sores can become infected by the bacteria. Tetanus is acquired from the environment; it is not transmitted person to person.

Etiology

The disease is caused by *Clostridium tetani*, a bacterium commonly found in soil. The bacillus becomes pathogenic when its spores enter the body through a puncture wound. Burns, surgical incisions, and chronic skin ulcers may also provide opportunities for *C. tetani* spores to enter the body, as may generalized conditions such as otitis media and dental infections. The spores produce a powerful toxin that attacks the central nervous system and that also acts directly on voluntary muscles to produce contraction.

Signs and Symptoms

The onset of symptoms may be either gradual or abrupt. Stiffness of the jaw, esophageal muscles, and some neck muscles is often the first sign of the disease. Later, in the most common manifestation of tetanus, the jaws become rigidly fixed (lockjaw), the voice is altered, and the facial muscles contract, contorting the individual's face into a grimace. Finally, the muscles of the back and the extremities may become rigid, or the individual may experience extremely severe convulsive muscle spasms. This final phase of the disease often is accompanied by high fever, profuse sweating, tachycardia, dysphagia, and intense pain.

Diagnostic Procedures

Tetanus is diagnosed on the basis of its classic symptomatology.

Treatment

Human tetanus immune globulin, administered intramuscularly within the first 24 hours, is the first course of treatment. The site of the wound or the point of infection must be thoroughly cleaned and debrided. Antibiotics to kill the bacteria are administered. Muscle relaxants may be prescribed. Meticulous care and support are required to maintain adequate nutrition and hydration and to avoid the development of decubitus ulcers. Tracheostomy is routinely performed in moderate to severe cases of tetanus to prevent choking.

Complementary Therapy

No significant complementary therapy is indicated.

⟳ CLIENT COMMUNICATION

The disease process can be frightening; however, education about tetanus helps alleviate anxiety and fears. It is important to follow clients carefully and watch for any complications. Special attention should be given to ensure a proper diet and ample fluids.

Prognosis

The disease usually runs its course in about 6 to 7 weeks, seldom producing any lasting disability. However, despite effective treatment measures, tetanus is frequently fatal, especially among unimmunized people, most often in developing countries. Death may result from asphyxiation, a host of possible complications, and sometimes from sheer exhaustion.

Prevention

Surprisingly enough, having tetanus does not confer future immunity to the disease. Immunization with DTaP should be routinely started at 3 months of age. Boosters are required periodically throughout life. The risk of contracting tetanus also can be minimized by wearing protective clothing and by promptly cleansing and caring for wounds and other skin lesions.

IMMUNIZATION

Immunizations are important for protection against certain communicable diseases. Medical personnel maintain accurate records of immunizations, but in the current mobile society and with the ever-present changes in primary care providers due to insurance restrictions within the United States, parents and guardians are advised to keep a separate and complete record of their child's and their own immunizations. Additional health immunizations are required for travel to certain other countries. County health departments have specific information on recommended or required immunizations for world travel.

Three excellent sources of information on immunizations are:

- Centers for Disease Control and Prevention (http://www.cdc.gov)
- Morbidity and Mortality Weekly Report (http://www.cdc.gov/mmwr)
- National Center for Health Statistics (http://www.cdc.gov/nchs)

The incidence of certain communicable diseases in the United States has steadily declined. Because of advances in medical knowledge, general improvements in living conditions, and government-mandated immunization programs, children and adolescents are no longer the routine victims of many diseases. For example, poliomyelitis (ICD-10: A80.9), once endemic, was eradicated in 1979 in the United States. However, its threat is again on the rise in war-torn countries throughout the world.

Caution cannot be thrown to the wind, however. A serious outbreak of rubeola occurred on a college campus, where a substantial number of students had not been vaccinated against the disease owing to their religious beliefs. In some areas of the United States, limited access to medical care, lack of knowledge, or a distrust of government-sponsored health outreach programs may leave significant numbers of children unprotected by vaccines. In the absence of the effective immunization provided by vaccines, communicable disease can still cause major epidemics.

A vaccine is a suspension of infectious agents, components of the agents, or genetically engineered antigens. It is given for the purpose of establishing resistance to an infectious disease. There are two general classes of vaccines:

- Live, generally attenuated, infectious agents (e.g., measles virus)
- Inactivated agents or products obtained through genetic recombination (e.g., acellular pertussis vaccines)

Both types are used in vaccines for many diseases (poliomyelitis and influenza).

Whatever its makeup, a vaccine stimulates the development of specific defense mechanisms that should result in permanent protection from the disease. Figure 4.6 is an immunization schedule that lists the vaccines

Figure 1. Recommended immunization schedule for persons aged 0 through 18 years – United States, 2015.
(FOR THOSE WHO FALL BEHIND OR START LATE, SEE THE CATCH-UP SCHEDULE [FIGURE 2]).
These recommendations must be read with the footnotes that follow. For those who fall behind or start late, provide catch-up vaccination at the earliest opportunity as indicated by the green bars in Figure 1. To determine minimum intervals between doses, see the catch-up schedule (Figure 2). School entry and adolescent vaccine age groups are shaded.

Vaccine	Birth	1 mo	2 mos	4 mos	6 mos	9 mos	12 mos	15 mos	18 mos	19–23 mos	2-3 yrs	4-6 yrs	7-10 yrs	11-12 yrs	13–15 yrs	16–18 yrs
Hepatitis B[7] (HepB)	1st dose	←---- 2nd dose ----→			←-------------------- 3rd dose --------------------→											
Rotavirus[7] (RV) RV1 (2-dose series); RV5 (3-dose series)			1st dose	2nd dose	See footnote 2											
Diphtheria, tetanus, & acellular pertussis[3] (DTaP: <7 yrs)			1st dose	2nd dose	3rd dose		←---- 4th dose ----→					5th dose				
Tetanus, diphtheria, & acellular pertussis[4] (Tdap: ≥7 yrs)														(Tdap)		
Haemophilus influenzae type b[5] (Hib)			1st dose	2nd dose	See footnote 5		3rd or 4th dose, See footnote 5									
Pneumococcal conjugate[6] (PCV13)			1st dose	2nd dose	3rd dose		←---- 4th dose ----→									
Pneumococcal polysaccharide[6] (PPSV23)																
Inactivated poliovirus[7] (IPV: <18 yrs)			1st dose	2nd dose	←-------------- 3rd dose --------------→							4th dose				
Influenza[8] (IIV; LAIV) 2 doses for some: See footnote 8					Annual vaccination (IIV only) 1 or 2 doses						Annual vaccination (LAIV or IIV) 1 or 2 doses		Annual vaccination (LAIV or IIV) 1 dose only			
Measles, mumps, rubella[9] (MMR)					See footnote 9		←---- 1st dose ----→					2nd dose				
Varicella[10] (VAR)							←---- 1st dose ----→					2nd dose				
Hepatitis A[11] (HepA)							←---------- 2-dose series, See footnote 11 ----------→									
Human papillomavirus[12] (HPV2: females only; HPV4: males and females)														(3-dose series)		
Meningococcal[13] (Hib-MenCY ≥ 6 weeks; MenACWY-D ≥9 mos; MenACWY-CRM ≥ 2 mos)				See footnote 13										1st dose		Booster

	Range of recommended ages for all children		Range of recommended ages for catch-up immunization		Range of recommended ages for certain high-risk groups		Range of recommended ages during which catch-up is encouraged and for certain high-risk groups		Not routinely recommended

This schedule includes recommendations in effect as of January 1, 2015. Any dose not administered at the recommended age should be administered at a subsequent visit, when indicated and feasible. The use of a combination vaccine generally is preferred over separate injections of its equivalent component vaccines. Vaccination providers should consult the relevant Advisory Committee on Immunization Practices (ACIP) statement for detailed recommendations, available online at http://www.cdc.gov/vaccines/hcp/acip-recs/index.html. Clinically significant adverse events that follow vaccination should be reported to the Vaccine Adverse Event Reporting System (VAERS) online (http://www.vaers.hhs.gov) or by telephone (800-822-7967). Suspected cases of vaccine-preventable diseases should be reported to the state or local health department. Additional information, including precautions and contraindications for vaccination, is available from CDC online (http://www.cdc.gov/vaccines/recs/vac-admin/contraindications.htm) or by telephone (800-CDC-INFO [800-232-4636]).

This schedule is approved by the Advisory Committee on Immunization Practices (http://www.cdc.gov/vaccines/acip), the American Academy of Pediatrics (http://www.aap.org), the American Academy of Family Physicians (http://www.aafp.org), and the American College of Obstetricians and Gynecologists (http://www.acog.org).

NOTE: The above recommendations must be read along with the footnotes of this schedule.

Figure 4.6   Recommended immunization schedule for persons aged 0–18 years—United States 2014. *(Department of Health and Human Services, Centers for Disease Control and Prevention; http://www.cdc.gov/vaccines/schedules/downloads/child/0-18yrs-schedule.pdf.)*

commonly administered during childhood and adolescence. The immunization schedules are generally based on the consensus of the Advisory Committee on Immunization Practices of the CDC, the American Academy of Pediatrics, and the American Academy of Family Physicians. For a list of the recommended adult immunizations, visit http://www.cdc.gov/vaccines/recs.

CLIENT COMMUNICATION

It is important that all individuals be given information related to the particular vaccine and any side effects that might occur. Respect must be given to those who refuse vaccinations; however, it can be helpful to make certain they are properly informed of the dangers of communicable diseases.

SUMMARY

Infectious and communicable diseases emerge and reemerge in our lives. One disease is eradicated, only to have another surface. Diseases once completely eradicated from the world are again becoming a threat. Infectious diseases that once responded to antibiotics are now resistant. The SARS and recent MERS outbreak make us look at a prevention method not practiced for many years—isolation and quarantine. The H1N1 viral outbreak in 2009 caused many individuals to change travel plans and wear protective masks in public. Frequent hand washing and careful handling of all materials that may be contaminated, coupled with available vaccinations, continue to offer the best protection against infectious and communicable diseases.

| For more resources and to sharpen your skills with interactive exercises, visit DavisPlus at http://davisplus.fadavis.com. Keyword Tamparo.

ONLINE RESOURCES

Antimicrobial Resistance
http://www.who.int/mediacentre/factsheets/fs194/en/

DEET (N,N-diethyl-3-methylbenzamide)
http://www.deet.com/faqs.html

Emergency preparedness and response/bioterrorism
http://emergency.cdc.gov

Emerging and Reemerging Infectious Diseases
http://www.niaid.nih.gov/topics/emerging/pages/default.aspx

HIV infection/AIDS
http://www.avert.org/worldstats.htm

MERS
http://www.cdc.gov/features/novelcoronavirus/

Morbidity and Mortality Weekly Report
http://www.cdc.gov/mmwr

National Center for Health Statistics
http://www.cdc.gov/nchs

Reportable diseases. Find greater detail on reportable infections, diseases, or conditions
http://www.in.gov/isdh/files/ReportableDiseaseList.pdf

West Nile Virus: Chicagotribune.com. 2014 West Nile Virus Season Update and Safety Tips.

CASE STUDIES

Case Study 1

Austin is a 40-year-old architect who has been fighting AIDS for 13 years. With the consent of his primary care provider, he removes himself from all medications. He improves. His appetite improves, and his stamina increases. He thinks about returning to work. Six months later, however, he returns to his provider weaker and sicker than before. At this point, Austin and his provider decide to seek complementary therapies.

Case Study Questions

1. What complementary therapies might be considered?
2. How will the integration of complementary therapies and the primary care provider's therapies be carried out?

Case Study 2

Peter travels the world in his position on the advance team for the secretary of state. He has likely visited as many as 20 different countries in 12 months' time and is frequently in areas where infectious diseases are far more common than in his home country, the United States. Using the CDC and the WHO as your resources, plan a strategy to keep Peter healthy.

Case Study Questions

1. What vaccinations are necessary for Peter?
2. Is there any prophylactic treatment or medications that might be identified prior to travel?
3. What other precautionary measures might be taken?
4. What economic and political factors are considered here?

REVIEW QUESTIONS

Matching

Match the following by placing the correct letter in the column.

_____ 1. Disease that is readily transmitted from one person to another

_____ 2. Contains DNA typical to avian, swine, and humans

_____ 3. A common cause of coryza

_____ 4. Estimated 20 million episodes occur every year in the United States

_____ 5. Should be maintained by health professionals *and* individuals

_____ 6. Formerly known as *hard* or *red measles*

_____ 7. Eradicated in 1979; still a potential weapon

_____ 8. Outbreak in Saudi Arabia spread to the United States

_____ 9. Prevents diphtheria, pertussis, tetanus

_____ 10. Causes inflammation of the parotid salivary glands.

a. Infectious

b. Rubeola

c. MERS

d. HINI virus

e. Infectious diarrheal disease

f. Communicable

g. Vaccination records

h. Rhinovirus

i. Rubella

j. Smallpox

k. Influenza

l. DTaP

m. Mumps

Short Answer

1. Koplik spots are characteristic of what childhood disease?

_____

2. What is the medical term for German measles?

_____

3. What is a common name for tetanus?

_____

4. The vaccine to prevent mumps is identified by what abbreviation?

_____

5. What is the infectious disease caused by parvovirus B19?

_____

6. What is difficult to treat and can progress to life-threatening blood, bone, or skin infections?

Multiple Choice

Place a checkmark next to the correct answer.

1. Which of the following statements is true about chronic fatigue syndrome?

_____ a. CFS is easily diagnosed with laboratory testing.

_____ b. CFS occurs more frequently in young adults.

_____ c. CFS is a debilitating illness with at least 6 months of unresolved fatigue.

_____ d. CFS is treatable and curable.

2. What is known about Lyme disease?

_____ a. Is caused by tiny, tick-transmitted spirochete

_____ b. Progresses in two stages

_____ c. Is treated by strict bed rest and a low-salt diet

_____ d. Is difficult to prevent

3. How are infectious diseases that can be used as weapons defined?

_____ a. Are listed in six categories

_____ b. Are reported to the FDA

_____ c. Incidence kept private to prevent panic in any outbreak

_____ d. Are easily disseminated or transmitted from person to person

4. What defines HIV infection and AIDS?

_____ a. They are curable.

_____ b. They can be treated with a new vaccine.

_____ c. They are showing evidence of a "superinfection."

_____ d. They are caused by a virulent bacterium that depresses the immune system.

5. What is *E. coli* O157:H7?

_____ a. It is a viral infection of the gastrointestinal tract.

_____ b. It is highly contagious from human to human.

_____ c. It is found in undercooked, contaminated ground beef.

_____ d. It is rarely fatal.

6. What are possible complementary therapies for the common cold?

_____ a. Acupuncture

_____ b. Antiviral medications

_____ c. Use of the Indian herb andrographis

_____ d. Use of antioxidants

Discussion Questions/Personal Reflection

1. Contact your county health department to ascertain which communicable diseases must be reported in your geographic location. List them.

_____

_____

_____

_____

_____

_____

_____

_____

_____

_____

_____

2. Contact a grade school or day-care center and compare their recommendations with those of your local health department for immunizations children must have when starting school.

_____

_____

_____

_____

_____

_____

_____

_____

_____

_____

3. Discuss what steps might be taken to reduce the risk of methicillin-resistant *Staphylococcus aureus* infection in local schools and gyms.

_____

_____

_____

_____

_____

_____

_____

_____

_____

_____

_____

_____

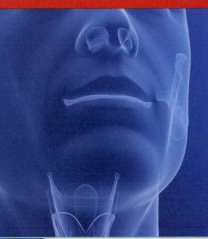

In the hour of adversity be not without hope, for crystal rain falls from black clouds.
—PERSIAN POEM

5

Cancer

● *key words*

Allogeneic (ăl″ō•jĕ•nē′ĭk)
Anaplasia (ăn″ă•plā′zē•ă)
Autologous (aw•tŏl′ō•gŭs)
Carcinogen (kăr•sĭn′ō•jĭn)
Carcinoma in situ
  (kăr″sĭn•ō′mă ĕn si′tū)
Dysplasia (dĭs•plā′zē•ă)
En bloc (ĕn blŏk′)

Epithelial (ĕp″ĭ•thē′lē•ăl)
Erythema (ĕr″ĭ•thē′mă)
Hyperplasia (hī″pĕr•plā′zē•ă)
Leukopenia (loo″kō•pē′nē•ă)
Leukoplakia (loo″kō•pla′kē•ă)
Mesothelioma
  (mĕs″ō•thē•lē•ō′mă)
Metastasis (mĕ•tăs′tă•sĭs)

Metastasize (mĕ•tăs′tă•sīz)
Palliative (păl′ē•ă•tĭv)
Radioisotope
  (rā″dē•ō•ī′sō•tōp)
Reed-Sternberg cell
  (rēd•stĕrn′•bĕrg sĕl)
Sarcomas (săr•kō′măs)
Syngeneic (sĭn•jĕ•nē′ĭk)

● *learning outcomes*

Upon successful completion of this chapter, you will be able to:

• Define key terms.
• Describe *neoplasm*.

• Compare benign and malignant tumors.
• Recall death statistics about cancer.
(learning outcomes continues)

(learning outcomes continued)

- List at least seven possible causes of cancer.
- Describe the main classifications for cancer.
- Recall signs and symptoms of cancer.
- Discuss how cancer is diagnosed.
- Identify the grading and staging of cancers and their use.
- Discuss six major forms of cancer treatment and their advantages and disadvantages.
- Identify at least seven suggestions for cancer prevention.
- Recall integrative and complementary therapies in cancer treatment.
- Recognize the warning signs of cancer.

CHAPTER EPISODE—PART I

Like many couples who decide their child-bearing years are over, 34-year-old Judd and his spouse decided shortly after their second child was born that a vasectomy was their best option. The procedure was successful with no problems. However, over a period of time, Judd observed that the scar tissue seemed thicker and denser. He wasn't too concerned but kept an eye on the scar. Much later, when the scar became larger, harder, and painful, he was concerned enough to go back to the urologist who performed the vasectomy.

- At this point, should Judd be worried? Justify your response.
- What might the urologist do to determine the cause of this change?

DESCRIPTION OF CANCER

Definitions

Some new growth in the body is necessary and advantageous; repair of bone and skin is an example. A *neoplasm* is a new growth that can be frightening, perplexing, and life-threatening. Neoplasm is a new formation or new growth that serves no useful purpose. The growth is uncontrollable and progressive, and it may be detrimental to other parts of the body. *Cancer*, a term most feared by individuals, is a group of diseases expressed by this uncontrolled growth and spread of abnormal cells that can cause death. The term *tumor*, a swelling or an enlargement, is used interchangeably with *neoplasm*.

A tumor may be benign or malignant, depending on its growth pattern, cell characteristics, potential for the cells to move from one part of the body to another (or **metastasis**), tendency to recur, and capacity to cause death.

A benign tumor is one that remains localized as a discrete mass. It has an excessive growth of cells but may grow slowly and is rarely fatal. A benign tumor can grow large enough to interfere with normal body function, however. Some benign uterine tumors have grown to be the size of a basketball, displacing adjacent organs and causing digestive problems. The benign tumor usually is encapsulated and does not infiltrate surrounding tissue; it does not tend to recur when surgically removed. A favorable recovery is likely.

A malignant tumor, by comparison, is invasive, grows rather rapidly, is sometimes **anaplastic** (has lost its cell definition and function), and can metastasize through the blood or lymph. Generally, the more virulent the tumor, the greater the chance of metastasis. These tumor cells are not normal; they are distorted in size, shape, and structure. If untreated, the malignancy progresses, and death may result. Malignant tumors are known as *cancer*, the disease on which this chapter focuses. Cancers are generally divided into three categories: carcinomas, **sarcomas,** and cancers of blood and lymph.

Statistics

Cancer is a focus of attention in American society because of its toll in lives, the suffering it causes, and the economic losses it produces. Cancer strikes people of all ages, both men and women, and is the second-leading cause of death in the United States, preceded only by heart disease. Cancer accounts for about 1 in every 4 deaths, more than 1,600 every day. According to the National Cancer Institute, 1,658,370 new cancer cases were expected to be diagnosed in 2015. About 77% of all cancers are diagnosed at age 55 or older. According to the American Cancer Society (ACS), the lifetime risk for men developing cancer is a little less than 1 in 2. For women, the risk is a little greater than 1 in 3. Childhood cancer is less common; however, approximately 1 in 285 children will be diagnosed with cancer by the age of 20. The National Cancer Institute's (NCI's) Surveillance Epidemiology and End Results website provides a table that lists the estimated new cancer cases and deaths by site and sex (go to http://seer.cancer.gov and search their statistics).

In the United States, more than 1.6 million new cases of cancer are diagnosed each year. Almost half of all deaths from cancer are from the four most frequently diagnosed kinds: lung and bronchus (ICD-10: C34.X*), prostate (ICD-10:C61), breast (ICD-10: C50.X), and colorectal cancer (ICD-10: C19). For males, prostate cancer is the most frequently diagnosed cancer; for women, breast cancer is the most frequently diagnosed. Lung and bronchus cancers remain the leading cause of cancer death for both men and women. Colorectal cancer occurs at about the same frequency in men and women.

One measure of the overall success of cancer treatment is how many individuals remain alive at specific time intervals (e.g., 5, 10, and 15 years) after they are diagnosed. The 5-year survival rate is a widely used marker. For all cancers combined, the 5-year survival rate has now reached 68%.

The number of cancer deaths is gradually declining. In fact, both incidence and death rates for all cancers combined have declined for both men and women since 1998. It is believed that the reduction is due largely to earlier screening, better treatment, and real gains in prevention of certain cancers. For example, the decline in smoking has resulted in fewer lung cancers. The incidence of lung cancer deaths dropped an average of 2.8% per year in California after the state placed a ban on smoking in public facilities. Other states have followed this practice. These numbers are quite significant because in 2015, nearly 480,000 cancer deaths were the result of tobacco use.

ETIOLOGY OF CANCER

Cancer can start in any body tissue and has no single cause. There are over 200 different types of cancer, and most are multifactorial, meaning that many factors contribute to the cancer. Research indicates that all cancers arise because of complex alterations in DNA that result in unrestrained cellular proliferation. These cell mutations alter gene chemistry enough to produce abnormal cells. It is suspected that mutations occur fairly frequently but that the body's immune response is able to destroy the abnormal cells as soon as they occur. Therefore, it is possible that a malignancy may represent a failure of the body's immune system.

This abnormal cell growth may take many years to occur in humans; it may stop at any point and occasionally is reversible. Generally, there is a progressive evolution of cancer cells through different states—**hyperplasia** (excessive growth of cells), **dysplasia** (abnormal growth of cells), **carcinoma in situ** (a cancerous growth that remains in place), and carcinomas that **metastasize** (spread through the circulatory system).

Carcinogens

The cell mutations often occur slowly over a period of time, even as long as 10 years, and can be caused by substances or agents that increase the risk of cancer development when humans are exposed to them. Such an element is termed a **carcinogen.** Carcinogens include many kinds of chemicals and certain kinds of high-frequency radiation such as ultraviolet and ionizing radiation that damage the DNA.

Tobacco use is a carcinogen that plays a significant factor in the cause of respiratory cancers, all of which could be prevented completely. A high incidence of colon cancer may be linked to a high-fat, low-fiber diet, which is very popular in American households. About 3 million skin cancers diagnosed could be prevented by protection from the sun's harmful rays.

A recent study of firefighters in San Francisco, Chicago, and Philadelphia showed that they have a higher incidence of certain cancers such as mesothelioma and cancers of the respiratory, digestive, and urinary systems than the general population. It is believed this increased rate is directly related to the exposure to contaminants such as combustion by-products like benzene and formaldehyde, asbestos, and burned debris from fires.

Other Factors That Influence Cancer Development

Not everyone who smokes gets lung cancer, and not everyone with high exposure to the sun's damaging rays

---

*The X represents the fourth digit that is often required and supplied once more detailed information about the disease or disorder is made known to the provider.

gets skin cancer. Other factors that can influence the development of cancer or help to prevent it are age, genetics, immune system response, body weight and diet, exercise and physical activity, environment, viruses, and even bacterial infections.

Age is a factor in that many cancers are more common as a person ages. This is because cell mutations often take a long time to develop into cancer cells. The longer a person lives, the greater the time for genetic mutations to occur in the cells. Approximately 55% of cancers are diagnosed after age 65.

Genetics implies that a person may be born with genetic mutations or have less ability to prevent the cells from mutating into cancer. A few examples deserve discussion. Cancer of the breast generally is more common in female relatives of affected women than in the general population. Women who have abnormal BRCA1 and BRCA2 breast cancer genes have a higher chance of developing breast cancer than those who do not carry the gene. The uncommon condition polyposis coli[1] (ICD-10: K63.5) is inherited through an autosomal dominant gene and eventually leads to carcinoma of the colon. Another rare cancer, retinoblastoma[2] (ICD-10: C69.2X), is inherited as a Mendelian dominant trait and usually is present at birth. Being born with a genetic predisposition to cancer does not mean that a person will get cancer; it only means that with a mutation present from birth, it is more likely that cancer will develop within a lifetime.

Individuals with depressed immune systems are more likely to have cancer. These individuals include those who received organ transplants and take antirejection drugs that suppress the immune system, persons with HIV or AIDS, and those born with rare medical problems that affect their immune response. The cancers related to immune system dysfunction are:

1. Caused by viruses such as those seen in cervical, liver, and stomach cancers and cancers of the genital or anal area.
2. Lymphomas, which can develop as the result of chronic infections or transplanted organs.

Body weight and diet also play a role in cancer development. In the United States, a large amount of red meat, cured meat, and food high in fat is consumed. Such large consumption of these foods, plus a diet that is lacking in fruits, vegetables, and whole grains, enables obesity and puts an individual at higher risk for cancer. Alcohol abuse is linked to liver, rectal, and breast cancers. Also, a combination of alcohol abuse and smoking greatly increases the incidences of cancers in the mouth and the respiratory organs.

Exercise and physical activity are believed to decrease the incidence of breast and colorectal cancer. It is thought that a healthy diet plus regular exercise and physical activity boosts the body's immune system. A healthy immune system is more apt to be able to prevent cell mutation and prolific cellular growth. Recent studies report, however, that much of the benefit of exercise and physical activity may be lost if there is insufficient sleep and rest.

Environment can play a role in cancer development. Harmful tobacco smoke (even secondhand) and the damaging sun rays have already been mentioned. Other environmental factors include natural and man-made radiation, asbestos, and some workplace hazards. Asbestos exposure increases the risk of **mesothelioma,** lung cancer, and cancers of the larynx and kidneys.

Viruses that can alter the cells' genetic makeup can cause some cancers. These viruses may include the human papillomavirus (HPV), the hepatitis B and C viruses, the Epstein-Barr virus (EBV), and HIV. These viruses cause cancer in only certain situations, and being infected with any of these viruses does not mean that cancer always results. There are similarities, however. Liver cancer is linked to chronic hepatitis B and C viral infections. Individuals who have EBV (very common) have an increased risk of lymphoma. In sub-Saharan Africa, EBV accompanied by repeated attacks of malaria cause a cancer called Burkitt lymphoma[3] (ICD-10: C83.7X). Individuals who received transplants and persons with AIDS who also carry EBV are at greater risk for lymphoma. HPV is linked directly to cervical cancers; however, a recently developed vaccine can prevent the types of genital HPV that cause most cases of cervical cancer.

Bacterial infections have recently been tied to cancer. Chronic infections are related to about 20% of cancers. Studies show that persons who have chronic *Helicobacter pylori* (bacterium related to stomach inflammation and ulcers) infection of the stomach are at greater risk of stomach cancer. Some kinds of digestive bacteria can increase the risk of both stomach and bowel cancer.

---

[1] *A highly malignant condition marked by multiple adenomatous polyps lining the intestinal mucosa, beginning about puberty.*

[2] *A tumor arising from retinal germ cells, malignancy of the eye in childhood.*

[3] *A malignant neoplasm composed of undifferentiated lymphoreticular cells that form a large osteolytic lesion in the jaw or an abdominal mass. It is seen chiefly in Africa.*

CHAPTER EPISODE—PART II

Judd's urologist is not too concerned but suspects this problem has little or nothing to do with the vasectomy. The urologist suggests an ultrasound and some blood work. There seemed to be no urgency, so it was a bit before Judd got in for the testing. The blood work came back perfectly normal. The ultrasound, however, showed a mass. A subsequent CT scan and further testing indicated testicular cancer, stage III with metastasis into the lymph nodes. Judd was dumbfounded.

- Why is Judd dumbfounded?
- Did the delay that took place in this episode have an impact on the outcome?

CLASSIFICATION OF CANCERS

Cancers are classified for diagnostic, treatment, and research purposes and to aid in reporting cancer statistics. One commonly accepted system classifies cancers according to the type of body tissue in which they appear.

Carcinomas

Carcinomas, the largest group, are solid tumors of **epithelial** tissue of external and internal body surfaces. These tumors are found in the breast, colon, liver, lung, prostate, and stomach and are often identified as such. For example, *colorectal carcinoma* refers to cancer of the colon and rectal area. Benign tumors of epithelial origin usually are named using just the suffix *-oma* added to the type of tissue involved. For example, an *adenoma* is a benign tumor of a gland. Malignant tumors of epithelial origin are named with the term *carcinoma* added to the type of tissue involved. For example, an *adenocarcinoma* is a malignant tumor of a gland. Such terminology often is confusing for the layperson, who may believe that *all* tumors are cancerous.

Sarcomas

Sarcomas, which are less common than carcinomas, arise from supportive and connective tissue such as bone, fat, muscle, and cartilage. Again, benign tumors of connective tissue are named by appending the suffix *-oma* to the type of tissue involved, and malignant tumors of connective tissue are named by adding the term *-sarcoma* to the type of tissue involved. Thus, osteoma (ICD-10: D16.X) is a benign tumor of bone, and osteosarcoma (ICD-10: C41.X) is a malignant tumor of bone.

Cancers of the Blood and Lymph

Cancers of blood and lymph include leukemias, Hodgkin disease, and non-Hodgkin lymphoma.

Leukemias arise from the body's blood-forming tissues within the bone marrow. The abnormal tissue proliferates, crowding out normal blood-forming cells and causing anemia, infections, and hemorrhage. Leukemias are further subdivided into chronic and acute forms. The chronic leukemias include chronic myelocytic leukemia (CML; ICD-10: 92.1X), chronic lymphocytic leukemia (CLL; ICD-10: C91.1X), and hairy cell leukemia (ICD-10: C91.4X). Survival rate for individuals with chronic leukemias is much higher than the rate for acute leukemias. The acute leukemias include acute myeloblastic leukemia (AML; ICD-10: C92.0X) and acute lymphocytic leukemia (ALL; ICD-10: C91.1X). If untreated, the acute leukemias can cause death in just weeks or months. Hodgkin disease or lymphoma is a cancer of the lymphatic system and is characterized by an unusual giant cell, the **Reed-Sternberg cell.** The disease greatly weakens the body's immune system and is evidenced by painless enlargement of lymph nodes or spleen.

Non-Hodgkin lymphomas, also known as *malignant lymphomas,* are more common than Hodgkin disease and are increasing in incidence, especially in clients with autoimmune disorders. They, too, are characterized by painless lymph node swelling. The many different types of non-Hodgkin lymphoma are often divided into two categories—those that are aggressive and fast growing and those that are slow-growing and indolent.

SIGNS AND SYMPTOMS OF CANCER

The symptoms are varied and will depend upon the kind of cancer; however, there are some basic guidelines that can be helpful to all individuals. Remember that your clients are likely the first ones to suspect a cancer. The basic symptoms follow, but keep in mind that these symptoms do not always indicate cancer:

- Unexplained weight loss of 10 pounds or more is often seen in cancers of the pancreas, stomach, esophagus, and lung.
- Fatigue that does not get better with rest can be a symptom of leukemia, cancers that cause blood loss, or any cancer that grows.
- Pain can be found in bone or testicular cancer. Serious headaches that do not go away with treatment might be a symptom of a brain tumor. Back pain may suggest colon, rectum, or ovary cancers. Metastasized cancers are more likely to exhibit pain also.
- Changes in the skin may be a sign of cancer. They include darker than normal skin pigmentation, jaundice or yellow skin and eyes, reddened skin

or erythema, itching or pruritus, and excessive hair growth.

- Change in bowel or bladder habits or blood in the stool or urine should be reported to a physician, as it might be a sign of bowel or bladder cancer.
- Sores that do not heal, scabs that flake off but then the sore returns.
- White patches inside the mouth or on the tongue may be a sign of **leukoplakia,** a precancerous area that's caused by frequent irritation. It's often caused by smoking or other tobacco use.
- Unusual bleeding or discharge. This might be coughing up blood, blood in the stool, abnormal vaginal bleeding, blood in the urine, or a bloody discharge from the nipple.
- Thickening or lump in the breast or other parts of the body such as the testicles, lymph nodes, or soft tissues of the body.
- Indigestion or trouble swallowing may be a sign of cancer of the throat, esophagus, or stomach.
- Recent change in a wart or mole or any new skin change, especially in size, shape, or color should be investigated.
- Nagging cough or hoarseness can be a sign of throat or larynx cancer.

CHAPTER EPISODE—PART III

Judd had an orchiectomy (removal of the testes), followed by "heavy-duty" chemotherapy. The treatment takes about 5 months out of Judd's life, causing serious side effects—neutropenia, loss of hair and sense of taste, and chemo fog. During this time, he made a "bucket list."

- What is a "bucket list"? Why did Judd make the list?
- What are Judd's chances of survival?

DIAGNOSTIC PROCEDURES FOR CANCER

Responsibility for early detection lies partly with the individual who knows his or her body, understands warning signs of cancer, and promptly seeks medical attention. Any delay in the diagnosis and treatment of cancer can significantly alter the disease course.

Any suspicion of a neoplasm or cancer should include a thorough medical history and a physical examination. Specific tests for early detection include blood chemistry analysis, ultrasonography, radiography, endoscopy, nuclear medicine scans, isotope scanning, computed tomography (CT) scanning, and magnetic resonance imaging (MRI). The single most helpful tool is probably the biopsy. Tissue samples can be taken for biopsy through curettage, fluid aspiration, fine-needle aspiration biopsy, dermal punch, endoscopy, and surgical excision.

Tumor markers are substances that can be found in abnormal amounts in the blood, urine, or tissues of some individuals with cancer. Tumor markers are also used to help diagnose cancer, predict an individual's response to certain therapies, check the response to treatment, or determine if cancer has returned. Generally, tumor markers are not used alone to diagnose cancer but are combined with other tests.

A tumor marker called carcinoembryonic antigen (CEA) may alert practitioners to malignancies of the colon, stomach, pancreas, lungs, and breasts. CEA most likely serves as a baseline during chemotherapy to determine tumor spread, to regulate drug dosage, to detect cancer recurrence, and to prognosticate after surgery or radiation. The prostate-specific antigen (PSA) tumor marker is probably the most widely used to detect and monitor prostatic cancer in a manner similar to the CEA. While tumor markers can be helpful in diagnosis, they are not the final prediction of cancer.

To help in the diagnosis of some cancers in women, a Papanicolaou test (or Pap) and a biopsy may be performed. This test was developed by Dr. George N. Papanicolaou (1883–1962) to detect cancer, commonly of the uterus and cervix. It is a simple test using an exfoliative cytology staining procedure, and it can be performed on any body excretion, such as urine and feces; any secretion, such as sputum, prostatic fluid, and vaginal fluid; or tissue scrapings, such as from the uterus or the stomach. The specimen sample is placed on a slide, stained, and studied under the microscope for abnormal cells. The Pap test is highly effective in detecting early cancer of the cervix or the uterus and HPV. For a person at average risk who has had two negative Pap tests 1 year apart, the ACS recommends subsequent Pap tests every 3 years until age 65.

Grading and Staging Cancer

Part of the diagnosis is the grading and staging of cancer. Pathologists grade cancers by studying the microscopic appearance of suspected tumor cells obtained through biopsy to determine their degree of **anaplasia.**

Grading helps in the diagnosis and in treatment planning, provides a possible prognosis, and allows for comparison of treatment results between different treatments. Usually, four grades are used:

- Grade 1: Tumor cells are well differentiated, closely resembling normal parent tissue.
- Grade 2: Tumor cells are intermediate in appearance, moderately or poorly differentiated.

- Grade 3: Tumor cells are very abnormal and poorly differentiated.
- Grade 4: Tumor cells are so anaplastic that recognition of the tumor's tissue origin is difficult.

Grading also is used when evaluating cells from body fluids in preventive screening tests, such as those found in the Pap smears of the uterine cervix.

Staging neoplasms involves estimating the extent to which a tumor has spread. Several types of staging methods are used. As with grading, staging is important in determining a proper course of treatment. The TNM classification stages tumors according to three basic criteria: *T* refers to the size and extent of the primary *tumor*, *N* refers to the number of area lymph *nodes* involved, and *M* refers to any *metastasis* of the primary tumor. The grading and staging system is specific and more greatly detailed according to the site of the disease.

Tumor (T):

- T0: No evidence of tumor
- Tis: Carcinoma in situ (limited to surface cells)
- T1–T4: Increasing tumor size and involvement

Node (N):

- N0: No lymph node involvement
- N1–N4: Increasing degree of lymph node involvement
- NX: Lymph node involvement cannot be assessed

Metastases (M):

- M0: No evidence of distant metastases
- M1: Evidence of distance metastases

A numerical system is also used to identify the extent of cancer disease:

Stage 0: Cancer in situ
Stage I: Cancer limited to primary site; evidence of cancer growth
Stage II: Unlimited local spread of cancerous cells but still inside primary site
Stage III: Extensive local and regional spread of cancerous cells
Stage IV: Distant metastasis

TREATMENT OF CANCER

In treating cancer, much depends on the stage of the cancer at the time it is diagnosed. A localized cancer is one in which the cancer cells have not yet spread from the site of the original tumor. In the regional stage, the cancer has spread to sites within the same region of the body. The cancer is said to be in the distant stage when cancerous cells have entered the bloodstream and have been carried to other sites in the body (metastasis). Successful treatment is more likely with localized tumors and least likely in the distant stage.

REALITY EPISODE

Rachael felt fine. If she had any complaint, it was that she felt a little tired, and she was in the midst of her second cold of the season. Routine blood work during her annual physical examination indicated problems with her white blood cell count. Further testing revealed that she had acute myeloid leukemia. All Rachael heard from the doctor's discussion with the family was that the only hope was a remission, and with a remission, she might have 2 years to live. Without treatment, she had only weeks. She chose treatment. Death came 6 months later. The 6 months of treatment were brutal. She had many bouts of nausea and vomiting, she needed to eat but did not want to because nothing tasted right, and she received 40 units of blood. She lost 50 pounds, all her hair, and her capacity to function normally.

Discuss Rachael's choices. What might you choose given the same options?

Treatment of cancer is continually changing as new technology develops. The treatment may offer symptomatic relief, be used in conjunction with some primary course of treatment, and perhaps cure the cancer. The major types of treatment against cancer are surgery, chemotherapy, radiation therapy, immunotherapy or biotherapy, hormonal therapy, and stem cell and bone marrow transplants. The primary care provider or specialist may recommend one or any combination of these treatments to combat a particular form of cancer.

Surgery

Surgery now is more precise because of improved diagnostic equipment and operating procedures and advances in preoperative and postoperative care. Surgery for cancer may be specific or curative, **palliative,** or preventive.

Specific or curative surgery is done to remove all of the cancerous tissue in the hopes of curing the person. The types of cancers that respond well to this type of surgery are those of the lung, skin, stomach, large intestine, and breast. Debulking surgery is done to remove as much of a tumor as possible without destroying an organ or tissues close by. This surgery is commonly used in advanced ovarian cancer.

Palliative surgery is done to sustain the individual with cancer or to alleviate the pain that directly or indirectly results from the cancer. Examples include treating complications of cancer, such as abscesses, intestinal perforation, and bleeding, or removing intestinal obstructions. Reconstructive surgery may also be used, especially in breast, skin, head, and neck cancers. In advanced cancers, palliative surgery may be done to sever nerves to alleviate pain.

Preventive surgery may be done to prevent the development of cancer. For example, polyps of the colon may be removed when they are thought to be precancerous. Women with a family history of breast cancer and the breast cancer gene BCRA1 or BCRA2 may choose prophylactic mastectomy prior to being diagnosed with cancer.

Types of surgery include excisional, or **en bloc,** which is removal of the primary tumor, lymph nodes, adjacent involved structure, and surrounding tissues. En bloc surgery is done during a radical mastectomy, colectomy, or gastrectomy.

Electrocautery is the burning of cancer tissue with electric current. This is the preferred method of treating cancers of the rectum. Laser surgery uses a powerful light source to cut through tissue or to vaporize cancers of the cervix, larynx, liver, rectum, or skin. Cryosurgery uses liquid nitrogen to freeze and kill cancer cells. This procedure is sometimes used in precancerous situations or in early stages of skin cancer. It is being researched for use in treatment of other cancers too. Mohs, or microscopically controlled surgery, shaves off skin one layer at a time until all the cells in a layer of skin removed look normal under the microscope. In other words, the skin cancer is removed one layer at a time.

Chemotherapy

Over 50 chemotherapy drugs may be used alone or in combination with other cancer treatments. Chemical agents are used to stop the growth of cancer cells. Chemotherapy is especially effective against cancers that spread, such as leukemias, some solid cancers, and Hodgkin disease. The goals of chemotherapy are to cure, to control, or to serve as a palliative agent. About half of all persons with cancer receive chemotherapy treatment. Many of the chemotherapeutic drugs are experimental and can be used only by oncologists. Chemotherapeutic drugs of similar action generally are grouped together.

Most of these drugs are toxic and have side effects on the gastrointestinal tract, skin, and bone marrow. The most common side effects of chemotherapy include nausea, vomiting, anorexia, anemia, **leukopenia** (an abnormal decrease in white blood cells), "chemo brain" or "chemo fog" (confusion, disorientation, memory issues), and loss of hair. The person receiving chemotherapy is monitored closely with laboratory testing and physical examination to evaluate the efficacy of the treatment and to detect potentially serious side effects.

Radiation Therapy

Radiation may be used alone or in combination with other forms of cancer treatment. Similar to chemotherapy, more than half of all persons with cancer receive some type of radiation therapy. Radiation may be used to cure, to control the disease, or to prevent malignant leukemias from infiltrating the brain or spinal cord. There are different types of radiation and different ways to deliver it. The radiation may be applied externally or internally. In the external mode, an x-ray machine or a radioactive form of an element called a **radioisotope** may be used. In the internal mode, a radioisotope is placed into catheters, beads, seeds, ribbons, or needles and implanted inside the body. Systemic radiation therapy uses radioactive materials that can be taken by mouth or injection. This process is sometimes used to treat thyroid and adult non-Hodgkin lymphoma. Radiation therapy can be received before, during, or after surgery, depending upon the cancer type.

The goal of radiation therapy is to destroy as much of the tumor as possible without affecting surrounding healthy tissue. Unfortunately, some cancers are situated where radiation would cause serious harm to surrounding tissues. Moreover, some cancers are *radioresistant,* meaning they are not affected by radiation within the safe dosage range.

The effects of radiation on the body include cell death, because ionizing radiation disrupts DNA and interferes with cell replication and growth. Recovery from radiation damage to normal tissue does occur between doses, but the degree varies depending on the radiosensitivity of the normal tissue. The radiation dose is determined by the size, type, and location of the tumor.

The side effects of radiation generally occur in the skin, mucous membranes, and bone marrow. Hair may begin to fall out; **erythema,** or redness of the skin, may develop; and eating may be difficult because of the nausea, vomiting, and mucosal damage to the mouth and stomach. These distressing side effects generally subside, either between radiation treatments or after the therapy is complete. Late effects of radiation therapy may be more severe and chronic, especially when combined with other treatment modalities. New developments in cancer radiology are continually appearing for both curative and palliative purposes.

Immunotherapy (Biotherapy)

A treatment that is often used in combination with radiation and chemotherapy is immunotherapy or biotherapy, or biological treatment of tumors. Immunotherapy stimulates or restores and strengthens the body's own immune system, allowing it to recognize, attack, and hopefully kill cancer cells. Immunotherapy is most effective in the early stages of cancer. The use of interferon, a naturally occurring body protein capable of killing cancer cells or stopping their growth in high-risk melanomas, has been useful. Immunotherapy also is approved for treatment of leukemias, lymphomas, and cancers of the kidney, prostate, breast, cervix, ovaries, rectum, colon, and lung.

Hormonal Therapy

Hormonal therapy is treatment that adds, blocks, or removes hormones. It is based on research showing that some hormones affect the growth of certain cancers. Surgical removal of glands that produce the hormones may be necessary, or administration of synthetic hormones may be able to block the body's natural hormones. In women, estrogen promotes the growth of about two-thirds of breast cancers, according to the ACS. Hence, hormonal therapy is aimed at blocking the effects of or lowering the estrogen levels in the treatment of breast cancer. After breast surgery, drugs such as tamoxifen or toremifene may be prescribed for 5 years. In metastatic prostate cancer, hormonal deprivation therapy is the main treatment, especially in men with less advanced prostate cancer. More and more drugs for hormonal therapy are available for use in the treatment of prostate cancer. Whether to consider hormonal therapy requires an assessment of the client's needs, including the stage and extent of the cancer, as well as the side effects and cost of the treatment.

Stem Cell and Bone Marrow Transplants

Bone marrow transplantation (BMT) has proven effective in restoring hematologic and immunologic properties in people with some cancers, such as Hodgkin disease and multiple myeloma. Other transplantations used include peripheral blood stem cell transplantation and cord blood transplantation. Healthy cell transplants are harvested from the individual client (**autologous**), from an identical twin (**syngeneic**), from a sibling or parent, or from an unrelated person (**allogeneic**). These cells are then transplanted into the recipient much like a blood transfusion.

The goal of transplantation therapy is to restore stem cells destroyed by high doses of chemotherapy or radiation. The transplanted cells travel to the bone marrow where they begin to produce new blood cells that ultimately replace the cancer cells. A problem may arise if the donor cells identify cells in the recipient's body as foreign and attack them. This can damage such organs as the skin, liver, and intestines. To prevent this kind of reaction, recipients are often given medications to suppress their immune system.

Measles Vaccine for Cancer Treatment

Research is currently under way investigating the use of the measles vaccine to treat cancers of the blood. The Mayo Clinic injected a patient, who had run out of all options for her cancer treatment, with enough measles vaccine to inoculate 10 million people. Her metastasized cancer went into complete remission.

Exploring Nanotechnology

Nanotechnology has the potential to become a new method of diagnosis and treatment of cancer. Nanodevices are from 100 to 10,000 times smaller than human cells. This size permits them to enter most cells and move out of blood vessels that circulate through the body. These nanodevices can provide quick detection of cancer-related molecules residing in a small percentage of cells for quick diagnosis. Treatment using nanotechnology has the potential for targeting malignant cells with chemotherapeutic agents or therapeutic genes without destroying surrounding healthy cells.

The NCI's Alliance for Nanotechnology in Cancer is researching technologies for:

- Imaging techniques to detect cancer in the earliest stages
- Providing data on real-time success or failure of treatment
- Using multifunctional nanodevices to bypass biological barriers in their delivery of therapeutic agents to cancer cells and tissues
- Assessing agents that can prevent precancerous cells from becoming malignant
- Seeking less invasive methods to treat cancer symptoms
- Researching methods to quickly identify precancerous cells and predict drug resistance

Researchers had known for some time that mass doses of intravenous viral therapy can kill cancer in mice, but this was the first time the therapy was used on a human. Time and continued research will determine the lasting effects of such a revolutionary approach to cancer treatment.

CHAPTER EPISODE—PART IV

Judd survived. He is alive and doing well nearly 4 years later. He was able to check off at least one event on his "bucket list"—to go into a boxing ring to spar with a professional. With the help of friends, and the willingness of a professional boxer, a match was organized to help raise awareness of the cancer center that had been so supportive and helpful in Judd's recovery. And Judd realized one of his goals.

- What did the bucket list do for Judd?
- What does Judd's action after his treatment tell you about his overall approach to cancer? Is this healthy? Justify your response.

Integrative and Complementary Therapy

Most individuals diagnosed with cancer have considered or participated in some form of complementary medicine therapy, and they spend billions of dollars per year, mostly out-of-pocket, for integrative and complementary medical treatment. In some circles, the debate rages on, with traditional therapies on one side and complementary on another. However, the two are increasingly being blended in cancer treatment. Refer to Chapter 2 for a more detailed discussion of these types of therapies.

Increased benefit may be achieved if persons with cancer carefully consider both traditional or conventional treatments and complementary treatment therapies. Many choose to embrace both simultaneously and will want to seek practitioners who are willing and able to offer both or to work cooperatively in an integrative way with the client's wishes in mind.

Integrative practitioners recognize all the major forms of conventional cancer treatment and understand the wisdom of each. Integrative oncology moves into another arena, however, in that it includes evidence-based therapy that can offer prevention, support, and antineoplastic treatment. Integrative oncology also addresses all levels of a person's being—body, mind, soul, and spirit—within their specific culture and natural world. Generally, there is no debate regarding prevention of cancers; both traditional and integrative practitioners agree on all the main preventive factors. Also, there is little disagreement in the "supportive" aspect for persons with cancer. However, integrative practitioners usually pay closer attention to that treatment area than do traditional practitioners, who often rush to aggressively treat the cancer before it has an opportunity to metastasize.

When chemotherapy and/or radiation is deemed necessary, complementary therapies can, in some cases, reduce many side effects or enhance the effectiveness of chemotherapy and radiation. Proponents of complementary therapies consider that cancer is a manifestation of an unhealthy body whose defenses are so seriously out of balance that they can no longer destroy cells that turn cancerous. The goal of integrative medicine is to strengthen the body's immune system. These therapies may include treatments that rely on biopharmaceutical, immune enhancement, metabolic, nutritional, and herbal nontoxic methods. Of these methods, mind–body techniques such as yoga, tai chi, meditation, and prayer or some form of spirituality have shown evidence of benefit to those with cancer. Also, eating a macrobiotic diet (mostly vegetables and whole grains), drinking green tea, and using more soy products in the diet appear to assist in enabling the body to destroy cancer cells. Also, acupuncture can reduce cancer-related pain. See Table 5.1 for a listing of complementary therapies that may help to reduce symptoms persons with cancer often experience.

Cancer is very complex and can be life-threatening. It requires professional medical care. Some complementary remedies may actually make cancer worse if not used properly, just as conventional methods can be so toxic that a person succumbs to the treatment rather than to the disease itself. Any complementary therapies should become a part of a total cancer treatment program that is guided and monitored by a qualified practitioner experienced in integrative medicine and treatment.

PREVENTING CANCER

There are numerous reports related to preventing cancer. Often the reports are conflicting. However, the following seven steps are consistent in nearly all prevention measures. This list is a compilation of information from the Mayo Clinic and ACS:

1. Do not use tobacco. Smoking cigarettes, cigars, pipes, chewing tobacco, inhaling chewing tobacco or snuff, and inhaling secondhand smoke puts you at risk for a number of different cancers.
2. Practice sun safety. Sun exposure is the most common cause of skin cancer. Avoid ultraviolet rays during the peak hours of 10:00 a.m. to 4:00 p.m., stay in the shade as much as possible, and wear sunscreen or protective clothing and a wide-brimmed hat. Stay out of tanning salons.
3. Eat a healthy diet. A diet that includes vegetables, fruits, whole grains, and legumes and that limits fat intake helps to reduce cancer risk. Drink alcohol only in moderation, if at all.
4. Exercise regularly and maintain a healthy weight. Exercise is helpful in prevention of obesity and may also lower risks of breast, colon, prostate, and uterine cancers.

Table 5.1	Complementary Therapy Used to Reduce Symptoms of Cancer Treatment	
COMPLEMENTARY THERAPY	**REDUCE SYMPTOMS**
Acupuncture, hypnosis, music therapy, aromatherapy	Nausea and vomiting
Acupuncture, hypnosis, music therapy, aromatherapy, meditation, prayer, massage, biofeedback	Pain and discomfort
Exercise, massage, relaxation, yoga	Fatigue and exhaustion
Aromatherapy, exercise, hypnosis, massage, yoga, tai chi, meditation, prayer	Worry and stress
Hypnosis, massage, meditation, prayer, relaxation	Anxiety
Exercise, relaxation, tai chi, yoga	Sleep disturbances

5. Get vaccinated. Certain cancers that are related to viruses can be prevented with vaccination. These include hepatitis A and B and HPV. There may be a vaccine for hepatitis C within the next few years.

6. Avoid risky practices. HPV, HIV, and hepatitis B and C can be passed through sexual contact and by sharing contaminated needles (for HIV and hepatitis B and C). Practice safer sex, never share needles, and seek treatment for substance abuse.

7. Practice self-examination and screening. Discovering cancer early saves lives. Be aware of any body changes. Regular screening should be done for the skin, mouth, colon, rectum, prostate, testes, breast, and cervix.

The ACS, NCI, and the U.S. Department of Health and Human Services recommend a mammogram every 1 to 2 years for women older than age 40. A sonogram is recommended if suspicious or abnormal results are found. Also, the Papanicolaou test should be performed on women (3 years after becoming sexually active or by age 21) at regular intervals—every 3 years for women ages 21 to 65. Men should be regularly checked for prostate cancer. This check includes a yearly digital examination for men older than 40, a blood test to detect PSA in men showing any symptoms, and ultrasonography if abnormal results are found. A rectal examination should be part of every medical checkup for men and women, and stool samples should be examined for blood, which may be an indication of colon cancer.

SUMMARY

Cancer is a life-threatening, sometimes preventable disease that can strike any person at any age. It can strike with or without warning and has been a recognized disease for more than 100 years. Prevention is the best line of defense. Early detection, diagnosis, and prompt treatment form the best course of action. If the spread is not controlled or checked, cancer can result in death; however, many cancers can be cured if detected and treated promptly. Integrative medicine may offer the best solution to enhance cancer treatment.

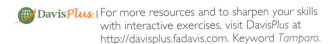 | For more resources and to sharpen your skills with interactive exercises, visit DavisPlus at http://davisplus.fadavis.com. Keyword *Tamparo*.

ONLINE RESOURCES

American Cancer Society
http://www.cancer.org/
http://www.cancer.org/cancer/cancerbasics/signs-and-symptoms-of-cancer

Cancer Facts and Figures
http://www.cancer.org/acs/groups/content/@research/documents/webcontent/acspc-042151.pdf

National Cancer Institute
http://www.cancer.gov

Measles Vaccine for Cancer Treatment
http://www.mayoclinic.org/medical-professionals/clinical-updates/neurosciences/update-measles-virus-novel-therapy-glioblastoma

U.S. Department of Health and Human Services
http://www.hhs.gov

CASE STUDIES

Case Study 1

Kai Simpson has surfed since he was a young teenager and up through his young adulthood years off the coast of Maui, where he was born and raised. Every time the surf was up and the sun was out, he was on his board. Twenty years later, he is diagnosed with malignant melanoma.

Case Study Questions

1. What protective measures might Kai have taken as a young surfer?
2. Identify possible treatment measures that might be taken.

Case Study 2

Juan was only 55 when he learned he had cancer. He was shocked. He saw his doctor for what he thought was a pulled muscle in his side, a nagging cough, and feeling tired all the time. A chest x-ray showed a mass in his lung. He had a CT scan at the nearest hospital and got sicker as he waited 10 days for the results. The results indicated the need for an oncologist—another wait of nearly 45 days. Juan's daughter went on the Internet to find a place where he might get treatment earlier.

A call was made to a cancer treatment center about 1,100 miles away. They asked for his records, called back in 24 hours, and made an appointment. The results were staggering. He had stage IV cancer with tumors in one of his kidneys, a lung, liver, and several lymph nodes.

Juan had a radical nephrectomy with removal of surrounding lymph nodes and the adrenal gland. This was followed by aggressive biotherapy for about 8 weeks. Today Juan has passed his 10-year mark cancer free.

Case Study Questions

1. Is Juan's experience waiting for treatment common? Why or why not?
2. What issues might Juan face having only one kidney and no adrenal gland? Search the Internet for your response.

REVIEW QUESTIONS

Matching

Match the terms below to their correct statements.

a. Carcinogens

b. Sarcomas

c. Mohs

d. Tis

e. Grading cancers

f. Debulking

g. Palliative

h. NX

i. Staging cancers

j. Chemotherapy

k. Radiation

l. Stage IV

1. _____ Substances that can increase the risk of cancer development

2. _____ Estimates the extent to which a tumor has spread

3. _____ Removes much of tumor without destroying nearby tissues

4. _____ Arise from supportive and connective tissue

5. _____ Removes skin cancer one layer at a time

6. _____ Carcinoma in situ

7. _____ Indicates distant metastasis

Short Answer

1. _____ is a new formation that serves no useful purpose; it is uncontrollable and progressive.

2. _____ is a new formation that may grow slowly and remains localized.

3. _____ is a new formation that is invasive, grows rather rapidly, is anaplastic, and is capable of metastasis.

4. Cancer of the _____ is the leading cause of cancer death in both men and women.

5. _____ is the most commonly diagnosed cancer in women.

Multiple Choice

Place a check next to the correct answer.

1. Which of the following is the single most helpful diagnostic tool of neoplasms?

_____ a. Breast self-examination

_____ b. Testicular self-examination

_____ c. Pap test

_____ d. Biopsy by needle aspiration, endoscopy, or surgical incision

2. Which of the following is treatment for cancers of leukemias, lymphomas, and some other tumors?

_____ a. Radiation

_____ b. Chemotherapy

_____ c. Immunotherapy/biotherapy

_____ d. Hormonal therapy

3. Where have stem cell and bone marrow transplants been most effective in treatment?

_____ a. High-risk melanomas

_____ b. Hodgkin disease and multiple myeloma

_____ c. Bone cancers

_____ d. Prostate cancers

4. What are the substances in the blood, urine, and tissues of individuals with cancer that are used in diagnosis and prediction of certain therapies?

_____ a. Genetic factors of the cancer

_____ b. Tumor markers of the cancer

_____ c. Viruses that can cause cancer

_____ d. Bacteria that can cause cancer

5. Can you name the surgery for cancer that is done to sustain an individual or alleviate pain?

_____ a. Palliative

_____ b. Curative

_____ c. Preventative

_____ d. En bloc

Discussion Questions/Personal Reflection

1. Discuss the reasons to include an integrated medicine approach to cancer treatment.

_____

_____

_____

_____

_____

_____

_____

_____

_____

2. Consider how you might personally prevent cancer in your life. Consider your family history and lifestyle.

_____

_____

_____

_____

_____

_____

_____

_____

_____

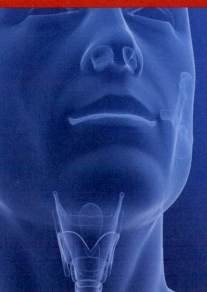

The last of the human freedoms is to choose one's attitudes.
—VIKTOR E. FRANKL

6

Congenital Diseases and Disorders

● *chapter outline*

DESCRIPTION

CARDIOVASCULAR SYSTEM DISEASES AND DISORDERS

Congenital Heart Defects

CIRCULATORY SYSTEM DISEASES AND DISORDERS

Sickle Cell Anemia

NERVOUS SYSTEM DISEASES AND DISORDERS

Neural Tube Defects: Spina Bifida, Meningocele, and Myelomeningocele

Hydrocephalus

Cerebral Palsy

DIGESTIVE SYSTEM DISEASES AND DISORDERS

Cleft Lip and Palate (Orofacial Clefts)

Tracheoesophageal Fistula and Esophageal Atresia

Pyloric Stenosis

Malrotation With Volvulus

Hirschsprung Disease (Congenital Aganglionic Megacolon)

Omphalocele

GENITOURINARY SYSTEM DISEASES AND DISORDERS

Undescended Testes (Cryptorchidism)

Congenital Defects of the Ureter, Bladder, and Urethra

MUSCULOSKELETAL SYSTEM DISEASES AND DISORDERS

Clubfoot (Talipes)

Congenital Hip Dysplasia

Duchenne Muscular Dystrophy

METABOLIC ERRORS

Cystic Fibrosis

Phenylketonuria

SYNDROMES

Down Syndrome (Trisomy 21)

Fetal Alcohol Syndrome

Tourette Syndrome

SUMMARY

ONLINE RESOURCES

CASE STUDIES

REVIEW QUESTIONS

key words

Acetabulum (ăs"ĕ•tăb'ū•lŭm)
Alveoli (ăl•vē'ō•lī)
Anastomosis (ă•năs"tō•mō'sĭs)
Anoxia (ăn•ŏk'sē•ă)
Arrhythmias (ă•rĭth'mē•ăz)
Atelectasis (ăt"ĕ•lĕk'tă•sĭs)
Auscultation (aws"kŭl•tā'shŭn)
Bronchioles (brong'kē•ŏlz)
Cardiomegaly
　(kăr"dē•ō•mĕg'ă•lē)
Chiari malformation
　(kē•ăr'ē măl•for•mā'shŭn)
Chyme (kīm)
Claudication (klaw•dĭ•kā'shŭn)
Cyanosis (sī•ăn•o'sĭs)
Ductus arteriosus
　(dŭk'tŭs ăr•tē"rē•o'sĭs)

Dystonia (dĭs•tō'nē•ă)
Epigastrium (ĕp'ĭ•găs'trē•ŭm)
Epistaxis (ĕp"ĭ•stăk'sĭs)
Excoriated (ĕk•skŏr'ē•āt•ĕd)
Fontanel (fŏn•tă•nĕl')
Ganglion (găng'lē•ŏn)
Hematuria (hē'mă•tū'rē•ă)
Hydronephrosis
　(hī"drō•nĕf•rō'sĭs)
Hydroureter (hī"drō•ū•rē'tĕr)
Hypertrophy (hī•pĕr'trŏ•fē)
Lumen (lū'mĕn)
Meconium (mĭ–kō'nē•ĕm)
Meninges (mĕn•ĕn'jēz)
Microcephaly (mī"krō•sĕf'ă•lē)

Nephrectomy (nĕf•rĕk'tō•mē)
Nevus (nē'vŭs)
Nystagmus (nĭs•tăg'mŭs)
Parasympathetic
　(păr"ă•sĭm"pă•thĕt'ĭk)
Peristalsis (pĕr•ĭ•stăl'sĭs)
Pylorus (pī•lŏr'ŭs)
Reflux (rē'flŭks)
Resection (rē•sĕk'shŭn)
Septum (sĕp'tŭm)
Tachycardia (tăk"ē•kăr'dē•ă)
Tachypnea (tăk•ĭp'nē•ă)
Teratogen (tĕr•ăt'ō•jĭn)
Toxemia (tŏk•sē'mē•ă)

learning outcomes

Upon successful completion of this chapter, you will be able to:

- Define key terms.
- Describe the two main causes for congenital abnormalities.
- Summarize the most common teratogens that contribute to birth defects.
- Compare and contrast the various congenital defects of the heart.
- List and describe the four defects of tetralogy of Fallot.
- Discuss prevention of congenital heart defects.
- Describe sickle cell anemia signs and symptoms.
- Identify the signs and symptoms of spina bifida, meningocele, and myelomeningocele.
- Recall the diagnostic procedures used for hydrocephalus.
- Describe the three types of cerebral palsy and their etiology.
- Compare and contrast the two main types of orofacial clefts and feeding techniques.
- Discuss tracheoesophageal fistula and esophageal atresia.

- Identify the etiology of pyloric stenosis and its classic symptom.
- Discuss symptoms of malrotation with volvulus.
- Discuss Hirschsprung disease.
- Recall the treatment for omphalocele.
- Define cryptorchidism and its diagnosis.
- Compare and contrast the congenital defects of the ureter, bladder, and urethra.
- List the four common forms of clubfoot.
- Recall the etiology of congenital hip dysplasia.
- Restate the diagnostic procedures for Duchenne muscular dystrophy.
- Describe the possible complications of cystic fibrosis.
- Restate the diagnostic procedures for phenylketonuria.
- Discuss the prognosis of Down syndrome.
- List possible signs and symptoms of fetal alcohol syndrome.
- Discuss complementary therapy for Tourette syndrome.

CHAPTER EPISODE—PART I

Hank and Melanie were expecting their first child. Everything was progressing normally and they were delighted when ultrasound showed they would have a son. Immediately they picked his name—Josh. The months flew by, the nursery was ready, and when labor began, they had no fears. In the hospital, Melanie struggled for 12 hours in labor before Josh was born close to 2:00 a.m. Both Hank and Melanie were elated to hear their son's first cry, to see him as the nurse handed him to Melanie. But quickly little Josh was taken to the other side of the room to be cleaned. They heard the nurse and obstetrician whispering. One of the nurses asked for the name of their pediatrician and then said they would take Josh to be weighed and checked. Hank and Melanie were a little concerned; they thought they would be able to hold him longer. Melanie was prepared and taken to her room. Hank was right beside her. The wait began for the staff to bring little Josh to them.

- Does this action on the part of the medical staff seem normal? Why or why not?

DESCRIPTION

Chapter 1 provided a basic description of genetic factors relating to the body's disease processes. Here, the term *congenital disease* refers to problems that are present at birth even if they do not exhibit until sometime later. Abnormalities can occur in any major organ or part of the body. Major abnormalities affect the way a person looks and generally require medical and/or surgical treatment. Minor abnormalities do not cause serious health or social problems. Congenital abnormalities or birth defects may have genetic causes, may be caused by exposure to some agent or **teratogen** during pregnancy that causes malformation, or may result from a combination of the two.

The most common teratogens are infectious diseases, physical agents such as radiation, drugs and chemicals, and maternal issues such as diabetes. Congenital defects usually occur during the first 3 months of pregnancy, many in the first 3 to 4 weeks of pregnancy before a woman suspects she is pregnant. Multiple birth defects that have a similar cause are known as a *syndrome*. An example is Down syndrome. Multiple birth defects that have no similar cause are called *associations*. Some abnormalities may be detected at birth; others are not apparent until later in infancy or childhood.

The Centers for Disease Control and Prevention (CDC) reports that 1 out of every 33 babies born has a birth defect. There are more than 3,000 possible abnormalities, including 21 that are considered major. All congenital abnormalities, however, require the attention of primary care providers (PCPs) and involve the entire family. Children with congenital abnormalities may require more medical care, more frequent hospitalizations, and increased educational services than children with no abnormalities.

The most common congenital abnormalities affect the cardiovascular system, followed by neural tube defects, and are identified first in this chapter.

Cardiovascular System Diseases and Disorders

CONGENITAL HEART DEFECTS

Description

Congenital heart defects can be broadly classified according to whether or not poorly oxygenated blood entering from the veins mixes in the heart with the freshly oxygenated blood reentering the systemic circulation. Acyanotic defects are those in which there is no mixing of poorly oxygenated blood with the blood reentering the systemic circulation. Cyanotic defects are those in which poorly oxygenated blood mixes with the blood reentering the systemic circulation.

The American Heart Association provides a fact sheet on congenital heart defects (go to http://www.heart.org). About 40,000 babies in the United States are born with congenital heart defects.

Acyanotic Defects

Acyanotic defects occur when the blood flows from the left side of the heart to the right side of the heart due to a hole in the interventricular septum. Acyanotic defects do not normally interfere with the oxygen or blood reaching the body's tissues. The most common acyanotic defects include the following:

- *Ventricular septal defect* (VSD; ICD-10: Q21.0) is the most commonly occurring congenital heart defect, where there is an abnormal opening between the wall, or **septum,** of the right and left ventricles (Fig. 6.1). The extent of the opening may vary from the size of a pin to a complete absence of the ventricular septum, creating one common ventricle. Blood from the left ventricle flows back into the right ventricle, causing too much blood to be pumped to the lungs. This results in lung congestion. This defect typically accompanies other congenital anomalies, especially Down syndrome, renal defects, or other cardiac defects.
- *Atrial septal defect* (ASD; ICD-10: Q21.1) is an abnormal opening between the right and left atria (see Fig. 6.2). The size and location of the opening determine the severity of the defect. If the hole is

Ventricular Septal Defect (VSD)

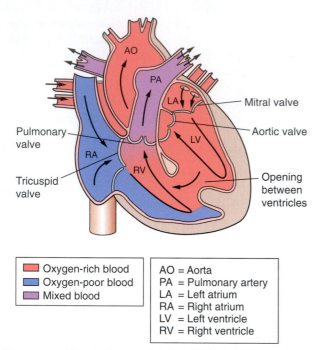

■ Oxygen-rich blood	AO = Aorta
■ Oxygen-poor blood	PA = Pulmonary artery
■ Mixed blood	LA = Left atrium
	RA = Right atrium
	LV = Left ventricle
	RV = Right ventricle

Figure 6.1 Ventricular septal defect (VSD). In VSD, a hole in the ventricular septum occurs, and blood from the left ventricle flows back into the right ventricle, due to higher pressure in the left ventricle. This backflow causes an extra volume of blood to be pumped into the lungs by the right ventricle, creating lung congestion.

Atrial Septal Defect (ASD)

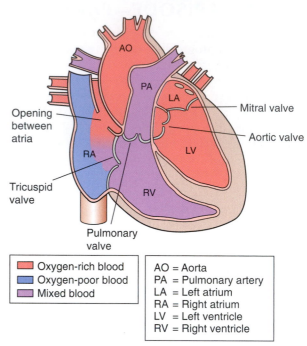

■ Oxygen-rich blood	AO = Aorta
■ Oxygen-poor blood	PA = Pulmonary artery
■ Mixed blood	LA = Left atrium
	RA = Right atrium
	LV = Left ventricle
	RV = Right ventricle

Figure 6.2 Atrial septal defect (ASD). In ASD, there is an abnormal opening between the two atria of the heart, causing an abnormal blood flow through the heart. Some infants have no symptoms and appear healthy. If the ASD is large and permits a large amount of blood to pass through the right side, symptoms will be noted.

large, a fair amount of oxygen-rich blood leaks back to the right atria and is then pumped back into the lungs, which are already rich in oxygen.

- *Coarctation of the aorta* (ICD-10: Q25.1) is a malformation in a portion of the aorta wall that causes narrowing of the aortal opening, or **lumen,** at the point of the defect (Fig. 6.3). Consequently, blood pressure is increased proximal to the defect and decreased distal to it. Congestive heart failure may result.

- *Patent ductus arteriosus* (PDA; ICD-10: Q25.0) is a defect resulting from the failure of the **ductus arteriosus,** a connection between the aorta and the pulmonary artery in the fetus, to close after birth (Fig. 6.4). During the prenatal period, much of the fetal circulation bypasses the lungs through this blood vessel, which connects the pulmonary artery to the aorta. When this fetal structure fails to close after birth, blood from the aorta flows back into the pulmonary artery. This defect is common in premature infants and puts a strain on the heart, causing **tachypnea,** or fast breathing.

Cyanotic Defects

Cyanotic defects cause the oxygen-rich blood and the oxygen-poor blood to mix, allowing less oxygen-rich blood to reach the body tissues. Often a bluish tint

to the skin results. The most common cyanotic defects follow:

- *Tetralogy of Fallot* (ICD-10: Q21.3) is a combination of four congenital heart defects: (1) pulmonary stenosis, a narrowing of the opening into the pulmonary artery from the right ventricle; (2) VSD, an abnormal opening in the septum between the left and right ventricles; (3) dextroposition of the aorta, in which the opening of the aorta bridges the ventricular septum, receiving blood from both the left and right ventricles; and (4) right ventricular **hypertrophy,** an increase in size or volume (Fig. 6.5).

- *Transposition of the great arteries* (TGA; ICD-10: Q20.3) is a condition in which the two major arteries of the heart are reversed, with the aorta arising from the right ventricle and the pulmonary artery from the left ventricle (Fig. 6.6). The result is two noncommunicating circulatory systems—one circulating blood in a closed loop between the heart and lungs and the other between the heart and systemic circulation.

- *Tricuspid atresia* (ICD-10: Q22.9) is a condition in which the valve between the right atrium and the right ventricle fails to develop (Fig. 6.7). This defect may be combined with ASD, VSD, and transposition of the great arteries.

Coarctation of the Aorta

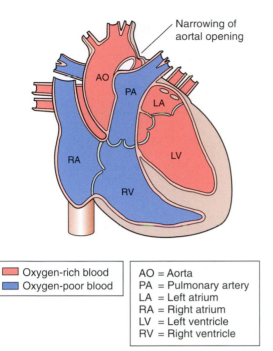

Figure 6.3 Coarctation of the aorta (coarct). In this condition, the aorta is narrowed or constricted, obstructing blood flow to the lower part of the body and increasing blood pressure above the constriction. Usually there are no symptoms at birth, but they can develop as early as the first week of life. If severe symptoms of high blood pressure and congestive heart failure develop, surgery may be considered.

Patent Ductus Arteriosus (PDA)

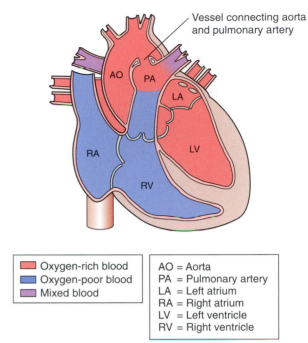

Figure 6.4 Patent ductus arteriosus (PDA). This defect normally occurs during fetal life. PDA short-circuits the normal pulmonary vascular system and allows blood to mix between the pulmonary artery and the aorta. Prior to birth, there is an open passageway between the two blood vessels that closes soon after birth. When it does not close, some blood returns to the lungs. PDA is often seen in premature infants.

Etiology

The etiology of congenital heart defects is mostly unknown, but there may be a genetic link. Predisposing factors may include maternal infections, use of certain drugs during gestation, diabetes, alcoholism, and poor maternal nutrition. In roughly 85% of cases, however, there is no one identifiable cause of a congenital heart defect. The abnormalities are thought to be multifactorial—both genetic and environmental. Clinical features vary with age and seriousness of the defect.

Signs and Symptoms of Acyanotic Defects

- *VSD:* The classic clinical feature is a loud, early systolic murmur heard during **auscultation,** or listening for sounds produced by the internal organs. The typical murmur is described as blowing or rumbling. There may be signs of rapid, heavy breathing; poor feeding; poor weight gain; and sweating.
- *ASD:* There are very few symptoms of ASD. The classic clinical feature is a crescendo-decrescendo type of systolic ejection murmur. A large hole can cause **arrhythmias** and congestive heart failure in middle age.
- *Coarctation of the aorta:* The clinical features vary with age. A murmur may or may not be present. An infant may exhibit dyspnea, pulmonary edema, **tachycardia** (an abnormally rapid heartbeat), and failure to

thrive. Symptoms appearing after adolescence may include dyspnea, **claudication** (lameness), headache, **epistaxis** (nosebleed), and hypertension.
- *PDA:* The clinical feature is a "machinery" murmur usually associated with an abnormal tremor accompanying a cardiac murmur or thrill and often accompanied by a widened pulse pressure. Respiratory distress and cyanosis are common.

Signs and Symptoms of Cyanotic Defects

- *Tetralogy of Fallot:* A bluish discoloration of the skin and mucous membranes, or **cyanosis,** is often evident at birth or within several months of birth and is considered the hallmark of the disorder. The infant may exhibit other signs of poor oxygenation, such as increasing dyspnea on exertion, diminished exercise tolerance, and delayed physical growth and development.
- *Transposition of the great arteries* (TGA): The infant is typically severely cyanotic at birth and has tachypnea. Signs of congestive heart failure and **cardiomegaly** (an increase in the volume of the heart or the size of the heart muscle tissue) follow.
- *Tricuspid atresia:* The extent of VSD and the relationship of the great arteries will determine the symptoms. The neonate will have low oxygen levels and cyanosis. There can also be tachypnea and poor feeding.

Tetralogy of Fallot (TOF or "Tet")

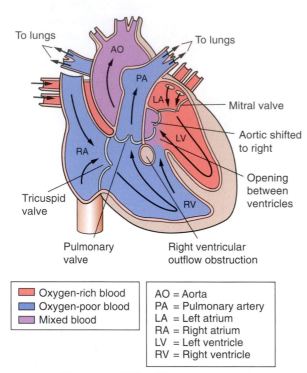

Transposition of Great Arteries

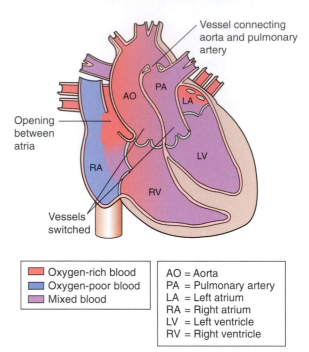

Figure 6.5 Tetralogy of Fallot. This condition is characterized by four defects: (1) An abnormal opening or ventricular septal defect that allows blood to pass from the right ventricle to the left ventricle without going through the lungs. (2) A narrowing or stenosis at or just beneath the pulmonary valve that partially blocks the flow of blood from the right side of the heart to the lungs. (3) The right ventricle is more muscular than normal. (4) The aorta lies directly over the ventricular septal defect. Tetralogy of Fallot results in cyanosis due to lack of oxygen.

Figure 6.6 Transposition of great arteries. With this congenital defect, the positions of the pulmonary artery and the aorta are reversed, thus the aorta originates from the right ventricle, so most of the blood returning to the heart from the body is pumped back out without first going to the lungs, and the pulmonary artery originates from the left ventricle, so that most of the blood returning from the lungs goes back to the lungs again.

Diagnostic Procedures

Signs and symptoms often point to a diagnosis, but a history and physical examination are essential and may be all that are necessary to diagnose some congenital heart abnormalities. Other diagnostic procedures may include an echocardiogram, chest x-rays, an electrocardiogram (ECG), magnetic resonance imaging (MRI), pulse oximetry, and heart catheterization. Laboratory studies may be ordered to determine the degree of cyanosis and to detect possible acidosis.

Treatment

Some congenital heart defects require no treatment because there is spontaneous closure of the defects, or some medications may be effective in closing defects. If surgery is necessary, it usually is done during the first year of life. Surgery may include closing holes in the heart with patches or stitches, repairing or replacing heart valves, or widening arteries or openings to heart valves. When the defect is complex, however, more than one surgical procedure may be required. Some surgical procedures may be delayed until the child is old enough to better withstand the surgery. Heart catheterizations

are also used in treatment. A needle puncture is made in the skin to insert a catheter into a vein or artery to repair some defects. Because this procedure is much easier than surgery on an individual with a birth defect, it is the preferred treatment when possible.

Complementary Therapy

No significant complementary therapy is indicated.

➔ CLIENT COMMUNICATION

Any heart defect is frightening to all involved. Reassurance is important and should include explanations to the parents and caregivers of any procedures to be performed. The March of Dimes has a website that can be a quick reference for parents who are trying to understand what is happening and why: http://www.marchofdimes.com/4439.aspx.

Prognosis

The prognosis is dependent on the type of defect, its location, and its severity. If the defect is small and treatment is successful, the prognosis is quite good. Some defects, however, are so severe as to put the infant's life in immediate danger.

Tricuspid Atresia

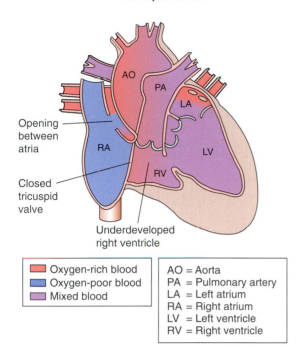

Opening between atria

Closed tricuspid valve

Underdeveloped right ventricle

■ Oxygen-rich blood
■ Oxygen-poor blood
■ Mixed blood

AO = Aorta
PA = Pulmonary artery
LA = Left atrium
RA = Right atrium
LV = Left ventricle
RV = Right ventricle

Figure 6.7 Tricuspid atresia. In tricuspid atresia, there is no tricuspid valve; therefore, no blood flows from the right atrium to the right ventricle. Tricuspid atresia defect is characterized by a small right ventricle, a large left ventricle, diminished pulmonary circulation, and cyanosis. A surgical shunting procedure is often necessary to increase the blood flow to the lungs.

Prevention

The best prevention begins prior to pregnancy and continues through the first trimester. The following steps are recommended:

- Confirm immunity to rubella.
- Take a daily multivitamin that contains folic acid.
- Avoid use of all recreational drugs.
- Avoid viral infections, especially of the upper respiratory tract.

 REALITY EPISODE

Expectant parents were shocked when they learned from their ultrasound at 30 weeks' gestation that their baby had a heart defect—tetralogy of Fallot. Fortunately, they had some time to prepare. They knew there would be a long hospital stay, transfer to a children's hospital 3 hours away, and surgery to correct the defect. They named their unborn child Rachael. Rachael was born just 3 weeks later.

Describe events or circumstances that Rachael's parents might not have expected or anticipated.

- Avoid alcohol.
- Do not take prescription medications, such as lithium or drugs that treat acne and seizures.[1]
- Avoid x-rays, strong chemicals, and solvents.
- Consider genetic counseling if another child or a relative has a congenital heart defect.

Circulatory System Diseases and Disorders

SICKLE CELL ANEMIA

ICD-10:D57.1

Description

Sickle cell anemia is a congenital issue of the circulatory system. It is a hereditary, chronic anemia in which abnormal sickle- or crescent-shaped red blood cells are present. These abnormally shaped red blood cells tend to clump together within capillaries, impairing circulation, damaging blood vessels, and causing chronic organ damage. The incidence of sickle cell anemia is highest among those of African descent and, to a lesser extent, those of Mediterranean or Middle Eastern ancestry and aboriginal tribes in India. It affects millions of people worldwide.

Etiology

The condition is due to the presence of an abnormal form of hemoglobin called *hemoglobin S* within the red cells. The defective hemoglobin is synthesized by individuals inheriting homozygous hemoglobin S genes.

If the individual is heterozygous for the hemoglobin S gene, then he or she possesses the *sickle cell trait*. This is a comparatively benign condition that typically produces no symptoms; however, the red blood cells of such individuals may "sickle" as a consequence of any condition that produces hypoxia. If two individuals with the sickle cell trait have offspring, then their children have a 25% chance of inheriting sickle cell anemia.

Signs and Symptoms

All individuals with sickle cell anemia are anemic. Signs and symptoms characteristic of sickle cell anemia are episodic attacks of intense pain (pain crises) in the arms, legs, or abdomen. The white of the eye, or sclera, is jaundiced. Recurrent bouts of fever, chronic fatigue, dyspnea, tachycardia, cardiac murmurs, and pallor may be additional manifestations of the disease. Infections, stress, and extremes in temperature may trigger the painful crises.

---

[1]*Women with diabetes or seizure difficulties are advised to consult their primary care provider prior to pregnancy to minimize risk to the fetus while maintaining proper management of their health issues.*

Diagnostic Procedures

If parents are known carriers of the sickle cell trait, it is recommended that the infant be screened for the condition. Individuals with the trait exhibit normal hemoglobin levels and normal hematocrit, whereas a person with sickle cell disease has a low hematocrit and sickle cells on smear. A positive family history and a physical examination will confirm the diagnosis. Hemoglobin electrophoresis is the laboratory test of choice; it can be done on an umbilical cord at birth.

Treatment

The goal is to relieve pain and prevent organ damage, infections, and stroke. Treatment of sickle cell anemia is symptomatic and typically involves the prescription of analgesics and the maintenance of adequate hydration. Bone marrow transplantation may be curative, but it is available for only a small number of people because of severe organ damage or lack of an available compatible donor. Hydroxyurea is used with some success but must be administered with careful medical follow-up. Studies are under way in the search for additional medications. Chronic transfusions may be ordered and are useful in decreasing the severity of the disease.

Complementary Therapy

Complementary therapies embraced by individuals with sickle cell disease include spiritual or energy healing, relaxation and imagery, exercise, and diet. Each seems to provide personal benefits not offered in traditional treatments.

 CLIENT COMMUNICATION

Infections must be avoided or treated immediately. Pain is ever present in varying degrees and must be treated while trying to maximize the person's ability to function. Proper hydration is important, too.

Prognosis

The prognosis is highly variable. Sickle cell anemia is a life-threatening disease. Many affected individuals die in childhood; however, because of improvements in the care of sickle cell clients, some live into the middle years. Complications include infections, stroke, renal failure, pulmonary hypertension, leg ulcers, orthopedic disorders, cerebral hemorrhage, shock, and the formation of gallstones in the gallbladder or bile duct, a condition called *cholelithiasis*.

Prevention

There is no prevention for sickle cell anemia other than genetic counseling for those at risk. However, a number of factors can decrease the incidence of pain crises. They include eating a healthy and balanced diet; taking vitamins, including a folic acid supplement; drinking plenty of fluids; avoiding extremes in temperature; and getting moderate exercise and plenty of rest.

Nervous System Diseases and Disorders

NEURAL TUBE DEFECTS: SPINA BIFIDA, MENINGOCELE, AND MYELOMENINGOCELE

Description

The neural tube defects (NTDs) spina bifida (ICD-10: Q05.8), meningocele (ICD-10: Q05.X*), and myelomeningocele (ICD-10 Q05.7) are developmental defects of the first month of pregnancy (Fig. 6.8). They are characterized by incomplete closure of the bones encasing the spinal cord. Spina bifida occulta is the most common and least severe of these defects. It is marked by an incomplete closure of one or more vertebrae, with no protrusion of the spinal cord or the membranes covering the brain and spinal cord, called the **meninges.** In meningocele, the incomplete closure of the vertebra is accompanied by a protrusion of the spinal fluid and meninges into an external sac. Myelomeningocele results when the external sac contains meninges, cerebrospinal fluid, and a portion of the spinal cord or its nerve roots.

Etiology

Between 20 and 23 days' gestation, the neural tube should be complete except for the opening at each end. What causes the failure to close or a later reopening is essentially unknown. There may be genetic factors. Research has identified a lack of folic acid in the pregnant woman's diet. NTDs may be isolated birth defects, or they may result from exposure to a teratogen that adversely affects normal cellular development in the embryo or fetus.

Signs and Symptoms

Spina bifida occulta may show no visible signs or may be manifested by a dimple in the skin, hair tuft, or a **nevus** (port-wine birthmark along the posterior surface of the body) in the midline above the buttocks. In general, spina bifida occulta does not cause neurological dysfunction, although there may be associated foot weakness or bowel and bladder disturbances. With meningocele and myelomeningocele, a saclike structure protrudes from the spinal area. A meningocele may cause little or no neurological deficit, or there may be partial paralysis and bladder and bowel dysfunction. A myelomeningocele

---

The X represents the fourth digit that is often required and supplied once more detailed information about the disease or disorder is made known to the provider.

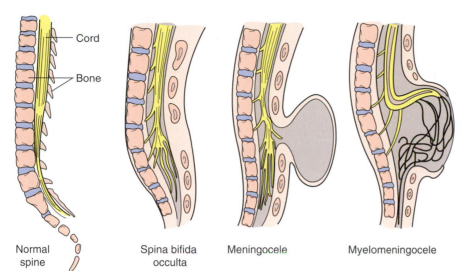

Normal spine

Spina bifida occulta

Meningocele

Myelomeningocele

Figure 6.8 Neural tube defects.

frequently results in permanent neurological difficulties. This includes paralysis, bladder and bowel dysfunction, twisted or abnormal legs and feet (club foot), and **Chiari malformation.** Chiari malformation is when the back portion of the brain is pushed through the hole in the bottom of the skull into the cervical spinal canal, limiting the flow of cerebrospinal fluid.

Diagnostic Procedures

NTDs are often diagnosed during pregnancy either through imaging or laboratory testing. A "triple screen" blood test is used to determine an elevated level of alpha-fetoprotein (AFP), human chorionic gonadotropin (HCG), and estriol. All are an indication for a higher risk of NTDs. This test generally is done during the second trimester. X-rays, MRIs, and computed tomography (CT) scans can look for spinal defects and excess fluid.

Prenatal detection of some open NTDs is possible through ultrasonographic examination between the 14th and 16th weeks of gestation or through the use of amniocentesis, which shows high levels of acetylcholinesterase. An unusually high measurement of the maternal serum alpha-fetoprotein (MSAFP) between 16 and 18 weeks' gestation will also detect most cases of NTDs. After birth, meningocele and myelomeningocele are obvious on examination. Spina bifida occulta may not be evident on visual inspection. Accordingly, x-ray, pinprick examination of the legs and trunk, and myelography are other procedures used to diagnose the condition and to show the level of sensory and motor involvement.

Treatment

There is no cure. Spina bifida occulta usually requires no treatment. Meningocele and myelomeningocele require surgical repair of the sac and closure of the bone defect and supportive measures to promote independence and to decrease the possibility of complications. Surgical repair, however, cannot restore the permanent nerve damage.

Complementary Therapy

No complementary therapy is known.

CLIENT COMMUNICATION

Refer prospective parents to agencies where information and support are given. Encourage the use of prenatal vitamins and folic acid supplements. After birth, parents will benefit from the assistance of rehabilitation professionals, social workers, and physicians.

Prognosis

The prognosis is dependent on the extent of neurological deficit that accompanies the condition. The prognosis is worse for individuals with large open spinal lesions, neurogenic bladder, or leg paralysis and is much better for those with only spina bifida occulta, with many individuals able to live a normal life. In the most severe cases of NTDs, waist supports, leg braces, and management of fecal incontinence and neurogenic bladder are necessary.

Prevention

Prevention of NTDs includes administering folic acid to pregnant women. Because spinal cord defects occur more often in offspring of women who have previously had a child with a similar defect, genetic counseling may be helpful.

HYDROCEPHALUS

ICD-10: Q03.X CONGENITAL
ICD-10: G91.1 ACQUIRED
ICD-10: G91.0 COMMUNICATING

Description

Hydrocephalus is a condition marked by too much cerebrospinal fluid (CSF) in the ventricles of the brain. The condition is congenital if hydrocephalus occurs before the cranial sutures have fused. The ventricles expand beyond the point of obstruction, the cranial sutures separate, the head expands, and the **fontanels,** commonly called *soft spots* of the skull, bulge. Acquired hydrocephalus can develop at birth or anytime afterward and is usually caused by disease or injury. The condition is called *noncommunicating hydrocephalus* when there is an obstruction in CSF flow. If the problem is faulty absorption of CSF, the condition is called *communicating hydrocephalus*.

Etiology

Hydrocephalus may be the result of a genetic defect or a developmental disorder such as those associated with NTDs. It may be caused by traumatic head injury, diseases such as meningitis or tumors, or intraventricular or subarachnoid hemorrhages.

Signs and Symptoms

The symptoms of hydrocephalus vary with age. An infant's skull can more easily accommodate increased CSF, but the head will become enlarged. Hydrocephalic infants often have high-pitched cries and abnormal muscle tone in their legs. Projectile vomiting likely occurs. Infants may also be irritable and/or very sleepy. Older children and adults will have a headache; nausea; vomiting; blurred or double vision; and problems with balance, coordination, and walking.

Diagnostic Procedures

A clinical neurological assessment is done. The head circumference is often measured, as an abnormally large head may indicate the diagnosis. However, MRI and CT scanning confirm the diagnosis.

Treatment

Surgical correction is the treatment of choice for hydrocephalus. A shunt is usually placed from the affected ventricles of the brain into the peritoneal cavity or into the right atrium of the heart, where the excess fluid makes its way into the venous circulation.

Complementary Therapy

No significant complementary therapy is indicated.

⊙ CLIENT COMMUNICATION

Help parents and caregivers focus on rehabilitation after surgery, building on the child's abilities and potential. Information about what to watch for in shunt malfunction is essential. The shunt may have mechanical failure, an infection may develop, or an obstruction may occur—all requiring medical attention.

Prognosis

The prognosis is difficult to predict but may remain guarded even with early detection and surgical correction. There can be both cognitive and physical developmental difficulties, vision loss, and impaired motor function. Without surgery, the mortality rate is high.

Prevention

Regular prenatal care helps to reduce premature birth, which puts an infant at risk for hydrocephalus. Also, tell parents to protect infants and children from head injuries with child safety seats and equipment that meets all safety standards

CEREBRAL PALSY

ICD-10: G80.X

Description

Cerebral palsy (CP) is permanent, bilateral, symmetrical, nonprogressive paralysis resulting from developmental defects of the brain or from trauma during or after the birth process.

Etiology

CP is caused by central nervous system damage that occurs before, during, or after birth. About 70% to 80% of CP incidences occur prior to birth. The causes can include maternal rubella (especially in the first trimester), maternal diabetes, **anoxia** (absence of oxygen), or **toxemia** or preeclampsia (pregnancy-induced hypertension). About 10% of causes relate to the birth process and include trauma during delivery, prematurity, or asphyxia from the umbilical cord becoming wrapped around the infant's neck. Postnatal causes include head trauma, meningitis, or poisoning. There are three types of cerebral palsy: spastic, athetoid, and ataxic.

Signs and Symptoms

Spastic cerebral palsy affects about 70% of children with CP and is characterized by hyperactive reflexes, rapid muscle contraction, muscle weakness, spasticity, and underdevelopment of limbs. Children with this form of CP typically walk on their toes, crossing one foot in front of the other.

Athetoid cerebral palsy affects 20% of children with CP and is characterized by involuntary muscle movements that are generally slow and writhing and impaired muscle tone, or **dystonia.** The arms are affected more often than the legs, and speech may be difficult. The body movements in athetoid CP are increased during times of stress and are not apparent during sleep.

Roughly 10% of children with CP show signs of *ataxic* CP. They have difficulty with balance, depth perception, and coordination. They show signs of rhythmic, involuntary movement of the eyeball, or **nystagmus;** muscle weakness; and tremor. Sudden movements are almost always impossible.

A few children exhibit signs of all three types of CP. Decreased intellectual ability occurs in about 40% of children with CP. Seizure disorders, impaired motor function, and impaired speech or vision often are present. Many may have dental abnormalities and vision and hearing defects.

Diagnostic Procedures

Careful neurological assessment, including examination and history, is necessary. Ultrasound, CT scan, and MRI all can be used to detect abnormalities in the brain. The spontaneous movement and behavior of the child are observed for characteristic signs, such as inability to suck or keep food in the mouth, difficulty in voluntary movements, difficulty in separating the legs during diaper changes, and use of only one hand or both hands but not the legs.

Treatment

CP has no cure, and treatment is directed toward helping children overcome any functional or intellectual disability. Treatment may include the use of braces and special appliances, range-of-motion exercises, orthopedic surgery, and medications to decrease seizures and spasticity. Physical, speech, and occupational therapies may be very helpful. The treatment process typically involves the entire family. Recently, administering human fetal stem cells intravenously and subcutaneously to a client with CP has shown remarkable results. The stem cells search out and attempt to repair any damage, release growth factors, and stimulate the body's repair mechanisms. It can take 3 to 6 months to see improvement.

Complementary Therapy

Equestrian therapy is helpful in that riding a horse is often able to improve muscle tone, give the head and trunk greater control, and enhance equilibrium. Some studies show that acupuncture can increase the flow of energy.

⊕ CLIENT COMMUNICATION

Parents and caregivers can benefit from the assistance of PCPs, social workers, and other healthcare professionals for the child's rehabilitation.

Prognosis

The prognosis varies. If impairment is mild, a near-normal life may be possible. If impairment is severe, lifelong care is necessary.

Prevention

Early prenatal care and good maternal health are the only preventive measures known.

CHAPTER EPISODE—PART II

Hank and Melanie waited for an hour before they called the nurse to ask where their son was. The answer seemed vague, but they were assured that he would be in soon. Melanie's and Hank's parents arrived to see the new baby. When they came into the room, they said Josh was not in the nursery. Hank was furious; Melanie was frightened and began to cry. Her mother comforted her and told her not to worry and to try to get some sleep.

At about 5:00 a.m., the pediatrician came into the room, followed by the obstetrician. He commented about how cute the baby was but then began to describe some physical symptoms. Melanie and Hank only heard the words *trisomy 21*, or Down syndrome.

- What most likely are the reactions of these new parents?
- What are the main concerns of the pediatrician? Of the obstetrician?

Digestive System Diseases and Disorders

CLEFT LIP AND PALATE (OROFACIAL CLEFTS)

ICD-10: Q37.9

Description

Cleft lip (ICD-10: Q36.9) is a congenital birth defect in which there are one or more clefts in the upper lip. Cleft palate (ICD-10: Q35.9) is a birth defect characterized by a hole in the middle of the roof of the mouth. The cleft may extend completely through the hard and soft palates into the nasal area. The defects appear singly or together and vary in severity. Major problems for the infant are difficulty in sucking and the infant's facial appearance (Fig. 6.9).

Etiology

Orofacial clefts are thought to represent a multifactorial genetic disorder that results in a failure in the embryonic development of the fetus. The CDC reports that women who smoke during pregnancy, women who are diabetic, and women who take certain medications for epilepsy are more likely to have an infant with cleft lip and palate. The combination of cleft lip and cleft palate occurs in approximately 1 in 1,000 births.

Signs and Symptoms

The described physical symptoms are apparent at birth.

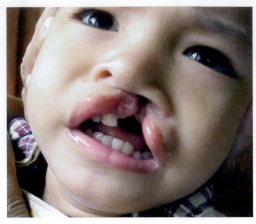

Figure 6.9 An infant with cleft lip and palate *(Key Kid Foundation.org, http://www.keykidfoundation.org/facefix/KyranPalubon1d.jpg, with permission.)*

Diagnostic Procedures

Cleft lip and palate can be diagnosed during pregnancy by a routine ultrasound. After birth, symptoms confirm the diagnosis and may include observing formula or the mother's milk come through the nose of the infant.

Treatment

Surgery is the treatment of choice and usually is done as soon as possible because sucking can be difficult. Some deformities require that surgery be performed in stages. Special feeding devices and techniques can be tried. A team of practitioners is likely to be required. Specialists, such as plastic surgeons, neurosurgeons, orthodontists, otolaryngologists, speech pathologists, and audiologists, are likely to be involved even into adulthood.

Complementary Therapy

No significant complementary therapy is indicated.

⊕ CLIENT COMMUNICATION

It will help parents to understand the condition and that clefting occurs often before a woman knows she is pregnant. Instructions will be given on feeding the infant. Breastfeeding may be easier because the breast has the capacity to mold to the shape of the infant's oral cavity. If bottle-feeding is necessary, a convenient mnemonic to remember the method is ESSR (*e*nlarge, *s*timulate, *s*wallow, and *r*est). Enlarge the nipple hole, allowing the infant to receive the formula in the back of the throat. Stimulate the infant by rubbing the nipple on the lower lip to engage the sucking reflex. The nipple is inserted into the mouth, and then the bottle is inverted. The infant swallows the fluid normally. The last step is a rest. If an infant is about to choke or

gag, his or her facial expressions will change. This is a signal to take a short rest, allowing the infant to finish swallowing formula that is already in the mouth. Remove the nipple slowly and gently from the mouth. Burp the infant often. Repeat the steps until normal amounts of formula have been given.

Prognosis

The prognosis is good with corrective surgery. Children may need speech therapy as they begin to talk.

Prevention

There is no known prevention. It is best for women to avoid smoking during pregnancy and to speak to their PCP regarding their diabetes or any medications for epilepsy.

TRACHEOESOPHAGEAL FISTULA AND ESOPHAGEAL ATRESIA

ICD-10: Q39.X

Description

Tracheoesophageal fistula (TEF) is an abnormal connection between the esophagus and the trachea, where there are normally two separate canals. When the infant swallows, liquid is passed into the lungs rather than the stomach. This can cause pneumonia and other complications. Esophageal atresia often accompanies TEF. In this condition, the esophagus does not form completely, creating two canals—one connected to the throat and the other connected to the stomach. The infant's food cannot get to the stomach. About 1 in 4,000 infants are born with one or both of these problems.

Etiology

In about the fourth to eighth week of fetal development, a single tube separates into two distinct tubes—the esophagus and the trachea. No one fully understands what causes the normal development to fail and the difficulties to occur. While these two problems are likely not inherited, they appear about 50% of the time with other birth defects that are genetic related. Cause is essentially unknown.

Signs and Symptoms

Symptoms are quickly realized. There may be frothy white bubbles in the mouth, vomiting, coughing or choking when feeding, cyanosis, and difficulty breathing.

Diagnostic Procedures

Physical examination, imaging studies, and x-rays are used for diagnosis. A tube can be placed into the mouth or nose of the infant and guided into the esophagus.

Using x-ray images, it will be obvious if there is an incomplete or abnormal connection.

Treatment

Surgery is the best treatment within a few days of birth. Until surgery can be performed, an infant is fed through a stomach tube.

Complementary Therapy

No complementary therapy is known.

Prognosis

Sometimes infants with esophageal atresia will have long-term digestive difficulties. There can be problems moving food through the esophagus, and there may be gastroesophageal reflux.

Prevention

Proper prenatal care is recommended.

PYLORIC STENOSIS

ICD-10: K31.1

Description

Pyloric stenosis is narrowing of the **pylorus** (pyloric sphincter), the lower opening of the stomach leading into the upper part of the intestine, or duodenum. This condition prevents **chyme** (the nearly liquid mixture of partially digested food and gastric secretions) from flowing into the small intestine. Pyloric stenosis is more common in male infants.

Etiology

The cause is unknown, but the disease may be hereditary. It is one of the most common developmental abnormalities of the digestive system.

Signs and Symptoms

The classic symptom is projectile vomiting, beginning about the second to fourth week after birth. The infant may eject vomitus a distance of 3 to 4 feet. Signs of dehydration and starvation may be evident if the pyloric sphincter closes completely. There may be decreased elasticity of the skin, abdominal distention, and a palpable tumor in the **epigastrium,** the region of the abdomen over the pit of the stomach.

Diagnostic Procedures

The history and physical examination may suggest the condition. Other studies may include upper gastrointestinal (GI) x-ray and laboratory tests, the latter being used to detect dehydration and electrolyte imbalances. Pyloric stenosis must be distinguished from feeding

difficulties associated with colic or disturbed mother-child relationships.

Treatment

The standard treatment is incision and suture of the pyloric sphincter. The procedure, called *pyloromyotomy*, is relatively simple, safe, and effective.

Complementary Therapy

No significant complementary therapy is indicated.

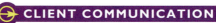

CLIENT COMMUNICATION

This disorder can be particularly unnerving for parents and caregivers; projectile vomiting is frightening. Reassurance is important. Prepare the family for the infant's surgery and necessary follow-up care.

Prognosis

The prognosis is excellent with proper care and surgical correction.

Prevention

There is no known prevention.

MALROTATION WITH VOLVULUS

ICD-10: Q43.3

Description

In the developing fetus, the intestine (a long straight canal) becomes a part of the abdomen at about the 10th week of pregnancy and makes two turns. If the turns do not occur, malrotation results. The cecum (lower end of the small intestine) will not develop normally, and both it and the appendix will stay in the upper right side of the abdomen. Bands of tissue form between the cecum and the intestinal wall, creating a blockage in the duodenum (the beginning of the small intestine). If the intestine becomes twisted, blocking the blood flow, damage to the intestine occurs. This is called a *volvulus.* These problems cause an obstruction that prevents food from being digested normally. Malrotation with volvulus occurs in about 1 in every 500 births.

Etiology

The cause is unknown. However, about 70% of infants with this defect have one or more congenital abnormalities of the heart, spleen, or liver.

Signs and Symptoms

Symptoms may include abdominal pain that causes an infant to draw up the legs, vomiting of a digestive fluid known as *bile,* a swollen abdomen, tachycardia and tachypnea, and bloody stools. A child can dehydrate quickly.

Diagnostic Procedures

Physical examination is followed by imaging studies that may include abdominal x-ray, CT scan, upper GI testing, and a contrast enema, which are important in diagnosis. Blood tests to check for electrolytes are also important.

Treatment

The extent of the problem will determine treatment. Malrotation may not be evident until volvulus occurs. A volvulus is life-threatening because the intestine can die without adequate blood supply. To untwist the intestine, surgical repair is performed as quickly as possible. A portion of the intestine may have to be removed if the damage is significant.

Complementary Therapy

No complementary therapy is known.

Prognosis

The majority of children have no residual problems following surgical repair. However, if a major portion of the intestine is removed, there may be long-term consequences. Adequate nutrition and fluids normally absorbed from food in the small intestine may be hindered, making high-calorie nutritional supplements necessary. Sometimes these may need to be given intravenously.

Prevention

There is no known prevention.

HIRSCHSPRUNG DISEASE (CONGENITAL AGANGLIONIC MEGACOLON)

ICD-10: Q43.1

Description

Hirschsprung disease is the obstruction and dilation of the colon with feces because the large intestine lacks nerve cells to create adequate intestinal motility. Feces are not moved past the aganglionic segment of the colon. Pressure from accumulating feces then distends the preceding portion of the colon. The amount of intestinal wall affected varies; involvement may be limited to the internal sphincter or may extend to the entire colon. The disease is more common in males and occurs in about 1 in 5,000 births. Hirschsprung disease may occur with other congenital anomalies such as trisomy 21. Get more information about this disease at http://digestive.niddk.nih.gov/ddiseases/pubs/hirschsprungs_ez.

Etiology

The cause of the disease is unknown, but it appears to be a hereditary, usually familial disease. The condition is due to an absence of autonomic **parasympathetic** (involuntary) **ganglion** cells (masses of nervelike cell bodies in the colorectal walls) resulting in the absence of **peristalsis** (involuntary wavelike contractions) in the affected portion.

Signs and Symptoms

Clinical manifestations typically appear during infancy, but they may not appear until adolescence. In infancy, the neonate fails to pass the first feces, or **meconium,** within 48 hours of birth. Signs and symptoms include severe abdominal distention and feeding difficulties. After the neonatal period, symptoms may include fever, failure to thrive, and explosive watery diarrhea. In adolescence, symptoms may include chronic constipation and abdominal distention. The child also may be anemic and appear poorly nourished.

Diagnostic Procedures

Diagnosis is confirmed with a rectal biopsy that reveals the absence of ganglion cells in the colorectal wall. In older infants and adolescents, a barium enema x-ray or rectal manometry (inflation of a small balloon within the rectum to check muscle pressures) may be ordered.

Treatment

Surgical treatment generally involves a two-stage procedure. First, a temporary colostomy is created in the normal bowel. The colostomy allows the infant to evacuate feces, allows the bowel to rest, and allows the infant to gain weight. The second-stage surgery is a pull-through procedure wherein the affected segment of the bowel is resected or removed and the normal bowel is anastomosed to the rectum. During this second stage, the colostomy is also closed. More recently, a one-stage procedure has been used with the pull-through, as described, but without a temporary colostomy. The benefits of a one-stage surgical procedure is that it involves only one operation and requires no colostomy care. Another type of procedure is called a laparoscope-assisted pull-through. In this procedure, a laparoscope is put through the anus, allowing the surgeon to pull the affected bowel segment through the opening. In all of these procedures, fluid and electrolyte balance must be maintained. Antibiotics may also be prescribed to reduce intestinal flora.

Complementary Therapy

No significant complementary therapy is indicated.

⊙→ CLIENT COMMUNICATION

See the Client Communication in the "Pyloric Stenosis" section. Impress upon parents and caregivers that immediate treatment is necessary.

Prognosis

With prompt treatment, the prognosis is good. If untreated, death is likely from enterocolitis or infection of the intestines, severe diarrhea, and shock.

Prevention

There is no known prevention.

OMPHALOCELE

ICD-10: Q79.2

Description

An omphalocele is a birth defect in which the infant's intestines or other abdominal organs poke through the navel when the abdominal wall (umbilical ring) does not close properly. These organs are covered with a thin layer of tissue but can easily be seen. About 30% of infants with an omphalocele have other congenital abnormalities.

Etiology

The cause is unknown, but omphaloceles seem to occur more frequently with increased maternal age.

Signs and Symptoms

The symptoms are obvious because the intestines poke through the navel area. An omphalocele may be large enough that the liver or spleen protrude out of the body as well.

Diagnostic Procedures

Prenatal ultrasounds often detect this defect prior to birth. At that time, additional screening may be performed to detect any other birth defects. Otherwise, physical examination is the only diagnosis necessary.

Treatment

Surgery is the treatment of choice but may not be done immediately if there are other pressing medical problems. The protective sac holds the intestine and other organs in place until surgery is performed. To repair, the sac will be covered with a special synthetic material and then stitched in place. Over time, the abdominal contents are pushed into the abdomen. When the contents are fully returned to the abdomen, the synthetic material is removed and the abdomen is sutured closed.

Complementary Therapy

No complementary therapy is known.

Prognosis

Complete recovery of an omphalocele can be expected. Complications occur if there is death of the intestinal tissue or an infection. Without prompt treatment, the condition can be life-threatening.

Prevention

There is no known prevention for an omphalocele.

Genitourinary System Diseases and Disorders

UNDESCENDED TESTES (CRYPTORCHIDISM)

ICD-10: Q53.9

Description

This congenital condition is the failure of the testes to descend into the scrotal sac from the abdominal cavity. The condition may be unilateral or bilateral; it more commonly affects the right testis. The testes can be either retractable or ectopic. A retractable testis is descended but readily retracts with examination or physical stimulation, whereas an ectopic testis is found outside the normal path of descent. It can be in the groin, perineum, or abdominal wall. Cryptorchidism is a common birth defect affecting about 1 in 125 male infants.

Etiology

The cause is unknown, but it may be linked to inadequate or improper hormone levels in the fetus. The testes normally descend into the scrotal sac during the eighth month of gestation, so the condition is most often seen in premature births and neonates with low birth weight.

Signs and Symptoms

When the condition is unilateral, the testis on the affected side is not palpable in the scrotum. In bilateral cryptorchidism, the scrotum will appear to be underdeveloped.

Diagnostic Procedures

Physical examination reveals cryptorchidism. A serum gonadotropin test will confirm the presence of testes because it assesses the level of circulating hormone produced by the testes. Ultrasound may be used to determine their location.

Treatment

In many cases, the testes descend during the infant's first year. Otherwise, the treatment of choice is surgical correction between ages 2 and 4. Human chorionic gonadotropin may be tried to stimulate descent of the testes.

Complementary Therapy

No significant complementary therapy is indicated.

CLIENT COMMUNICATION

The goal of this communication is to offer information to caregivers to help alleviate any fear or anxiety about treatment or lack thereof. Answering questions about concerns regarding sexuality or fertility is paramount.

Prognosis

The prognosis is good with proper attention. Corrected cryptorchidism generally does not cause sexual dysfunction later in life. Testes that have not descended by the time of adolescence will atrophy, causing sterility, but testosterone levels remain normal. A child with undescended testes has a 20% to 44% increase in risk for developing a malignant testicular tumor in adulthood.

Prevention

There is no known prevention.

CONGENITAL DEFECTS OF THE URETER, BLADDER, AND URETHRA

ICD-10: 60.X

Description

The March of Dimes reports that birth defects of the ureter, bladder, and urethra are common, affecting as many as 1 in 10 infants. Some abnormalities cause few if any symptoms; others are painful and may cause urinary tract infections and kidney disease.

Etiology

The causes of congenital defects of the ureter, bladder, and urethra are unknown. Some of the problems are obvious at birth; others are not apparent until later, when they produce symptoms. The following is a brief discussion of the most common congenital urinary tract anomalies, together with their symptoms and possible treatments.

Duplicated ureter means that each kidney has two ureters rather than one. Sometimes the two ureters join before they enter the urinary bladder. The common symptoms may include frequent urinary infections, urinary frequency and urgency, diminished urine output, and flank pain. Surgery is the treatment of choice to remove the unnecessary ureter.

Retrocaval ureter occurs when the right ureter passes behind the inferior vena cava before entering the urinary bladder. The symptoms may include **hydroureter** (swelling of the ureter with urine), right flank pain, urinary tract infection, renal calculi, and **hematuria** (blood in the urine). Surgical **resection** and formation of a connection called **anastomosis** of the ureter constitute the treatment of choice.

Ectopic orifice of the ureter occurs when the ureteral opening inserts into the vagina in females or into the prostate or vas deferens in males. The symptoms may include urinary obstruction, **reflux** of urine, incontinence, flank pain, and urinary urgency. Resection and ureteral reimplantation into the bladder are necessary for correction.

Stricture or stenosis of the ureter means that one of the ureters is tightened or partially closed. The affected ureter may become enlarged, and **hydronephrosis** (swelling of the renal pelvis of the kidney with urine) may result. Surgical repair is necessary. **Nephrectomy** may be required if severe renal damage has occurred as a result of hydronephrosis.

Ureterocele is the bulging of the ureter into the urinary bladder, sometimes almost filling the bladder. Urinary obstruction difficulties and recurrent urinary tract infections occur. Surgical excision or resection of the ureterocele is necessary.

Exstrophy of the bladder is a congenital malformation in which the lower portion of the abdominal wall and the anterior wall of the bladder are missing. Consequently, the inner surface of the posterior wall of the bladder is everted through the opening in the abdominal wall. In effect, the bladder appears turned inside out. The skin covering the hole in the abdominal wall is easily **excoriated,** or roughened by accumulating urine, and infection typically results. Surgical closure of the defect is necessary. Reconstruction of the bladder and abdominal wall is required, and urinary diversion may be necessary.

Congenital bladder diverticulum is caused by a diverticulum or pouching out of the bladder wall. Fever, urinary frequency, and pain on urination are common. Surgery is the treatment of choice to correct the herniation and reflux.

Hypospadias is an abnormal opening of the male urethra onto the undersurface of the penis or of the female urethra into the vagina. Epispadias is an abnormal opening of the male urethra onto the upper surface of the penis or of the female urethra through a fissure in the labia minora and clitoris. In all these instances, normal urination is difficult or impossible. Surgical repair is almost always necessary.

Diagnostic Procedures

Diagnostic tests include an x-ray of the urinary tract after the introduction of a contrast medium, or excretory urography; voiding cystoscopy; cystourethrography; urethroscopy; and ultrasonography.

Complementary Therapy

No significant complementary therapy is indicated.

CLIENT COMMUNICATION

It is important to support parents during the diagnosis, treatment, and recovery phases of these congenital defects. Providing adequate information and education is essential.

Prognosis

With prompt treatment and surgical repair, most individuals live a normal life with little or no long-term complications.

Prevention

There is no known prevention.

Musculoskeletal System Diseases and Disorders

CLUBFOOT (TALIPES)

ICD-10: Q66.89

Description

Clubfoot is a nontraumatic, frequently occurring congenital deformity in which the foot is permanently bent. The four basic forms are (1) talipes varus, an inversion or inward bending of the foot (Fig. 6.10); (2) talipes valgus, an eversion or outward bending of the foot; (3) talipes equinus, or plantar flexion, in which the toes are lower than the heel; and (4) talipes calcaneus, or dorsiflexion, in which the toes are higher than the heel. An individual also may have a combination of these basic forms: for example, talipes equinovarus, in which the toes point downward and the body of the foot bends inward.

Etiology

The exact cause is unknown, but a combination of genetic and environmental factors in utero has been implicated. A Mendelian pattern of inheritance is suspected. It is twice as common in boys as in girls.

Signs and Symptoms

Clubfoot varies greatly in severity; however, in all cases the talus is deformed, the Achilles' bursa is shortened, and the calcaneus is flattened and shortened. It is painless.

Diagnostic Procedures

The deformity is usually obvious at birth.

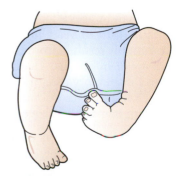

Figure 6.10 An infant with talipes varus clubfoot. There is a bending inward of the feet.

Treatment

Treatment is aimed at correcting the deformity and maintaining the corrected position. Simple manipulation and casting may be done and repeated several times. Corrective surgery may be required. Maintenance treatment includes special exercises, night splints, and orthopedic shoes. Close follow-up observation is essential.

Complementary Therapy

No significant complementary therapy is indicated.

⊕ CLIENT COMMUNICATION

Parents can be taught how to care for an infant with casts, splints, or orthopedic shoes. Exercise may be ordered, so show parents how to perform the exercises at home.

Prognosis

The prognosis is good with prompt treatment. There are usually no long-term complications.

Prevention

There is no known prevention.

CONGENITAL HIP DYSPLASIA

ICD-10: Q65.89

Description

Hip dysplasia, also known as *developmental dysplasia of the hip* (DDH), is an abnormality of the hip joint that may take three forms: (1) unstable hip dysplasia, in which the hip can be dislocated manually; (2) incomplete dislocation, in which the femoral head is on the edge of the **acetabulum,** the rounded cavity on the outer surface of the hip bone that receives the femur; and (3) complete dislocation, in which the femoral head is outside the acetabulum. It is more common in females.

Etiology

The cause is not known; however, it tends to run in families. Hip dislocation may result if the fetus is not positioned correctly within the uterus before and during birth.

Signs and Symptoms

Physical examination shows asymmetric folds in the thigh of neonates with limited abduction of the affected hip. A shortening of the femur is noted when the knees and hips are flexed at right angles. The signs are typically quite obvious when children attempt to walk, if the condition has not been discovered before that time.

Diagnostic Procedures

Observations during physical examination may suggest the diagnosis, but a positive Ortolani sign will confirm the diagnosis. Ortolani sign is the "clunk" felt when an examiner abducts (draws away from the body) and lifts the femurs of a supine infant. The "clunk" indicates a partial or an incomplete displacement of the hip. X-ray may be used.

Treatment

It is important for treatment to begin as soon as possible. Before 3 months of age, treatment requires closed reduction of the dislocation, followed by the use of a splint-brace or cast for 2 to 3 months. If the child is much older, open reduction followed by casting may be necessary.

Complementary Therapy

No significant complementary therapy is indicated.

➔ CLIENT COMMUNICATION

Families will need support and teaching on how to care for an infant or a child with a cast or splint, if necessary.

Prognosis

When treatment occurs before age 5, the prognosis is excellent. If not treated promptly, abnormal development of the hip and permanent disability may result.

Prevention

There is no known prevention for congenital hip dysplasia.

DUCHENNE MUSCULAR DYSTROPHY

 ICD-10: G71.0

Description

Duchenne muscular dystrophy is a congenital disorder characterized by progressive bilateral wasting of skeletal muscles; the symptoms of the disorder do not include neural or sensory defects. It generally strikes during early childhood and can cause death within 10 to 15 years of onset. Because of the way the disease is inherited, far more males than females develop symptoms. Duchenne muscular dystrophy occurs in about 1 in 3,600 males.

Etiology

The disease is the result of an X-linked recessive disorder, which is usually inherited but may also be due to mutation. Normally, the gene on the X chromosome produces dystrophin, a protein found in muscle tissue that provides strength and flexibility. Because the inheritance of one faulty X chromosome results in the absence of dystrophin, males rather than females have the disease. Females are carriers. The exact mechanism by which the genetic defect produces muscle wasting is not known.

Signs and Symptoms

Manifestations of Duchenne muscular dystrophy begin between ages 3 and 5. Without the protein dystrophin, muscles become weak and are easily damaged. Fatigue and weakness is a common complaint. The disease affects the leg and pelvic muscles before spreading to involuntary muscles. The affected child may have a characteristic waddling gait, may engage in toe-walking, and may have lordosis or other spinal deformities. The child may have difficulty running and climbing stairs and may tend to fall easily. Muscle deterioration is progressive, and contractures typically develop. By age 12, the child usually loses the ability to walk.

Diagnostic Procedures

A family history of the disease together with the clinical picture of characteristic symptoms suggests the diagnosis. A muscle biopsy showing characteristic connective tissue and fat deposits will confirm the diagnosis. Electromyography can rule out muscle atrophy that is neurological in origin. Tests of urine creatinine and serum levels of creatine phosphokinase (CPK) and transaminase are usually ordered.

Treatment

No known treatment is successful in curing Duchenne muscular dystrophy, but procedures to correct or preserve mobility are helpful. These include orthopedic appliances, exercise, physical therapy, and surgery.

Complementary Therapy

There is no known complementary therapy.

Prognosis

The prognosis is poor for a child with Duchenne muscular dystrophy. Children with this condition are usually confined to a wheelchair by ages 9 to 12. Formerly it was believed that within 10 to 15 years of the onset of the disease, death commonly resulted from cardiac or respiratory complications or infections. Thanks to advances in both cardiac and respiratory care, men with the disease are living much longer lives—some even into their 40s and 50s—and are married and have families.

Prevention

Carriers of the genetic defect known to cause muscular dystrophy may receive genetic counseling regarding the risks of transmitting the disease.

Metabolic Errors

CYSTIC FIBROSIS

ICD-10: E84.X

Description

Cystic fibrosis (CF) is a life-threatening congenital disorder of the exocrine glands characterized by the production of copious amounts of abnormally thick mucus, especially in the bronchus and lungs. The mucus clogs the pancreas, stopping the important enzymes that help the body break down and absorb food. There are over 30,000 children and adults living with CF in the United States, and nearly 1,000 new cases are diagnosed each year.

Etiology

The disease is caused by an underlying biochemical defect transmitted as an autosomal-recessive trait. If both parents are carriers of the recessive gene, the offspring have a 25% chance of having the disease.

Signs and Symptoms

The signs of CF may appear soon after birth or take some time to develop. Because all exocrine glands can be affected, the symptoms can be quite numerous. The sweat glands and respiratory and GI functions are those most commonly affected. The sweat glands typically express increased concentrations of salt in sweat. Respiratory symptoms may include wheezy respirations, a dry cough, dyspnea, tachypnea, and frequent lung infections, all stemming from accumulations of thick secretions in the smaller passages conveying air within the lung (**bronchioles**) and the air sacs (**alveoli**) of the lungs. GI symptoms may include intestinal obstruction, vomiting, constipation, electrolyte imbalance, and the inability to absorb fats. Fibrous tissue and fat slowly replace the normal saclike swellings found in the pancreas, resulting in pancreatic insufficiency characterized by insufficient insulin production. Some individuals with CF have only respiratory symptoms; others have only digestive problems. Still others have both respiratory and digestive symptoms.

Diagnostic Procedures

The Cystic Fibrosis Foundation has developed the following criteria for a definitive diagnosis: two positive sweat tests using a sweat inducer and one of the following: obstructive pulmonary diseases, confirmed pancreatic insufficiency or failure to thrive, and a family history of CF. DNA testing may be done prenatally to diagnose the disease. Chest x-rays and pulmonary function tests may be ordered to diagnose and evaluate respiratory function.

Treatment

The treatment for CF is designed to help a child lead as normal a life as possible. Antibiotic therapy to ward off lung infections is helpful. Mucus-thinning drugs and bronchodilators can help keep airway passages clear. Client management includes chest physical therapy to combat pulmonary dysfunction, loosening and removing mucopurulent secretions, and oxygen therapy. Vitamin and oral pancreatic supplements are often given to accompany a high-calorie diet. Some individuals may be candidates for lung transplants. The Cystic Fibrosis Foundation identifies developing therapies that may continue to help in the treatment of clients with CF:

- *Gene therapy* that may correct the defective cystic fibrosis transmembrane conductance (CFTR) protein made by the CF gene. This would allow chloride and sodium to move through the cells in the lungs and other organs.
- *Restore airway surface liquid* is an approach that targets proteins to assist in moving salt in and out of cells and to hydrate the mucus so it clears more easily.
- *Anti-inflammatory medications* to assist in reducing inflammation in CF lungs.
- *Anti-infective medications* to fight acute and chronic lung infections.

Complementary Therapy

One study showed that long-term treatment with omega-3 supplementation helped to decrease lung infection.

> ➤ **CLIENT COMMUNICATION**
> Genetic counseling may be advisable in families known to be at risk for CF.

Prognosis

The prognosis for CF is poor. There is no cure, but the average life expectancy has increased to 38 years or older. Serious, often fatal, respiratory complications include pneumonia, emphysema, and **atelectasis** (collapsed lung). GI complications include rectal prolapse and malnutrition.

Prevention

There is no known prevention for CF.

PHENYLKETONURIA

ICD-10: E70.0

Description

During normal metabolic processes, the enzyme phenylalanine hydroxylase converts the amino acid phenylalanine to tyrosine, another amino acid. In phenylketonuria (PKU), this enzyme is not produced by the body, so phenylalanine accumulates in the blood and urine and is toxic to the brain. Permanent intellectual disability results if the condition is not quickly corrected.

Etiology

PKU is an autosomal-recessive defect resulting in an error in phenylalanine metabolism.

Signs and Symptoms

The infant not diagnosed at birth is typically asymptomatic until about 4 months of age, when signs and symptoms of hyperactivity, personality disorders, **microcephaly** (a smaller-than-normal head), and irritability begin to appear. There often is a characteristic musty odor to the child's perspiration and urine due to the presence of phenylacetic acid, a metabolite of phenylalanine.

Diagnostic Procedures

The presence of an elevated blood phenylalanine level and a urine phenylpyruvic acid level after the infant has received dietary protein for 24 to 48 hours after birth confirms the diagnosis. A heelstick is generally used to obtain the blood sample. Repeated testing may need to be done using the infant's urine to detect PKU.

Treatment

Treatment consists of following a protein-restrictive diet for life. Most natural proteins need to be restricted, because phenylalanine is a component of most proteins. Serum phenylalanine levels need to be monitored to determine the efficacy of the diet.

Complementary Therapy

No significant complementary therapy is indicated.

 CLIENT COMMUNICATION

Provide parents and caregivers with diet and nutritional assistance in how to maintain a protein-restricted diet for their infant. The skills of a dietitian can be beneficial.

Prognosis

The sooner the protein-restrictive diet is started, the better is the prognosis. If the disease is detected and treated before age 2, the chances of the child achieving normal intelligence are good. The protein-restrictive diet will not reverse any existing intellectual disability, but it will prevent further progression.

Prevention

There is no known prevention for PKU.

Syndromes

DOWN SYNDROME (TRISOMY 21)

ICD-10: Q90.9

Description

Down syndrome is the most common single cause of congenital abnormalities. It is also called trisomy 21 because the infant has three chromosomes 21 rather than the usual pair. Every cell in the body will have an extra copy of chromosome 21. Down syndrome involves a number of birth defects that affect the heart, vision and hearing, facial features, and some degree of intellectual ability. Approximately 1 in 691 infants are born with Down syndrome. The name Down syndrome comes from a physician of the same last name who first described the condition in 1866. However, more recently the term *trisomy 21* is being used.

Etiology

Trisomy 21 occurs when there is an extra copy of chromosome 21. The extra chromosome causes problems in body and brain development. The incidence of trisomy 21 increases with the age of the mother.

Signs and Symptoms

Symptoms vary with each individual, but there are characteristic features. The head can be smaller and abnormal in shape. The inner corner of the eyes is rounded. There may be a flat nose and excessive skin in the nape of the neck. The tongue may be large and may protrude. Ears and mouth are small, and the hands are short with short fingers. Rather than three creases in the palm of the hand, there will only be two. Generally, there is low muscle tone.

Diagnostic Procedures

Screening tests can estimate the chance of the fetus having Down syndrome while diagnostic tests can give a definitive diagnosis with almost 100% accuracy. Blood tests can provide information on chromosomal genetic markers from the fetus that are circulating in the maternal blood. They are used in conjunction with ultrasound to determine possible Down syndrome. Chorionic villus sampling (CVS) and amniocentesis are nearly 100% accurate in diagnosing Down syndrome. Amniocentesis is usually performed in the second trimester after 15 weeks of gestation, and CVS is done in the first trimester between 9 and 11 weeks. At birth, physical features may be the only necessary diagnosis. A blood test can confirm the extra chromosome. Other tests to check for additional congenital difficulties include the echocardiogram, electrocardiogram, and x-rays of the chest and GI tract.

Treatment

There is no one specific treatment for trisomy 21; rather, treatment will pertain to specific difficulties and problems. GI blockage and heart defects may require surgery. There is an increased risk of visual or hearing impairment that may be treated with corrective devices. Speech therapy and physical therapy may be prescribed. Children with trisomy 21 are at increased risk for all types of infection. They require regular medical attention.

Complementary Therapy

No complementary therapy is known.

Prognosis

A number of issues must be faced. Decreased intellectual ability is likely and may be slight or severe. About half of children are born with heart defects. Some have an increased risk of leukemia. There usually is a weakness of the back bones at the top of the neck and a greater risk of compression injuries to the spinal cord. The good news, however, is that individuals with trisomy 21 are living much longer and are able to have productive lives, especially with early intervention programs.

Prevention

The only prevention is genetic counseling. There is a maternal age risk to consider. From the maternal age 25 to 29, the risk is 1 in 1,250. By age 45 and older, the risk increases to 1 in 30.

CHAPTER EPISODE—PART III

After the initial shock and tears, Hank and Melanie learned that the doctors had one piece of good news. The baby's heart seems perfectly normal. As they leave, the nurse brings Josh to his parents. He is bundled tightly and has a beautiful blue cap on his head. To Hank, Melanie, and their parents, he looks perfect and love overflows in their hearts.

- What is positive about this response?
- Does there appear to be a family support system here?

FETAL ALCOHOL SYNDROME

ICD-10: Q86.0

Description

This syndrome, formally described in 1968, is also known as *fetal alcohol spectrum disorder,* or FASD. This is an umbrella term for a number of problems that may occur when the mother drinks excessive amounts of alcohol during her pregnancy. These problems may include physical, mental, behavioral, and learning disabilities with possible lifelong implications.

Etiology

An infant born with FASD had a mother who consumed alcohol during pregnancy. Dependence and addiction to alcohol in the mother causes the fetus to become addicted. At birth, when the alcohol ceases, the infant's overstimulated central nervous system (CNS) causes withdrawal symptoms. The majority of children diagnosed with FASD had mothers who consumed at least eight to ten drinks a day. Women who drank four to six drinks a day had children with subtle signs of FASD. Drinking less than two drinks a day did not seem to harm the fetus.

Signs and Symptoms

Signs and symptoms include characteristic facial features, growth deficiencies, and CNS difficulties. The following characteristics may occur:

- Small stature in relationship to peers
- Mild facial abnormalities, including small eyes, flat nose, microcephaly, underdeveloped upper lip, and flat cheekbones
- Poor coordination
- Hyperactive behavior
- Poor reasoning and judgment skills
- Speech and language delays

Diagnostic Procedures

The minimal criteria for FASD are small size and weight before and after birth, at least two of the facial abnormalities listed, and evidence of development delay, intellectual impairment, or neurological abnormalities. This information and the mother's history of alcohol use confirm the diagnosis.

Treatment

There is no one treatment for FASD. Treatment is symptomatic. There are some specific medications that can be used to treat symptoms of withdrawal in infants with FASD. See Figure 6.11 for a description of the brain structures most sensitive to prenatal alcohol exposure.

Complementary Therapy

There is no known complementary therapy.

CLIENT COMMUNICATION

Pregnant women who are addicted to alcohol pose a special problem. Some may not reveal their addiction; others recognize the risk of the alcohol use to the fetus and seek help. Factual information accompanied by sensitivity on the part of healthcare providers can be the key to helping pregnant women abstain from alcohol.

Brain Structures Most Sensitive to Prenatal Alcohol Exposure

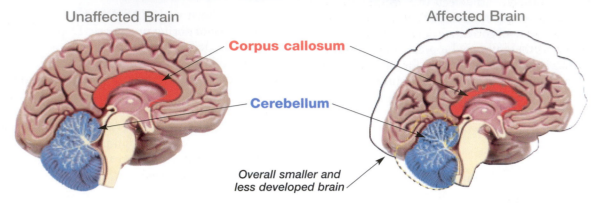

Unaffected Brain   Affected Brain

Corpus callosum

Cerebellum

Overall smaller and less developed brain

Brain Structure	Function	Prenatal alcohol exposure may result in problems with:
Corpus callosum	Communicates motor, sensory, and cognitive information between the two hemispheres of the brain	Storing and retrieving information, problem solving, attention, and verbal memory
Cerebellum	Processes input from other areas of the brain to coordinate motor and cognitive skills	Controlling movements, maintaining balance and fine motor skills

National Organization on Fetal Alcohol Syndrome (NOFAS)
1.800.66NOFAS or visit www.nofas.org

Figure 6.11 Brain structures most sensitive to prenatal alcohol exposure. *(National Organization on Fetal Alcohol Syndrome [NOFAS]: http://www.nofas.org/healthcare.)*

Prognosis

The prognosis depends on the severity of the FASD. Lifelong treatment may be necessary for severe cases of FASD.

Prevention

FASD can be prevented when women refrain from excessive use of alcohol during pregnancy. Even though scientifically it appears that drinking fewer than two drinks a day during pregnancy does not harm the fetus, a "better-safe-than-sorry" approach is suggested. Therefore, having no alcohol during pregnancy is the best prevention. Inform clients about the warning label on all alcoholic beverages in the United States that says, "According to the surgeon general, women should not drink alcoholic beverages during pregnancy because of the risk of birth defects."

TOURETTE SYNDROME

ICD-10: F95.2

Description

Tourette syndrome is a disorder of the nervous system that causes an individual to make repeated involuntary sounds or tics and movements. Tourette syndrome is named for Georges Gilles de la Tourette, who first described the disorder in 1885.

Etiology

The disorder is thought to be autosomal dominant; however, no specific gene has been identified. The disorder also may be linked to chemicals in the brain (dopamine, serotonin, and norepinephrine) that facilitate communication among nerves. It is four times more likely to occur in males.

Signs and Symptoms

Facial tics usually surface in early childhood. Other tics may follow and include arm thrusting, throat clearing, jumping, eye blinking, or shoulder shrugging. The use of curse words or inappropriate phrases occurs in only a small number of individuals. While the tics can be controlled for a period of time, to do so is uncomfortable. When the voluntary control ceases, the tics return with increased intensity for a period of time.

Diagnostic Procedures

A diagnosis of Tourette syndrome requires the following:

- Started the tics prior to age 1.
- No other brain problem that might cause the symptoms.
- Tics must occur nearly every day, several times a day, for at least 1 year.
- Both motor and vocal tics must be present.

Treatment

If symptoms are mild, there may be no treatment. Antipsychotic medications that may be used to lessen the symptoms often have side effects worse than the symptoms, causing cognitive fog and movement issues. Clonidine, a blood pressure medication, has been used to reduce the tics. Tetrabenazine is a common medication used for Tourette syndrome, but it is linked with movement problems and depression.

Complementary Therapy

Some individuals respond to relaxation techniques, belly breathing exercises, and going to a private room to scream, yell, swing arms, and "let off some steam." There is some thought that quiet-mind computer games, crossword puzzles, and other high-concentration activities may lessen the symptoms.

⊕ CLIENT COMMUNICATION

It is important to educate and encourage clients with this syndrome. The public is not very accepting, may even be fearful, of someone with obvious tics. Clients are able to live a normal life and can learn how to minimize their symptoms as well as the public's reaction. The Tourette Syndrome Association may be of help: http://www.tsa-usa.org.

Prognosis

Symptoms of Tourette syndrome sometimes lessen with age. The disorder tends to be lifelong and chronic, but it is not degenerative. There is a normal life expectancy and normal intelligence in individuals with the syndrome.

Prevention

There is no known prevention for Tourette syndrome other than genetic counseling for those at risk.

CHAPTER EPISODE—PART IV

As the time passes, Josh grows fairly normally but has some physical and developmental delays. He does not walk, talk, or play like most children. He was almost impossible to potty train. He has no heart abnormalities, but he does have digestive issues, including Hirschsprung disease; poor vision; and poor hearing. His language skills, when they do develop, are poor and he is hard to understand. Speech therapy helps.

- What services will this family most likely need in Josh's life?
- What is the future for Josh?

SUMMARY

The introduction stated that congenital diseases and disorders affect the entire family and all caregivers. Health-care professionals tend both to the afflicted and to the parents and caregivers. There is a tendency, especially in congenital problems, for guilt. Also, treatment and care are often arduous and lengthy. Referrals to appropriate support systems may be especially helpful. With increased medical knowledge and understanding of genetic difficulties, more and more disorders appear to have a genetic link. Throughout the remainder of this text, a number of other diseases and disorders will note a possible genetic link.

 DavisPlus | For more resources and to sharpen your skills with interactive exercises, visit Davis*Plus* at http://davisplus.fadavis.com. Keyword *Tamparo*.

ONLINE RESOURCES

American Heart Association
http://www.heart.org

Cleft Palate Foundation
http://www.cleftline.org

Cystic Fibrosis Foundation
http://www.cff.org

Muscular Dystrophy Association
http://www.mda.org/disease/DMD.html

National Down Syndrome Society
http://www.ndss.org

National Organization on Fetal Alcohol Syndrome
http://www.nofas.org

Spina Bifida Association
http://www.spinabifidaassociation.org

United Cerebral Palsy
http://www.ucp.org

CASE STUDIES

Case Study 1

Nathan, who was born with a cleft lip and palate, is abandoned by his drug-dependent mother and unknown or unidentified father shortly after birth. Social services personnel place the infant in a foster home where the caregivers have experience with special needs children. In a short time, specialists rule that surgery is necessary. After three operations, Nathan's congenital defect is very difficult to detect.

Case Study Questions

1. What might have happened if Nathan's mother had kept him?
2. What future complications might Nathan's caregivers anticipate?

Case Study 2

Alison and Jordan are considering having their first child. Close friends of theirs have a child who was born with serious heart defects. They have some fears about birth defects and the costs of any necessary treatment.

Case Study Questions

1. What resources could you recommend for them to read?
2. Would you advise that they speak to a specialist?
3. How might they research their health-care insurance coverage?

REVIEW QUESTIONS

Matching

Match each of the following definitions with its correct term.

Spinal cord defects

_____ 1. Incomplete closure of one or more vertebrae

_____ 2. Incomplete closure of vertebrae with protrusion of spinal fluid and meninges into the sac

_____ 3. External sac that contains meninges, cerebrospinal fluid, and a portion of the cord and nerve roots

a. Meningomyelocele

b. Meningocele

c. Spina bifida occulta

Congenital defects of the heart

_____ 4. Abnormal opening between the two atria

_____ 5. Failure of the fetal ductus arteriosus to completely close

_____ 6. Abnormal opening between the right and left ventricles

_____ 7. Localized narrowing of the aorta

a. Ventricular septal defect

b. Atrial septal defect

c. Coarctation of the aorta

d. Patent ductus arteriosus

e. Tetralogy of Fallot

Short Answer

1. What are the two types of orofacial clefts?
   _____ and _____

2. What is the characteristic symptom in pyloric stenosis? _____

3. The abbreviation TEF is used for what disorder?
   _____

4. What does PKU stand for? _____
   Describe the treatment.
   _____
   _____

5. Can you name at least three congenital defects of the ureter, bladder, and urethra?
   _____
   _____

6. What are the four most common forms of clubfoot or talipes?
   _____
   _____

7. What are the three forms of congenital hip dysplasia?
   _____
   _____

8. What is the term used to identify Down syndrome that names the congenital defect?
   _____
   _____

9. What is the congenital disease that affects only males?
   _____
   _____

10. What is the classic symptom of Tourette syndrome?
    _____
    _____

Multiple Choice

Place a check next to the correct answer.

1. What do you recall about cerebral palsy?

   _____ a. It is caused by defective spinal cord development prior to birth.

   _____ b. It is marked by too much cerebrospinal fluid on the brain.

   _____ c. A neurological assessment is the first common diagnostic tool.

   _____ d. The condition is curable.

2. Can you name the signs and symptoms of cystic fibrosis?

   _____ a. Intestinal obstruction and wheezy respirations

   _____ b. Diarrhea and muscle aches

   _____ c. Tachycardia and skin infections

   _____ d. Productive cough and shallow breathing

3. What is known about cleft lip and palate?

_____ a. The defect may occur singly or together and vary in severity.

_____ b. It occurs in 1 in 10,000 births.

_____ c. The defect almost always occurs when the mother has diabetes.

_____ d. The defect is usually corrected in one surgery.

4. How might you best describe an omphalocele?

_____ a. It is a birth defect in which the umbilical cord comes out of the navel.

_____ b. It seems to occur more frequently during teenage pregnancy.

_____ c. It may be detected prior to birth through ultrasound.

_____ d. It is surgically repaired once the infant is about 3 months old.

5. What do you know about fetal alcohol syndrome?

_____ a. It is the result of the mother being addicted to street drugs.

_____ b. There will be almost no symptoms in a child.

_____ c. With treatment it can be quickly corrected with no complications.

_____ d. It is totally preventable.

Discussion Questions/Personal Reflection

1. What can individuals and/or families do to help prevent congenital diseases?

_____

_____

_____

_____

_____

_____

_____

_____

_____

_____

2. Discuss the difficulty that arises in prevention of fetal alcohol syndrome. How might health-care providers lessen the abuse of alcohol in pregnant women?

_____

_____

_____

_____

_____

_____

_____

_____

_____

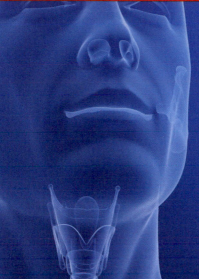

7

Mental Health
Diseases and Disorders

● *key words*

Alogia (ă•lŏ'jē•ă)
Amygdala (ă•mig'dă•lă)
Avolition (ă•vō•lĭsh'ŭn)
Catatonia (kăt"ă•tō'nē•ă)
Decompensate
  (dē•kŏm'pĕn•sāt)

Delusion (dē•loo'zhŭn)
Echolalia (ĕk•ō•lā'lē•ă)
Folate (fō'lāt)
Gustatory (gus'tă•tōr•ē)
Hallucination (hă•loo•sĭ•nā'shŭn)
Heritability (her"ĭ•tă•bĭl'ĭ•tē)

Intoxication (ĭn•tŏk"sĭ•kā'shŭn)
Intromission (ĭn"trō•mĭ'shŭn)
Mutism (mū'•tĭzm)
Serotonin (sēr"ō•tōn'ĭn)
Tolerance (tŏl'ĕr•ăns)
Withdrawal (wĭth•drăw'ĕl)

Upon successful completion of this chapter, you will be able to:

- Define key terms.
- Review the integration of health care and mental health care.
- Discuss the cost of mental health care.
- Explore stigma and safety in those with mental health disorders.
- Discuss the use of the *Diagnostic and Statistical Manual of Mental Disorders*, fifth edition (*DSM-V*).
- Define *mental status examination* (MSE).
- Discuss the use of the MSE tool.
- Describe the difference between nature and nurture.
- Recall the influence of culture, age, and gender in mental disorders and diseases.
- Compare the different types of depressive disorders.
- Review the affects of gender and age in depressive disorders.
- State the complementary therapies of depressive disorders.
- Compare and contrast two types of bipolar disorders.
- Name and discuss the different types of schizophrenia.
- Review the differences between a delusion and a hallucination.

- Define the four different types of anxiety disorder.
- Discuss the treatment of obsessive-compulsive disorder.
- Recall the impact of post-traumatic stress disorder on veterans.
- List the *DSM-V* criteria for a diagnosis of personality disorder.
- Discuss the difference between substance-use disorders and substance-induced disorders.
- Contrast the seven different drug classes of substance-related and addictive disorders.
- Assess the complementary therapies for substance-related and addictive disorders.
- Review the cause of intellectual disability (intellectual developmental disorder).
- Describe the symptoms of autism spectrum disorder.
- Recall incident rates for attention deficit-hyperactivity disorder (ADHD).
- Compare anorexia nervosa and bulimia nervosa.
- Compare and contrast the three different categories of sexual disorders for men and women.

CHAPTER EPISODE—PART I

Matt is a 24-year-old male who lives in Seattle, Washington. He is a college graduate but lost his job and is living at home. He has no health insurance but is currently a temporary employee at a construction site. He seems distant and withdrawn at times. After work, he comes home and isolates himself in his room. Matt's mother notices a hand tremor that he appears to be trying to control. He barely eats and is often upset when asked what he is doing. His friends call and say that they would like to see him, but he dismisses them. He does not seem to care that he has missed some job interviews. His mother offers to pay for him to see their primary care provider (PCP), believing that there could be something wrong with her son. Matt accepts.

- As a parent, would you be concerned or just think this is a phase Matt is experiencing? Explain your response.
- What is the PCP most likely to do during the examination?

INTEGRATION OF HEALTH CARE AND MENTAL HEALTH CARE

In the not too distant past, primary care providers and mental health specialists (psychiatrists, psychologists, nurse practitioners, physician assistants, social workers, and mental health counselors) had little in common and often did not agree on treatment protocols for anyone with a mental health problem. There seemed to be a total separation of the body from the mind in determining the etiology and establishing a diagnosis. The result has been a proliferation of community and professional organizations that have established family advocacy programs, substance abuse rehabilitation clinics, stress management seminars, school counseling, bereavement counseling, support systems, life coaching, and shelters for abused and battered women along with educational systems that provide training and information.

Today, primary care providers (PCPs) and mental health specialists work collaboratively in hospitals, community mental health centers, and family medical centers. This collaboration helps in diagnosing, treatment, and recovery. Mental health specialists readily recommend a physical examination from a PCP before treating a client with a mental disorder. Likewise, PCPs are more willing to refer clients to a mental health specialist in areas where counseling or psychotherapy is indicated. Specialists from the many community mental health resources are turning to both PCPs and mental health specialists for guidance and assistance. Additionally, there are a number of complementary therapies used in the treatment for many mental health disorders today. Always, these are best discussed among the primary care provider, the mental health specialist, and the client. Prior to taking any supplements or vitamins, it is especially important that the client first consult with the PCP and mental health specialist.

COST OF MENTAL HEALTH CARE

The National Institute of Mental Health (NIMH) reports 26.2% of the U.S. population is diagnosed with a mental health disorder each year. The World Health Organization (WHO), the World Bank, and Harvard University reported in the Global Burden of Disease Study in 2005 that mental health disorders will account for over 15% of the total burden of disease in 2020. According to WHO, those with a mental health disorder such as depression or schizophrenia will have a 40% to 60% higher rate of mortality than those without. This information alone suggests the same need for integration of health care between PCPs and mental health specialists as is suggested here in this text for traditional and nontraditional medical therapies.

State and local representatives, with little understanding of the issues involved and with no training to make wise decisions regarding mental health, have decreased funding of mental health programs. Concerns arise about the legitimacy of mental health and the discrimination or stigma of those with mental health disorders. One issue is that fewer health insurance programs provide adequate coverage for clients suffering with mental health issues. In an effort to fill this gap, some employers offer Employee Assistance Programs (EAP), separate from what insurance programs offer, to help employees seek mental health treatment. Also, communities, religious and spiritual institutions, schools, hospitals, colleges, and some businesses have developed resources and support for those with mental health issues in their families.

Currently, mental health focuses on "recovery" rather than "cure," as is found in most medical health care. *Recovery* is the term often used with drug and alcohol addiction but has now found its place within the treatment for most mental health disorders. Recovery is a way to express that clients are never fully cured from a mental health issue but have developed skills to successfully live in and contribute to their environment and social support network, allowing them to lead functional lives in society with the help of PCPs. Recovery is often lifelong, creating a financial burden quite unlike the "cure" method of medical treatment.

Mental Health Insurance Coverage

Mental health disorders are treatable; however, insurance benefits for mental health vary among plans and employers as well as within states, which may provide only standard and/or minimal coverage for treatment of mental health disorders or substance abuse and dependence. According to a recent study by the National Alliance on Mental Illness (NAMI), only 17% of respondents indicated that their insurance covered mental health adequately. Mental health care usually incurs higher deductibles and copays for coverage on certain types of disorders. Changes are being made, however.

As of 2014, the Mental Health Parity Act (MHPA), established in 1996 and updated in 2008, requires that mental health and addiction issues have the same insurance benefits as medical and surgical benefits. In January 2014, enrollment for insurance coverage provided medical, mental health, and substance-abuse treatment due to the MHPA. However, over 6 million people in the United States, due to states choosing to not participate in the MHPA, still are uninsured and are not allowed access to these insurance benefits today. Under the Federal Patient Protection and Affordable Care Act of 2010, "mental health and substance use disorder services, including behavioral health treatment" are to be considered "essential health benefits." These benefits would include ambulatory client services, hospitalizations, and prescription drugs. There are likely changes in how Medicare and Medicaid clients will receive mental health coverage, yet over 4 million citizens do not have access to the new Medicaid Expansion program mostly because not all states in the United States participated in the program. There are some ways to increase insurance coverage by exploring medical savings accounts (MSAs), health savings accounts (HSAs), and flexible spending accounts as options for nonmedical needs, such as mental health and substance abuse and dependence treatment needs.

Stigma, Safety, and Access to Mental Health Treatment

Mental health issues are commonly reported in the media and usually associated with a stigma and violence. *Stigma* is defined as a negative belief around a personal trait, such as a mental health disorder or substance-abuse disorder. Those who have mental health issues are often stigmatized because there is a belief that they cannot accomplish certain tasks or are violent/dangerous and because of ignorance of the disorder. It is important to know that violence may be increased with those who suffer from a mental health issue, and the potential for violence may be increased in those who suffer both a mental health disorder and a substance-related disorder. However, people diagnosed with a mental health disorder are up to 11 times more likely the victims of violence than those who do not suffer from a mental health disorder.

Mental health disorders can be treated in mental health communities and medical facilities as well as inpatient settings specifically designed to help those who cannot be safe or take care of themselves in the community. These inpatient settings provide both voluntary and involuntary treatment and medication to help in recovery and to stabilize a client. Even though inpatient settings can provide an appropriate level of care for clients unable to care for themselves, access to inpatient treatment is currently seriously limited, and it falls primarily to community mental health programs, hospital emergency rooms, and community medical clinics to provide structure and safety. Many cities in the United States are lacking available inpatient beds for mental health clients to receive the treatment necessary to ensure stabilization and safety. It is important to remember that it is more common for those with mental health issues to harm themselves than others.

DIAGNOSTIC PROCEDURES

Diagnostic procedures identified in this chapter are brief and are not intended to provide specific procedures such as those detailed in the *Diagnostic and Statistical Manual of Mental Disorders*, fifth edition (*DSM-V*). This text, published by the American Psychiatric Association (APA), provides a helpful guide with diagnostic criteria and classifications that enable clinicians and investigators to diagnose, communicate about, study, and treat people with various mental disorders using a common foundation. Since the *DSM-V* was published in May 2013, there have been impacts on insurance claims due to changes in the diagnosis and criteria for some mental health and substance-related disorders. The *DSM-V* contains both ICD-9-CM and ICD-10-CM coding.

MENTAL STATUS EXAMINATION

Primary care providers, mental health specialists, and complementary therapy practitioners use a mental status examination (MSE) in their assessment of clients with a suspected mental disorder. The MSE is a set of observations and impressions of the client obtained during a short question-and-answer examination. The general components of an MSE are summarized here:

- Appearance: gender, age, ethnicity, apparent height and weight, any physical deformities, grooming, hygiene, gait, motor coordination, posture, noteworthy mannerisms
- Speech: speed, volume, amount, clear, coherent, includes profanity, animated/excited, difficulty finding words, poor articulation
- Motor activity: movement, ability to move, and type of movements
- Manner and approach: interpersonal characteristics, such as congenial, guarded, open/candid, cooperative, withdrawn, distant, annoyed, engaging, hostile, shy, relaxed, cautious, resistant, defensive, English as primary language, other languages used
- Mood: happy, sad, despondent, irritable, anxious, depressed, hopeless
  - Suicide assessment is part of this section, if a client's mood is hopeless; if a suicide assessment is warranted, an inquiry is made if the client has a plan and the ability to implement the plan.
- Affect: emotional presentation, such as constricted, blunted, labile, flat (appropriate, strength, duration, range)
- Perceptions: the way a client views his or her environment and/or situation
  - **Hallucinations,** or false perceptions (perceiving something or someone that is not really there)
- Thought content: subjects of a client's thoughts
  - **Delusions,** or false beliefs (beliefs held in the face of strong contradictory evidence)
- Thought process: patterns, if any, of a client's thoughts
- Level of consciousness: orientation, cognitive ability
  - Assesses three specific areas: Is the client oriented to person (What is your name?), place

(What city are we currently in?), time (What is today's date?)
- Memory: the ability to recall and/or retain information
- Level of concentration and calculation: ability to perform basic calculations
- Information and intelligence: educational level, literacy
- Judgment: decision-making and relationships with other people and things

These components help identify signs and symptoms that can be related to a mental health diagnosis. MSEs can be very useful in multiple settings and can be used throughout interactions to assess a client's ability to accept and understand the information that is given.

NATURE VERSUS NURTURE

In the past decade, increased research points to a biological or genetic cause of many mental health illnesses. DNA research is still in its infancy, but increased evidence shows the importance of nature and genetics in many of the diseases and disorders presented here. NIMH reports that a recent study found there were chromosomal variations leading to **heritability** (genetic or inheritable trait) in five mental health disorders: schizophrenia, bipolar disorder, major depressive disorder, autism spectrum disorders, and attention deficit-hyperactivity disorder. This research suggests that it is common for people who have been diagnosed with schizophrenia to also receive a diagnosis of other mental health disorders, including anxiety, depression, and substance-related and addictive disorders. This evidence does not negate the importance of nurture, however. How a child is nurtured, what traumatic events that child experienced, and how those events were dealt with by family members and caregivers have lasting effects on children. Children's minds are an open vessel for every event that is recorded in their brain for future reference. For example, if a child is reared in an environment where there is a great deal of anxiety, the child is likely to show symptoms of stress or to express anxious behavior. *Nature* or *genetic makeup* is already determined and is still difficult or impossible to alter. *Nurture*, however, is continually influenced by other individuals and their own influences and preferences.

CULTURE, RACE, AGE, AND GENDER

Probably more than in other diseases and disorders, culture and its influence are critical to individuals with mental health issues. Individuals with a mental health

disease or disorder can benefit from individuals, including family members, who understand their ethnic background. Immigrants coming to the United States from another country often settle in clustered groups of similar populations. While this may be beneficial for support, it only delays their integration into the whole of society and can make any required treatment more difficult. Within specific cultures, the presentation of symptoms often reflects the culture and belief systems. Access to proper treatment may be additionally influenced by culture and race, stigmatizing the disorder or viewing that it is unnecessary. Age knows no limits in mental illness. Alcohol and drug problems are seen as early as age 8. Mental health issues in the elderly are often ignored in the belief that treatment would be difficult and that most expect to have some mental health issues as they grow older. Many of the diseases and disorders reflect gender bias; many afflict women more often than men. Men are more likely to restrict their access to appropriate treatment because they perceive a stigma attached to mental health care. Whether it is culture, age, or gender, each has an impact on the client's accessibility and response to treatment.

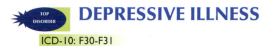

Mental Health Disorders

DEPRESSIVE ILLNESS

ICD-10: F30-F31

Description

Nearly 22 million U.S. adults have a depressive illness. WHO predicts that by 2020 depression will be the second leading cause of disability worldwide. The economic cost of depression is enormous, but the cost in human suffering is beyond estimation. Depressive disorders affect the body, a person's moods, and thoughts. They are not a passing "blue mood." They are not a sign of personal weakness, and people cannot merely "pull themselves together." There are various types of depressive disorders, but they are characterized by sadness, emptiness, lack of motivation, and inability to function well. Most people who suffer from depression do not seek treatment, but those who do, even those with severe depression, can be helped. Many years of fruitful research have introduced new medications and psychosocial therapies that help ease the pain of depression.

One form of depressive disorder that is commonly diagnosed is major depressive disorder (*DSM-V: F32.X*, F33.X**), which causes individuals to have feelings of worthlessness, despair, guilt, and hopelessness. They have difficulty in working, studying, sleeping, and

*The X represents the fourth digit that is often required and supplied once more detailed information about the disease or disorder is made known to the provider.

enjoying life's pleasures. Major depression occurs in up to 16.5% of adults and affects all racial and ethnic groups and both genders. Average age of onset is 32 years old. About one-half of depressed clients have only a single episode of depression; the rest have more than one occurrence. Major depressive disorder can profoundly affect all facets of a person's life. The most serious consequence of this form of depression is suicide, which occurs when the feelings of despair are so great that an individual believes is no longer a reason to go on living.

The following are specific major depressive disorder types, each with unique signs and symptoms, during a specific time or situation:

- *Major depressive disorder with peripartum onset* was previously known as *postpartum* or *paternal postnatal depression* (PPND). PPND affects roughly 14% of the population during and following childbirth. It generally affects women more than men. Yes, fathers suffer from postpartum depression, too, often in isolation, because many health-care providers are not aware of the problem. Some studies indicate that 10% of men have major depressive disorder with peripartum onset. Rare forms of psychosis, including delusions or hallucinations, can occur. Generally, symptoms occur over weeks and months rather than during a brief period of time after childbirth and include mild to severe symptoms of loss of appetite, lack of joy in life, insomnia that creates an overwhelming fatigue, loss of interest in sex, difficulty bonding with the baby, thoughts of harming the baby or self, and feelings of guilt or shame.
- *Major depressive disorder with seasonal pattern* (previously known as *seasonal affective disorder [SAD]*) is believed to affect 5% of the population in its severe form. The seasonal pattern affects women more than men. In its milder form, depressive disorder with seasonal pattern affects about 14% of the population. Symptoms of SAD increase in fall and winter, decrease in spring and summer, and correspond with season changes. Clients complain that they sleep too much, have little energy, and crave sweets and starchy foods. They may also feel depressed. Scientists believe that a lack of sunlight, especially during winter when daylight is shorter, may be the cause. Exposure to a special type of light therapy for 30 minutes every day often helps.
- *Persistent depressive disorder (dysthymia) (DSM-V: F34.1)* is a less severe form of depression that involves long-term, chronic symptoms that last for at least 2 years. While the symptoms do not disable a person, they keep him or her from feeling good or from functioning well. Many people with this form of depression also suffer major depressive episodes at some time in their lives.

Suicide

In 2010, suicide was the 10th leading cause of death in the United States, yet suicides are less common than suicide attempts. For every 25 suicide attempts, there is one suicide. Suicide attempts are gestures toward harming oneself that can potentially lead to a person's death. Suicide and suicide attempts are more commonly seen in depression but are prevalent in other disorders, such as substance abuse. In 2010, suicide was more common in those who were between the ages of 45 and 64 years old, followed by those who were over age 85. Lastly, suicide has decreased in those between 15 and 24 years old. Suicide attempts are to be treated carefully and appropriately because a suicide attempt increases the likelihood of another attempt or an actual suicide. The Centers for Disease Control and Prevention (CDC) reports that suicide in men is four times more common than in women.

Etiology

There are many possible causes of depression. Major depression is often associated with changes in brain structure and function and seems to occur through generations, possibly making a genetic connection. Research has shown that a gene that helps to regulate **serotonin,** a chemical messenger in the brain, plays a role in depression. Decreased serotonin increases the likelihood of feeling depressed. Other possibilities include biochemical, physical, psychological, and social causes. Depression may be secondary to a medical condition, such as those seen with metabolic disturbances, endocrine disorders, nervous disorders, cancers, cardiovascular disorders, and many chronic or degenerative diseases. Some prescription drugs can cause depression. Anxiety, borderline personality disorder, and substance-related disorders can also cause depression.

Signs and Symptoms

The primary symptom is a predominantly sad mood, along with a loss of interest in pleasurable activities that lasts more than several days. Individuals may seem unhappy and apathetic, have difficulty concentrating, and be unable to finish tasks. Fatigue and insomnia can occur. Some individuals lose their appetite; others may want to eat all the time. Hallucinations or delusions can also occur. Other symptoms of major depressive disorder are catatonia, anxiety, and melancholy.

Diagnostic Procedures

For a diagnosis, at least five of the following symptoms must be present over a 2-week period and must represent a change from previous functioning:

- Persistent, sad, anxious, or depressed mood
- Diminished interest or pleasure in most activities

- Significant weight loss or weight gain
- Insomnia or excessive sleep nearly every day
- Agitated or reduced psychomotor activity
- Fatigue or loss of energy
- Inappropriate guilty feelings or feelings of worthlessness, hopelessness
- Diminished ability to concentrate, make decisions, remember
- Thoughts of death or suicide
- Persistent physical symptoms that do not respond to treatment

Depression in Women

Women experience depression about twice as often as men; hormonal factors are thought to be a major contributor to this increased rate. Menstrual cycle changes, pregnancy, miscarriage, postpartum period, perimenopause, and menopause are considered important factors. Stressful life events, additional work and home responsibilities, caring for children and aging parents, abuse, and poverty also may trigger depression. For example, 20% of women experience rape or attempted rape in their lifetime. Research indicates that women, more so than men, respond to stressors in a way that prolongs their feelings of stress, increasing their risk of depression.

Depression in Men

Men are less likely than women to admit to depression. The rate of completed suicide in men is nearly five times that in women and is even higher after age 70, reaching its peak after age 85. NIMH indicates that more than 6 million men have depression each year. Depression in men is often masked by the use of alcohol and drugs or by socially acceptable habits such as working excessively long hours. Men are more likely to exhibit symptoms of irritability, anger, and being discouraged.

Depression in Adolescents

Depression in this age group can be a response to many situations and stressors. Conflict with parents, fluctuating hormones, reaction to a disturbing event, feelings of low self-esteem, lack of self-identity, and feelings of no control in their lives or that "life sucks" all can be triggers to a depressive mood. Suicide attempts are more common in adolescents than in other groups (women, men, and elderly people). The CDC reports that suicide is rising in youth who identify as lesbian, gay, bisexual, or transgender. In 2001, the CDC conducted an investigation of suicide in schools and found that roughly 15% of high school students had thought about suicide. Only in the past two decades has depression in children and adolescents been taken very seriously.

Depression in Older Adults

The older adult population is increasing exponentially in the United States, currently accounts for 12% of the population. Diagnosis is difficult because some ordinary symptoms of depression, such as fatigue, loss of appetite, and sleep difficulties, may represent symptoms associated with the normal aging process. In general, depression often occurs with a medical issue, regardless of its severity. Depression in older adults, however, is a widespread problem and often goes undiagnosed and untreated. Treatment is focused on coordinating with PCPs and medical facilities, as well as reaching out to family members.

Treatment

Depression is difficult to treat, especially in children, adolescents, and older adults. A good diagnostic evaluation is necessary to determine the presence of depression and its appropriate treatment; this includes a complete physical examination and a review of the client's history and any symptoms presented. Treatment depends on the evaluation, but the primary treatments are drug therapy, psychotherapy, and in some cases, electroconvulsive therapy (ECT).

The primary medications used are the following antidepressants: selective serotonin reuptake inhibitors (SSRIs), serotonin and norepinephrine reuptake inhibitor (SNRIs), norepinephrine and dopamine reuptake inhibitor (NDRIs), atypical antidepressants, tricyclic antidepressants (TCAs), and monoamine oxidase inhibitors (MAOIs). The SSRIs have fewer side effects than the TCAs, but SSRIs must be used with caution because recent research indicates a higher risk of suicide rates and aggressive behavior due to clients' failure to follow the prescribing recommendations, causing an increase in neurotransmitter serotonin. Sometimes it takes a variety of antidepressants before an effective medication is found to treat the disorder. Sometimes dosages must be increased; in general, antidepressants must be taken regularly for 3 to 6 weeks before the full therapeutic effect occurs. Often individuals take themselves off the medication too soon, either because they are feeling better or because they think the drug is not working. Antidepressants should be taken and stopped only under the direct supervision of a qualified primary care provider or mental health specialist.

Individuals with depression may do well with psychotherapy or a combination of antidepressants and psychotherapy. Many therapists believe the best results are achieved with a combination of individual, family, and group therapy. "Talking" therapies help individuals gain insight into and resolve their own problems through verbal exchanges with the therapist or with others. Behavioral therapists help individuals learn how to obtain more satisfaction and rewards through their own actions and how to unlearn the behavioral patterns that contribute to or result from their depression. ECT is useful for individuals whose depression is severe or life-threatening or who cannot take antidepressants. In recent years, ECT has been much improved. A muscle relaxant is given to the client, and the ECT is administered under brief anesthesia. Electrodes are placed at precise locations on the head to deliver electrical impulses. The stimulation causes about 30 seconds of seizure within the brain. The person receiving ECT does not consciously experience the electrical stimulus. Typically, several sessions of ECT are given at the rate of 3 per week; each session may include multiple monitored treatments within 1 session for up to 12 treatments or 4 weeks.

Complementary Therapy

There has been extensive research of complementary therapies and treatments for depression, including exercise, yoga, acupuncture, meditation, and lifestyle changes. Simple use of light boxes and full-spectrum lightbulbs in light therapy has shown improvement of SAD symptoms during the fall and winter months where sunlight is not as prevalent. A new approach called transcranial magnetic stimulation (TMS) is similar to ECT; however, the client remains awake and does not need any form of anesthesia. TMS stimulates the left prefrontal cortex where depression has been isolated in the brain. A coil transmits a pulse only centimeters into the scalp and brain in specific areas to stimulate neurons in the brain that affect mood and affect. The treatment can take several weeks; however, it is not yet covered by health insurance. TMS may also be used in the treatment of other mental health disorders.

St. John's wort is an herb that has been used extensively in the treatment of mild to moderate depression in Europe. It should be noted, however, that the Food and Drug Administration (FDA) has issued a public health advisory that St. John's wort is contraindicated for any individuals who are taking medications for such conditions as AIDS, heart disease, depression, seizures, certain cancers, and rejection of transplants. Any herbal supplement should be taken only after consultation with a primary care provider.

The National Center for Complementary and Integrative Health (NCCIH) reports that the use of lavender as an aromatherapy may decrease depressive symptoms. The herbal supplement 5-hydroxytryptophan has shown some positive results in decreasing depression symptoms by affecting the serotonin level in the body.

Lifestyle changes can be done through incorporating healthy living, such as eating a well-balanced diet, exercising, encouraging sleep hygiene, and creating a routine for daily living. It may be done in conjunction with medications and psychotherapy, but some individuals find initial benefit from attempting to change their lifestyle in order to cope with their depressive symptoms. Reducing or stopping alcohol or drug use is important. Sleep hygiene is used to maintain a wake and sleep pattern by regulating when you fall asleep and when you wake. Developing a routine can help stabilize emotions and create a sense of purpose to help alleviate hopelessness, focus, and memory issues. Self-hypnosis has also been an effective treatment of mild to moderate depression.

 CLIENT COMMUNICATION

Appropriate diagnosis and treatment are important. Individuals are encouraged to continue treatment until symptoms abate. Regular follow-up care should be provided so that adjustments can be made in treatment as necessary. Individuals suffering from depression require understanding, patience, affection, and encouragement. A depressed person may need diversion or companionship, but too many demands can increase feelings of failure.

Prognosis

Good results can be obtained with the proper treatment of mild and moderate depression. Major depression may require long-term or lifelong treatment, but improved quality of life is possible. Suicide is an ever-present risk, especially in severe cases, and all precautions should be taken to prevent it.

Prevention

Some episodes of depression can be avoided by practicing effective stress management techniques, avoiding drugs and alcohol, exercising regularly, and maintaining good sleep habits. These practices increase the activity levels and socialization of clients, which help reduce isolation and hopelessness, the main symptoms of depression. These preventative techniques also enhance generalized physical health and functioning. Many episodes of depression are not preventable, however. Treatment, including medications and psychiatric intervention, may prevent recurrences.

BIPOLAR

ICD-10: F31.X

Description

Bipolar disorder, also called *manic-depressive disorder*, is characterized by cycling mood changes from severe highs (mania) to severe lows (depression). Sometimes the mood switches are dramatic, but more often they are gradual. From high to low, from recklessness to listlessness—these are the extremes associated with bipolar disorder, a mental illness that can be serious and disabling. These mood swings may last for weeks or months, causing great disturbances in the lives of those affected and those of family and friends. The suicide rate is very high among those with bipolar disorder; studies show that roughly 15% to 50% of those diagnosed with bipolar disorder will attempt suicide.

Bipolar disorder is classified in two main subtypes:

- Bipolar I disorder (*DSM-V:* F31.X): Clients have at least one manic episode with or without previous episodes of depression.
- Bipolar II disorder (*DSM-V:* F31.81): Clients have at least one episode of depression and at least one hypomanic episode that is not as severe or long-lasting as a manic episode. In hypomania, clients generally continue to function in their daily routine. In bipolar II disorder, the periods of depression are typically much longer than the periods of hypomania.

Etiology

The cause of bipolar disorder is essentially unknown. However, biochemical brain activity, genetic tendencies, and environmental influences are suspect in the cause and triggering of bipolar episodes. Brain scans show that the biochemical activity in the brain of a person with bipolar disorder is different than those without. The prefrontal cortex, used to regulate emotions and decision-making, is shown to function less than those who do not have bipolar disorder. Bipolar often is genetic and runs within families, yet within studies of twins, with obviously shared genetic material, one may develop bipolar while the other does not. This leads researchers to believe that there is an increased environmental factor contributing to the development of bipolar disorder. Environmental influences in bipolar disorder can include stress and seasonal patterns.

Signs and Symptoms

Symptoms are exhibited by an alternating pattern of emotional highs (mania) and lows (depression). The intensity of symptoms varies from mild to severe; there can be periods when there are no symptoms. A more severe form of bipolar disorder is rapid-cycling bipolar disorder, which is diagnosed as having four or more episodes of depressive or manic symptoms in a year.

When in the depression cycle, an individual can have all of the symptoms of a depressive disorder. These include insomnia, fatigue, sadness, hopelessness, anxiety, guilt, loss of interest in activities, irritability, and suicidal thoughts or behavior.

In the manic cycle, the individual may be overactive, talk too much, have enormous energy, have an inflated self-esteem, become aggressive or agitated, express an increased sexual desire, and experience an inability to concentrate. Mania can affect thinking, judgment, and social behavior in ways that can cause serious problems and embarrassment. For instance, the individual in this phase may make unwise business decisions or create grand schemes that are difficult to fulfill and create financial burdens due to not thinking clearly. Manic individuals report minimal sleep or inability to sustain sleep for long, but this can also be a trigger for manic symptoms as well. Untreated, mania may worsen to a psychotic state.

Diagnostic Procedures

The depressive episode of bipolar disorder is diagnosed the same as for depression and is dependent on the following: a distinct period of abnormally elevated, expansive, or irritable mood lasting at least 1 week. Three (or more) persistent symptoms must also be present, such as inflated self-esteem or grandiosity, decreased need for sleep, unusual talkativeness, racing thoughts, distractibility, increase in goal-directed activity, and engagement in pleasurable activities with a high potential for painful consequences. It can also be reviewed by keeping mood charts and sleep and wake patterns to determine if or what type of bipolar disorder is diagnosed. Another component is to rule out other disorders and review substance-related and addictive disorders to ensure proper diagnosis.

Treatment

The primary goal of treatment is to decrease the episodes of both depression and mania. It is important to gain awareness of when a person moves between depressive and manic symptoms by watching for triggers, such as life stressors and environmental factors. Treatment may involve family and support systems to help recognize these shifts in moods and help to reinforce the need for treatment, as mania can be seen as positive in patients with bipolar disorder. Creating systems for monitoring mood shifts, suicidal thoughts, and risky behaviors is another way to help the individual gain control over his or her bipolar treatment. Treatment is lifelong and includes maintenance treatment during periods of remission. Major treatment includes medications (often taken for life), psychotherapy, and ECT. Medications include mood stabilizers, atypical antipsychotics, and antidepressants. Atypical antipsychotics and antidepressants are often used in conjunction to reduce mood swings. Psychotherapy is aimed at educating the individual on their mood swings and to help create a system to reduce stressors and develop coping strategies. Sometimes, clients are admitted for inpatient treatment to help stabilize their moods and identify medications that decrease symptoms.

Complementary Therapy

See "Depression."

CLIENT COMMUNICATION

Encourage clients to remain on their medications or stay involved in their designed treatment plan. It is a myth that clients do not take medications because they do not want to recover. Clients who have bipolar disorder have positive feelings associated with the initial "high" of manic symptoms, such as heightened energy, positive self-esteem, and increased sexual drive; therefore, they do not want to take medications and follow their treatment. It can also be difficult for families and support systems to cope with these behaviors and they may withdraw as the problems increase. Problems often arise when individuals stop all treatment during a remission cycle.

Prognosis

Left untreated, clients may suffer severe emotional and even legal and financial problems in their lives. Complications include suicide, substance and alcohol abuse, legal and financial problems, poor school or work performance, and difficulties in relationships.

Prevention

There is no known prevention for bipolar disorder. However, treatment at the earliest sign of difficulties can help prevent bipolar disorder from worsening.

SCHIZOPHRENIA

ICD-10: F20.XX

Description

Schizophrenia spectrum disorders (*DSM-V:* F20.XX) involve altered sensory perception with physical and psychological changes that affect brain functioning, behavior patterns, and all five senses. In the United States, approximately 2.4 million adults have schizophrenia. It is the most chronic and disabling of the severe mental illnesses. People with schizophrenia often experience frightening symptoms, such as hearing internal voices (hallucinations) or believing that others are controlling their thoughts or plotting to harm them (delusions). Schizophrenia generally is diagnosed during adolescence or in the early 20s or 30s. A "first break" is described as those who experience a hallucination or delusion at the initial onset of schizophrenia. Overall, men are more affected than women. Schizophrenia appears at an earlier age in men than in women. It is rarely diagnosed in children.

One unique form of schizophrenia is schizophrenia with catatonia. **Catatonia** (a marked psychomotor disturbance) is marked by extreme negativism, **mutism** (not speaking), and excessive motor activity that does not make sense or have purpose and is not necessarily influenced by any external stimuli. They experience **echolalia,** which is a pathological, senseless repetition of a word or phrase just spoken; it is a parrotlike repetition. During some periods, affected persons will need close supervision because they can harm themselves or others. Another form of schizophrenia is schizoaffective disorder (*DSM-V:* 295.70), where persons may not exhibit all the symptoms of schizophrenia and mood disorders but are psychotic with or without a mood component, such as bipolar or depressive type.

Etiology

Possible etiologic theories of schizophrenia include the following:

- *Genetic theory:* The actual genetic defect has not been identified, but it is believed that a potential location is on chromosomes 13 and 6. Predisposing genetic factors include intrauterine starvation, viral infections, and perinatal complications. Studies of families, twins, and adoptive parents show increased risk for the disease in people with first-degree relatives (biological parents and siblings) with schizophrenia. In fact, a person with a parent or sibling with schizophrenia has an approximately 10% risk of developing the disorder compared with a 1% risk for a person with no family history.
- *Psychodynamic neurobiological theory:* Research studies of living and postmortem brains of people with schizophrenia show decreased brain volume and abnormal functioning. Neurochemical studies reveal alterations in neurotransmitter systems. In neurodevelopment, studies have shown that there are functional, structural, and chemical brain deviations in those with schizophrenia, and such deviations can be found long before the diagnosis is made. It is unknown if these are genetic or environmental in nature or a combination of both.
- *Diathesis stress theory:* This theory states that symptoms develop on the basis of a relationship between the amount of stress a person experiences and the individual's internal stress tolerance. Schizophrenia is a disorder that both causes stress and can be exacerbated by it.

Signs and Symptoms

Two or more of the following signs and symptoms must be present for at least 1 month, allowing for a significant amount of time for the diagnosis of schizophrenia to be made: delusions, hallucinations, disorganized speech, disorganized or catatonic behaviors, and negative symptoms. To accurately diagnose schizophrenia, a person must have delusions, hallucinations, or disorganized speech. The signs and symptoms are classified as both positive (those that are excessive or distortions of normal functions) and negative (those that reflect a loss of or decrease in normal functions). Positive symptoms include hallucinations, delusions, and disorganized speech; negative symptoms include flat affect, **alogia** (inability to speak owing to a mental condition or symptoms of dementia), attention deficit, and **avolition** (decreased motivation). Hallucinations are perceptions that no one else experiences. They affect one or several of the senses: auditory, visual, olfactory, tactile, **gustatory** (associated with the sense of taste or eating), and general somatic sensations. The most common hallucination is auditory, where the individual hears someone speaking to or around him or her.

People with schizophrenia are 90% likely to have a delusional component to their illness. Delusions can be bizarre and have a variety of themes. There are six different types of delusions: persecutory (belief of being harmed), referential (belief that everything pertains to them), grandiose (belief of heightened capability or fame), erotomanic (belief that someone is in love with them), nihilistic (belief that they do not exist), and somatic (belief that health is not normal).

Diagnostic Procedures

A thorough genetic and family history is required to aid in the diagnosis. Computed tomography (CT) scans of the head and other imaging techniques (magnetic resonance imaging (MRI) or positron emission tomography (PET) may identify some changes associated with the disorder and may rule out other neurophysiological disorders. Laboratory testing also rules out any abnormalities that may be contributing to the symptoms.

Treatment

Treatment includes psychotropic medications, psychotherapy, and counseling. Antipsychotic medications are primarily used to treat schizophrenia. Newer medications, called *atypical antipsychotics,* are effective in the treatment of psychosis, including hallucinations and delusions. There are oral and injectable forms of these medications. Some of the injectable forms are available on a bimonthly or monthly basis. Medication levels and dosages must be carefully monitored every 3 to 4 weeks. These medications may require as long as 1 month to show any improvements in symptoms. Long-term psychotherapy may be needed. Counseling focuses on establishing therapeutic relationships and educating clients on their disorder and on how they can cope. Stress and crisis management are essential, as is social skill development. People often suffer loss of employment and skills, and they suffer financially and in personal relationships. In order to have a better prognosis, treatment focused on assisting in these areas is key. Persons may identify an agent (a trusted person) to act on their behalf when they **decompensate** (failure or inability to act

appropriately in acute episodes of mental illness) or are hospitalized.

An advance directive may be formed with the client and caregivers so that clients, while at a maximum level of psychological health and well-being, can have a say in their course of treatment. Such directives are individual care plans for people with schizophrenia and are an effective way to not only involve clients in self-care but also provide the motivation for clients to continue with their care plan.

In the treatment of persons with schizophrenia, it is imperative that there is collaboration between medical and mental health practitioners. All health practitioners must focus on clients' rights while providing care that addresses their diverse communities and lifestyles.

Complementary Therapy

Acupuncture has proved useful in paranoid schizophrenia. In fact, in one study, hospital stays decreased after the initiation of acupuncture. Biofeedback, relaxation, and guided imagery are helpful in reducing stress associated with schizophrenia. If histamine levels are low, complementary therapists prescribe **folate** (a form of vitamin B complex) and nutrients. If histamine levels are high, calcium is given to help release excess histamine from body cells. New research from the Agency for Healthcare Research and Quality under the U.S. Department of Health and Human Services reports that significant findings show decreased symptoms of schizophrenia in participants who ingest foods with omega-3 fatty acids, such as various fish, nuts, and plants.

➔ CLIENT COMMUNICATION

Education of schizophrenia symptoms and treatment is critical. Clients must be taught the importance of strict adherence to the treatment regimen, especially taking the medications as prescribed. Clients may do well in a support system or day-care treatment. Encourage families to become involved in the client's care and treatment. Because of the chronic nature of the condition, it is important to educate clients about their illness, possible complications, and their specific treatment plan. It is important that clients understand their medications and trials of medications as well as to coordinate requests for changes in medications with their primary care provider or mental health specialist.

Prognosis

Recognizing the early signs and symptoms of schizophrenia improves prognosis. The prognosis varies; most improve with medication, but many experience functional disability and are at risk for repeated acute episodes.

Prevention

It is important to monitor the medication dosage and to encourage the client to continue the medication as prescribed—this is the best prevention. Continued participation in community support systems and vocational counseling is definitely beneficial. Some persons remain too disabled to live independently, requiring group homes or other long-term structured living situations.

CHAPTER EPISODE—PART II

Matt almost missed the appointment and would have if his mother did not remind him and bring him. Matt does not want his mother to be present in the appointment. Dr. Hart obtains a basic health history and reviews current issues. Matt reports no medical issues but says he smokes about 10 cigarettes a day. He also says he drinks about a six-pack or more of beer "every once in a while" and some hard liquor but "just to relieve stress." He tells the doctor he uses alcohol to relax. Dr. Hart notes that Matt appears slow to respond to questions, has difficulty recalling important facts, and sometimes loses track of time. The doctor also notices trembling and some agitation. Dr. Hart orders blood and urine tests for Matt and suggests he consider nicotine-cessation treatments and stop drinking to see if the tremors cease. Matt takes the information but declines treatment.

- What are the signs and symptoms that Matt is presenting?

ANXIETY

ICD-10: F40.XX

Description

Anxiety disorders are the most common mental health problem, affecting about 40 million adults in America. Women are more likely to develop anxiety symptoms and disorders, and anxiety disorders generally appear more commonly in people between the ages of 30 and 44 years old. Anxiety is rooted in the anticipation of a fear. Anxiety disorders can be terrifying and crippling and can affect a person's relationships with others and how they relate to their environment.

Etiology

Research shows that a combination of psychological and biological factors influence the development of an anxiety disorder. The causes may be unknown, but some theorists believe that conflict, whether intrapsychic, sociopersonal, or interpersonal, promotes an anxious state. Distressful events and major depression may also be causes. Anxiety disorders tend to run within families.

Signs and Symptoms

Anxiety disorders can be specific to an object, as is often seen in phobias, or they can be less specific, as in generalized anxiety and panic disorders. The following are types of anxiety disorders and their symptoms:

- *Generalized anxiety disorder* (GAD; *DSM-V:* F41.1): excessive and unrealistic worry lasting 6 months or longer with accompanying physical symptoms that might include muscle tension, gastrointestinal upset, heart palpitations, or headaches. Women are twice as likely as men to be afflicted.
- *Panic disorder* (*DSM-V:* F41.0): recurrent episodes of intense apprehension, terror, or impending doom. This is anxiety in its most severe form. Heart palpitations, chest pain, sweating, trembling, and a feeling of choking are a few of the symptoms. Women are twice as likely as men to be afflicted.
- *Obsessive-compulsive disorder* (OCD; *DSM-IV-TR:* F42): persistent, recurring thoughts that reflect exaggerated fear. Some thoughts are violent; others include worrying about contamination with dirt, germs, or feces. Some people perform ritualistic, repetitive, involuntary, and compulsive behaviors, such as counting, touching, hand washing, and repeated "checking" to make certain something is in place. Women are twice as likely as men to be afflicted.
- *Specific phobia:* a persistent and irrational fear of an object, an activity, or a situation that compels a client to avoid the perceived hazard. Individuals know the fear is irrational but are unable to control the fear. Phobias are one of the most common psychiatric disorders, affecting between 7% and 15% of the population. Severe anxiety occurs when a client is confronted with the feared object or situation. Some clients report dizziness, loss of bladder or bowel control, tachypnea, feelings of pain, and shortness of breath. Women are twice as likely to be afflicted.
- *Social anxiety disorder (social phobia):* fear of embarrassing oneself in most all public or social situations where someone may judge or observe them. People may avoid public situations where others may observe them, or they may isolate or restrict their functioning, as they cannot do basic, everyday tasks outside of their home. Men and women are affected equally but differ in the types of social situations that trigger the anxiety.
- *Agoraphobia:* a fear of being in one of five situations: public transportation, open spaces, enclosed places,

standing in line or a crowd, or being outside of the home alone. These situations are then avoided, as they provoke fear and the fear that they cannot escape the situation. It is more common in women than in men.

- *Hoarding disorder:* difficulty letting go of or getting rid of possessions due to the inaccurate belief that they will use, need, or want them. Hoarding can include hoarding of animals. It is beyond what is considered collecting or a collection of items that people will display. It is common for people to not believe this is a problem; however, issues around sanitation and safety can compromise a person's ability to function in life.

Diagnostic Procedures

Symptoms and other conditions must be evaluated. Anxiety disorders must be determined by a person's inability to function properly in society (i.e., difficulty with work, relationships, and normal daily activities for a persistent period of time).

Treatment

Anxiety disorders are highly treatable, yet only about one-third of those with the disorder receive treatment. Singly or in combination, psychotherapy, cognitive behavioral therapy (CBT; a therapy to identify the relationship between emotions, behaviors, and cognitive responses), and medication therapy are effective treatments. Some clients also have depression, substance abuse, or both, which further complicates treatment. The goal of treatment is to help individuals function effectively. Antianxiety medications, antidepressant medications (SSRIs, tricyclics, and MAOIs), and beta blockers may help to relieve symptoms. Psychotherapy, specifically CBT, has proven effective in identifying triggers and ways to lessen the anxiety response to the triggers. Therapy may desensitize a person to the object that promotes anxiety. Many times people stop treatment as they believe they have failed, but patience is required in order to find the right combination of medications or psychotherapy.

Complementary Therapy

Practicing meditation and deep-breathing exercises may be helpful. Hypnotherapy is often beneficial. NCCIH reports that the kava plant has been shown to provide relief from some anxiety symptoms; however, the FDA reports that kava increases the potential for liver damage. Therefore, it is important that the client consults the primary care provider or mental health specialist before taking herbs or supplements. Kava may be taken in capsules, mixed as a powder in water or fruit juice, or steeped as a tea.

 CLIENT COMMUNICATION

It is helpful if a partner or close friend is supportive and encouraging of the person with an anxiety disorder. It is not helpful to tease or poke fun at an anxious individual. Recognize the anxiety as real and approach the person unhurriedly. Encourage active diversion through activities such as whistling, humming, counting, jogging in place, or using a stress ball to divert unwanted thoughts.

Prognosis

The prognosis is good when clients can learn to cope with their anxiety by finding diversions or becoming effectively desensitized to the stimuli through therapy and treatment.

Prevention

There is no known prevention other than avoidance of the stimuli.

TRAUMA- AND STRESSOR-RELATED DISORDERS

Description

In the United States, 8% of the population will develop a trauma and stressor-related disorder. These disorders occur when there is distress after a traumatic event. One reviewed here is post-traumatic stress disorder (PTSD; *DSM-V:* F43.10 or F43.12). PTSD is the psychological consequences that persist for at least 1 month after a traumatic event outside the realm of usual human experiences. Examples of traumatic events include events of war, terror attacks, serious accidents, physical assault, and rape. The types of trauma vary between men and women. Men are more common to experience assaults, combats, and disasters, whereas women are more likely to experience sexual assault or childhood abuse.

REALITY EPISODE

It is time for school. The school bus will arrive in 5 minutes. Kelsey, an 11-year-old, cannot decide whether to wear sneakers or loafers. Mom presses her about the time, but instead of making the choice and snatching her jacket off the hook by the door, she has a temper tantrum that quickly escalates into a full-blown panic attack. She misses the bus; Mom is going to be late for work.

This 11-year-old has obsessive-compulsive disorder (OCD). One of the issues in children with OCD is that they often are quite indecisive about fairly simple decisions.

What can Mom do now? Is there treatment for OCD?

Veterans and PTSD

PTSD is common among veterans. During their military service, veterans can experience a wide array of mental health disorders. PTSD is the most common mental health issue; it is found in about 20% of returning military personnel. Only half of those will seek treatment. In a 2008 study, The Mayo Clinic reported that the frequency of PTSD increases with multiple tours of combat. In 2007, NIMH reported that "male veterans have doubled the suicide rate of civilians." According to the Veterans Administration (VA) study in 2012, roughly 18% of those who committed suicide in the United States were veterans; however, roughly 23% of the total population could not be ruled out as veterans, so the low percentage is assumed to be higher. Those directly active in a war zone as well as military personnel in support roles outside the war zone can experience PTSD. The VA provides mental health assessments and evaluations for current military personnel; however, a number of difficulties are reported with its program. The following facts are identified by Veterans for Common Sense and Veterans United for Truth:

- Of the 24 million veterans in the United States, only about 8 million are enrolled in the VA.
- On any given night, there are as many as 154,000 homeless veterans on the streets of America—most suffering from PTSD.

Etiology

Obviously PTSD occurs when a person experiences some form of trauma, but the cause of why it hinders a person to the point of difficulty with functioning in life is not clearly known. Researchers are looking at genes and brain areas for help in identifying the causes and risks for those who may develop it. Several chemicals in the body are used in the brain to signal, produce, or create a fear response in the brain—serotonin, stathmin (a protein), and gastrin-releasing peptide. The **amygdala** in the brain is where emotional reactions are formed; it is being researched as to how these fear reactions and trauma reactions affect it to cause PTSD symptoms.

Signs and Symptoms

Symptoms may not occur for weeks or months after a traumatic incident and are common to start around the third month after exposure to trauma. Symptoms can vary in duration and severity. Individuals suffer flashbacks or nightmares, avoidance of the place related to the trauma, emotional numbing or detachment from others, and changes in emotional responses. Another piece of PTSD is dissociation or feeling detached from oneself. Some people report dissociative symptoms as though they are walking in a dreamlike state or blacking out, not remembering how they got to a specific place.

Diagnostic Procedures

To be diagnosed, a person must have at least one flashback or nightmare, at least three avoidant symptoms, and at least two changes in emotional responses. Symptoms must reach a level of difficulty functioning in many everyday tasks. Suicidal thoughts are common, as well as depression, excessive drug or alcohol use, or other related anxiety disorders.

Treatment

The primary treatments are use of psychotherapy, medications, or both. Psychotherapy is primarily "talk" therapy, which can be done individually with a therapist or psychiatrist or in group settings. Individually, people can learn coping skills and learn to identify symptoms, whereas in group therapy people can normalize and relate to others who have experienced similar symptoms and reactions. CBT can be done through exposure therapy, cognitive restructuring, or stress inoculation therapy. CBT's primary function is to learn to identify the fear and learn ways to cope with it. Eye movement desensitization and reprocessing (EMDR) has also been used to effectively treat PTSD symptoms. EMDR uses eye movements to help a client process and react to past trauma. Medication therapy includes antidepressants, antianxiety medications, and prazosin. Antidepressants that are primarily used are SSRIs, which are approved by the FDA for the treatment of PTSD. Antianxiety medications are used to help a person stabilize, sleep, and treat other anxiety symptoms related to PTSD, but they are not given long-term. Prazosin (Minipress) can help with insomnia and nightmares. It is not currently FDA approved but is being prescribed for PTSD symptoms and is used for treatment in community mental health and the VA.

Complementary Therapy

NCCIH indicates many complementary treatments for PTSD: meditation, such as chanting and development of mantras; acupuncture; yoga; or massage. The University of Maryland Medical Centers reports the effectiveness of emotional freedom technique (EFT), which includes tapping on acupuncture points. In addition, herbal supplements, such as omega-3 fatty acids, a daily multivitamin, coenzyme Q10, L-theanine, and melatonin can be helpful to some.

Prognosis

If the symptoms occur longer than 3 months, PTSD is considered chronic. If chronic, symptoms can lessen; however, it is unlikely for a complete recovery.

Creating a network of family and friends, effective coping strategies, and following a treatment regime when symptoms increase is essential to its prognosis.

Prevention

There is no known prevention. Researchers have been trying to identify medications to help target and prevent PTSD symptoms. They are comparing those who experience a shared or similar traumatic event but do not have shared PTSD symptoms.

PERSONALITY DISORDERS

ICD-10: F60.XX

Description

Personality disorders are a set or pattern of behaviors and experiences that prevent a person from maintaining healthy relationships with others and from adapting to the everyday situations in their environment. There is a persistent inability to cope with the demands and expectations of self, others, and life. The pattern is pervasive and continuous rather than episodic or of short duration. Personality is believed to be developed in early childhood and adolescence; therefore, onset of personality disorders occurs generally in childhood or adolescence, but it can occur in early adulthood as well. Symptoms can be moderate and functional to severe and dysfunctional in the way a person interacts with others and their environment. There is no known difference in most personality disorders between men and women (see "antisocial personality disorder" as the exception below) and race. In the general population, 10% have a diagnosed personality disorder. There are 12 specific types of personality disorders. Following are four of the personality disorders more commonly found in ambulatory care:

- *Antisocial personality disorder* (*DSM-V*: F60.2): pattern showing disregard for rights of others and violating those rights, lying, seduction, and manipulation. Roughly 1% of the population has antisocial personality disorder. It is found more often in men than women.
- *Borderline personality disorder* (*DSM-V*: F60.3): patterns of attention seeking and excessive emotions, self-destructive behavior, and profound mood shifts. Borderline personality disorder is found in 5.6% of the population. No notable difference between men and women.
- *Narcissistic personality disorder* (*DSM-V*: F60.81): pattern of lack of empathy, need for admiration and grandiosity. Roughly 6% of the population is diagnosed with narcissistic personality disorder.
- *Avoidant personality disorder* (*DSM-V*: F60.6): pattern of feelings of inadequacy, hypersensitivity

to negative criticism, social inhibition. Roughly 5% of the population has been diagnosed with avoidant personality disorder.

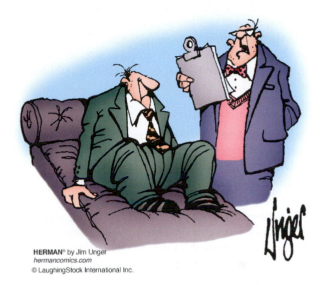

HERMAN® by Jim Unger
hermancomics.com
© LaughingStock International Inc.

"You are two completely different personalities. That'll be $100 each."

HERMAN© is reprinted with permission from LaughingStock Licensing Inc., Ottawa, Canada. All rights reserved.

Etiology

It is unclear what causes personality disorders; however, it is thought to be multiple factors. The etiologic theories are neurobiological factors, developmental factors, and sociocultural factors. Many researchers believe there is a genetic susceptibility or inherited biological link, especially in some of the more severe personality disorders. One study shows some structural brain dysfunction; other studies have shown a link to alcohol and drug abuse. The developmental factors indicate that early separation from parents, disturbed parental involvement, and child abuse may predispose a child to develop a personality disorder; however, child abuse and neglect by themselves are not sufficient to invoke a diagnosis. In fact, theories of family impact on personality disorders are highly controversial. It is known that sociocultural factors can influence a person's ability to establish and maintain relationships. Immigrants who move to another country may experience loneliness and alienation. Sometimes people form their own close-knit groups to help create relationships but may, in fact, erect barriers to the outside world, further alienating themselves.

Signs and Symptoms

Individuals with personality disorders are inflexible and maladaptive in their environment and have very few strategies for forming and maintaining relationships. Their patterns of behavior and communication evoke negative reactions from others. They lack resilience in day-to-day life and are often unable to adapt to changes in their world. As a consequence, they experience loneliness, withdraw, and become dependent on their jobs and their homes for their solace. Each specific type of personality disorder has its unique set of signs and symptoms in addition to those listed in the "Description" section.

Diagnostic Procedures

For a diagnosis to be made, the person must exhibit difficulties in at least two of the following areas: cognitive, affectivity, impulse control, and interpersonal functioning. It is important to establish a pattern of behavior from childhood or adolescence if a personality disorder is determined. A person's ethnic, cultural, and social background must be taken into account when diagnosing the disorder to ensure the patterns are indeed markedly deviant. In children younger than age 18, the signs and symptoms must be present for at least 1 year for a diagnosis to be made (except for antisocial personality disorder, as it cannot be diagnosed prior to age 18). Most clients with personality disorder also have depression, substance-abuse disorder, or both.

Treatment

Treatment is difficult and requires a trusting relationship among the client, primary care provider, and mental health specialist. The type of treatment is dependent on the client's signs and symptoms and their severity. In general, clients seek treatment for depression, anxiety, alcoholism, or difficulties at work or in their relationships. Several therapies are prominent. Moral recognition therapy is used in the treatment of antisocial personality disorder by raising a client's awareness of his or her decision-making process. Dialectical behavior therapy is effective for the treatment of borderline personality disorder by allowing clients to recognize their emotions and to develop skills to regulate them. Medication is generally not prescribed because it does not affect personality; however, if acute signs and symptoms or other mental health issues are present, medication can provide some relief. The goal of treatment is to help clients change their behavior and thinking that result from their personality traits or patterns. Whatever the treatment, it needs to be consistent and structured. The treatment will encourage expression of feelings, self-analysis of behavior, and accountability for actions. Family and other support persons need to be involved to address the maladaptive social responses. A treatment team approach is also best and would include a client's primary doctor, psychiatrist, therapist, social worker, pharmacy, family, support network, and others

involved in their treatment. In some forms of personality disorder, clients need protection from harming themselves.

Complementary Therapy

Some nutrients may be deficient; hence, complementary therapy practitioners may supplement those nutrients in consultation with the primary care provider. Biofeedback, relaxation, and guided imagery may prove useful to address the stress that clients experience.

⟶ CLIENT COMMUNICATION

Family members need to be involved in the treatment of clients. It is important to provide a supportive atmosphere and encourage clients to follow the individualized plan. Watch for signs of suicide or self-harm, and seek appropriate medical attention as needed. Remembering good boundaries and ethics guidelines is important when working with clients with personality disorders because the relationships they form can be tenuous and manipulative.

Prognosis

The prognosis depends on the type and severity of the personality disorder. Some personality disorders diminish as the person ages, whereas for others, lifelong treatment is required. If clients can learn to adapt to their environment and maintain appropriate relationships with a support system, prognosis is good. A variety of reports indicate that 15% to 30% of suicide attempts related to a personality disorder more commonly occur in women diagnosed with borderline personality disorder.

Prevention

There is no known prevention for personality disorder.

SUBSTANCE-RELATED AND ADDICTIVE DISORDERS

Description

Addictions to alcohol or psychoactive drugs are serious and chronic diseases that can be life-threatening. Both interfere with physical and mental health, family and social relationships, and occupational responsibilities. Addiction is a physical and psychological dependence on or need for a potentially harmful drug or alcohol. Addiction cuts across all social and economic groups, involves both genders, and occurs at all stages of the life cycle, beginning as early as elementary school. Table 7.1 provides a list of addictive substances. There are two groups: substance-use disorders and substance-induced

Table 7.1   Commonly Abused Substances

DRUG CLASS	DESCRIPTION	EXAMPLES
Opiates and narcotics	Powerful painkillers with sedative and euphoric qualities	Heroin Opium Codeine Meperidine Demerol Hydromorphone (Dilaudid) OxyContin Fentanyl
Central nervous system (CNS) stimulants	Stimulating effects and can produce tolerance	Amphetamines Cocaine Dextroamphetamine Methamphetamines (meth, speed, crank) Methylphenidate (Ritalin) Caffeine Nicotine Crack cocaine (crack)
CNS depressants	Produce a soothing sedative and anxiety-reducing effect and can lead to dependence; includes many prescription drugs	Barbiturates (amobarbital, pentobarbital, secobarbital) Benzodiazepines (Valium, Ativan, Xanax) Chloral hydrate Paraldehyde Alcohol Ephedrine Nitrous oxide Halothane Flunitrazepam (Rohypnol) Gamma hydroxyl butyrate Amyl nitrate Methaqualone
Hallucinogens	Hallucinogenic properties and can produce psychological dependence	Lysergic acid diethylamide Mescaline Psilocybin/psilocin Phencyclidine (PCP or "angel dust") 3,4-methylenedioxy-methamphetamine (MDMA) (ecstasy) Ketamine
Inhalants	Volatile solvents, gases, and nitrates that can be sniffed, huffed, bagged, or snorted to produce an effect	Nail polish remover Lighter fluid Gasoline Embalming fluid Markers Paint Paint thinner Glue Rubber glue Waxes Varnishes
Anabolic steroids	Any drug or hormonal substance chemically and pharmacologically related to testosterone (other than estrogens, progestins, and corticosteroids) that promotes muscle growth	Boldenone Fluoxymesterone Methandriol Methyltestosterone Oxandrolone Oxymetholone Trenbolone
Tetrahydrocannabinol (THC)	Although used for their relaxing properties, THC-derived drugs can also lead to paranoia and anxiety	Cannabis Marijuana Hashish

disorders. Substance-use disorders are a combination of symptoms related to cognitive, behavioral, and physiological symptoms. Two main features of substance-use disorders are **tolerance** (increased substance use to achieve previous effects) and **withdrawal** (negative physical symptoms that occur after periods of abstinence). Substance-induced disorders include two conditions: **intoxication** (recent ingestion of substance, significant behavioral or psychological changes) and withdrawal. Within the groups, there are specific substances that can be broken down into the following categories:

- *Alcohol-related disorders:* includes alcohol use disorder, alcohol intoxication, and alcohol withdrawal (*DSM-V:* F10.20). Drinking is most prevalent between the ages of 21 and 34, but about 19% of 12- to 17-year-olds have a serious drinking problem. Men are five times more likely than women to abuse alcohol. Alcohol abuse is a factor in approximately 41% of all traffic accidents.
- *Psychoactive drug disorders:* abuse of opiates or narcotics, tobacco, caffeine, stimulants, sedatives/hypnotics or anxiolytic (also known as *depressants*), tetrahydrocannabinol (THC), hallucinogens, and inhalants (see Table 7.1). Other drugs of abuse include over-the-counter (OTC) medications (i.e., cough syrup, antihistamines) and anabolic steroids.

The most dangerous form of any addiction or abuse is when users mix multiple drugs simultaneously—including alcohol. Also significantly lethal is the use of drugs and alcohol while taking prescribed medications that may have heightened side effects due to their combined use.

Understanding Fetal Alcohol Spectrum Disorder

Fetal alcohol spectrum disorder (FASD) is a condition caused by prenatal exposure to alcohol. FASD affects 2% of neonates born in the United States, which is roughly 84,000 children each year. FASD includes fetal alcohol syndrome (FAS), alcohol-related neurodevelopmental disorder (ARND), and alcohol-related birth defects (ARBD). FAS is the most typical form of the spectrum, whereas ARND and ARBD are less common and have some of the signs and symptoms of FAS. FAS is diagnosed by distinctive facial features, growth deficiencies, and brain damage as well as other behavioral or cognitive problems. Associated with FAS are learning disabilities (refer to "Disorders Generally Diagnosed During Childhood or Adolescence" later in this chapter). There is no known safe quantity or level of alcohol use to prevent or reduce the probability of FASD. The only proven prevention is abstinence from alcohol use. (Refer also to Chapter 6.)

Etiology

Numerous biological, psychological, and sociocultural factors appear to be involved in alcohol and psychoactive drug abuse. Biological factors may include genetic or biochemical abnormalities, nutritional deficiencies, endocrine imbalances, and allergic responses. It is estimated that about 50% to 60% of the variance in alcohol dependence is due to genetic factors. Individuals with alcohol-related disorders are six times more likely than nonalcoholic persons to have blood relatives who have alcohol-related disorders. Psychological factors may include the urge to drink or experiment with drugs to reduce anxiety or avoid the responsibilities of family, life, and work situations. There is also the desire to experience the temporary euphoria or "feel-good" state that allows individuals to experience pleasure. Individuals with addiction to alcohol and psychoactive drugs may have low self-esteem, experience peer pressure, and possess inadequate coping skills. Individuals tend to hide their dependence on either alcohol or drugs and may temporarily maintain function in their lives only to gradually have that ability disappear as dependence becomes greater. Sociocultural factors of addiction stem from cultural and societal norms and expectations; an example is peer pressure. Alcohol is commonly used in religious ceremonies and familial celebrations in many cultures; therefore, addictions can grow out of availability and acceptance of use for many people. There is also research linking violence and alcohol use; specifically, 67% of domestic violence cases have used alcohol prior to or during the incident.

Signs and Symptoms

- *Alcohol-related disorders:* Individuals are unable to control their drinking even when it becomes the underlying cause of serious harm, including medical disorders, marital difficulties, job loss, and traffic accidents. Individuals dependent on alcohol develop a craving that must be satisfied. They experience impaired control and are unable to stop drinking once they start. When they stop drinking after a period of heavy use, they experience unpleasant physical withdrawal symptoms that include nausea, sweating, shaking, and anxiety. They drink to stop these symptoms and thereby develop a greater tolerance for alcohol.
- *Psychoactive drug disorders:* Signs and symptoms of drug addiction depend on the particular drug and can include needle marks, scars from skin abscesses, rapid heart rate, constricted pupils, and a relaxed or euphoric state. Symptoms of nervous system stimulant dependence are similar except the pupils are dilated and the individual may be restless and hyperactive. Symptoms of hallucinogen dependence include anxiety, frightening hallucinations, paranoid delusions, blurred vision, dilated pupils, and tremor.

Diagnostic Procedures

Generally alcohol and drug use is not easily detected or indicated, as the goal of many users is to keep the use hidden or secret. Diagnosis can come from a PCP suspecting use and requesting that a client complete a client history evaluating use. A client history may reveal past substance abuse. Family can suspect use and will often encourage clients to seek treatment even prior to diagnosis. Self-report is another method of identifying a psychoactive drug or alcohol addiction. Another aspect is the use of prescription pills and running out too quickly of the prescription, thus implying overuse, which can lead to an addictive disorder. Toxicology screens on blood and urine can confirm the presence of alcohol and drugs in the body. In regular users, some drugs can be detected in urine up to 28 days.

Treatment

Total abstinence from alcohol and drugs is the only effective treatment. There are many programs aimed at detoxification, rehabilitation, and aftercare that can be helpful to both clients and involved families. Long-term successful treatment will also depend on individuals in recovery filling the place that alcohol or drugs once occupied in their life with something constructive. Research has shown that it may take multiple attempts for recovery, recognizing that each attempt toward recovery may lead to longer periods of abstinence. There are multiple types of treatment. They include hospitalizations, inpatient treatment centers, outpatient treatment centers, and support groups for addictions. A combination of medications and therapies is the most effective treatment. There are medicinal treatments for alcohol dependence such as naltrexone, acamprosate, and disulfiram, or those that reduce the pleasurable effects of alcohol or cause a negative reaction to its use. The National Institute on Drug Abuse reports methadone treatment reduces heroin use by 69%. Methadone and other medicinal treatments are controversial; some believe it is replacing one drug with another. The main component of methadone and medicinal treatments that is different from drugs of abuse is that tolerance and withdrawal factors are not associated with methadone and similar drugs. Other treatments for opioids are buprenorphine and naltrexone, but they are effective only in some people.

Some medications prescribed focus on the treatment of withdrawal symptoms and are temporarily used. For tobacco treatments, there are nicotine replacement therapies to help cut down cravings and reduce use of tobacco. Therapies such as cognitive behavioral therapies, motivational interviewing, and motivational incentives are the primary therapeutic treatments. Cognitive behavioral therapies focus on allowing a person to recognize, build skills, and avoid situations that may trigger use. Motivational interviewing focuses on the person's readiness to change their addictive behaviors that stop them from seeking treatment. Incentives are used in motivational incentives therapy to promote abstinence or reduce use. Treatments should include assessment of infectious diseases, such as HIV, hepatitis B and C, and tuberculosis, as well as education around risks and ways to reduce the potential for acquiring infectious diseases.

Complementary Therapy

Recent research in the field of addiction suggests that excessive craving for any substance indicates an allergic condition in relation to that substance. Therefore, abstinence is advised. Acupuncture has proven effective in treating cocaine, heroin, and crack addictions. It is most effective when used in conjunction with other therapies, including psychological counseling. Biofeedback and neurofeedback may be useful to bring about significant behavioral changes in the addictive personality. Some herbal medications may be useful in treating the symptoms of withdrawal. Yoga, specifically the components of mindfulness and self-discipline, has been used as a therapy approach to help those with substance-abuse issues.

➤ CLIENT COMMUNICATION

Substance abuse affects the entire family. Perhaps the best advice that can be given is to have everyone receive as much information as possible on substance abuse, its possible causes, and its treatments. There are support groups where families and other supports can learn about the disorder and also normalize their situations. Blame, shame, and guilt only worsen the problem.

Prognosis

Clients can recover with total abstinence from alcohol and drugs, but there is no cure. Fewer than 25% of those with alcohol dependence seek treatment for this disease. For all addictions, including alcohol, only 11% receive any treatment. Relapse after treatment is common, between 40% and 60%, so it is important to maintain support systems to cope with any slips and to ensure that they do not turn into complete reversals. Treatment programs have varying success rates, but many people with alcohol and psychoactive drug dependency make a full recovery.

Prevention

Abstinence from alcohol and drugs and replacement of the substance with constructive activities are essential. Support and encouragement of family members and a support group can be helpful, but ultimately a person in recovery knows that he or she alone is responsible for abstinence.

CHAPTER EPISODE—PART III

Dr. Hart asked Matt to return in 2 weeks for blood and urine test results and to check how he was doing. Dr. Hart's medical assistant, Andrea, has Matt complete a health questionnaire that includes questions about his drinking and tobacco use. Andrea notes that Matt appears to be sweating and anxious while completing the questionnaire. He finishes the questionnaire and the lab work.

- Do you see any reason to be alarmed about Matt? Justify your response.

Disorders Generally Diagnosed During Childhood or Adolescence: Neurodevelopmental Disorders

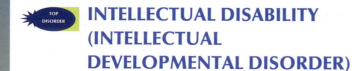

INTELLECTUAL DISABILITY (INTELLECTUAL DEVELOPMENTAL DISORDER)

ICD-10: F81.X

Description

Intellectual disability, also known as *cognitive disability* or *intellectual developmental disability* (*DSM-V:* F70, F71, F72, F73, F79), is a condition of significantly below-average intellectual functioning with concurrent deficits in adaptive behavior that exhibits itself generally before age 8. The IQ is approximately 70 or below on an individually administered test. It is the most common developmental disability, and it is estimated that 1% to 3% of the general population have intellectual disability to some degree. There are four types of developmental disability, defined by their degree of severity:

- *Mild intellectual disability:* 85% percent of those with intellectual disability fall into this category. Usually, these children develop their communication and social skills during preschool. On completion of high school, they usually achieve only at the sixth-grade level. This intellectual disability generally will be noticed in elementary grade schools. As adults, they can work but will need support to address social and economic stresses.
- *Moderate intellectual disability:* 10% of intellectually disabled persons are in this category. They achieve

second-grade level in education. Moderate supervision is required to take care of their personal needs, and additional support is needed for vocational training. They have difficulty in social and relationship situations. In adulthood, they can function in supervised settings.

- *Severe intellectual disability:* About 3% to 4% of those with intellectual disability fall into this category. During their early childhood years, they acquire little to no communication skills. In school, they learn elementary skills to care for themselves and learn to talk. In adult life, they live in group homes or with their families.
- *Profound intellectual disability:* About 1% to 2% of intellectually disabled individuals fall into this category. They generally have a neurological disorder that accounts for their intellectual disability. They display sensory motor function deficiencies in early childhood and require a caregiver and constant supervision.

Etiology

The exact cause of intellectual disability is known only in a small percentage of people. For example, in profound intellectual disability, a neurological problem is responsible, whereas the cause in the others forms may be a combination of factors. Other possible reasons include:

- prenatal causes such as hydrocephalus;
- chromosomal abnormalities such as in Down syndrome;
- metabolic causes such as phenylketonuria or Tay-Sachs disease;
- environmental causes such as cultural-familial retardation
- nutritional causes such as malnutrition;
- gestational causes such as prematurity
- infection, as seen in rubella
- intoxication such as exposure to lead poisoning, alcohol, cocaine, amphetamines, and other drugs;
- psychiatric disorders such as autism spectrum disorder;
- trauma such as mechanical injury, especially to the head.

According to the American Association of Intellectual and Developmental Disabilities, over 50% of intellectual disabilities have no known etiology.

Signs and Symptoms

In general, parents or pediatricians are first to note delays in the child's development. The child may show deviations in adaptive behaviors, experience learning disabilities, or have severe cognitive and motor skill impairment. Parents may be frustrated and exhausted with the child's lack of progress and development in communication, sensory, and motor skills. It is more common in males than in females.

Diagnostic Procedures

There are no laboratory tests to detect intellectual disabilities other than tests for the suspected neurological problem causing the disability. A psychological evaluation and an adaptive behavior evaluation are needed. The diagnosis is positive if a child is deficient in any two of the following areas: self-care, home living, communication, social/interpersonal skills, ability to use community resources, self-direction, functional academic skills, work, leisure, health, and safety. The diagnosis generally is given before the child reaches age 18.

Treatment

Treatment requires a team approach that builds on the client's strengths. The treatment focus is to develop skills in adaptive skills, communication, social, and motor areas. Special education classes are available, and many community resources can benefit families who have a child with intellectual disability. A good support network and socialization are important for treatment.

Complementary Therapy

No significant complementary therapy is indicated.

✈ CLIENT COMMUNICATION

Parents may be overwhelmed with caring for an intellectually disabled child, so support of the parents is essential. They also may need financial resources. If the child has an associated disability, special education may be necessary, and a referral should be made when the disability is first noted. The earlier education and training are available, the better the prognosis, in most cases. If the child is severely intellectually disabled, the family may need counseling, education, and support for the home care required for the child or possible institutional placement as the child ages and functioning decreases.

Prognosis

The prognosis depends on the client's degree of disability, motivation and skill level, availability of training opportunities, and any associated neurological problems. Many people with intellectual disabilities live productive, happy lives.

Prevention

Prenatal screening and genetic counseling are advised for high-risk families. Where the cause is unknown, there is no known prevention.

AUTISM SPECTRUM DISORDERS

ICD-10: F84.0

Description

Autism spectrum disorders (ASD; *DSM-V:* F84.8 or F84.5) are pervasive development disorders that affect over 2 million children in the United States. In the *DSM-IV,* the diagnosis for ASD includes autistic disorder (autism), Asperger's disorder, childhood disintegrative disorder, and pervasive developmental disorder. These disorders have the following common characteristics: deficits in social aspects of their lives and restricted repetitive behaviors. ASDs generally affect children before age 3 and continue throughout the life span.

Also included is a rare form of ASD: Rett syndrome. In Rett syndrome, normal early development is followed by loss of purposeful use of the hands, slowed brain and head growth, and gait abnormalities. It affects females almost exclusively.

Etiology

ASD has no direct known cause. Several generalized factors may contribute to its diagnosis. Genes have been identified as being involved in autism. In studies of twins, it has been shown that if one has ASD, the other has a 90% chance of also having ASD symptoms. If one sibling has ASD, the other siblings have a 35% likelihood of also having ASD. Other factors contributing to ASD are environmental, such as general health problems, viral infections, and air pollutants. Issues related to labor and delivery of the child may also contribute to ASD. Vaccinations have been discussed as possibly causing autism, but research does not support this belief.

Signs and Symptoms

ASD is usually noted early in childhood because a child with ASD may have delays in the areas of socialization and communication. ASD includes three levels of severity, with level 1 being the least severe and level 3 being the most severe. Severity is determined by the impact of the symptoms on a child's development and growth as well as the impact on relationships and the child's environment. Symptoms may include poor eye contact, inability to play, repetitive behaviors, hearing impairment (at times), lack of emotional response, echolalia, inability to regulate emotions, precocious language, sensory problems, learning disabilities, intellectual disabilities, sleep difficulties, gastrointestinal problems, or seizures. Each child diagnosed with an ASD has a unique group of symptoms and pattern of behavior.

As clients progress with ASD, they may become more engaged and their symptoms may lessen. Development of skills may be slower than in children without ASD;

however, children with ASD have normal to high intelligence overall.

Diagnostic Procedures

Through screening by the parents, family, and PCP, a child can be observed and concerns identified. Screening can begin as early as 18 months, and the potential for diagnosis by age 2 has resulted in marked improvements with treatment, but it is generally not diagnosed until age 2 to 3.

Treatment

There are multiple treatments that can be used in conjunction or separately to provide a positive result for ASD. NIMH reports that "intensive early intervention in optimal educational settings for at least two years during the preschool years results in improved outcomes for most young children with ASD." Structured educational programs can promote successful integration of children with ASD. Intensive behavioral therapies to teach them how to act and react in social situations and communication therapies to build communication skills can benefit ASD symptoms. Medications are to be used only for individualized symptoms, such as coexisting mental health conditions like depression and anxiety, rather than for communication and socializations skills.

Complementary Therapy

A special diet, gluten-free specifically, has been suggested for the treatment of some ASD symptoms. Tell the parents or caregiver to consult with the PCP and a dietitian before changing to any special diet. Sensory therapies or creative therapies, such as music or art therapy, can help to decrease sensory issues. A treatment that has not been shown to be effective but is noted in research to be recommended by some doctors is chelation therapy, a treatment to remove mercury from the blood.

⊙ CLIENT COMMUNICATION

Family members coping with a child with an ASD, such as Asperger or autism, will want to provide a structured living environment for the child to promote growth and socialization. A structured environment includes routines for sleep, eating, play, and activities out of the home. It is important to provide a calm and positive environment for the child with ASD as well as for other children in the home not diagnosed with ASD. Families need to become educated and to seek support from other families and friends with children who have the same disorders.

Prognosis

There is no known cure for ASD. Early diagnosis and intervention increase the likelihood of positive socialization and ability to manage and maintain symptoms. It will continue into adulthood, and therapies and treatment may need to be changed and monitored.

Prevention

There is no known prevention for ASD.

ATTENTION DEFICIT-HYPERACTIVITY DISORDER

ICD-10: F90.1, F90.2, or F90.9

Description

Attention deficit-hyperactivity disorder (ADHD; *DSM-V:* F90.1, F90.2, F90.0, or F90.9); is the most common neurobiological disorder in children. It occurs in adults as well, although there is limited research on adult ADHD. The person with ADHD is inattentive, impulsive, and hyperactive and has difficulties with gratification. People with ADHD are on a roller coaster because of their impulsiveness and emotional overarousal. Many times they receive more negative reinforcement and feedback because of their behavioral patterns.

ADHD is found in about 11% of the general population. Unfortunately, it is estimated that fewer than one-half of these individuals are appropriately diagnosed. In the general population, the disorder is twice as likely in males than in females. About 50% to 80% of children with ADHD carry their symptoms into adulthood.

There are three types of ADHD: ADHD with a combined presentation, ADHD with a predominantly inattentive presentation, and ADHD with a predominately hyperactive/impulsive presentation. A general discussion of all three is given.

Etiology

It is believed that environmental factors such as lead poisoning, genetic factors, socioeconomic factors, food additives, and prenatal and perinatal complications all play a part in the development of the disorder. Most support a neurobiological basis as well. In ADHD, the brain areas that control attention use less glucose, indicating that they are less active. The conclusion is that a lower level of activity in the brain may cause inattention and other ADHD symptoms. Other causes may be brain injury, alcohol and tobacco use during pregnancy, premature delivery, or low birth weight. Research has shown that ADHD does run in families. Contrary to popular belief, ADHD is not caused by bad parenting, poor teachers, family problems, food allergies, or too much sugar. The family may experience conflict and parenting problems, although the latter may be a result of the child's behavior.

Signs and Symptoms

The classic symptoms include distractibility, impulsivity, and hyperactivity. These symptoms must be excessive, long-term, and across the life span, occurring before age 12 and continuing for at least 6 months. The behaviors must create a real hardship in at least two of the following areas: home, school, or social settings.

The person with ADHD seems to not listen, avoids difficult tasks, talks excessively, is careless, and has difficulty following through. In general, the person is forgetful, fidgety, and has a difficult temperament. People with ADHD often interrupt other speakers and do not like waiting for their turn.

Diagnostic Procedures

Many times, the diagnosis of ADHD is not made until the child starts school, as parents tend to tolerate the expressed behaviors better than do others. In school, the behaviors interfere with the child's academic performance and peer relationships. Many earlier indicators generally are present, however. A comprehensive evaluation that includes a complete individual and family history, ability tests, achievement tests, and a collection of observations of those closest to the individual.

Treatment

The treatment of the disorder encompasses the client and the entire family and includes medication to improve brain function. Most of the time, psychotropic medications used as stimulants are prescribed, but antidepressants, antihypertensives, or tricyclic antidepressants may be prescribed. Adjusting the medication dosage is a challenge in children because they metabolize and eliminate drugs more rapidly than adults. Encouraging safe practices around the use of medications can reduce the risk of abuse and addiction that come from using these stimulant medications.

Behavior management, social skills development, and cognitive therapy are initiated in conjunction with medication to help the child learn problem-solving and communication skills. Parents are educated about the disorder and the child's individual treatment plan. Art therapy, children's games, and storytelling help children deal with their feelings, relieve their distress, and learn new coping skills. Children may need continued counseling with or without their family. It is imperative that the treatment plans continue, and children may require day treatment programs as well as intensive in-home programs.

In adults, medication is prescribed along with behavior management and cognitive therapy. Work may pose challenges requiring mental health counseling.

Complementary Therapy

Some practitioners recommend that the client eat every 2 hours and restrict foods high in sugar to combat symptoms of hyperglycemia. Others recommend that clients take high-potency nutritional supplements with the approval of the PCP. If food allergies are a problem, avoid the allergens. Any herbal tea that has a calming or relaxing effect may be tried. Yoga and exercise are also relaxation techniques that can reduce symptoms of ADHD.

 CLIENT COMMUNICATION

Those closest to the individual with ADHD will want to provide a supportive environment and to teach organizational, study, and memory skills. Basic time management and learning how to be self-aware need to be reinforced. A structured environment and consistency within home, school, and extracurricular activities are important for children with ADHD. Whether at work or at school, it is important to investigate what kind of environment best suits them so that they can be productive. Proper diet and sleep are essential, especially because of the side effects of some medications that might be prescribed.

Prognosis

By the time the child is diagnosed with ADHD, other mental health problems may have surfaced, such as low self-esteem and poor socialization. If the child has associated mental health problems, the prognosis is not as good. ADHD will continue into adulthood in one-half to one-third of those affected. Obviously, this impacts their job, family, and social relationships. ADHD is recognized as a disability under the Americans with Disabilities Act and as such requires reasonable accommodation in school and at work. This helps ADHD clients to live more productive lives.

Prevention

There is no known prevention for ADHD.

Feeding and Eating Disorders

ANOREXIA NERVOSA

ICD-10: F50.00

Description

Anorexia nervosa (*DSM-V:* F50.00) is a complex psychogenic feeding and eating disorder. The key feature is self-imposed starvation and an irrational fear of gaining weight, even when the individual is already emaciated. The disorder, primarily affecting young women, occurs in 13% of the population around the age of puberty. White women from middle-class backgrounds are affected most frequently. The reported incidence of anorexia in men is low, but anorexia appears to be occurring more in adult men and women.

Etiology

The cause of anorexia nervosa is not known, although most health-care professionals believe it is essentially a mental health disorder. It is believed to stem from biological, psychological, or environmental circumstances. Research has connected serotonin, linked to depression, to be decreased in those diagnosed with anorexia. Some theorists believe the refusal to eat is a subconscious effort to exert control over one's life. Attitudes in society that equate slimness with beauty play some role in provoking the disorder. A client's socioeconomic status, family background, and cultural conditioning may be predisposing factors in development of the condition.

Signs and Symptoms

Anorexia nervosa is marked by weight loss, clinical evidence of semistarvation, amenorrhea, and an alteration in body image. A loss of at least 25% of original body weight, in the absence of any detectable underlying medical disorder, may suggest a diagnosis of anorexia nervosa. Evidence of food avoidance, vomiting, and excessive exercise also suggest the diagnosis. In severe cases, a host of secondary symptoms may be evident as a result of metabolic and hormonal disturbances resulting from malnutrition. The affected individual also may tend to deny feelings of hunger and will typically claim to be overweight despite physical evidence to the contrary. It is common to have associated mental health issues, including depression, or substance abuse and dependence disorders.

Diagnostic Procedures

Careful interpretation of clinical data is important to rule out other disorders that cause physical wasting. No specific diagnostic tests exist for anorexia nervosa, but a physical evaluation to review basic functioning and height-to-weight ratio, as well as blood testing may reveal associated nutritional anemia and vitamin or mineral deficiencies.

Treatment

Medical treatment of anorexia nervosa is aimed at reversing the effects of malnutrition and improving control for individuals who may also have the compulsion to binge and purge. Noncooperation on the part of the affected individual, however, typically makes treatment of this disorder difficult. Aggressive medical management, nutritional counseling and coaching, and individual, group, and family psychotherapy are recommended. Hospitalization may be required in the event of severe weight loss and malnutrition.

Complementary Therapy

For both anorexia nervosa and bulimia nervosa, hypnotherapy may be beneficial. Some practitioners believe the absence of zinc may be a contributing factor in the disease; any zinc supplement should be given only under the supervision of a qualified practitioner. A well-balanced diet high in fiber may be established. The use of acupuncture, massage, yoga, and meditation has been helpful in those with anorexia symptoms.

 CLIENT COMMUNICATION

It may be necessary to stay with the individual during and after meals and to give rewards for satisfactory weight gain. Referring the client and family members to the National Association of Anorexia Nervosa and Associated Disorders for additional information and support can be beneficial.

Prognosis

The prognosis varies. Relapses are frequent. Death may occur from malnutrition and complications, such as hypothermia and cardiac disturbances, in as many as one-fourth of diagnosed cases, especially when the person is not anxious to overcome the disorder.

Prevention

There is no known specific prevention for anorexia nervosa, but it seems helpful that an individual develop a sense of self-esteem that is not dependent on the thin, "model-like" body image so prized in today's society. Family support can be beneficial, as can nutritional education and medical support to help establish positive and healthy routines in families and young adults.

BULIMIA NERVOSA

ICD-10: F50.2

Description

Bulimia nervosa (*DSM-V:* F50.2) is a psychogenic eating disorder characterized by repetitive gorging with food followed by self-induced vomiting. The condition also may involve laxative abuse, the use of diuretics, and fasting. The individual with anorexia nervosa seems obsessed with becoming even thinner; the person with bulimia has a morbid fear of becoming fat. Other behavioral abnormalities include obsessive secrecy about the condition and sometimes food stealing. The disorder principally affects young women and may occur simultaneously with anorexia nervosa.

Bulimia nervosa affects 1% to 3% of the population, and only 5% to 15% of the population with bulimia nervosa is male.

Etiology

The cause of bulimia is not known. Psychosocial factors, such as family conflict, sexual abuse, and a cultural overemphasis on physical appearance, may be contributing factors. There may be a struggle for self-identity and a history of depression, anxiety, phobias, and OCD. Some people may be genetically susceptible to bulimia nervosa when there is a family member diagnosed with the same issue or with another type of eating disorder.

Signs and Symptoms

Most persons with bulimia hide the behavioral evidence of their condition, and they are often of normal weight or even slightly overweight on diagnosis. They may still exhibit signs of malnutrition, however, because the "binge" diet of a bulimic individual is often wildly unbalanced, usually consisting of junk foods, such as donuts, ice cream, and candy. Owing to the high sugar content of the binge diet and the subsequent reflux of gastric juices during vomiting, the bulimic person typically has a high incidence of dental decay. Reflux of gastric secretions also can produce a chronic sore throat. Menstrual irregularities are much less common in bulimia than in anorexia nervosa. Chronic depression, low tolerance for frustration, anxiety, self-consciousness, and difficulty expressing feelings such as anger are common. The client is apt to possess an exaggerated sense of guilt and have difficulty controlling impulses.

Diagnostic Procedures

Physical examinations, laboratory testing, psychological examinations, and other medical examinations, including x-rays, may help to diagnose the eating disorder. Serum electrolyte studies may reveal the diagnosis. Electrocardiograms may reveal cardiac arrhythmias or evidence of renal dysfunction.

Treatment

Long-term psychotherapy is usually indicated. The bulimic person knows that the eating patterns are abnormal but is unable to control them. Nutritional therapy, coaching, and education are also important. As with the anorexic person, noncooperation on the part of the bulimic client generally makes treatment difficult and frustrating. Treatment concentrates on interrupting the binge-purge cycle and helping the client regain control over eating behavior. Medications such as antidepressants, specifically Prozac, are used for the treatment of bulimia, even in those who do not suffer from depression.

Complementary Therapy

Inositol, a naturally grown isomer, has shown effectiveness compared with placebo medications when injected over 12 weeks in those with bulimia nervosa. Inositol produced complete remission for several months. Some studies have shown that massage, meditation, yoga, biofeedback, hypnosis, and acupuncture can be effective in treating bulimia as a complementary approach. Also, see "Anorexia Nervosa."

 CLIENT COMMUNICATION

See "Anorexia Nervosa."

Prognosis

The prognosis is guarded unless the client responds to therapy. Persons with bulimia have twice as high an incidence of suicide as do anorexics. Other complications may include pneumonia, anemia, heart problems, gastrointestinal difficulties, rupture of the esophagus or stomach, and pancreatitis.

Prevention

There is no known specific prevention for bulimia nervosa.

Sexual Dysfunctions

Sexual dysfunctions are characterized by physiological and psychological changes that disturb the sexual desire and sexual response cycle and cause difficulties among sexual partners.

Etiologic factors generally are believed to be psychological and some medical conditions may also be a factor, although the condition by itself may not necessarily cause the disorder. Some primary considerations are the couples' relationship versus each individual's own factors, such as communication, self-esteem of each individual, and any other preexisting mental health or medical conditions that can interfere with the relationship. In the diagnosis and treatment phases, it is important to consider the individual's ethnic, cultural, religious, and social background, all of which may affect the client's attitude, perception, desire, and expectations about performance.

An important consideration in the treatment of any sexual disorder is a sensitivity to open communication about the problem. Both the client and the PCP may have difficulty raising questions regarding sexual functions. If this occurs, disorders may go undetected and untreated.

All health-care professionals need to be alert to an individual's signals and questions that may indicate a sexual concern. Clients often feel more comfortable asking a question with someone other than the

PCP; therefore, it is important that the PCP include a detailed sexual history as part of the medical history. It is helpful if all health-care professionals feel comfortable initiating questions about sexual function. Health care in which the total person is treated cannot ignore the human sexual response and its function or dysfunction.

GENITO-PELVIC PAIN/ PENETRATION DISORDER

ICD-10: R37

Description

Genito-pelvic pain/penetration disorder, or painful intercourse (*DSM-V:* F52.6), previously known as *dyspareunia,* refers to pain associated with sexual intercourse. It occurs in women during, before, or after sexual intercourse, but the disorder affects roughly 15% of women in the general population. The disorder includes difficulties with vaginal penetration during intercourse, increased pain during vaginal intercourse, heightened anxiety around vaginal penetration, or tensing of the pelvic floor during vaginal penetration.

Etiology

The cause of the pain may be anatomic or physiological, including but not limited to lesions of the vagina, retroversion of the uterus, urinary tract infection, lack of lubrication, scar tissue, or abnormal growths. More commonly the cause may be psychosomatic, which can include fear of pain or injury, feelings of guilt or shame, ignorance of sexual anatomy and physiology, and fear of pregnancy.

Signs and Symptoms

For a diagnosis to be made, the person must experience persistent genital pain. The disturbance causes interpersonal difficulty and marked distress. The individual may experience mild to severe discomfort before, during, or after intercourse.

Diagnostic Procedures

A detailed sexual history is important to help reveal any psychological factors that may be causing the disorder. A pelvic examination, and possibly a pelvic ultrasound, may be indicated.

Treatment

Individuals may be instructed to use creams or water-soluble jellies for lubrication before intercourse. Hygiene is important, as is avoiding products with scents or minerals that may irritate the skin. Medications may be prescribed if any infections are detected. Check to see if the client is taking any medications that could cause increased vaginal dryness. Excision of any

scars and gentle stretching of the vaginal orifice may be needed. Education about the sexual response and counseling or short-term psychotherapy may be indicated.

Complementary Therapy

No significant complementary therapy is indicated.

 CLIENT COMMUNICATION

Teach clients who have sexual partners how to listen to one another, learn foreplay techniques, and be patient. Open communication is important.

Prognosis

The prognosis is good with adequate treatment, proper education, and sensitivity on the part of both sexual partners.

Prevention

Preventive measures include prompt treatment of any infections or inflammatory diseases of the genitourinary tract.

ERECTILE DISORDER

ICD-10: F52.21

Description

Erectile disorder (*DSM-V:* F52.21) is the inability of a man to achieve or sustain an erection sufficient to complete sexual intercourse. Erectile disorder increases with age and affects nearly one-third of men during their life.

Etiology

Erectile disorder may be psychological or physiological. Psychological causes account for 50% to 60% of the cases and include anxiety or depression, feelings of inadequacy, and rejection of others. Physiological causes include certain pharmacological agents; drug and alcohol abuse; heart disease; obesity; low testosterone; diabetes mellitus; surgical complications; spinal cord and disk injuries; and neurological, endocrine, or urological disorders.

Signs and Symptoms

Erectile disorder may occur when a person is unable to achieve any erection, is able to achieve an initial erection and then loses it, or is able to achieve an erection only during masturbation. There is also a noted reduction in sexual desire. The erectile disorder must occur at least for 6 months and at least 75% to 100% of the time in sexual activities.

Diagnostic Procedures

The diagnostic procedures help to differentiate between physiological and psychological causes of the erectile disorder. They typically include a physical examination, medical history, and detailed sexual history. There are several noninvasive medical procedures, such as an ultrasound, urinalysis, neurological examinations, and dynamic infusion cavernosometry cavernsonography (dye injected into the penile blood vessels to monitor flow), to better help diagnose erectile dysfunction. A psychological examination may be done or an overnight sleep test to determine if it is psychological or physiological.

Treatment

The aim of treatment of erectile disorder is to correct any underlying physiological disorders and provide counseling or psychotherapy to alleviate psychological problems. The surgical implantation of a penile prosthesis is a treatment option for individuals when erectile dysfunction is due to untreatable neurological or vascular disorders. The drugs sildenafil (Viagra), tadalafil (Cialis), and vardenafil (Levitra) have proved successful in some men with erectile disorder. The drugs enhance the effect of nitric oxide, the chemical released into the penis during sexual arousal, allowing the increased blood circulation necessary for an erection. Other medications that are used are alprostadil self-injections or suppositories, or possibly testosterone replacement.

Complementary Therapy

Complementary health-care practitioners identify Arginine supplements that work like Viagra to improve a man's ability to achieve an erection. The supplement should not be taken without a PCP's supervision. Ginkgo biloba boosts circulation to the penis, thus helping to reverse erectile disorder. Tantric yoga teaches techniques for improving sexual performance. Two methods are "holding the wand" and "tapping into pleasure." These methods involve grasping the penis, manipulating it as if it were a wand, gently rubbing the head across the clitoris, and tapping the penis against the lips of the vagina and the clitoris. Dehydroepiandrosterone is a steroid hormone that can help increase testosterone levels in men with deficiencies. It is banned from athletics, however. Acupuncture has also been shown to reduce erectile dysfunction.

⊙ CLIENT COMMUNICATION

It is important to help the client talk about his sexuality and his sexual disorder.

Prognosis

The prognosis is variable, depending on how long the client has suffered from the disorder and its severity.

Prevention

Prompt treatment and management of any physiological cause is important, as well as living a healthy lifestyle.

FEMALE SEXUAL INTEREST/ AROUSAL DISORDER

ICD-10: F22.22

Description

Female sexual interest/arousal disorder (*DSM-V:* F22.22) is an inability to achieve orgasm. It is characterized by the lack of desire for sexual activity and arousal.

Etiology

Female arousal disorder may be caused by physiological factors, especially diseases that produce nerve damage, such as diabetes mellitus or multiple sclerosis. Drug reactions, pelvic infections, hormonal imbalance, and vascular disease also may be the cause. More commonly, however, female sexual interest/arousal disorder is due to psychological factors, such as anxiety, depression, stress, and fatigue; sexual misinformation; inadequate or ineffective stimulation; and early traumatic sexual experiences. The prevalence of female sexual arousal disorder is probably more common in younger women; however, once a woman reaches orgasm, she is not likely to lose the ability to do so unless she has a traumatic experience or a relationship conflict.

Signs and Symptoms

A woman with sexual interest/arousal disorder may express a loss of sexual desire or report slow sexual arousal. She may lack the vaginal lubrication and vasocongestive response of sexual arousal. The woman with orgasmic disorder has an inability to achieve orgasm totally or under certain circumstances.

Diagnostic Procedures

A physical examination, a medical history, and a detailed sexual history are needed to differentiate physiological causes from psychological causes. Associated mental health issues may occur and may need to be assessed, such as depression and anxiety.

Treatment

The treatment of arousal disorder is directed toward correcting underlying physiological disorders or alleviating any psychological problems. Psychological problems may involve sex therapy for both partners. The goal of treatment for sexual interest/arousal disorder is to eliminate involuntary inhibition of the orgasmic reflex. Treatment may include short-term psychotherapy or behavior modification. Possibly using lubricants or a clitoris stimulator can be another recommended treatment. Medication treatments may be used to regulate hormones, such as estrogen or androgen therapy.

Complementary Therapy

No significant complementary therapy is indicated.

⊕ CLIENT COMMUNICATION

It is important that the woman understand her sexuality and experiences surrounding it and to be patient in this process. Counseling with a sexual partner is helpful.

Prognosis

In the absence of nerve damage, the prognosis is good if the woman has had some pleasurable sexual arousal previously. Psychological causes require more lengthy treatment.

Prevention

Early treatment of any physiological or psychological problem is the best prevention.

PREMATURE EJACULATION

ICD-10: F52.4

Description

Premature ejaculation (*DSM-V:* F52.4) is the persistent or recurrent onset of orgasm and expulsion of seminal fluid roughly 1 minute after vaginal penetration. It generally occurs immediately after the beginning of sexual intercourse or before the person wishes to ejaculate.

Etiology

Psychological factors of premature ejaculation include anxiety or guilty feelings about sex. Negative sexual relationships, such as may exist when a man unconsciously dislikes women or seeks to deny his partner's need for sexual gratification, also may induce premature ejaculation. Physiological factors are rare, but when they occur, they may be linked to abnormal hormone levels, thyroid problems, degenerative neurological disorders, urethritis, or prostatitis.

Signs and Symptoms

Ejaculation during masturbation, foreplay, or as soon as **intromission** (insertion of one part into another) occurs is a classic symptom. It is believed to be lifelong or considered to occur over time.

Diagnostic Procedures

Physical examination and laboratory tests may be ordered to rule out any physiological causes. A detailed sexual history is important to adequately assess this disorder. A person may be referred to a urologist or a mental health professional for an accurate diagnosis. The disorder causes marked distress or interpersonal difficulty. Premature ejaculation can be diagnosed for those who experience symptoms over 75% of the time in sexually related activities.

Treatment

The goal of treatment is to allow the person to control when they have an orgasm during sexual activity. An intensive program of sex therapy may be necessary. It is important that both partners be involved in the treatment to learn the technique of delaying ejaculation and to understand that the condition is reversible. The use of antidepressants such as Prozac or other SSRIs are prescribed to help with any psychological distress associated. In some cases use of medications for erectile dysfunction may help.

Complementary Therapy

Practitioners recommend the scrotal pull. During self-stimulation, the man gently pulls down on his scrotal sac before orgasm. During the sexual act, either partner may pull on the scrotal sac. Eventually the pull is no longer needed. Another technique is to squeeze the muscles in the anal area as if trying to stop the flow of urine. The exercise is repeated several times and strengthens the muscles used during sexual intercourse, especially those used during ejaculation. Another common technique is to use distraction as a way to prolong ejaculation.

⊕ CLIENT COMMUNICATION

Learning how to deal with self-doubt or guilt may be necessary. The disorder may cause marked distress or interpersonal difficulty. Encourage partners to seek treatment and therapy together.

Prognosis

The prognosis is excellent with proper treatment and understanding on the part of both partners. A positive self-image should be encouraged by explaining that premature ejaculation is a disorder that does not reflect on one's masculinity.

Prevention

There is no known prevention for premature ejaculation.

CHAPTER EPISODE—PART IV

Matt returns to the follow-up appointment with Dr. Hart. Matt has allowed his mother to attend the appointment. All laboratory tests have returned and Dr. Hart shares his concerns. The doctor asks Matt if he has stopped drinking. Matt reports, "I thought about it, but I like to drink; I don't think the drinking is causing the trembling. I feel fine." The doctor reports that the results of his laboratory tests and questionnaire indicate that Matt is underreporting his drinking. Matt laughs at the doctor. The doctor reports that his blood alcohol level was significantly high on the urinary drug test and the urinalysis showed liver and kidney concerns. Dr. Hart also found that the questionnaire indicates that Matt has been drinking at a high level for the last 2 years, since his unemployment. Dr. Hart tells Matt, "You are likely experiencing withdrawal from the alcohol use, as well as depression symptoms from the loss of your job. Your health is likely dependent upon further consultation and treatment." Dr. Hart is complimentary of Matt's family support and encourages Matt to include them in the treatment process.

- What possible mental health disorder(s) specifically related to alcohol use and depression symptoms could be explained by the symptoms presented?
- What kinds of treatment might the PCP recommend for Matt?
- How would you recommend including family support in the treatment process?

SUMMARY

This chapter covers the most commonly recognized mental health diseases and disorders found in primary care settings, hospitals, and communities in the United States in adults and children—from mental disorders, such as schizophrenia, depression, and autism spectrum disorders, to substance-related and addictive disorders. It also discusses sexual disorders because a significant amount of research associates sexual disorders of both men and women with an individual's mental health. Evaluation tools and primary symptoms are listed to provide awareness and to promote accurate assessments. Both primary care recommendations and complementary therapy recommendations are presented. Health insurance or the lack thereof, with regard to mental health, is assessed and reviewed as well. Nature versus nurture is also discussed in relation to mental illness and its cause. The chapter looks into how a client's culture, race, age, and gender play a role in the diagnosis and treatment of mental health disorders.

The chapter offers resources that can be accessed in the health-care setting or through the Internet. The case studies and review questions help to incorporate the chapter objectives, while challenging evaluation skills and knowledge.

 Davis*Plus* | For more resources and to sharpen your skills with interactive exercises, visit Davis*Plus* at http://davisplus.fadavis.com. Keyword *Tamparo*.

ONLINE RESOURCES

Anxiety and Depression Association of America
http://www.adaa.org

Autism Society
http://www.autism-society.org

Autism Speaks
http://www.autismspeaks.org/index.php

Centers for Disease Control and Prevention
http://www.cdc.gov/

Children and Adults with Attention-Deficit/Hyperactivity Disorder
http://www.chadd.org

National Alliance on Mental Illness
http://www.nami.org

PTSD: National Center for PTSD
http://www.ptsd.va.gov/index.asp

National Institute of Mental Health
http://www.nimh.nih.gov/index.shtml

Substance Abuse and Mental Health Services Administration
http://www.samhsa.gov

CASE STUDIES

Case Study 1

Grenda Castillo is a 25-year-old woman who has been diagnosed with PTSD. She recently returned from three tours with the army infantry in Afghanistan and Iraq. Her mother invited her to live at home with her two younger sisters until she finds a job and a new residence. Grenda is found in the living room or on the porch early in the morning asleep. She states that she is unable to sleep in her bed. Her youngest sister has awakened to hear Grenda screaming and yelling in her sleep. Her sister wakes her up to find her crying and shaking. Grenda will not explain why she wakes up with such a fright, but it continues to happen night after night. Grenda barely eats and hardly gets out of the house when her friends call. Her mother has offered to get her counseling, but Grenda states it won't help.

Case Study Questions
1. Discuss the implications this case has on each family member.
2. Review any complementary treatments that may be used.
3. What long-term consequences are there in this situation?

Case Study 2

Gabrielle Hart, an African American woman, is 34 years old and gave birth to twin boys 2 weeks ago. Gabrielle's husband reports that she is easy to anger and cries easily. Gabrielle refuses to pick up the baby at times and then feels guilty for her lack of attachment. Gabrielle has a history of depression but reports that this is not her being depressed. She is not sleeping well and sometimes not at all. She is not social with her friends and begins to resent their attempts at connecting with her and her new babies.

Case Study Questions

1. What might be the mental health issue Gabrielle is experiencing?
2. What treatment might be suggested?
3. Will Gabrielle be able to return to her previous pattern of functioning?

Case Study 3

Earl and Suzie have been married for a number of years and have three children. There is unhappiness, however, in their lives. Earl has premature ejaculation every time sexual intercourse is attempted, and Suzie is nonorgasmic. Suzie refuses to seek counseling. Earl is embarrassed and does not like the idea that there might be something "abnormal" about his sexual performance, but he would like to correct the problem.

Case Study Questions

1. What recommendations might be made to Earl and Suzie?
2. Discuss the meaning of sexual health.
3. What is the prognosis for these two different disorders?

REVIEW QUESTIONS

Matching

Match the following by placing the correct letter in the column.

_____ 1. Considered the most chronic and disabling mental health disorder

_____ 2. Senseless repetition of words or phrases

_____ 3. A marked psychomotor disturbance

_____ 4. Autism spectrum disorder

_____ 5. Fear of being alone or in open spaces

_____ 6. Decreased motivation

_____ 7. Need for more substance to achieve previous effects

_____ 8. Pattern of lack of empathy

_____ 9. Treatment for borderline personality disorder

_____ 10. Common among veterans

a. Schizophrenia

b. Substance use disorder

c. Tolerance

d. Agoraphobia

e. Dialectal behavior therapy

f. PTSD

g. Echolalia

h. Narcissistic personality disorder

i. Rett syndrome

j. Catatonia

k. Avolition

Short Answer

1. Persons might receive _____ for depression if they cannot take antidepressants and their depression is severe and life-threatening.

2. The personality disorder that does not respect the rights of others is _____.

3. There is _____ funding for mental health care from community, state, and federal agencies.

4. According to the World Health Organization, by the year 2020, depression will be the _____ leading cause of disability.

5. Bipolar is primarily diagnosed due to having both _____ and _____ symptoms.

6. Contrary to popular belief, _____ is not caused by bad parenting or poor teaching.

7. Whereas *nature* refers to factors that are already determined and difficult to alter, _____ refers to factors determined by individual preferences and outside influences.

8. The two different types of bipolar disorder are _____ and _____.

9. A _____ is a persistent and irrational fear of an object.

10. Symptoms of _____ are weight loss, semistarvation, amenorrhea, and an alteration of body image.

Multiple Choice

Place a check mark next to the correct answer.

1. Which of the following is a drug of abuse and addiction?

_____ a. Crack cocaine

_____ b. St. John's wort

_____ c. Folate

_____ d. Glucosamine

2. Which of the following statements is true of obsessive-compulsive disorder?

_____ a. Found in about 20% of the general population

_____ b. More common in females than in males

_____ c. Shown in those with fears around contamination

_____ d. Easily preventable

3. Which of the following is a disorder defined by below-average intellectual functioning with current deficit adaptive behaviors?

_____ a. ADHD

_____ b. Personality disorder

_____ c. Schizophrenia

_____ d. Intellectual disability

4. Which of the following statements is false?

_____ a. The *DSM-V* is published by the American Psychiatric Association.

_____ b. Major depression affects all ethnic groups and both genders.

_____ c. Delusions and hallucinations can occur in depression.

_____ d. St. John's wort is not contraindicated with some mental disorder medications.

5. What is the major cause of intellectual disability?

_____ a. Tobacco use

_____ b. Neurological disease

_____ c. Obesity

_____ d. Chemical imbalance

Discussion Questions/Personal Reflection

1. Discuss the implications of insurance coverage for mental health disorders in comparison to those of medical diseases. Relate to individual situations.

_____

_____

_____

_____

_____

_____

_____

_____

_____

_____

2. Discuss the implications on the family when a family member is diagnosed with one of the schizophrenia disorders.

_____

_____

_____

_____

_____

_____

_____

_____

_____

_____

_____

3. Brainstorm and identify possible socially acceptable activities that replace the time and the energy put into abusing alcohol or drugs.

_____

_____

_____

_____

_____

_____

_____

_____

_____

_____

_____

> *I'd get a tattoo if I had any skin tight enough to draw on.*
> —MAXINE

8

Skin Diseases and Disorders

● *chapter outline*

● *key words*

Abrade (ă•brād')
Bacteremia (băk•tĕr•ē'mē•ă)
Bulla (pl. bullae) (bŭl'lă)
Comedo (kŏm'ă•dō)
Debridement (dĭ•brēd•mĭnt')
Electrodesiccation (ē•lĕk"trō•dĕs"ĭ•kā'shŭn)

Induration (ĭn'dū•rā"shŭn)
Keratin (kĕr'ă•tĭn)
Keratolytic (kĕr"ă•tō•lĭt'ĭk)
Melanin (mĕl'ă•nĭn)
Mohs micrographic surgery (mōz mī"krŏ•grăf'ĭk sŭr'jĕr•ē)
Papule (păp'ūl)

Pustule (pŭs'tūl)
Pyoderma (pī•o•dĕr'mă)
Raynaud phenomenon (rĕ•nō' fĕ•nŏm'e•nŏn)
Rhinophyma (rī•nō•fi'mă)
Stratum corneum (strā'tŭm kŏr•nē'ŭm)

Upon successful completion of this chapter, you will be able to:

- Interpret key terms.
- Describe the anatomy and physiology of the integumentary system.
- Compare and contrast seborrheic dermatitis and psoriasis.
- Describe the etiology of contact and atopic dermatitis.
- Compare the life of a normal skin cell with that of a psoriatic skin cell.
- Identify the signs and symptoms of urticaria.
- Discuss the progression that occurs when a comedo becomes an acne pustule or papule.
- Name at least five causes of alopecia.
- Restate the sources of infection of herpes simplex.
- Describe the etiologic process of herpes zoster.
- Restate the prognosis and prevention for impetigo.
- Compare and contrast furuncle and carbuncle.

- Name the three common locations for pediculosis.
- Discuss the prevention of decubitus ulcers.
- Identify the five areas where dermatophytosis is likely to occur.
- Describe the diagnosis and treatment for scabies.
- Recall the treatment for corns and calluses.
- Identify the etiology of warts.
- Name the five causes of rosacea.
- Identify the three types of vitiligo.
- Restate the prognosis for scleroderma.
- Recall the areas affected by keratosis pilaris.
- Identify the two most common types of skin cancers.
- Identify the four types of malignant melanomas.
- Name at least four common symptoms of skin diseases and disorders.
- Identify reconstructive skin procedures.

CHAPTER EPISODE—PART I

Amanda is a 25-year-old female who loves spending her summers outdoors. She enjoys swimming, going on her parents' boat on the Chesapeake Bay, and sunbathing whenever the sun shines. Recently she fell asleep on the beach for an entire afternoon and has been feeling a great amount of discomfort since.

- What could be causing Amanda her discomfort?
- What should she do?

INTEGUMENTARY SYSTEM ANATOMY AND PHYSIOLOGY REVIEW

The integumentary system is composed of the skin; accessory structures, such as the hair and glands; and the subcutaneous tissue below the skin. Skin is considered an organ because it is made up of several different kinds of tissue. The integumentary system protects the body against infection, trauma, and toxic compounds. Skin contains the receptors for touch and other sensations that are important to individual well-being from birth to death. It also helps regulate body temperature and synthesizes vitamin D when exposed to sunlight. Additionally, skin serves as an excretory organ by allowing the skin to excrete water, excess salt, and small amounts of waste, such as urea and lactic acid. Figure 8.1 illustrates the structure of the skin.

Skin consists of three layers: the epidermis, the dermis, and the subcutaneous layer. The epidermis, or outer layer, is made of several layers of epithelial cells that contain the hard, fibrous protein **keratin,** which gives skin flexibility, creates a seal that prevents dehydration, and forms a protective barrier. This layer also contains melanocytes that produce the pigment **melanin,** which gives the skin its color. The dermis, or middle layer, consists of fibrous proteins that give the skin strength

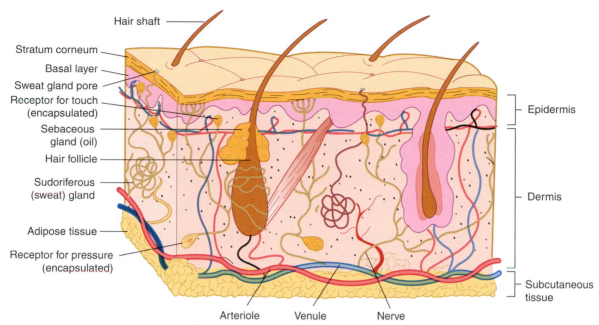

Figure 8.1 Structure of the skin and subcutaneous tissue.

and elasticity. This layer contains the nerves, hair follicles, glands, and blood vessels. The subcutaneous layer consists mostly of fat, which connects the skin to the muscle beneath and provides insulation from trauma and heat loss.

Hair, nails, and glands are also part of the integumentary system. All of these structures are made of epithelial cells, which are specialized to meet the function of the structure.

Hair sparsely covers the body except on the soles of the feet, palms of the hands, lips, nipples, and parts of the external reproductive organs. The eyelashes and eyebrows protect the eyes from dust and perspiration, and the nasal hairs prevent dust from entering the pharynx and the lungs. The hair on the scalp keeps the head warm. All hairs grow from a root within a follicle. As the hair lengthens, the epithelial cells thicken and keratinize like the epidermis.

Nails give limited protection to the nerve endings of the hands and feet. Each nail grows from a nail matrix, and as the cells push away from the matrix, they fill with keratin to form a flexible covering for the tip of each finger and toe.

Skin contains two types of glands: sebaceous (oil) and sudoriferous (sweat). These are exocrine glands that excrete substances through ducts. The sebaceous glands secrete sebum, an oily substance that lubricates and helps waterproof the hair and skin and inhibits the growth of bacteria on the skin's surface. During the aging process, the production of sebum decreases, which generally accounts for dryer skin and brittle hair in elderly people.

The sudoriferous glands secrete sweat, an odorless, watery substance that aids in cooling the body. In the axillary and genital regions, these glands produce sweat that reacts to the bacteria in these areas, producing a distinctive odor. Modified sweat glands are the mammary glands and the ceruminous glands. The mammary glands are located in the breasts and secrete milk; the ceruminous glands are located in the ears and secrete cerumen, or earwax. Cerumen provides lubrication and helps prevent microorganisms and insects from entering the ear.

Skin Lesions

Skin diseases frequently manifest due to alterations in the skin surface called lesions. Most skin diseases produce a specific type of lesion or set of lesions, and diagnoses are often made on the basis of the lesions' appearance. Figure 8.2 illustrates nine basic types of skin lesions. Refer to this figure as you study the signs and symptoms of the various skin diseases discussed throughout the chapter. Table 8.1 identifies the characteristics of skin lesions and gives examples.

PSORIASIS

ICD-10: L40.X*

Description

Psoriasis is a chronic, noninfectious, inflammatory skin disease marked by the appearance of discrete pink or

*The X represents the fourth digit that is often required and supplied once more detailed information about the disease or disorder is made known to the provider.

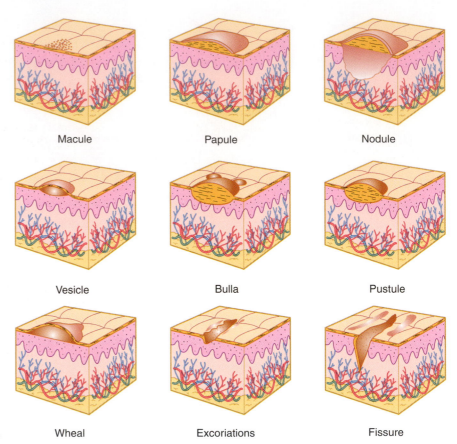

Macule   Papule   Nodule

Vesicle   Bulla   Pustule

Figure 8.2 Skin lesions.   Wheal   Excoriations   Fissure

red lesions surmounted by a characteristic silvery scaling (Fig. 8.3). The epidermal cells are produced six to nine times faster than normal. The disease may appear in a person of any age but occurs more frequently between the ages of 15 and 50.

Etiology

Psoriasis affects nearly 8 million Americans. Its cause is not known, but it appears to be an autoimmune disorder that is often genetically determined. Precipitating factors may include trauma, infections, and hormonal

Table 8.1	Skin Lesions	
TYPE *Flat Lesions*	**CHARACTERISTICS**	**EXAMPLES**
Macule	Flat, discolored, circumscribed lesion of any size	Freckle, flat mole, hyperpigmentation
Elevated Lesion		
Papule	Solid elevated lesion, less than 1 cm in diameter	Nevus, warts, pimples
Nodule	Palpable circumscribed lesion, larger than a papule, 1–2 cm in diameter	Benign or malignant tumor
Wheal	Dome-shaped or flat-topped elevated lesion, slightly reddened and often changing in size and shape, usually accompanied by intense itching	Hives
Vesicle and bulla	Elevated lesion that contains fluid; a bulla is a vesicle greater than 0.5 cm	Blister, herpes zoster, second-degree burn
Pustule	Elevated lesion containing pus that may be sterile or contaminated with bacteria; small abscess on the skin	Acne, pustular, psoriasis
Scale	Excessive dry exfoliation shed from upper layers of the skin	Psoriasis, ichthyosis
Cyst	Elevated, encapsulated mass of dermis or subcutaneous layers, solid or fluid filled	Sebaceous cyst
Tumor	Swelling; well-demarcated, elevated lesion greater than 2 cm in diameter	Fibroma, lipoma, steatoma, melanoma, hemangioma
Depressed Lesion		
Fissure	Small cracklike sore or break exposing the dermis; usually red	Athlete's foot, celosias
Ulcer	Loss of epidermis dermis within a distinct border	Pressure sore, basal cell carcinoma

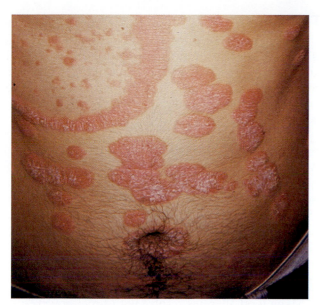

Figure 8.3 Psoriasis. *(From Goldsmith, LA, Lazarus, GS, and Tharp, MD: Adult and Pediatric Dermatology: A Color Guide to Diagnosis and Treatment. Philadelphia: F.A. Davis, 1997, p 258, with permission.)*

changes such as those occurring during pregnancy, emotional stress, or even changes in climate.

Signs and Symptoms

A high rate of skin cell turnover produces the thick, flaky scaling that is characteristic of psoriasis. The affected areas of skin typically appear dry, cracked, and encrusted with a buildup of skin that is composed of both living and dead tissue. Pruritus is a common complaint. In some individuals, psoriasis spreads to the nail beds, causing thickened, crumbling nails that separate from the skin. Arthritis is associated with psoriasis in 10% to 35% of cases.

There are five types of psoriasis:

- *Plaque psoriasis* is characterized by inflamed, raised, red lesions covered in white scaly patches. These lesions are typically found on the elbows, knees, scalp, and lower back. Plaque psoriasis is the most common type of psoriasis with about 80% of clients presenting with these symptoms.
- *Guttate psoriasis* appears as small, red spots found most often on the torso and limbs.
- *Inverse psoriasis* develops as smooth, shiny, red lesions in the armpits, groin, between the buttocks, under breasts, and in skin folds.
- *Pustular psoriasis* is characterized by white, pus-filled blisters surrounded by reddened skin. This type primarily affects adults.
- *Erythrodermic psoriasis* is a generalized inflammation characterized by fiery-red skin that peels in sheets. Inflammation is accompanied by severe pain, itching, tachycardia, and intermittent fever.

Diagnostic Procedures

Observation of the skin, a careful medical history, or a skin biopsy may suggest the diagnosis, although a skin biopsy may be of little value.

Treatment

There is no cure for the disease, and the treatment is only palliative. Any aggravating or precipitating factors need to be identified and removed, if possible. The scales may be gently removed after they are softened with petroleum jelly or a preparation containing urea. Exposure to ultraviolet (UV) A or UV-B light may reduce the cell reproduction. Corticosteroid creams, nonsteroidal creams, low-dosage antihistamines, oatmeal baths, and coal tar preparations may be applied to affected areas. Open, wet dressings may also be ordered. Careful skin hygiene is important. Biological agents such as alefacept (Amevive; suppresses the immune system) and etanercept (Enbrel; helpful with psoriatic arthritis) block the immune response and have shown promise in providing a convenient treatment that can be used continuously. Intralesional therapy includes injections of triamcinolone acetonide. Some systemic drugs may be ordered.

Complementary Therapy

Foods high in omega-3 fatty acids and some vitamin supplements may be recommended. Topical applications of aloe vera may be helpful but are not to be used without the approval of the primary care physician (PCP). Frequent exercising, deep breathing, and relaxation techniques may reduce stress.

CLIENT COMMUNICATION

It is important for clients to understand that although there is no cure for the disease, it can be controlled and requires lifelong management. Avoidance of any over-the-counter medications for psoriasis is paramount because they can exacerbate the disease. Educate clients not to pick at the skin, to avoid stressful situations when possible, and to seek psychological help if needed.

Prognosis

Psoriasis is controllable, but remissions and exacerbations frequently occur. The unsightly lesions that characterize the disease may cause psychological distress. The disease may progress to an exfoliative psoriatic state in which the person is acutely ill and experiences fever, chills, and electrolyte imbalance.

Prevention

There is no known prevention for psoriasis.

URTICARIA (HIVES)

ICD-10: L50.X

Description

Urticaria (hives) is an episodic inflammatory reaction of the capillaries beneath a localized area of the skin.

Etiology

Urticaria most frequently results after ingesting certain foods such as shellfish, nuts (especially peanuts), soy, wheat, and eggs. The condition also may result from allergic reactions to insect stings or some inhalants such as animal dander. Heat, cold, water, and sunlight may be predisposing factors of urticaria. Food allergies are the most common cause of urticaria in children.

Signs and Symptoms

The condition is characterized by the eruption of pale, raised wheals on the skin, possibly surrounded by erythema (Fig. 8.4). The lesions usually form and then resolve quite rapidly, often moving from one area of the body to another. This vascular reaction usually is accompanied by intense itching.

Diagnostic Procedures

The client's medical history should cover topics such as medications used, frequently ingested foods, environmental factors, and psychological status. The appearance of the inflamed area and its history should help pinpoint a diagnosis of urticaria. Sensitization testing may help to identify the causative agent.

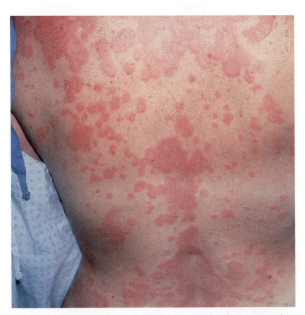

Figure 8.4 Urticaria (hives). These huge wheals occurred on a client allergic to penicillin. *(From Goldsmith, LA, Lazarus, GS, and Tharp, MD: Adult and Pediatric Dermatology: A Color Guide to Diagnosis and Treatment. Philadelphia: F.A. Davis, 1997, p 209, with permission.)*

Treatment

Urticaria usually subsides when the offending stimulus is removed. Antihistamines are often useful in controlling an ongoing attack. Epinephrine may be injected to control severe reactions. Hydrocortisone creams or lotions are helpful in providing symptomatic relief from itching.

Complementary Therapy

After food allergens are identified, they are to be avoided while still maintaining a varied diet. Sometimes two bicarbonate tablets put in water and taken every 15 minutes for 2 hours can reduce symptoms. A topical solution of calamine lotion with beta-carotene can be placed over the affected area.

⊙→ CLIENT COMMUNICATION

Many food allergies resolve with time; however, it is important to teach clients to avoid the offending food. Having the client keep a diary of food intake and activities may prove helpful in diagnosing the cause of urticaria.

Prognosis

The prognosis for an individual with this uncomfortable disorder generally is good, especially once the offending cause is removed. Repeated exposure to the offending allergen may lead to an anaphylactic reaction. If urticaria is chronic, emotional factors are to be considered, which may make one more susceptible to the inflammation.

Prevention

Avoiding the causative agent is the best means of preventing urticaria.

ACNE VULGARIS

ICD-10: L70.X

Description

Acne vulgaris is a very common inflammatory disease of the sebaceous glands and hair follicles that affects 85% of Americans at some time in their lives. It is characterized by the appearance of **comedos** (blackheads or whiteheads), **papules** (solid elevation less than 1 cm), and **pustules** (small, raised areas of the skin filled with pus). It is more common in adolescents and young adults between ages 12 and 35, but the lesions can appear at an earlier or a later age, too.

Etiology

The underlying cause of acne vulgaris is a genetic predisposition. The condition is inherited in an autosomal dominant pattern and may skip a generation. The focus of research is on follicular occlusion and androgen-stimulated sebum production. Predisposing factors include disturbances in hormonal balances affecting the activity of the sebaceous glands. Precipitating factors may include endocrine disorders, the use of corticosteroid drugs, or psychogenic factors. Bacteria also play a large role in acne development, as indicated by successful results of low-dose antibiotic therapy.

Signs and Symptoms

The acne plug often appears first as an open comedo (blackhead) or a closed comedo (whitehead) (Fig. 8.5). The color in the blackhead is caused by the melanin produced by the hair follicle, not by dirt. Eventually, an enlarged plug may rupture or leak, spreading its contents to the dermis. This results in inflammation and acne pustules or papules. Scars can develop in cases of chronic irritation.

Diagnostic Procedures

A medical history and observation of the characteristic lesions are usually all that is necessary to confirm the diagnosis.

Treatment

The treatment goals are to reduce the bacterial count, decrease sebaceous gland activity, and prevent the follicle from becoming inflamed. Therapy may include the use of topical antibacterial treatments, orally administered antibiotics, or both. Topically applied cleansing and peeling, or **keratolytic** agents, may prove useful to some, but in general, the skin should be kept as clean and dry as possible. It is important to prevent scarring and eliminate predisposing factors.

Complementary Therapy

A diet that emphasizes vegetables is helpful. Reducing saturated fats and increasing fiber may prove beneficial. Fresh air and daily exercise are important. Clients should avoid sunburn and use only non-oil-based makeup. Facial masks containing egg whites followed by a rinse with filtered water may be helpful.

CLIENT COMMUNICATION

A good balanced diet is helpful in the treatment and prevention of acne. Remind clients to be cautious about sun exposure and all makeup should be washed off each night. Effective over-the-counter medication contains salicylic acid and benzoyl peroxide. Some people, however, may be sensitive to these ingredients. If clients are on antibiotics, advise them to watch for possible oral or vaginal candidiasis, a yeastlike fungal infection. Inform clients that treatment may be needed for years.

Prognosis

Acne vulgaris is a persistent, often emotionally upsetting problem that usually requires prolonged treatment before it subsides. The ultimate prognosis for most acne sufferers is good. For a few, though, the disease can produce permanent scarring and disfigurement.

Prevention

There is no known prevention for acne vulgaris.

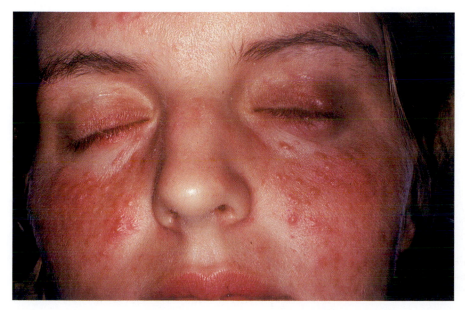

Figure 8.5 Acne vulgaris. *(From Goldsmith, LA, Lazarus, GS, and Tharp, MD: Adult and Pediatric Dermatology: A Color Guide to Diagnosis and Treatment. Philadelphia: F.A. Davis, 1997, p 277, with permission.)*

ROSACEA

ICD-10: L71.X

Description

Rosacea is a chronic inflammatory condition that causes erythema (flushing or redness) and the formation of red pustules on the face (Fig 8.6). This condition is often misdiagnosed as acne vulgaris.

Etiology

The cause of rosacea is unknown, but it may be a combination of genetic predisposition and environmental factors, such as sunlight, stress, spicy food, hot or cold temperatures, wind, corticosteroids, alcohol, and drugs that dilate the blood vessels. Rosacea occurs in those with fair complexions between the ages of 30 and 50. Women, especially those who are menopausal, are more likely than men to develop rosacea.

Signs and Symptoms

The appearance of rosacea may differ among clients. Some may have a flushing of the cheeks, forehead, nose, or chin. For others, small red pustules form on the same areas, and the skin of the cheeks, forehead, and nose may thicken. The nose may also enlarge and become misshapen, resulting in a condition called **rhinophyma.** Eye problems, such as redness, burning, dryness, and excessive tearing, occur in 50% of rosacea cases.

Rosacea appears in three phases: (1) Pre-rosacea is a tendency to blush or flush easily, (2) vascular rosacea occurs when the skin becomes sensitive and small vessels on the cheeks and nose swell, and (3) inflammatory rosacea marks the appearance of small red pustules on the cheeks, nose, forehead, and chin. Rosacea symptoms are variable and can heal without treatment but reoccur. The symptoms tend to progress and worsen over time.

Diagnostic Procedures

A physical examination of the affected area and a medical history are usually sufficient to make a diagnosis.

Treatment

Reduction of inflammation using topical creams or lotions containing tretinoin, benzoyl peroxide, and azelaic acid is the goal of treatment. Oral antibiotics, such as tetracycline, erythromycin, and minocycline, may be administered because they tend to reduce inflammation faster than other topicals. Laser surgery may reduce the appearance of blood vessels and remove excess tissue.

Complementary Therapy

No significant complementary therapy is indicated.

➔ CLIENT COMMUNICATION

Instruct clients to avoid skin care products that contain alcohol, acids, and other irritants.

Prognosis

Rosacea is a chronic condition, but with early treatment the prognosis is good.

Prevention

The only prevention for rosacea is to reduce flare-ups by encouraging clients to wear sunscreen, protect their faces from wind, and avoid overheating. Gentle facial cleansers are recommended. Advise clients to refrain from drinking alcohol, which can cause vasodilation.

KERATOSIS PILARIS

ICD-10: Q81.9 or Q82.8

Description

Keratosis pilaris is a common skin disorder that appears as painless, skin-colored bumps that may redden and form rough patches of skin (Fig 8.7).

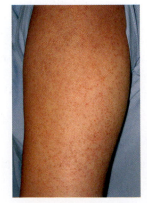
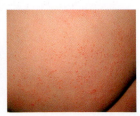

Figure 8.7　Keratosis pilaris. *(From Barankin, B, and Freiman, A:* Derm Notes: Clinical Dermatology Pocket Guide. *Philadelphia: F.A. Davis, 2006, p 106, with permission.)*

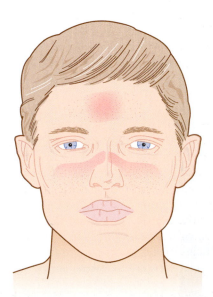

Figure 8.6　Rosacea.

Etiology

This disorder occurs in 50% to 80% of adolescents and 40% of adults worldwide. Age of onset is usually before age 10 and tends to worsen with puberty. Many clients find the condition improves with age and may clear when they reach adulthood. Those with dry skin tend to have more severe symptoms; the skin can improve in the summer and reappear or exacerbate in the winter.

Signs and Symptoms

Keratosis pilaris occurs from hyperkeratinization of the stratum corneum. The excess skin is slow to shed and clogs the hair follicles, forming skin-colored plugs that may become inflamed. These plugs appear as small, evenly spaced papules on the upper arms, thighs, buttocks, and sometimes the face. The skin may feel coarse and rough. Often the papules are mistaken for acne vulgaris.

Diagnostic Procedures

Keratosis pilaris is often considered a cosmetic condition but not associated with medical complications, a dermatologist is most likely to be sought for consultation. A physical examination of the affected area and a medical history is sufficient for diagnosis.

Treatment

Removal of the buildup of keratin to improve the appearance of the skin is the most effective treatment. Lotions, creams, or ointments containing ammonium lactate, alpha hydroxy acid, urea, glycolic acid, or salicylic acid can be used to exfoliate the skin. Topical retinoids promote cell turnover. Hyperpigmentation of the affected areas can occur after recurrent bouts of flare-ups and healing. Certain types of keratosis pilaris respond well to laser therapy.

Complementary Therapy

No significant alternative therapy is indicated.

 CLIENT COMMUNICATION

Advise clients to not use harsh methods to exfoliate the skin, such as scrubbing, pumice stones, or picking at the bumps. This can lead to infection and scarring.

Prognosis

With treatment prognosis is good, but if treatment is discontinued, keratosis pilaris will return.

Prevention

There is no known prevention for keratosis pilaris.

ALOPECIA AREATA

ICD-10: L63.8 or L63.2

Description

Alopecia areata is the absence or loss of hair, especially on the head. The two types are (1) scarring alopecia, where there is fibrosis, inflammation, and loss of hair follicles, and (2) nonscarring alopecia, where the hair shafts are gone but the hair follicles are preserved, making this type of alopecia reversible.

Etiology

Current evidence indicates that alopecia areata is the result of an abnormal immune response. Scarring alopecia may result as a consequence of certain systemic illnesses, such as lupus erythematous and cutaneous metastases, as well as some forms of dermatitis. Nonscarring alopecia is caused by the use of certain drugs and may occur as a consequence of chemotherapy or radiation therapy (causing total loss of all body hair), a hormonal imbalance, or trauma. Causes of trauma include mechanical pulling of the hair, use of rollers or rubber bands, braiding, or exposure to heat and chemicals. In some cases, alopecia is not related to any specific pathological process. Among men, alopecia seems to be part of the aging process. This form of the condition, called *male pattern baldness,* seems to be related to levels of the hormone androgen and may be genetically determined. In infants, alopecia is a common, temporary physiological condition.

Signs and Symptoms

Alopecia may occur gradually with advancing age, or it may be more sudden, occurring all at once or in patchy spots (Fig. 8.8).

Diagnostic Procedures

The visual examination may be all that is necessary, but the cause must be determined, too. A detailed health history will be taken. A complete examination of the skin and oral mucosa may be combined with a biopsy and direct immunofluorescence microscopy.

Treatment

Treatment varies with the cause of alopecia. There is no treatment for scarring alopecia. In nonscarring alopecia, spontaneous regrowth may occur, requiring no treatment in about 50% of cases. If the cause is a change in androgen levels, medications may be ordered. Minoxidil preparations may be used to treat male pattern baldness. The oral medication finasteride can prevent the shrinkage of hair follicles and prevent hair loss. Another treatment is surgical redistribution of hair follicles by autografting.

Complementary Therapy

Advise clients to massage the scalp with their fingers daily. A mixture from one part rosemary oil and two

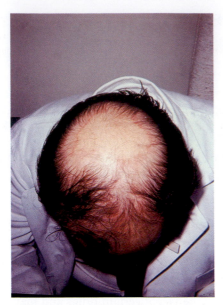

Figure 8.8   Alopecia areata. Well-defined areas of complete hair loss. *(From Goldsmith, LA, Lazarus, GS, and Tharp, MD: Adult and Pediatric Dermatology: A Color Guide to Diagnosis and Treatment. Philadelphia: F.A. Davis, 1997, p 473, with permission.)*

parts almond oil may be used. The oils of cedarwood, lavender, and thyme also show promise.

⊖ CLIENT COMMUNICATION

Alopecia is visual; therefore, it is important to help clients psychologically handle comments or stares, if they are bothersome. A referral to specialty shops that fit wigs and toupees may be helpful to those who are especially sensitive about their baldness. Today, male baldness is quite popular.

Prognosis

The prognosis depends on the cause. Alopecia due to scarring is permanent.

Prevention

There is no known prevention for some forms of alopecia. For others, early treatment of any disease known to cause alopecia is essential.

FURUNCLES AND CARBUNCLES

ICD-10: L02.02 or L02.03

Description

A furuncle, or boil, is an abscess involving the entire hair follicle and adjacent subcutaneous tissue. A carbuncle consists of several furuncles developing in adjoining hair follicles with multiple drainage sinuses (Fig. 8.9). The most common sites of these lesions are hairy parts of the body exposed to irritation, pressure, friction, or moisture.

Etiology

Infection by staphylococcal bacteria is the most common cause. Predisposing factors include diabetes mellitus, nephritis, hematologic malignancies, debilitation, and an infected wound elsewhere in the body. Both furuncles and carbuncles are more common in clients who live in hot climates.

Signs and Symptoms

Affected portions of skin may be extremely tender, painful, and swollen. The abscess may eventually enlarge, soften, and open, discharging pus and necrotic material. Erythema and edema may persist at the site for days or weeks. A mild fever may accompany this condition.

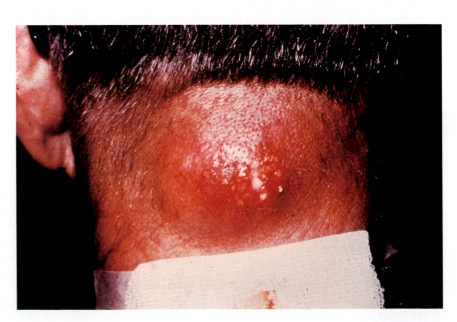

Figure 8.9   Carbuncle. *(From Goldsmith, LA, Lazarus, GS, and Tharp, MD: Adult and Pediatric Dermatology: A Color Guide to Diagnosis and Treatment. Philadelphia: F.A. Davis, 1977, p 364, with permission.)*

Diagnostic Procedures

Diagnosis is made on the basis of the appearance of the characteristic lesion. There may be slight leukocytosis, as evidenced through a complete blood count (CBC). Gram stains of the purulent content will reveal the causative organism.

Treatment

The boil should never be squeezed, because doing so destroys the protective wall that localizes the infection. The infected area must be cleansed with soap and water, and hot, wet compresses should be applied. Antibiotic agents are frequently prescribed. Surgical incision and drainage by the PCP may be necessary after the lesion is mature. If the buttock is the affected area, bed rest may be required for healing.

Complementary Therapy

It may be beneficial for clients to eat plenty of green, yellow, and orange vegetables. Encourage clients to increase fluid intake, especially water with an added teaspoon of fresh lemon juice. Garlic, beta-carotene, and vitamin A supplements may be ordered. Oils from vitamins E and A, honey, and some zinc oxide may be beneficial as a topical application. Tea tree oil has been used for centuries as an antiseptic, antibiotic, and antifungal agent. It may help relieve discomfort and speed healing when applied to the lesion.

CLIENT COMMUNICATION

If topical ointments are ordered, instruct clients to wear gloves when touching the afflicted area. Cleanliness is paramount. Bedsheets, clothes, or soiled dressings that have drainage must be cleaned or disposed of properly. Further infection must be prevented. A good nutritional diet is recommended to promote healing.

Prognosis

The condition may recur for months or years. Complications from carbuncles may include **bacteremia,** a condition of bacteria in the blood.

Prevention

Prevention of furuncles and carbuncles includes good personal hygiene and prevention of any infectious process.

PEDICULOSIS

ICD-10: B85.X

Description

Pediculosis is skin infestation with lice, a parasitic insect affecting millions of individuals each year. The body

(pediculosis corporis), the scalp (pediculosis capitis—quite common in schoolchildren), and the pubic area (pediculosis pubis) are the typical sites for infestation to occur.

Etiology

The lice feed on human blood and lay their eggs, or nits, in body hair or clothing, and the eggs hatch, feed, and mature in 2 to 3 weeks. The louse bite injects a toxin in the skin. Pediculosis capitis is more common in people with long hair. Pediculosis is more common in people who live in overcrowded places with inadequate facilities. The lice thrive on clean hair, which allows lice to get a better hold. The parasite can be transmitted via infected clothing, hats, combs, bedsheets, and towels. Pubic lice may be acquired through sexual intimacy with an infested person.

Signs and Symptoms

Intense pruritus and evidence of nits (eggs) on hair shafts (Fig. 8.10) or lice on clothing or on skin are the most common signs and symptoms. There may be gross excoriation of patches of skin and **pyoderma,** an acute, pus-causing, inflammatory skin disease. Rashes or wheals may develop.

Diagnostic Procedures

Visual examination is typically all that is necessary to diagnose pediculosis. Nits can be found on the hair, body, or clothing.

Treatment

For scalp lice, permethrin cream rinse is rubbed into the hair for 10 minutes. This step is followed by the use of a fine-tooth comb to remove lice and nits. A shampoo containing lindane or pyrethrin compounds with piperonyl butoxide may be used. Resistant infestations can be treated with a lotion containing malathion. Body lice must be removed by washing with soap and water. All clothing and bedding must be washed or dry cleaned. The PCP will help clients decide if chemical treatment

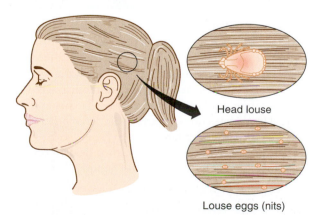

Figure 8.10 Head louse and louse eggs (nits).

is necessary. Pubic lice may be treated with creams, lotions, or shampoos.

Complementary Therapy

Substances that coat the lice, thereby trapping and suffocating them, also may be used. These substances include petroleum jelly, herbal oil, and mayonnaise. After this application, the nits and lice should be combed out with a small-toothed comb. This is best done by sectioning of the hair. Soaking the hair in a solution of equal parts water and white vinegar and then wrapping the wet scalp in a towel for at least 15 minutes may help facilitate removal.

Prognosis

The prognosis for pediculosis is excellent with treatment, but complications include severe pruritus, pyoderma, and dermatitis, which can be treated with antipruritics, systemic antibiotics, and topical corticosteroids.

Prevention

Prevention of pediculosis includes practicing good hygiene, avoiding contact with infested persons, and not sharing combs, brushes, or clothing.

⊙ CLIENT COMMUNICATION

With pediculosis capitis, it can be difficult to comb the hair with a fine-toothed comb; however, it must be done to remove all nits. Instruct clients that it may be necessary to pick off the nits with the fingernail, one by one. Because the condition spreads rapidly, it is important to start the treatment immediately and to inspect each family member daily for at least 2 weeks to check for infestation. All family members should be instructed in the control of infestation. Bedding and clothing should be washed in hot water or dry cleaned.

⊙ REALITY EPISODE

Karla is in second grade, and last week she brought home a letter from school alerting parents that head lice had been found on several students. When she came home from school yesterday, her mother noticed that Karla was frequently scratching her head. When her mother asked her what was wrong, Karla answered, "My head itches and feels crawly." Upon inspection of Karla's hair, her mother found what resembled grains of sand close to Karla's scalp. When she tried to brush the grains away, they held to the hair strand. Karla's scalp was also red and bumpy.

What condition does Karla have?
What should her mother do now?

DECUBITUS ULCERS

ICD-10: L89.XX

Description

A decubitus ulcer is a localized area of dead skin and subcutaneous tissue.

Etiology

These lesions are caused by impairment of the blood supply to the affected area as a result of persistent pressure against the skin surface. The condition is most frequently a consequence of prolonged immobilization and is often seen in debilitated, unconscious, or paralyzed individuals. Those with weak circulation, especially elderly persons, are at greatest risk for developing decubitus ulcers.

Signs and Symptoms

Early signs of decubitus ulcer include shiny, reddened skin, usually appearing over a bony prominence (stage 1). If not treated quickly, the ulcer may become more serious when skin is swollen and shows a blister (stage 2). A craterlike ulcer that goes deeper into the skin (stage 3) and a deep ulcer that goes into fat, muscle, or bone (stage 4) are very serious (Fig. 8.11). If the ulcer becomes infected, it will be foul-smelling and purulent. Pain may or may not accompany the lesion.

Diagnostic Procedures

Visual examination of the lesion usually is sufficient to establish the diagnosis. Wound culture and sensitivity testing may be performed to isolate the causative organism if infection is suspected.

Treatment

Skin pressure must be alleviated and excellent skin hygiene provided. The affected area must be kept clean and dry. Topical antibiotic powders may be prescribed. Surgery may be necessary in severe cases. Research is now being done using honey preparations, hyperbaric oxygen, and chemicals to stimulate cell growth.

Complementary Therapy

Apply a paste made with vitamin E oil, zinc oxide, and goldenseal powder to the affected area. Daily baths with gentle soaps containing aloe vera and exposure to sufficient natural light may be helpful.

⊙ CLIENT COMMUNICATION

It is important to discuss with clients proper positioning when sitting or lying to best alleviate pressure points. Frequent movement should be encouraged whether clients are in bed, in a wheelchair, or sitting for long periods of time. Advise clients to ambulate as often as possible and remain active. If there is

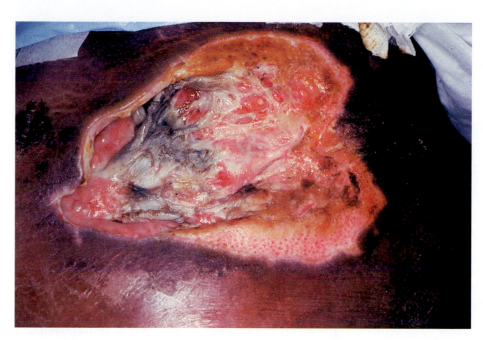

Figure 8.11 Deep decubitus ulcer over bony prominence. *(From Goldsmith, LA, Lazarus, GS, and Tharp, MD:* Adult and Pediatric Dermatology: A Color Guide to Diagnosis and Treatment. *Philadelphia: F.A. Davis, 1977, p 445, with permission.)*

decreased sensory perception, teach them how to observe for potential ulcer formation. Teach clients to rub or massage vulnerable areas if indicated. Minimize moisture formation whenever possible, because moist areas provide an environment conducive to bacterial formation.

Prognosis

The sooner the decubitus ulcer is diagnosed and treated, the better is the prognosis. The healing process generally is slow and tedious.

Prevention

Prevention includes frequent repositioning of clients who are immobilized and gentle massage of pressure areas to increase circulation. Pressure-relieving devices are proven to be helpful in prevention and include high-density foam, air, or liquid mattress overlays or soft moisture-absorbing padding.

CORNS AND CALLUSES

ICD-10: L84

Description

Corns are horny **indurations** (hardened tissue) and thickenings of the **stratum corneum,** the outermost or horny layer of the epidermis. Corns have a central keratinous core. Calluses are localized hyperplasia (increased growth) of the stratum corneum. A callus exhibits as a lesion with an indefinite border. Corns and calluses usually appear on areas of the body that receive repeated trauma, especially the feet.

Etiology

Both conditions may be caused by pressure or friction from ill-fitting shoes, orthopedic deformities, or faulty weight-bearing. Persons who expose their skin to repeated trauma, such as manual laborers or string instrument players, are prone to calluses. Also, individuals with diabetes, peripheral vascular disease, arteriosclerosis, or impaired circulation are more apt to develop corns and calluses. Corns occur on any toe, but more commonly the small toe or great toe are involved.

Signs and Symptoms

Tenderness and pain are common symptoms. Corns have a glassy core, are smaller and more clearly defined, and are more painful than calluses.

Diagnostic Procedures

A physical examination of the affected area along with a medical history are usually sufficient for diagnosing corns and calluses.

Treatment

Treating the underlying cause, if known, is essential. Treatment consists of relieving pressure or friction points along the skin as soon as possible. A keratolytic ointment may be used in the treatment of a callus. Orthopedic devices may be made to remove the pressure points. Surgical **debridement,** or the removal of dead or damaged tissue under local anesthetic, may be necessary. Local injections of corticosteroids to relieve pain may be tried. Metatarsal and corn pads may be worn to relieve pain and pressure.

Complementary Therapy

For corns on the feet, hot Epsom salt foot baths followed by rubbing the affected area with fresh lemon juice is helpful. Aloe vera and castor oil may be rubbed on the corns twice daily.

➔ CLIENT COMMUNICATION

It is important to educate clients about wearing well-fitting shoes that do not rub or hurt any corns presently on the feet. If the corn or callus is painful, soaking in warm water may help alleviate the pain. Keeping the feet dry after bathing or showering is helpful. Careful observation of reddened areas on the foot will help in prevention.

Prognosis

The prognosis for corns and calluses is good with proper care and if the causative factor is removed.

Prevention

Prevention of corns or calluses includes wearing well-fitting shoes and avoiding any trauma to the feet or hands.

DERMATOPHYTOSES

ICD-10: B35.X

Description

Dermatophytosis is a chronic, superficial fungal infection. It can occur in the scalp (tinea capitis), body (tinea corporis), nails (tinea unguium), feet (tinea pedis), or groin (tinea cruris).

Etiology

Dermatophytosis is caused by several species of fungi that have the ability to invade the keratinous structures of the body. The infection is transmitted by direct contact with the fungus or its spores. Infection is more likely if the skin is traumatized, or infection can occur through the use of fomites—inanimate objects on which disease-causing organisms can be carried. Common fomites are towels or shoes. Infection can occur when the skin is chaffed, roughened, or **abraded,** or in cases of poor hygiene. It is the most common superficial fungal infection in children, but it is rare in adults.

Signs and Symptoms

- *Tinea capitis* is a persistent, contagious, often epidemic infection occurring most frequently in children. The child may be asymptomatic or have slight itching of the scalp. The characteristic lesions are round, gray, and scaly (Fig. 8.12).
- *Tinea corporis,* or ringworm, occurs on exposed skin surfaces in persons with a history of exposure to

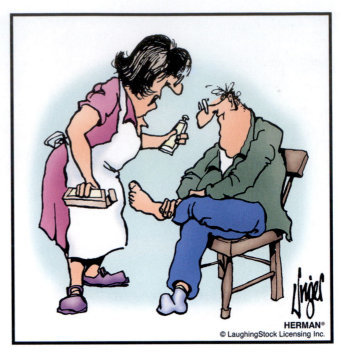

"You getting athlete's foot is about as ridiculous as a coal miner with sunstroke!"

HERMAN(c) is reprinted with permission from LaughingStock Licensing Inc., Ottawa, Canada. All rights reserved.

infected domestic animals, especially cats. The lesions are ringed and scaled with small vesicles.
- *Tinea unguium* is usually asymptomatic. The infection frequently starts at the tip of one or more toenails, with the affected nail appearing lusterless, brittle, and hypertrophic.
- *Tinea pedis,* or athlete's foot, causes intense, persistent itching—this is its most common presenting symptom. Burning, stinging, and pain may result. The entire sole may become inflamed and dry with exfoliation and fissuring.
- *Tinea cruris,* or jock itch, may be associated with tinea pedis and often occurs among male athletes. It is characterized by red, raised, sharply defined, itching lesions in the groin.

Diagnostic Procedures

Diagnosis is dependent on the location and appearance of the skin lesion. The suspected lesions may be cultured to isolate the fungus; however, this procedure is unnecessary because most superficial fungi are sensitive to topical and oral antifungal agents. The most sensitive test for superficial fungal infections is the potassium hydroxide (KOH) examination, which involves placing the hair or scales of the lesion on a microscopic slide with a few drops of KOH solution. The KOH dissolves the keratinous material for better visualization.

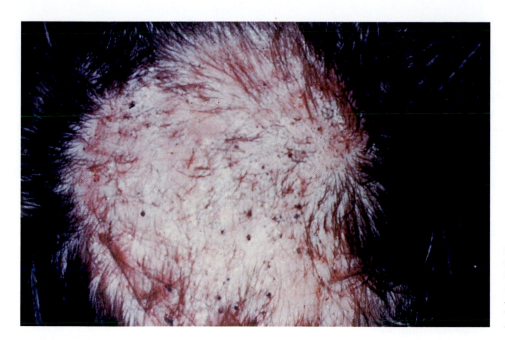

Figure 8.12 Patchy tinea capitis with broken hair stubs and spots of early inflammation, or kerion formation. *(From Goldsmith, LA, Lazarus, GS, and Tharp, MD:* Adult and Pediatric Dermatology: A Color Guide to Diagnosis and Treatment. *Philadelphia: F.A. Davis, 1997, p 174, with permission.)*

Treatment

It may be necessary to treat the lesions by applying a topical fungicidal medication. Extreme caution is necessary when applying such preparations because they are strong irritants. Some oral medications may be prescribed, but these must be taken with caution as well because of their side effects. The affected area of skin must be kept as dry and clean as possible. Loose-fitting clothing should be worn, and it should be changed frequently. Exercise and activity may need to be limited for a time to prevent excessive perspiration.

Complementary Therapy

It is recommended that clients keep affected areas exposed to fresh air and sunlight as much as possible and keep the areas clean and dry. Tea tree oil and liquid from grapefruit seed extract, available in health food stores, is a helpful remedy. Advise clients to apply a light coating of either mixture on the affected areas three to four times daily and add two cloves of raw garlic (that can be cut up and served in food), which is a known antifungal agent, to the daily diet.

⊖ CLIENT COMMUNICATION

Educate clients regarding the spread of fungal infections and how the infection can be avoided. Public showers or dressing rooms in gymnasiums may harbor fungal organisms. Remind clients to be cautious of their environment.

Prognosis

All forms of dermatophytosis tend to be chronic and persistent. Scrupulous management is required to resolve the condition. Even so, recurrences may be common.

Prevention

Following proper hygiene practices is the best means of preventing dermatophytosis.

SCABIES

ICD-10: B86

Description

Scabies is an age-old skin infection that is the result of infestation by the itch mite. It is endemic in some parts of the world, affecting about 300 million individuals, most commonly children younger than age 2.

Etiology

The infection is caused by the *Sarcoptes scabiei* var. *Hominis,* commonly called the *itch mite* or *sarcoptic mange.* Mites live their entire lives in the skin of humans, causing chronic infection. Scabies is transmitted through skin or intimate contact. The adult mite can survive outside a human host for only 2 to 3 days.

Signs and Symptoms

The itching intensifies at night. The lesions are usually excoriated and may appear threadlike. They are about 3/8 inches long and commonly appear between fingers, on wrists, on elbows, in the axilla, at the waist, on nipples and buttocks, and on genitalia.

Diagnostic Procedures

Visual examination of the area may be sufficient. A drop of mineral oil is placed over the burrow made by the mite, and superficial scrapings are taken. The scrapings can then be placed under a microscope to determine if ova or mite feces are indicated.

Treatment

The application of a pediculicide, such as permethrin, lindane cream, or crotamiton, left on for 8 to 12 hours a day for about 5 days is the treatment of choice. Antipruritics and oral antihistamines can reduce itching. Unfortunately, health-care agencies in developing nations may not be able to provide individuals with complete treatment.

Complementary Therapy

No significant alternative therapy is indicated.

 CLIENT COMMUNICATION

Instruct clients that the prescribed cream is to be applied from the neck down, covering the entire body. Clients should wait 15 minutes before dressing and not bathe for 8 to 12 hours. Contaminated clothing and bedding should be washed in hot water. Teach clients how to avoid contamination and to practice good hand-washing techniques.

Prognosis

With treatment, the prognosis for scabies is good. Intense scratching can lead to secondary bacterial infection, which may require antibiotic treatment.

Prevention

The best prevention of scabies is to practice good hygiene.

IMPETIGO

ICD-10: L40.1

Description

Impetigo is a contagious superficial skin infection marked by a vesicle (a small, fluid-filled blister) or a **bulla** (a large, fluid-filled blister) that becomes pustular, ruptures, and forms a yellow crust.

Etiology

The disease is usually caused by streptococcal or staphylococcal bacteria that enter the skin through a cut or lesion. Predisposing factors include poor hygiene, malnutrition, and anemia. Impetigo occurs more frequently in clients who live in warm climates. It is more common among infants and small children but can occur occasionally among older children and adults.

Signs and Symptoms

The lesions of impetigo begin as macules, vesicles, and pustules, usually accompanied by pruritus. The primary lesion ruptures, leaving a honey-colored serous liquid. The liquid hardens, and a thick, yellow crust eventually forms over the infected site. Impetigo can occur anywhere, but it is most common on the mouth, nose, neck, or extremities. Satellite lesions may appear as a result of autoinoculation. Erythema with ulcerations and scarring may result.

Diagnostic Procedures

The characteristics of the lesions assist in the diagnosis of impetigo. Viewing a Gram stain, which is a method of differentiating between bacteria, of the vesicle fluid under the microscope typically confirms the infection.

Treatment

Antibiotics are essential; topical and/or oral antibiotic treatment may be used. Thorough cleansing of the lesions is necessary two to three times daily. Impetigo is highly contagious and can spread to other parts of the body as well as other family members.

Complementary Therapy

No significant complementary therapy is indicated. However, it is noted that soaking the infected area with 1 tablespoon of white vinegar mixed in 1 pint of water for 20 minutes can help remove the scabs.

 CLIENT COMMUNICATION

Cleanliness is paramount. If topical treatment is ordered, it is important to bathe the skin with a soap solution at the lesion site before applying the medication. Instruct clients and family to wear gloves when applying the medication or bathing the skin. Each person should have a separate towel or washcloth. Limit direct contact with the infected person.

Prognosis

The prognosis for impetigo is good.

Prevention

Prevention of impetigo includes good hygiene and avoidance of infected persons.

WARTS

ICD-10: B07.X

Description

Warts (verrucae) are benign, circumscribed, elevated skin lesions resulting from hypertrophy of the epidermis (Fig. 8.13). Warts may be solitary or clustered, occurring most often on the exposed surfaces of the skin. There are five types of warts:

- *Common warts* appear most often on the hands, but they may be located anywhere on the body. They are rough, shaped like a dome, and gray-brown in color.

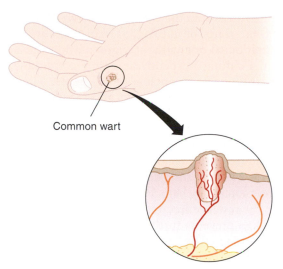

Figure 8.13   Common wart.

- *Plantar warts* grow on the soles of the feet. They look like hard, thick patches of skin and often cause pain when walking.
- *Flat warts* usually appear on the face, arms, or legs. They are smaller than a pencil eraser, are flat, and can be pink, brown, or yellow.
- *Filiform warts* are seen near the mouth, nose, or beard area. They are the same color as the skin and have growths looking like threads sticking out of them.
- *Periungual warts* grow under and around the toenails and fingernails. They are rough bumps with an uneven surface and can affect nail growth.

Children between ages 12 and 16 are affected most frequently.

Etiology

Warts are caused by infection from papillomaviruses, each tending to infect different parts of the body. In general, the mode of transmission is through direct contact or autoinfection (spreading infection from one area of the body to another).

Signs and Symptoms

Warts are usually asymptomatic except when they occur on weight-bearing areas. The size, shape, and appearance of warts vary widely. Tenderness and itching may accompany the lesions.

Diagnostic Procedures

Visual examination of the wart is usually sufficient for diagnosis.

Treatment

Warts may be removed with carbon dioxide–applied laser therapy, salicylic acid plasters, surgical excision, cryosurgery, or keratolytic (peeling) agents. Immunotherapy may be tried for resistant warts. Treatment can be tedious and often is painful.

Complementary Therapy

Twice daily, clients can apply a mixture of garlic oil, vitamin E oil, castor oil, and vitamin A with a drop of zinc oxide cream to the affected area. Cover the area after each application and have the client repeat this treatment for 10 days.

➔ CLIENT COMMUNICATION

Instruct clients to avoid irritation to the area, to not scratch or pick the warts, and to follow prescribed treatment.

Prognosis

Spontaneous cures occur in about 50% of cases, but warts may resist any treatment, and recurrences are frequent. Secondary infection and scarring are possible.

Prevention

Because warts can be transmitted via direct contact, the best preventative measure is to have clients avoid touching any warts.

VITILIGO

ICD-10: L80

Description

Vitiligo is a disorder in which the melanocytes, pigment-producing cells of the skin, are destroyed or cease producing melanin (Fig. 8.14). The result is depigmentation or white patches on the skin and mucous membranes. See the National Vitiligo Foundation at http://nvfi.org for more information.

Etiology

Vitiligo affects about 0.5% to 1% of the world population. There are 1 to 2 million cases in the United States. It affects both genders and all races equally, though it is more noticeable on people with darker skin tones. Half of those affected show the disorder before age 20, though most develop it before age 40. The cause of vitiligo is not known, but it appears to be genetically determined or an autoimmune disorder. Nearly 30% of people with vitiligo have a family member with the condition. Some autoimmune diseases, such as hyperthyroidism, adrenocortical insufficiency, and pernicious anemia, are associated with vitiligo.

Signs and Symptoms

Depigmentation or white spots on the skin appear most often on those areas exposed to sunlight, such as the face, lips, hands, and feet. White patches also commonly occur in the armpits, navel, groin, genital, and rectal areas. Vitiligo appears in three patterns: (1) focal pattern, which is limited to one or a few areas; (2) segmental pattern, which

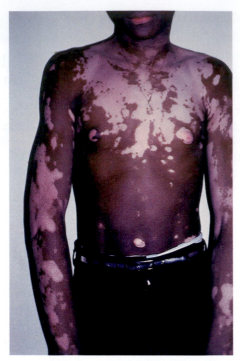

Figure 8.14   Vitiligo. *(From Gylys, BA, and Wedding, ME:* Medical Terminology Systems: A Body Systems Approach, *ed. 4. Philadelphia: F.A. Davis, 2009, p 87.)*

affects only one side of the body; and (3) generalized pattern, which is the most common type and occurs symmetrically on both sides of the body. Those with generalized vitiligo may have premature graying of scalp hair, facial hair, eyebrows, and eyelashes. Generalized vitiligo is usually progressive, and the rate can vary, either developing slowly over many years or occurring rapidly.

Diagnostic Procedures

A physical examination of the affected area and a medical history showing sunburn, trauma, premature graying, stress, or physical illness 2 to 3 months before depigmentation occurred and a family history of vitiligo or other autoimmune disease are sufficient to determine the condition. Skin biopsy with microscopic examination showing a lack of melanocytes confirms diagnosis. Blood tests to check for anemia, thyroid function, and a CBC are also performed.

Treatment

Treatment is generally an attempt to repigment the white areas. Topical corticosteroids may repigment the area but take at least 3 months to show results. Psoralen and ultraviolet A therapy repigment the skin by oral administration or topical application of psoralen followed by exposure of the skin to ultraviolet light. Side effects are severe blistering, sunburn, and increased risk of cataracts, especially in children under age 10. Clients may also experience nausea, vomiting, abnormal hair growth, and hyperpigmentation. For those with depigmentation on 50% or more of the skin, monobenzone is applied to

pigmented areas until they lighten to match depigmented areas. Skin grafts of autologous skin from an area of pigmentation to one without pigmentation can be attempted. Grafting is expensive and time-consuming, and results may not be acceptable to all clients. Micropigmentation or tattooing has shown good results, especially around the lip area.

Complementary Therapy

The client may take ginkgo biloba orally three times a day. Ginkgo is a potent antioxidant, anti-inflammatory, and immune-modulating herb. Research indicates that vitiligo may be the result of free-radical damage to the skin and that ginkgo prevents further damage. Ginkgo causes a blood-thinning effect in some individuals, so people on anticoagulant medication should avoid taking it unless under the direct supervision of a PCP. The use of ginkgo biloba should be reported prior to any surgical procedure.

CLIENT COMMUNICATION

Vitiligo can be emotionally and psychologically distressing, and it is important to reassure the client that there are ways to minimize the appearance of the depigmented skin. While treatment is being established, makeup and self-tanners can be used to cover and conceal areas of depigmentation.

Prognosis

Vitiligo is a chronic condition, and the prognosis is unpredictable. For less than one-third of clients, the depigmentation stops progressing and remains stable for a lifetime. Spontaneous repigmentation of the skin may occur in 30% of those with the condition. Even with treatment, vitiligo may not be fully reversed.

Prevention

There is no known prevention for vitiligo.

SCLERODERMA

ICD-10: M34.X

Description

Scleroderma, also called *systemic sclerosis,* is a progressive, chronic, connective tissue disease characterized by diffuse fibrosis of the skin and internal organs. In systemic scleroderma, both skin and internal organs are involved. The disease exhibits degenerative and fibrotic changes in skin, blood vessels, skeletal muscles, and internal organs, such as the esophagus, gastrointestinal (GI) tract, thyroid, lungs, and heart.

Etiology

The specific cause is unknown, but scleroderma appears to be an autoimmune disorder. Women are more frequently affected than men, especially those ages 30 to 50. It can be mild or severe.

Signs and Symptoms

Raynaud phenomenon (discoloration of the fingers or toes after exposure to changes in temperature) is usually the first symptom, followed by pain, stiffness, and swelling of the fingers and joints. Calcium deposits appear in connective tissue. The skin becomes thick, shiny, and taut.

Contractures eventually develop. GI symptoms include heartburn, reflux, diarrhea, constipation, weight loss, dysphagia, and malabsorption. In the late stage, cardiac and pulmonary fibrosis cause arrhythmias and dyspnea.

Diagnostic Procedures

The typical cutaneous clinical picture helps pinpoint the disease. Hand, chest, and GI x-rays may show systemic changes. Blood studies show an elevated erythrocyte sedimentation rate (ESR) and a positive antinuclear antibody test. Urinalysis may indicate renal involvement. A skin biopsy may be done.

Treatment

Treatment is palliative. Chemotherapy with immunosuppressive drugs may be tried. Corticosteroids and colchicine have shown some success in stabilizing symptoms. Raynaud phenomenon may be treated with vasodilators and antihypertensive drugs. Any digital ulcerations require immediate treatment.

Complementary Therapy

Physical and occupational therapy can help clients manage pain and increase their mobility and strength. Relaxation and meditation have been helpful in reducing the stress levels.

⊕ CLIENT COMMUNICATION

Remind clients not to have fingerstick blood tests because of poor blood circulation. Air-conditioning may aggravate Raynaud phenomenon.

Prognosis

The disease course is quite variable. The prognosis is poor, with death usually resulting from renal, cardiac, or pulmonary failure. About 30% of individuals with the disease die within 5 years of diagnosis. There is no cure for scleroderma.

Prevention

There is no known prevention of scleroderma except to prevent complications of the disease. The client is to avoid cold, stress, and trauma.

Dermatitis

Dermatitis is a common inflammation of the skin manifested by itching, redness, and the appearance of various skin lesions. The disease may be acute, subacute, or chronic. The following forms of dermatitis are considered here: seborrheic dermatitis, contact dermatitis (including latex allergy), atopic dermatitis, and neurodermatitis.

Complementary Therapy

The complementary therapies for the three forms of dermatitis are quite similar and are included here. Identifying any food allergens may be the first step. Common allergens are milk and wheat products. Many people also have allergic reactions to certain fabrics such as wool, to metals in jewelry, or to any number of chemicals found in makeup and body lotions and creams. There are toxic plants, such as poison ivy or poison oak, to consider. Once the offending allergens are found, they should be avoided.

Nutritional therapy may be useful and is likely to include vitamin B complex, acidophilus, zinc, and magnesium. Probiotic supplements have shown promise. Cold compresses can help control pain and itching. A mix of vitamin E, vitamin A, unflavored yogurt, a little honey, and zinc oxide may be applied on the affected area. Evening primrose oil applied directly to the cracks and sore areas in the folds of the elbows and behind the knees may promote healing, too. Aloe vera gel may be beneficial on irritated skin. Adults can take 500 mg of black currant oil twice a day for about 6 to 8 weeks to reduce dermatitis. Phototherapy is often used with success.

SEBORRHEIC DERMATITIS

ICD-10: L21.X

Description

Seborrheic dermatitis is a chronic functional disease of the sebaceous glands marked by an increase in the amount and often alteration in the quality of the sebaceous secretion. When the disease occurs in infancy, it is called *cradle cap* and usually clears without treatment by age 8 to 12 months. Seborrheic dermatitis also is common in the diaper area, where it can be confused with other forms of dermatitis.

Etiology

Seborrheic dermatitis is an idiopathic disease. It may occur when individuals have a disease of the nervous system, such as Parkinson disease. Persons with a stressful medical condition such as having had a heart attack also may develop this problem.

Signs and Symptoms

The disease is characterized by skin eruptions on areas of the scalp, eyelids, cheeks, beard, chest, axillae, groin, or trunk that produce dry, moist, or greasy scales (Fig. 8.15). The lesions are brown-yellow or red. Such scaling produced by the scalp is commonly called *dandruff*. The affected area of the skin frequently itches and may appear reddened.

Diagnostic Procedures

The diagnosis is usually made on the basis of the medical history and observation of the characteristic lesions. The disease must be differentiated from psoriasis (see the "Psoriasis" section in this chapter).

Treatment

Gentle shampooing with a mild shampoo is helpful in treating cradle cap. Shampoos containing tar, salicylic acid, or zinc pyrithione are often helpful in controlling the scaling. Hydrocortisone creams may be prescribed to relieve redness and itching.

 CLIENT COMMUNICATION

Scrupulous skin hygiene and keeping the skin as dry as possible are essential.

Prognosis

Seborrheic dermatitis is a chronic condition; however, the prognosis is good, given effective treatment that controls the disease. The presence of secondary infections may complicate treatment.

Prevention

There is no known prevention for seborrheic dermatitis.

CONTACT DERMATITIS

ICD-10: L24.X

Description

Contact dermatitis is any acute skin inflammation caused by the direct action of various irritants on the surface of the skin or by contact with a substance to which an individual is allergic or sensitive. These allergens are harmless to most people, but some individuals are born with or develop a hypersensitivity to certain allergens.

Etiology

A wide variety of animal, vegetable, and mineral substances may induce contact dermatitis. These may include drugs, acids, alkaline, and resins from such plants as poison ivy, poison oak, or poison sumac. Some individuals are even sensitive to the composition of certain metals and may experience contact dermatitis as a consequence of wearing jewelry. Others may develop dermatitis as a result of wearing latex gloves or wool fibers.

Signs and Symptoms

The symptoms include erythema and the appearance of small skin vesicles that ooze, scale, itch, burn, or sting. The affected area may be hot and swollen.

Diagnostic Procedures

Diagnosis is usually made on the basis of the appearance of the inflamed skin. A medical history revealing prior outbreaks of the condition and the location of the affected area of skin may help in isolating the specific irritant or allergen. A patch test with the offending agent may be done to determine the exact irritant.

Treatment

The skin surface must be thoroughly cleansed of the suspected irritant. Topical corticosteroid lotions or creams may be the treatment of choice.

 CLIENT COMMUNICATION

Explain to clients the importance of avoiding all contact with any particular allergen. This awareness necessitates careful label reading.

Prognosis

Contact dermatitis is generally self-limiting. The problem tends to recur if the individual is re-exposed to the

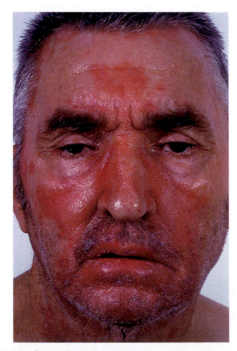

Figure 8.15 Seborrheic dermatitis. *(From Goldsmith, LA, Lazarus, GS, and Tharp, MD: Adult and Pediatric Dermatology: A Color Guide to Diagnosis and Treatment. Philadelphia: F.A. Davis, 1997, p 90, with permission.)*

particular irritant or allergen. It can take 2 to 4 weeks to resolve.

Prevention

The best prevention for contact dermatitis is avoidance of known allergens or irritants.

LATEX ALLERGY

ICD-10: T65.81XX

Description

Latex allergy is identified specifically here because so many health-care professionals are faced with this immune reaction. However, it generally is not thought of as a major form of dermatitis in the medical community; rather it is treated as contact dermatitis. This allergy is a hypersensitivity to products containing latex derived from the rubber tree. The reaction can range from local dermatitis to the very serious anaphylactic shock.

Etiology

Individuals with a history of asthma or other allergies, especially to bananas, avocados, and tropical fruits, seem to be at higher risk. Anyone with frequent contact with latex-containing products is at risk. The risk increases with each exposure. Medical and dental professionals are especially at risk because of their wide use of latex gloves.

Signs and Symptoms

The mild signs and symptoms are itchy skin, swollen lips, nausea and diarrhea, and red, swollen eyes. Signs of anaphylactic shock include hypotension, tachycardia, difficulty breathing, and bronchospasm. Anaphylactic shock is a medical emergency.

Diagnostic Procedures

A blood test for latex sensitivity that measures specific immunoglobulin E (IgE) antibodies against latex can confirm the diagnosis. Anyone reporting even mild irritation from activities such as inflating a balloon or wearing latex gloves should be suspected of having the allergy.

Treatment

The best treatment is avoidance of any products containing latex. Common nonmedical products include balloons, cervical diaphragms, condoms, disposable diapers, elastic stockings, glue, latex paint, bottle nipples and pacifiers, rubber bands, and adhesive tape. Medical and dental professionals should carefully read the labels on items used in their practice, although the use of latex within medical environments is reducing. Latex is a common ingredient in many items.

Complementary Therapy

No significant complementary therapy is indicated other than avoidance of the known allergen.

⊙ CLIENT COMMUNICATION

Teach clients how to identify latex items, what the dangers are, and how to prepare themselves and family members for the possibility of anaphylactic shock. Instructions should be given on the use of an epinephrine autoinjector. It is recommended that clients at risk wear a medical identification tag. If undergoing a medical procedure, advise clients to seek a latex-free environment.

Prognosis

The prognosis for latex allergy is good with proper attention to avoidance of latex-containing products.

Prevention

Avoidance of latex-containing products, wearing a medical identification tag, and being prepared to use an epinephrine autoinjector, if necessary, are essential.

ATOPIC DERMATITIS (ECZEMA)

ICD-10: L20.XX

Description

Atopic dermatitis is an inflammation of the skin accompanied by intense itching, of unknown etiology. The disease occurs in 3% to 5% of the population, mostly up to age 5.

Etiology

Although the condition is idiopathic, it appears to have allergic or hereditary components. It is more common in whites and Asians. For approximately 70% of cases, there is a family history of this disease, asthma, or allergic rhinitis.

Signs and Symptoms

There will be pruritus and often severe characteristic lesions on the face, neck, upper trunk, and bends of the knees and elbows (Fig. 8.16). Atopic dermatitis may cause vesicular and exudative eruptions in children and dry, leathery vesicles in adults.

Diagnostic Procedures

Observation of the skin and a medical history revealing a family tendency toward developing atopic dermatitis assist in diagnosing the condition. Serum IgE levels may be elevated.

Treatment

Local and systemic agents may be prescribed to prevent itching. Careful daily skin care and total avoidance of known irritants are important. In addition,

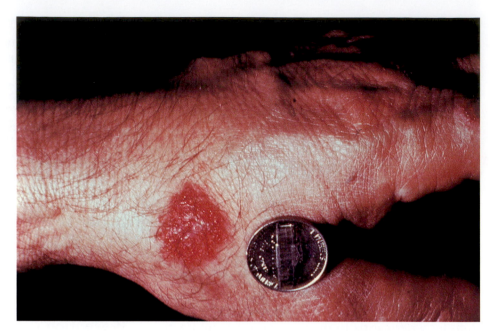

Figure 8.16 Nummular eczema. *(From Goldsmith, LA, Lazarus, GS, and Tharp, MD:* Adult and Pediatric Dermatology: A Color Guide to Diagnosis and Treatment. *Philadelphia: F.A. Davis, 1997, p 294, with permission.)*

topical corticosteroid creams and ointments may be prescribed. Skin moisturizer may be beneficial. Maintaining high humidity with a room humidifier may help. Phototherapy often helps reduce recurrences.

Complementary Therapy

It might be helpful to eliminate all milk and milk products from the client's diet. Adults can take black current oil twice a day; children should take only one-half of an adult dose. This regimen may take 6 to 8 weeks to produce the desired results. Aloe vera gel and calendula lotion or cream may be applied to irritated skin.

➔ CLIENT COMMUNICATION

Teach clients and family members to watch for any secondary infection. Discourage the use of laundry additives, and suggest ways to avoid offending irritants.

Prognosis

The prognosis is good, but the disorder itself can be frustrating to control, as it may have to be dealt with throughout most of the individual's life. Eczema can become infected with bacteria and, less commonly, with viruses.

Prevention

The best prevention for eczema is avoidance of known irritants.

NEURODERMATITIS

ICD-10: L28.1 or L28.0

Description

Neurodermatitis, or lichen simplex chronicus or scratch dermatitis, is a stubborn skin condition that

occurs when individuals excessively scratch an area of skin. Scratching makes the individual itch more, so the scratching continues until the affected skin becomes thick and leathery. This condition is more common between the ages of 30 and 50 and is seen more in women than men.

Etiology

The cause of neurodermatitis is unknown. The problem begins when an irritant aggravates the skin and triggers an itch. As the individual scratches, the itch intensifies, forcing prolonged bouts of scratching. Eventually, the individual is unable to stop the itch-scratch cycle. This cycle may be less of a problem during activities when the client is distracted and less aware of the itching and may be more irritating at rest when the client is not distracted and can refocus on scratching. Anxiety and stress can make itchiness worse.

Signs and Symptoms

The signs and symptoms of neurodermatitis include skin that itches in a particular area and then becomes leathery or scaly. The area may have a raised and rough patch that is darker than the rest of the skin.

Diagnostic Procedures

Patch testing may be helpful to determine any allergens. Otherwise, visual examination of the skin's appearance is all that is necessary for diagnosis.

Treatment

Oral corticosteroids and/or antihistamines can reduce inflammation and relieve the itching. Wet dressings applied to the affected area may be used. Antianxiety medications or antidepressants may help individuals "quiet" their tendencies to scratch.

Complementary Therapy

Black cumin oil or black seed oil can be applied topically several times a day and has been shown to lessen itching and heal the skin.

⊖ CLIENT COMMUNICATION

Advise clients that with treatment and stress relief, neurodermatitis can be treated, but it may take many months for the skin to return to a normal appearance.

Prognosis

If the itch-scratch cycle is not stopped, bacterial skin infection can occur.

Prevention

The best preventative measure includes a cool bath with baking soda or colloidal oatmeal to help break the itch-scratch cycle. Advise clients to wear comfortable, nonirritating clothing, to keep stress under control as much as possible, and to choose mild soaps.

Herpes-Related Skin Lesions

COLD SORES AND FEVER BLISTERS

ICD-10: B00.X

Description

Cold sores (see Chapter 14) and fever blisters are skin eruptions occurring around the perimeter of the mouth, lips, and nose or on the mucous membranes within the mouth. Sometimes tingling and numbness may precede or follow these eruptions. The condition affects people of any age.

Etiology

These lesions are produced by the herpes simplex virus type 1 (HSV-1). It is estimated that 9 out of 10 persons have been exposed to HSV-1. This virus may lie dormant within the body for extended periods, reactivating during times of lowered resistance or emotional and physical stress. Cold sores may erupt following a rise in body temperature, such as during a common cold or even preceding menstruation. In some instances, however, they may occur before the onset of illness or for no apparent reason at all.

Signs and Symptoms

The characteristic lesions are small, pale vesicles appearing individually or in clusters, especially on the lips or about the mouth. The lesions may also be seen elsewhere (Fig. 8.17). The affected area may burn and sting. The lesions may eventually break, forming ulcers or crusts. Over time the crust will fall off and the redness goes away. The whole process can take about 10 to 14 days.

Diagnostic Procedures

The diagnosis is made on the basis of the individual's characteristic lesions. The virus may need to be isolated by histological examination of the scrapings.

Treatment

Treatment is strictly symptomatic. The drug valacyclovir will shorten the outbreak and lessen recurrence. The lesions should be kept as dry and clean as possible and protected from trauma. Topical analgesics or ointments containing docosanol or benzalkonium chloride may be applied to relieve burning and itching and increase healing. Antibiotic ointments may be recommended to prevent secondary infection of open lesions.

Complementary Therapy

There may be some relief from the use of L-lysine 500 mg, an amino acid, found in the vitamin section of any drugstore. As soon as clients feel the burning or tingling, they should take three or four tablets a day for 2 days and then two tablets until the blisters

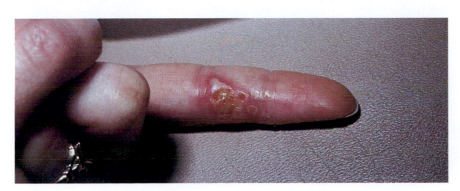

Figure 8.17 Herpes simplex. Primary infection in adult seen on a forefinger. *(From Reeves, JRT, and Maibach, H:* Clinical Dermatology Illustrated: A Regional Approach, *ed. 3. Philadelphia: FA Davis, 1998, p 64, with permission.)*

dry. (Instruct clients not to take L-lysine on an empty stomach.) Vitamin E oil may dry the sores within 5 to 7 days.

➔ **CLIENT COMMUNICATION**

HSV-1 is spread via close contact, such as kissing or sharing drinking glasses, eating utensils, and lipstick. Even towels should not be shared with someone who has an outbreak. This virus can be spread to the genitals by oral-genital contact. Outbreaks of HSV-1 in the genital area tend to be less severe than those caused by HSV-2, which is a strain of genital herpes (see Chapter 16). HSV-1 can spread from person to person even when the infected individual has no outbreak.

Prognosis

Cold sores and fever blisters usually resolve within 1 to 3 weeks. The HSV-1 resumes dormancy, however, and may reappear given favorable conditions. Sometimes another infection or exposure to wind or sun can reactivate the virus.

Prevention

There is no specific prevention other than avoiding intimate contact with persons with visible cold sores.

HERPES ZOSTER (SHINGLES)

ICD-10: B02.XX

Description

Herpes zoster (shingles) is an acute inflammatory eruption of highly painful vesicles on the trunk of the body or occasionally on the face. Adults over age 50 are primarily affected.

Etiology

Shingles is caused by reactivation of the varicella zoster virus, the same virus that causes chickenpox. What triggers this reactivation is not known. The lesions occur on a segment of skin lying above the course of a nerve that has been infected by the virus.

Signs and Symptoms

The first symptom is pain along the affected nerve, usually occurring 1 to 3 days before appearance of the lesions. The skin eruption begins as an erythematous maculopapular rash that develops quite rapidly into vesicles. The site of these lesions is usually on one side of the trunk of the body, but if nerves supplying the face are involved, lesions may also appear on one side of the face, mouth, or tongue or around one eye (Fig. 8.18). The region around the affected site is often intensely painful.

Diagnostic Procedures

The condition is diagnosed by its characteristic pattern of painful lesions. Confirmation of the diagnosis can be made by isolating the virus in cell cultures grown from scrapings of the lesions or by detecting varicella zoster antibodies in the blood.

Treatment

Antiviral drug therapy is the treatment of choice. With an early diagnosis, valacyclovir has shown success in preventing the progression of the rash and visceral complications. Sedatives, analgesics, and antipruritics may be prescribed. If the vesicles are infected, antibiotics may be given to prevent secondary infection.

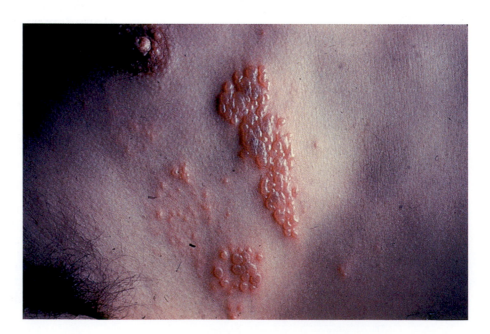

Figure 8.18 Herpes zoster (shingles).
(From Reeves, JRT, and Maibach, H: Clinical Dermatology Illustrated: A Regional Approach, *ed. 3. Philadelphia: F.A. Davis, 1998, p 255, with permission.)*

Complementary Therapy

A gel made from licorice root appears to be a helpful topical application in pain and inflammation. The application of transcutaneous electrical nerve stimulation (TENS) to affected nerves is also helpful to relieve more nerve pain.

 CLIENT COMMUNICATION

Teach clients how to keep the area dry and clean and how to prevent infection. Adequate rest and diversionary and relaxation activities are helpful.

Prognosis

The prognosis is usually good. Shingles runs its course within 7 to 10 days; however, recurrent bouts of severe pain may persist for weeks or months after the lesions have resolved. The disease may cause serious damage to the structure of the eye if nerves supplying the eye are involved. Shingles can recur.

Prevention

For those over age 60, a vaccine made from weakened chickenpox virus is recommended, though it may not protect all recipients.

CHAPTER EPISODE—PART II

Amanda can't handle the pain anymore and decides to take ibuprofen for relief. Her skin is extremely reddened. She is unable to move well without feeling the stiffness of her skin, and she starts to notice little blisters along the tops of her shoulders.

- What should Amanda do now?
- Should she seek medical attention? Explain your response.

Cancer

SKIN CARCINOMAS

ICD-10: C44.XX

Description

According to the American Cancer Society, the annual rates of all forms of skin cancer are increasing at an alarming rate. It is estimated that nearly half of all Americans who live to age 65 will develop skin cancer at least once. The most common skin cancers are basal cell carcinoma and squamous cell carcinoma. Basal cell carcinomas arise from the basal cell layer of the epidermis or hair follicles; are locally invasive, slow-growing, and destructive; and very rarely metastasize. Basal cell carcinoma is the most common form of skin cancer, accounting for about 90% of cases. It occurs more frequently in blond, fair-skinned individuals. Squamous cell carcinomas also arise from the epidermal layers above the basal layer. These cells lose the ability to keratinize and slough off, so they continue to grow outward. Squamous cell carcinoma is the more serious of the two because of its tendency to metastasize. This carcinoma occurs more frequently in fair-skinned men over age 60. See Skin Cancer Gallery at www.cancer.org.

Etiology

Repeated overexposure to the sun's ultraviolet rays is the most important etiologic factor in skin carcinomas. Other causes include radiation exposure, chronic skin irritation and inflammation, and exposure to carcinogens.

Signs and Symptoms

Cancerous skin lesions may appear anywhere on the body, but the common sites are sun-exposed areas, such as the face, chest, back, ears, forearms, and back of hands. Initially, both forms are painless. Basal cell carcinomas are classified as noduloulcerative lesions, superficial basal cell, and sclerosing basal cell. Squamous cell carcinoma is characterized by rough or red visible scales. Both carcinomas often ulcerate and form a crust.

Diagnostic Procedures

A medical history; careful observation of the skin, noting characteristic lesions; and biopsy of the lesions are necessary for diagnosis.

Treatment

The goal of treatment is to completely eradicate the lesions. The size, shape, location, and invasiveness of the carcinoma determine treatment. Methods of treatment include surgery (used in 90% of the cases), radiation therapy, curettage, cryosurgery, laser therapy and **electrodessication,** and **Mohs micrographic surgery.** Treatment of skin carcinomas may involve chemotherapeutic agents for persistent or recurrent lesions.

Complementary Therapy

Any alternative therapy for cancer (see Chapter 5) is best approved and integrated with the therapy suggested by traditional PCPs.

 CLIENT COMMUNICATION

Remind clients that it is necessary to avoid excessive sun exposure and to use sunscreen to prevent disease recurrence.

Prognosis

The prognosis for carcinomas of the skin is good, with a 90% cure rate if they are detected and treated in the early stage. Although basal cell carcinomas rarely metastasize, when untreated they may result in the loss of an ear, a nose, or a lip. Because squamous cell carcinomas may metastasize, individuals should be followed closely for a minimum of 5 years to detect new lesions or metastasis.

Prevention

The best prevention is to avoid overexposure to the sun. Sun damage to the skin is cumulative, so sunscreens and protective measures should be used throughout life. Warn clients to stay out of tanning booths.

MALIGNANT MELANOMA

ICD-10: C43.XX

Description

A malignant melanoma is a neoplasm composed of abnormal melanocytes appearing in both the epidermis and dermis. Malignant melanoma appears in one of four forms: (1) superficial spreading melanoma occurs on any body site and is the most common form of melanoma; (2) lentigo maligna melanoma occurs on exposed skin areas, especially the head and neck, and is a slowly evolving pigmented lesion; (3) nodular melanoma occurs on any site and directly invades tissue below the dermis; and (4) acral lentiginous melanoma occurs where hair follicles are absent (palms of hands, soles of feet, nail beds) and appears as irregular, pigmented macules that develop into nodules and become invasive early. Melanomas may appear suddenly without warning or can develop from or near a mole. The incidence of melanoma has more than tripled in individuals with pale complexions during the last 20 years and causes more deaths than all other skin diseases.

Etiology

Although ultraviolet rays are suspect, the etiology of malignant melanoma is unknown. The persons at greatest risk have fair complexions, blue eyes, red or blond hair, and freckles. Excessive childhood sun exposure, blistering childhood sunburns, an increased number of common and dysplastic moles, a family history of melanoma, and older age greatly increase the risk of melanoma.

Signs and Symptoms

Malignant melanomas are characterized by lesions having irregular borders and a diversity of colors. The lesion of superficial spreading melanoma tends to be circular, flat, and visibly or palpably elevated. Color variations include tan, brown, black mixed with gray, bluish black, or white. There may be a whitish pink color in a small area within the lesion. The lentigo maligna melanoma appears as a brown or black flat lesion that undergoes changes in size and color with time (Fig. 8.19). The nodular melanoma is generally blue-black in color, resembling a "blood blister" that fails to resolve. The lesion is spherical with a relatively smooth surface. The acral lentiginous melanoma appears as a dark brown flat lesion or a blue-black or brown-black raised lesion.

Diagnostic Procedures

Suspicious skin lesions must undergo biopsy to determine the diagnosis. Then the melanoma is staged on a scale of 1 to 4. Staging determines treatment. See http://www.cancerhelp.org and search stages of melanoma for

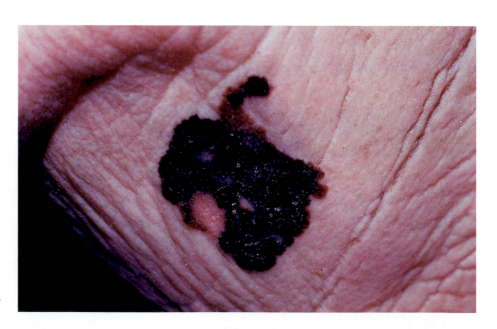

Figure 8.19 Dark lentigo maligna on cheek and in sideburn. Apparently clear area between the sites was probably involved in the past but is resolved. Seborrheic keratosis is present at upper edge of lower lesion. *(From Reeves, JRT, and Maibach, H:* Clinical Dermatology Illustrated: A Regional Approach, *ed. 3. Philadelphia: F.A. Davis, 1998, p 338, with permission.)*

a detailed description of this staging process. Physical examination, paying close attention to the lymph nodes, and review of other body systems can help determine metastasis.

Treatment

The level of invasion and measure of the melanoma's thickness determine the appropriate treatment. Surgical excision of the lesion is the most common treatment modality, and it may be necessary to remove nearby lymph nodes. Chemotherapy may be recommended. Radiation therapy is usually reserved for metastatic disease. Melanoma vaccines, a type of specific active immunotherapy, are in current clinical trials for advanced stages of the disease (III and IV); trials aimed at prevention are not yet available.

Complementary Therapy

See "Skin Carcinomas."

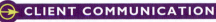

CLIENT COMMUNICATION

See "Skin Carcinomas."

Prognosis

The prognosis is related to the level of the dermal invasion and the thickness of the lesion. The prognosis is poorer if the melanoma grows vertically rather than horizontally. If metastasis occurs, it can affect every organ of the body. If the melanoma is detected and treated early, there is a good rate of survival. Statistics show that more than 10% of recurrence develops more than 5 years after the primary lesion is treated.

Prevention

Avoiding overexposure to the sun and ultraviolet rays and seeking prompt treatment for any suspected lesions or changes in the skin are the best prevention.

Reconstructive Skin Procedures

Reconstructive procedures (including surgery) are a necessary part of treatment and recovery for a number of disorders affecting the skin. For example, skin grafting is often required in the treatment of serious burns. In the past decade, however, cosmetic or plastic surgery has grown in popularity.

Cosmetic surgery was at one time a luxury for the rich and famous. As society has become more health conscious and youth oriented, the stigma once associated with cosmetic surgery has all but disappeared. Surgical techniques have improved, and the number of specialists certified to perform them has increased. While medical insurance plans do not cover elective cosmetic surgery, the cost involved has also dropped to a more obtainable price for the average person. Reasons for choosing cosmetic surgery vary. Many look to cosmetic surgery to change some aspect of their physical appearance in an attempt to gain self-esteem and a better body image. Others wish to make themselves into the culturally acceptable image of beauty that is unobtainable otherwise. Cosmetic surgery has gained in popularity not only to change appearance but also to maintain it. A youth-centric society has turned to cosmetic surgery to keep or recapture a youthful appearance. In a highly competitive job market, many people are using the rejuvenation of cosmetic procedures as a way to stay competitive with younger job seekers.

In 2014 the American Society for Aesthetic Plastic Surgery reported that nearly 14.6 million people in the United States had either a cosmetic surgical or nonsurgical procedure performed and spent more than $12 billion for the second year in a row.

Of the top five surgical procedures and the top five nonsurgical procedures sought by clients, liposuction is the most common surgical procedure, and Botox is the most popular nonsurgical procedure. Rounding out the surgical procedures, breast augmentation is a close second, followed by blepharoplasty (eyelid surgery), abdominoplasty, and rhinoplasty. The other nonsurgical procedures are laser hair removal, which has gained in popularity for second place, followed by hyaluronic acid, which is used as a wrinkle filler; chemical peel; and laser skin resurfacing.

Women account for the vast majority of cosmetic surgery clients, commonly receiving liposuction, breast augmentation, blepharoplasty, abdominoplasty or tummy tuck, and rhinoplasty. The most popular procedures with men were liposuction, followed by rhinoplasty, blepharoplasty, breast reduction, and ear shaping. For nonsurgical procedures, men and women were more similar in their choices. Botox was the number one nonsurgical treatment for both sexes, followed by hyaluronic acid, laser hair removal, microdermabrasion, and chemical peel.

Risks associated with cosmetic surgery are the same as for any surgical procedure. When general anesthesia is used, there are risks of heart arrhythmia, blood clots, heart attack, stroke, nerve damage, brain damage, infection, blood loss, and death. The mortality rate for cosmetic surgery clients is 1 in 57,000. Risks associated with cosmetic surgery can be decreased, but not alleviated, by using licensed and certified physicians and surgeons.

CHAPTER EPISODE—PART III

When Amanda has little or no relief from the pain, she decides to see her doctor. Her medical records indicate that she has been to her PCP's office a handful of times with the same complaint of "painful skin related to being in the sun."

- What lifestyle changes might Amanda's doctor suggest to her?
- What sun safety tips might be suggested to Amanda?
- Describe the warning signs of skin cancer to educate Amanda.

COMMON SYMPTOMS OF SKIN DISEASES AND DISORDERS

Individuals may present with the following common complaints, which deserve attention from health-care professionals:

- Skin eruptions
- Pruritus
- Erythema
- Pain
- Swelling
- Inflammation

SUMMARY

Many of the skin diseases and disorders are visually obvious and sometimes embarrassing to individuals. Health-care professionals can play an important role when this embarrassment occurs. There are varied complementary therapies for many skin diseases that work well with the traditional therapies. Clients should inform each practitioner of all treatments being used so that none are conflicting. Advances are continually being made in treatment of skin diseases and disorders; hence, the prognoses are improving.

 | For more resources and to sharpen your skills with interactive exercises, visit DavisPlus at http://davisplus.fadavis.com. Keyword *Tamparo*.

ONLINE RESOURCES

Warts
http://www.nlm.nih.gov/medlineplus
http://www.surgery.org/media/statistics

Skin cancer gallery
http://www.cancer.org

CASE STUDIES

Case Study 1

You have three preschool children. The mother of a neighborhood playmate calls to tell you that her child has impetigo.

Case Study Questions

1. What signs and symptoms should you look for?
2. What actions should you take with your children? What should you do in relation to the other neighborhood children?
3. What is the cause of impetigo?

Case Study 2

Marge Hallet requests an appointment to have her PCP examine a growth on her neck. She is 60 years old, blond, fair-skinned, and an avid tennis player. She did not call when she first noticed the growth, and it has now grown since then. The growth is raised, darkened, and irregular around the edges. The growth is removed. Biopsy indicates malignant melanoma.

Case Study Questions

1. What factors likely have contributed to this disease in Marge?
2. What treatment is indicated?
3. What might the prognosis be in this situation?

REVIEW QUESTIONS

Matching

Match each of the following definitions with its correct term:

_____ 1. Seborrheic dermatitis

_____ 2. Contact dermatitis

_____ 3. Atopic dermatitis

_____ 4. Psoriasis

_____ 5. Urticaria

_____ 6. Acne vulgaris

_____ 7. Alopecia

_____ 8. Herpes simplex virus type 1

_____ 9. Herpes zoster

_____ 10. Impetigo

a. Shingles

b. Hives

c. Inflammatory disease of sebaceous glands and hair follicles

d. Appears to have allergic or hereditary components

e. Produces dry, moist, or greasy scaling

f. Characterized by high rate of skin cell turnover

g. Cold sores or fever blisters

h. Baldness

i. Contagious streptococcal or staphylococcal skin infection

j. Causes erythema and small skin vesicles

k. Boil or abscess

l. Bedsore

Short Answer

1. A _____ or boil is an abscess involving the hair follicle and subcutaneous tissue. A _____ consists of several boils developing in adjoining hair follicles with multiple drainage sinuses.

2. Pediculosis is skin infestation with _____.

3. Dermatophytosis is caused by _____ infections of the skin.

4. A skin disorder you might find on a person who is elderly, debilitated, or paralyzed is _____.

5. Warts, or verrucae, are caused by the _____.

Multiple Choice

1. Which of the following is/are treatment(s) for psoriasis?

_____ a. Soften the scales with petroleum jelly or a preparation containing urea.

_____ b. Take a strong bacterial agent to combat infection.

_____ c. Administer antihistamines during the acute episodes.

_____ d. Wash or dry clean all clothing or bedding.

2. What are the cause(s) of urticaria?

_____ a. Ingestion of shellfish, nuts, wheat, soy, or eggs

_____ b. Hormonal changes

_____ c. Too much sunlight

_____ d. Streptococcal or staphylococcal bacteria

3. Where are corns and calluses likely located on the body?

_____ a. On the scalp, especially when always wearing a cap

_____ b. On the toes, especially the great toe, often from ill-fitting shoes

_____ c. Elbows because they receive the most pressure and friction

_____ d. On the knees, especially those working in construction

4. Which of the following dermatophytosis matches is correct?

_____ a. Scalp and tinea capitis

_____ b. Body and human capitis

_____ c. Feet and tinea corporis

_____ d. Groin and tinea unguium

5. Which of the following statements about latex allergy is correct?

_____ a. The allergy is more apt to occur in those suffering from asthma.

_____ b. A latex allergy can cause either local dermatitis or very serious anaphylactic shock.

_____ c. A blood test with an elevated ESR is the best diagnostic tool.

_____ d. Once diagnosed and treated, repeated exposures to latex will not cause symptoms.

Discussion Questions/Personal Reflection

1. Skin eruptions of any kind are often as personally embarrassing as they are difficult to treat or cure. Identify ways to help your clients overcome this embarrassment.

_____

_____

_____

_____

_____

_____

_____

_____

_____

2. Identify a number of reasons why skin cancer is more prevalent today than it was 10 years ago.

_____

_____

_____

_____

_____

_____

_____

_____

_____

_____

_____

Seeing yourself as you want to be is the key to personal growth.
—ANONYMOUS

9

Musculoskeletal Diseases and Disorders

● key words

Ankylosis (ăng″kĭ•lō′sĭs)

Blepharoptosis (blĕf″ă•rō•tō′sĭs)

Contracture (kŏn•trăk′chūr)

Crepitation (krĕp•ĭ•tā′shŭn)

Dysphagia (dĭs•fā′jē•ă)

Dysphasia (dĭs•fā′zē•ă)

Embolism (ĕm′bō•lĭzm)

Luxation (lŭks•ā′shŭn)

Paresthesia (păr″ĕs•thē′zē•ă)

Raynaud phenomenon (rĕ•nō′ fĕ•nŏm′e•nŏn)

Tinel sign (tĭn•ĕl′ sīn)

Tophus (pl. tophi) (tō′fŭs, tō′fī)

Virulence (vĭr′ū•lĕns)

Upon successful completion of this chapter, you will be able to:

- Interpret key terms.
- Review anatomy and physiology of the musculoskeletal system.
- Compare/contrast three spine deformities.
- Identify the common symptoms of and diagnostic tests for intervertebral disk herniation.
- Recall the incidence and treatment of osteoporosis.
- Describe osteomyelitis and its diagnosis.
- Discuss the complications and prognosis of Paget disease.
- List at least three diagnostic procedures used specifically for determining bone disorders.
- Identify the difference between a luxation and a subluxation.
- Illustrate at least four kinds of fractures with a simple drawing.
- Compare and contrast osteoarthritis and rheumatoid arthritis.

- Recall the description and symptoms of gout.
- Compare and contrast strains and sprains.
- Describe the treatment process for bursitis and tendonitis.
- Discuss prevention of carpal tunnel syndrome.
- Describe the prognosis for systemic lupus erythematosus.
- List the description and etiology of plantar fasciitis.
- Describe myasthenia gravis and identify the treatment.
- Recall the signs and symptoms of polymyositis.
- Discuss the signs and symptoms for fibromyalgia.
- List the main neoplasms of the musculoskeletal system.
- Recall at least four common symptoms of the musculoskeletal system.

CHAPTER EPISODE—PART I

Janet was not feeling well. She was exhausted, never felt refreshed when she awoke in the mornings, and had a lot of pain. Janet didn't think too much of the pain because every weekend she and her spouse would hike over 15 miles in the mountains nearby. She thought she was just a little out of shape. She also had a flare-up of her ulcerative colitis, even though she was taking medication for it. Finally, her family had enough and made certain Janet called her internist to see what was going on.

- As you read through the diseases/disorders of this chapter, remember this scenario and try to determine what her internist might suspect.
- Without reading the chapter, what diseases/disorders might you guess these symptoms identify?

MUSCULOSKELETAL SYSTEM ANATOMY AND PHYSIOLOGY REVIEW

The musculoskeletal system consists of bones, joints, ligaments, muscles, and tendons. The skeleton gives shape to the body, provides physical support and protection for the organs, stores minerals, is responsible for blood cell formation, and provides sites for muscle attachment. The muscles hold the skeleton upright and create physical movement of the body. Any disease or disorder of this system greatly affects activities of daily living.

The skeletal system consists of bones formed from osseous tissue that provide structure and function to the overall body. Also included in the skeletal system is the cartilage that forms the joints between bones and the ligaments that hold bones together at the joints. Bones can be subdivided into long bones (arms, legs, hands, and feet), short bones (wrists, ankles, and kneecaps), flat bones (ribs, sternum, shoulder blades, hip bones, and cranial bones), and irregular bones (vertebrae and facial bones).

The adult skeletal system (Fig. 9.1) has two divisions: the axial skeletal system and the appendicular skeletal system. The axial skeleton is the center portion of the body and includes the bones of the skull, hyoid bone, bones of the middle ear, vertebral column, and rib cage. The appendicular skeleton is composed of the bones of the appendages or limbs and includes the bones of the arms and legs, the shoulders, and the pelvic girdle.

There are two types of bone: compact and spongy. Compact bone is the dense, hard tissue found in the shafts of long bones. Yellow marrow, which is composed of fat, is stored in these bones. Spongy bone, or *cancellous bone,* is less dense and is found at the ends of long bones and in the other bones of the body.

The muscular system (Figs. 9.2 and 9.3) holds the body upright and moves the skeletal system. Muscles

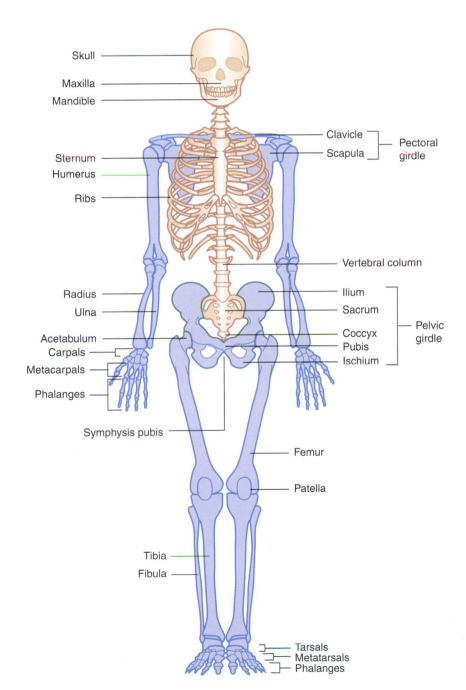

Figure 9.1 Skeleton (anterior view). *(From Thompson, GS: Understanding Anatomy & Physiology: A Visual, Auditory, Interactive Approach, ed. 1. Philadelphia: F.A. Davis, 2013, p 95.)*

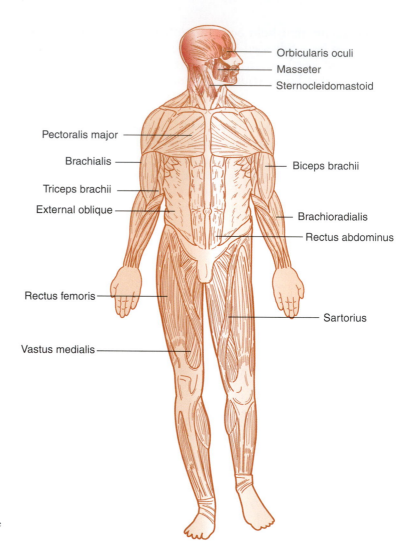

Figure 9.2 Anterior view of muscles. *(From Thompson, GS:* Understanding Anatomy & Physiology: A Visual, Auditory, Interactive Approach, *ed. 1. Philadelphia: F.A. Davis, 2013, p 136.)*

have specialized cells for contraction wherein they shorten and pull a bone to produce movement. Muscle movement creates heat that helps to regulate body temperature. There are three types of muscles:

1. *Skeletal muscle* is also called *voluntary muscle* because it is attached to the skeleton and its movement is consciously controlled. The cells of this type of muscle are elongated and have the ability to stretch and return to their previous shape.
2. *Smooth muscle* is also called *involuntary* or *visceral muscle* because it is found in the walls of organs, and its function is not consciously controlled. This type of muscle has shorter cells with tapered ends and cannot stretch as much as skeletal muscle.
3. *Cardiac muscle* is found only in the heart. This muscle is a combination of skeletal and smooth muscle. It is involuntarily controlled but has the ability to contract.

Diseases and Disorders of Bones

DEFORMITIES OF THE SPINE: LORDOSIS, KYPHOSIS, AND SCOLIOSIS

ICD-10: M40.40 (LORDOSIS)
ICD-10: M40.00 or M40.209 (KYPHOSIS)
ICD-10: M41.20 (SCOLIOSIS)

Description

Lordosis is an abnormal inward curvature of the lumbar or lower spine. This condition is commonly called *sway-back*. Kyphosis is an abnormal outward curvature of the upper thoracic vertebrae. Commonly, this curvature is known as *humpback* or *round back*. Scoliosis is an abnormal sideward curvature of the spine to either the left

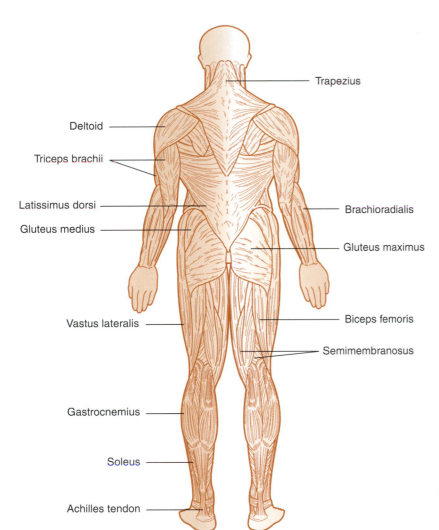

Trapezius

Deltoid

Triceps brachii

Latissimus dorsi

Gluteus medius

Brachioradialis

Gluteus maximus

Vastus lateralis

Biceps femoris

Semimembranosus

Gastrocnemius

Soleus

Achilles tendon

Figure 9.3 Posterior view of muscles. *(From Thompson, GS:* Understanding Anatomy & Physiology: A Visual, Auditory, Interactive Approach, *ed. 1. Philadelphia: F.A. Davis, 2013, p 137.)*

or right. Some rotation of a portion of the vertebral column may also appear. Scoliosis often occurs in combination with kyphosis and lordosis (Fig. 9.4). These three spinal deformities can affect children and adults.

Etiology

Lordosis, kyphosis, and scoliosis may be caused by a variety of problems, including congenital spinal defects, poor posture, a discrepancy in leg lengths (especially in scoliosis), and growth retardation or a vascular disturbance in the epiphysis of the thoracic vertebrae during periods of rapid growth. Kyphosis may be the result of collapsed vertebrae from years of poor posture, degenerative arthritis, or following a history of neuromuscular conditions. Obesity and osteoporosis can be contributing factors for lordosis. These three spinal deformities may also result from tumors, trauma, infection, osteoarthritis, tuberculosis, endocrine disorders such as Cushing disease, prolonged steroid therapy, and degeneration of the spine associated with aging. Lordosis, kyphosis, and scoliosis may also be idiopathic.

Signs and Symptoms

The onset of lordosis, kyphosis, and scoliosis is frequently insidious. Signs and symptoms may include chronic fatigue and backache. Scoliosis is often detected by individuals when they notice that their clothing seems longer on one side than on the other. Or they may notice when looking in a mirror that the height of their hips and shoulders appears uneven.

Diagnostic Procedures

Physical examination and anterior, posterior, and lateral x-rays of the spine are the most commonly used procedures to detect these spinal deformities. A magnetic resonance imaging (MRI) scan may be ordered if a tumor or infection is suspected.

Treatment

Treatment varies according to the nature and severity of the spinal curvature, the age of onset, and the underlying cause of the disorder. The goal is to slow the progression of the disease. Physical therapy, exercise, and

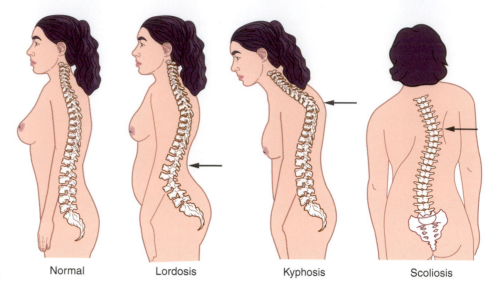

Figure 9.4 Spinal curvatures.

Normal   Lordosis   Kyphosis   Scoliosis

back braces may all play a role in the treatment of these conditions. Spinal bracing, if closely watched and properly constructed and fitted, may be able to halt the progression of the curve in scoliosis. Surgery may be necessary, however, in cases of adolescent scoliosis if the curvature seriously interferes with mobility or breathing. Spinal fusion, using bone grafts and metal rods, is sometimes performed to straighten the spine in this situation. Surgery is rarely necessary for correction of kyphosis. Analgesics may be prescribed to alleviate the pain that frequently accompanies these disorders.

Complementary Therapy

Kyphosis may respond well to therapeutic massage. Physical therapy and exercises to strengthen abdominal muscles can decrease lumbar lordosis. Hamstring stretches can reduce muscle **contractures,** or a permanent shortening of muscle. Yoga and acupuncture are helpful to some.

⊖ CLIENT COMMUNICATION

Emotional support is essential. Stress proper posture. Instruct clients on the use of any brace and to avoid vigorous sports. Meticulous skin care is important to prevent irritation and skin breakdown due to the brace rubbing against the skin. In scoliosis, it is helpful for individuals to turn their whole body, rather than just their head, when looking to the side.

Prognosis

The prognosis of an individual with lordosis, kyphosis, or scoliosis depends on the underlying cause of the particular disease, how early it is detected, and whether it responds to treatment. In some cases, a spinal deformity

may be arrested but not corrected. Pulmonary insufficiency, degenerative arthritis of the spine, and sciatica may arise as complications of spinal deformities.

Prevention

Prevention of lordosis, kyphosis, and scoliosis includes correction of any underlying cause and maintaining good posture. Weight loss can reduce the risk of lordosis. Scoliosis screening in public schools is mandated by law in some states.

HERNIATED INTERVERTEBRAL DISK

TOP DISORDER

ICD-10: M51.9

Description

An intervertebral disk is a saclike cushion of cartilage. One is found between each of the 33 vertebrae. Within each intervertebral disk is the nucleus pulposus, a soft, gelatinous mass that helps each disk cushion the movements of the vertebrae. A herniated intervertebral disk occurs when the nucleus pulposus protrudes through the wall of the disk and into the spinal canal, where it presses on spinal nerves and causes pain and disability (Fig. 9.5). The condition is commonly called a *slipped* or *ruptured disk*. The most common sites for herniated disks are between the fourth and fifth lumbar vertebrae or between the fifth lumbar and the first sacral vertebrae. The condition is more common in men.

Etiology

A herniated disk may be related to intervertebral joint degeneration. In this case, a minor trauma may result in a disk herniation. A herniated intervertebral disk is likely caused by spinal trauma from a fall, straining, or

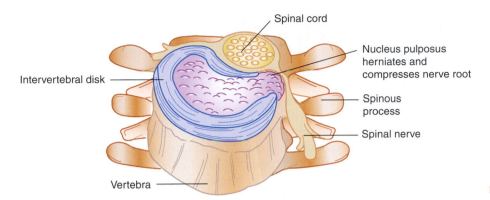

Spinal cord

Nucleus pulposus
herniates and
compresses nerve root

Intervertebral disk

Spinous
process

Spinal nerve

Vertebra

Figure 9.5   Herniated spinal disk.

heavy lifting. The herniation may occur at the time of the trauma or sometime later. Aging and excessive weight may be contributing factors.

Signs and Symptoms

Symptoms depend on the particular site of herniation, but severe back pain that worsens with motion is common. Sensation of numbness, prickling, tingling known as **paresthesia,** and restricted mobility of the neck often occurs. Coughing, sneezing, or bending intensifies the pain and discomfort. The sciatic nerve may be painful on the application of pressure. The sciatic pain may begin as a dull ache and progress to severe pain. The term *sciatica* is often used when considering symptoms of a herniated disk. A bad leg cramp that lasts for weeks before it goes away is often referred to as sciatica because the herniated (or even swollen) disk presses directly on nerve roots that become the sciatic nerve.

Diagnostic Procedures

Obtaining a thorough client history is important to rule out other causes of back pain. The diagnosis is confirmed if the individual complains of sciatic pain when a straight-leg-raising test is performed. In addition, spinal x-rays, computed tomography (CT) scans, and MRI may be ordered to confirm the diagnosis and to determine the level of herniation. Myelography may show the point of spinal compression caused by the herniated disk.

Treatment

Bed rest, alternating application of heat and cold to the affected portion of the spine, and salicylate analgesics may be prescribed. Muscle relaxants may be helpful. Traction of the lower extremities and a back brace may be beneficial in the event of a herniated lumbosacral disk. If conservative treatment is not successful, surgical removal of the herniated disk may be necessary (laminectomy). Endoscopic microdiscectomy is an alternative to the open removal of the disk if only small fragments of the vertebra need to be removed. With this procedure, a small incision is made and a camera is

inserted to locate the fragments of bone. Special instruments are used to remove the fragments with minimal damage to surrounding tissue. Spinal fusion may be necessary to stabilize the spine.

Complementary Therapy

Prolotherapy has shown some success. This type of therapy involves the injection of natural substances into the ligaments to stimulate growth of collagen to strengthen damaged joints, tendons, ligaments, or muscles. It is a nonsurgical treatment modality. Acupuncture and massage can provide short-term relief of lower back pain.

CLIENT COMMUNICATION

Remind clients not to expect an "instant fix" for a herniated disk. Bed rest is essential but not easily achieved and often frustrates clients. A referral to a physical therapist who can assist in proper movement, body mechanics, and exercise may also be made. Prepare the client for surgery if necessary.

Prognosis

About 1 in 50 people will experience a herniated disk. Often the symptoms last longer than 5 weeks. Approximately 80% to 90% of people get better over time. However, when there is still disabling pain after 3 months or more of treatment, surgery is considered.

Prevention

The use of proper lifting techniques may help prevent herniated intervertebral disks.

OSTEOPOROSIS

ICD-10: M81.0

Description

Osteoporosis is a metabolic bone disease affecting more than 10 million Americans. About 34 million Americans have low bone mass, which puts them at risk for developing the disease. Each year, an estimated 1.5 million fractures occur because of osteoporosis. In particular, it affects women who are over age 50, postmenopausal, small boned, or who come from a Northern European, especially Scandinavian, background. The total bone mass for someone affected by osteoporosis is less than expected for the individual's age and sex. The proportion of bone mineral to bone matrix is normal, however, and there usually is no detectable abnormality of bone composition. Bones become brittle, porous, and vulnerable to fracture because of the decreased calcium and phosphate in bones (Fig. 9.6).

Etiology

Recent research indicates that heredity plays a role in osteoporosis. Genes influence bone density. In some instances, osteoporosis is a manifestation of another disease, prolonged steroid therapy, alcoholism, lactose intolerance, or hyperthyroidism. Possible contributing factors to osteoporosis include low lifetime intake of calcium, a diet high in protein and fat, a sedentary lifestyle, poor or declining adrenal function, faulty protein metabolism due to estrogen deficiency, vitamin D deficiency, cigarette smoking, and amenorrhea. In men, low testosterone levels, especially in those who smoke cigarettes, increase the risk of osteoporosis.

Signs and Symptoms

Sometimes called the "silent disease," osteoporosis may go undiscovered until there is a presenting fracture, mostly because the disorder has long been considered a "traumatic" condition. Symptoms include bone pain, especially in the lower back and in the weight-bearing bones. The vertebrae, hips, and wrists are particularly susceptible to osteoporotic fractures. Over time, clients may notice a loss of height and/or kyphosis.

Diagnostic Procedures

Dual-energy x-ray absorptiometry (DEXA) is a diagnostic scan that primary care providers (PCPs) use to measure bone mineral density at sites especially susceptible to fracture. This test allows for a diagnosis of osteoporosis before any fracture occurs. Blood tests are run to measure levels of phosphorus, alkaline phosphatase, total protein, albumin, and creatine. Excretion of calcium, phosphate, creatinine, and hydroxyproline also may be monitored through urinalysis. X-rays are helpful but may be difficult to interpret in cases of osteoporosis because the density of skeletal parts may appear to be similar to that of soft tissue. A bone scintiscan, bone biopsy, or CT scan may be ordered if more specific diagnostic data are necessary.

Treatment

The goal is to prevent fracture and control pain. The treatment depends on the cause. Increased dietary calcium, phosphate supplements, and multivitamins may be prescribed. Bisphosphonates that slow or prevent the breakdown and resorption of bone are now the first treatment of choice for both men and women with osteoporosis. Long-term use of these medications is to be discussed with a PCP. The thyroid hormone calcitonin may be prescribed subcutaneously or via nasal spray to decrease bone resorption. Exercise helps minimize osteoporosis by slowing loss of mineral calcium, but if the bones have become brittle, exercise may need to be modified to prevent injury. Analgesics and muscle relaxants may be needed if pain or muscle spasms are a problem. Frequent rest periods are advised if bone pain is severe.

Complementary Therapy

Supplements of natural sources of calcium are the focus of complementary therapy. Natural sources of calcium include milk, yogurt, cheese, ice cream, sardines, clams, oysters, and salmon. Balancing the body's hormone production, regulating diet, and getting proper exercise can be helpful. It is recommended that clients stop smoking. A diet high in protein, sugar, soft drinks,

Normal Bone

Osteoporosis

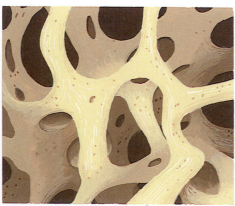 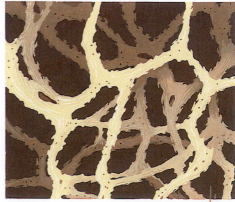

Figure 9.6 (A) Normal spongy bone, as in the body of a vertebra. (B) Spongy bone thinned by osteoporosis. *(From Scanlon, VC, and Sanders, T: Essentials of Anatomy and Physiology, ed. 4. Philadelphia: F.A. Davis, 2003, p 107, with permission.)*

A   B

caffeine, alcohol, and fried foods has an acidifying effect on the body and causes calcium to be drawn from the bones. Vitamins B, C, and D, as well as magnesium, zinc, and phosphorous, are also important for bone health.

⊙ CLIENT COMMUNICATION

Teach clients about a balanced diet that is not overly high in protein. Proper body mechanics are important to reduce possible fractures. Weight-bearing exercise, such as running and strength training, is essential for building bone but may need to be modified for some clients.

Prognosis

The prognosis for osteoporosis is mostly dictated by the cause. The major problem is the risk of fractures. That risk grows exponentially as an individual's age increases and bone mass weakens. Drugs are now available that can help restore lost bone and reduce the risk of fracture. Osteoporosis can cause permanent disability.

Prevention

Prevention of osteoporosis includes a calcium-rich diet. Premenopausal women need at least 1,000 mg of calcium and 800 mg of vitamin D daily. Women over age 65 should increase the dosage of calcium to at least 1,500 mg daily. A person at risk may need to take more calcium and vitamins and to exercise 20 minutes daily. The U.S. Preventive Services Task Force recommends DEXA screening for women age 65 and over. Table 9.1 lists the risk factors for osteoporosis.

OSTEOMYELITIS

ICD-10: M86.XX

Description

Osteomyelitis is an acute or chronic infection of the bone-forming tissue. Such infections are characterized by inflammation, edema, and circulatory congestion of the bone marrow. As the infection progresses, pus may form and sustained inflammatory pressure may cause fracturing of small pieces of bone. Osteomyelitis usually begins as an acute infection, but it may evolve into a chronic condition. The disease is more common in children, especially boys, in whom it often begins in the acute form.

Etiology

Osteomyelitis is most often caused by trauma resulting in hematoma formation and an acute bacterial infection, particularly *Staphylococcus aureus*. Viruses and fungi somewhere else in the body also may cause the condition. The infectious microorganisms may reach the bone marrow through the blood or by spreading from infected adjacent tissue; they can also be introduced directly into the bone tissue following physical trauma or surgery. Infection commonly affects the long bones in the arms and legs. The spine and pelvis may also be involved. Diabetes mellitus may predispose an individual to osteomyelitis because of poor circulation, as may the presence of prosthetic hardware (screws, plates, rods) within the bone. Individuals on hemodialysis, those with their spleen removed, and those who illegally inject drugs are also at high risk.

Signs and Symptoms

Specific signs and symptoms depend on which bone or bones are affected and the **virulence** (strength) of the infecting microorganism. Generalized symptoms may include the sudden onset of fever, chills, malaise, sweating, pain, and tenderness and swelling over the affected bone. In the acute phase, fever is abrupt and children can show irritability and fatigue. The chronic phase may exhibit drainage or seeping from an open wound near the infection site, and the client may have intermittent fever and chronic fatigue. Both the acute and chronic forms of osteomyelitis may exhibit the same clinical picture, although the chronic form may persist for years before it is detected following a flare-up due to minor trauma.

Diagnostic Procedures

A physical examination reveals bone tenderness, redness, and possibly swelling. Blood cultures or aspiration and culture of fluid from the infection site are essential to isolate the causative microorganism. X-rays, bone scans, and MRI may prove helpful in determining the site and extent of the infection. However, a bone biopsy may be necessary to reveal the type of bone infection.

Treatment

The goal of treatment is to eliminate the infection. Bed rest and parenterally administered antibiotics often suffice. If not, surgical drainage to remove pus and dead bone may be necessary. Tissue and/or bone grafts may be needed to restore blood flow to the site. Immobilization of the affected body part and analgesics may be required.

Table 9.1 Risk Factors for Osteoporosis

- Over age 50
- Female
- Family history of osteoporosis
- Thin, small-framed body
- Caucasian or Asian
- History of broken bones after age 50
- Low estrogen levels
- Smoking
- Alcohol (three or more drinks per day)
- Inactive lifestyle
- Certain medications (e.g., corticosteroids)
- Eating disorders
- Celiac disease

Complementary Therapy

No significant complementary therapy is indicated.

 CLIENT COMMUNICATION

> The goals are to control the infection and to protect the bone from injury. Teach clients how to avoid spreading infection by immediate cleaning and bandaging of any scrapes or cuts. Remind those at risk how to better protect themselves from injury.

Prognosis

With today's therapeutic options, osteomyelitis frequently resolves favorably. If the acute form of the disease progresses to a chronic form, the prognosis is less favorable. There can be bone and joint deformities and impaired bone growth in children. Resistant or extensive chronic osteomyelitis may result in amputation, especially in persons with diabetes or with poor blood circulation. Clients often experience a fair amount of pain and require lengthy hospitalization.

Prevention

Extreme care must be taken during surgery or following trauma to prevent contamination so that the disease does not have a chance to develop. Wounds should be cleaned and bandages replaced. The site should be checked often for signs of infection. Prompt and complete treatment of infections is helpful.

PAGET DISEASE (OSTEITIS DEFORMANS)

ICD-10: M88.9

Description

Paget disease is a chronic metabolic skeletal disease. In the initial phase, it is marked by a high rate of bone turnover. Bone is rapidly resorbed and replaced with bone of a coarse, irregular consistency. Consequently, the affected bone becomes enlarged and thicker but more porous and weaker. A later phase of the disease is characterized by the replacement of normal bone marrow with highly vascular fibrous tissue. The disease may occur in only one bone or at numerous sites throughout the skeletal system. It is more frequent in the spine, pelvis, femur, skull, and humerus. The disease appears primarily in men over age 40, and it becomes increasingly common with advancing age. It is estimated that 1% of American adults have Paget disease.

Etiology

The cause of Paget disease is not known. One theory is that early viral infection causes a dormant skeletal infection to erupt many years later as Paget disease. Recent research has found that genes appear to be associated with the disorder, but a definitive link has not been proven.

Signs and Symptoms

Many individuals with early Paget disease are asymptomatic. The nature of symptoms that do appear depends on the extent of the disease and which bone or bones are affected. Some individuals may first notice a swelling or other deformity in one of the long bones of the body or a need to increase their hat size if the bones of the skull are involved. The gradual onset of dull but persistent pain around the area of the affected bone may be the first symptom in some individuals. The pain may become severe enough to be disabling. Nerves may be pinched by enlarged bones, and tingling or numbness may be felt. The skin is often warm to the touch over the affected area. Headache and vision loss may occur due to enlargement of the skull, and gradual hearing loss may occur if the ossicles or nearby skull bones are involved.

Diagnostic Procedures

Bone scintiscans, x-rays, and bone marrow biopsies may help to diagnose the disease. Blood analysis and urinalysis are helpful in the diagnosis. The high rate of bone turnover that is characteristic of the disease is indicated by high levels of alkaline phosphatase in the blood together with high levels of hydroxyproline in the urine.

Treatment

Four methods of treatment are identified: (1) physical therapy to improve muscle strength, (2) pharmacological therapy using bisphosphonates or calcitonin, (3) pain management with analgesics, and (4) surgery. Bisphosphonates suppress or reduce absorption by osteoclasts. Calcitonins are used when clients are unable to tolerate bisphosphonates. Pain that is not managed by pharmacological therapy may respond to acetaminophen or NSAIDs. Surgery may involve repairing fractures and performing knee and/or hip replacements.

Complementary Therapy

The use of heat and massage can be helpful. Encourage clients to take adequate levels of vitamin D and calcium.

 CLIENT COMMUNICATION

> Remind clients to report any new areas of pain or deformity. Serum calcium phosphate levels should be monitored.

Prognosis

For severe forms of Paget disease, the prognosis is poor. Complications may include frequent fractures, hypercalcemia, kidney stones, deafness, blindness, and spinal cord injuries. Congestive heart failure may occur due to increased body mass. An especially serious complication is a transformation of the bone that becomes cancerous.

Prevention

There are no preventive measures for Paget disease.

FRACTURES

ICD-10: M84.XX

Description

A fracture is a break or crack in a bone. The more common types of fractures are illustrated in Figure 9.7 and are explained here:

- *Closed simple fracture:* a break in the bone with no external wound to the skin
- *Open or compound fracture:* a break in the bone in which there is an open wound leading down to the site of the fracture or in which a piece of broken bone protrudes through the skin
- *Simple fracture:* a break in the rib that is broken into two parts; likely occurs from a blow or direct shock to the thorax
- *Comminuted fracture:* a break in which the bone is broken or splintered into pieces, often with fragments embedded in surrounding tissue
- *Impacted fracture:* a break in which the bone is broken with one end forced into the interior of the other
- *Incomplete partial fracture:* a break in which the fraction line does not include the whole bone (stress fracture)
- *Greenstick fracture:* a break in which the bone is partially bent and split, as a green stick or twig does when bent; this type of fracture occurs most frequently in children, especially those who have rickets, or among adults with soft bones

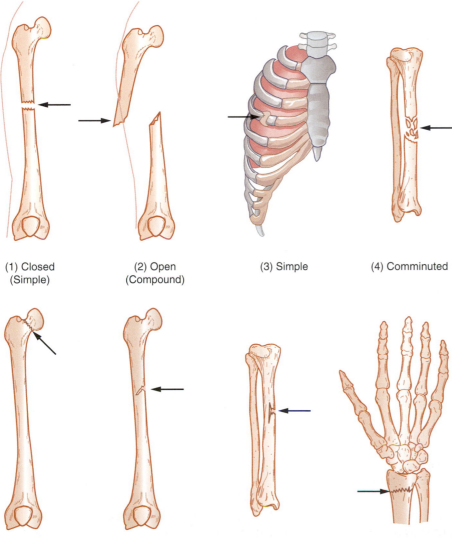

(1) Closed (Simple)

(2) Open (Compound)

(3) Simple

(4) Comminuted

(5) Impacted

(6) Incomplete

(7) Greenstick

(8) Colles fracture   **Figure 9.7** Common types of fractures.

• *Colles fracture:* a break in the end of the radius causing the wrist to extend and shorten; often occurs when the wrist is extended to break a fall

Etiology

Bone fractures are usually caused by physical trauma. Children are more likely to fracture arms from a fall; teens tend to fracture long bones in sports or motor vehicle crashes. A host of pathological processes, though, may occasion a bone fracture after only minimal trauma or following normal muscular contractions. Examples of diseases or conditions that may include fractures are bone neoplasms, osteoporosis, Paget disease, osteomalacia, osteomyelitis, and nutritional and vitamin deficiency disorders.

Older adults may be particularly susceptible to fracture as their bones become more brittle. Sometimes a traumatic incident is unnecessary for a hip or femur fracture.

Signs and Symptoms

Common symptoms of fractures include acute pain at the affected site, deformity, swelling, discoloration, loss of limb function, muscle spasm, and perhaps hemorrhage and shock. Bone may protrude through the skin.

Diagnostic Procedures

A history of traumatic injury assists in diagnosis. X-rays are used to locate the fracture and determine its severity. A bone scintiscan may be ordered to detect hairline fractures.

Treatment

Immobilization of the affected parts and control of any bleeding are paramount. Open or closed reduction may be needed to place the parts in their normal position for proper healing. Open reduction is accomplished by surgery, followed by external fixation such as casting or by internal fixation with the use of metal plates, screws, or rods. Closed reduction consists of manipulation and casting without a surgical incision. Traction may be used, especially for fractures of the leg bones, when a splint or cast fails to maintain reduction, until healing takes place or until internal fixation can be performed. Traction helps to reduce pain and further damage as the muscles stretch, bone fragments separate, and alignment is maintained. Rib fractures may require no treatment, or the chest may be bandaged or taped for support and pain control. Analgesics or muscle relaxants may be ordered to ease the pain accompanying many types of fractures.

Complementary Therapy

No significant complementary therapy is indicated.

➔ CLIENT COMMUNICATION

Reassuring clients and easing the pain are essential. Teach good cast care and remind clients to drink plenty of fluids. Teach proper use of crutches, if indicated. Physical therapy may be necessary following cast removal.

Prognosis

The prognosis depends on the severity of the fracture, the amount of tissue and vascular damage, and the age of the individual. The existence of an underlying pathological process worsens the prognosis by complicating the healing process. Other complications can occur in any type of fracture and may include **embolism** (clot), infection, delayed union or nonunion of the fracture, and complications resulting from immobilization.

Prevention

The best prevention of fractures is conscientious adherence to safety rules at work and in play.

DISLOCATIONS

ICD-10: S13.1X

Description

A dislocation or **luxation** occurs when a bone is separated from a joint. A subluxation is a partial dislocation. Any joint can become dislocated, but the shoulder and vertebral column are more likely to be luxated.

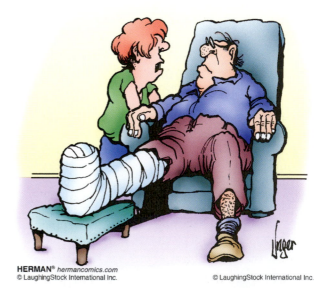

HERMAN® hermancomics.com
© LaughingStock International Inc.   © LaughingStock International Inc.

"If you were a horse, we would have shot you!"

HERMAN© is reprinted with permission from LaughingStock Licensing Inc., Ottawa, Canada. All rights reserved.

Etiology

Luxations and subluxations occur from a sudden impact to the joint, such as from a fall, a contact sports injury, an automobile crash, or other impact. Other dislocations can be attributed to obesity, poor sleeping postures, repetitive movement, and complication of other diseases, such as Paget disease or arthritis. Many children under age 5 suffer from "nursemaid's elbow," which is a dislocation of the elbow joint. This dislocation can occur from seemingly untraumatic events like someone lifting a child by the hand or swinging a child by the arm, or if the child falls onto his or her hands.

Signs and Symptoms

Because of the similarity in symptoms, a dislocation may be difficult to distinguish from a fracture. The bone may be visibly out of alignment or position and have a deformed appearance. Movement is limited, and the surrounding area may swell or bruise. Pain at the joint is severe, especially when in use.

Ligaments, muscle, and nerves can also be affected by a dislocation. The two areas that can have additional damage to more than the joint are the spine and shoulder. The vertebral column surrounds the spinal cord and has a pair of nerves attached to each individual vertebra. Either luxation or subluxation can result in nerve impairment, commonly called a *pinched nerve*. This impairment inhibits conduction of impulses from the spinal cord to the brain. Shoulder dislocation often involves tearing of the cartilage and the rotator cuff muscle. Blood vessels and nerves may be torn or impaired.

Diagnostic Procedures

Often, visual examination along with a patient history is all that is needed to determine a dislocation. X-rays are done to ascertain the dislocation and any fractures that may be present. An MRI may be ordered to determine if any soft tissue is damaged.

Treatment

Some dislocations can be manually reduced or realigned. Others may need surgical reduction as well as repair of torn muscles, ligaments, or vessels. Medication for pain and muscle relaxants are prescribed. Immobilization of the injured joint lasts for several weeks, depending on the location and severity of the dislocation. Physical therapy after healing gradually restores the range of motion.

Complementary Therapy

Complementary therapy may include the services of a physical therapist or sports medicine specialist. A number of modalities may be suggested, depending on the site of the dislocation. Water therapy, Pilates, resistance band exercises, and massage may be recommended during and after the healing process.

 CLIENT COMMUNICATION

Advise clients that immobilization of the joint is imperative for healing, as is refraining from activities that may aggravate the injury. Slowly returning to normal activity after removal of the splint or sling will increase the chances of full recovery and decrease the risk of a reoccurrence of the dislocation.

Prognosis

Prognosis is excellent with prompt and proper treatment, though dislocations can reoccur. Shoulder dislocations have an especially high reoccurrence, with 90% of those who had a dislocation before age 20 having a second dislocation at a later time. In these cases, surgical repair may be needed if it was not done at the first reduction.

Prevention

Dislocations are preventable in many situations. By adhering to proper lifting techniques, wearing protective clothing and gear when playing sports, and preventing falls, the risks of dislocation can be decreased.

Joints

TOP DISORDER OSTEOARTHRITIS

ICD-10: M15.X through M19.X (code is site specific)

Description

Osteoarthritis, also called *degenerative joint disease,* is a chronic inflammatory process of the joints and bones that results in degeneration of joint cartilage and the formation of new bone. The disease may affect any joint in the body, but weight-bearing ones, such as the knee and hip, are most often affected. It is the most common form of arthritis, and it occurs with equal frequency in both sexes until after age 55, when it is more common in women. In fact, after age 70, most individuals show evidence of some osteoarthritis on x-ray, although they may be asymptomatic.

Etiology

The cause of osteoarthritis is not known, but autoimmune factors may play a role. Chemical, genetic, metabolic, and mechanical factors are also possible. It seems to be related to aging. Secondary osteoarthritis generally occurs after trauma or a congenital abnormality such as dysplasia. Obesity is a risk factor.

Signs and Symptoms

The onset of osteoarthritis typically is insidious. The first symptom may include deep, aching joint pain that usually is relieved by rest. There may be stiffness and some swelling, especially in the morning, and aching during weather changes. There usually is minimal inflammation. **Crepitation,** a crackling sound due to the grating of bones, may be heard on joint movement. Deformity may be minimal in some cases, but bony enlargement can occur.

Diagnostic Procedures

A thorough medical history and examination will confirm symptoms. Skeletal x-rays from various angles may be necessary to indicate the changes in the joint and bone. Bone scans or MRI may be necessary for diagnosis.

Treatment

Because osteoarthritis cannot be cured, the goal of treatment is to minimize pain and inflammation, to maintain joint function, and to minimize disability. NSAIDs may help. Physical activity restrictions, rest, and the use of crutches or a cane may be necessary. Local heat, such as a paraffin bath for the hands, and weight reduction may be helpful. Physical therapy, especially warm-water exercise, often proves beneficial to improve muscle strength and the motion of stiff joints. Artificial joint fluid can be injected into a joint to provide temporary pain relief for up to 6 months. If the condition is severe, various forms of orthopedic surgery may help to relieve pain and improve joint function. These surgeries include debridement of loose or torn cartilage, bone realignment, bone fusion, or joint replacement. The hip and knee joints are the most common joints to be replaced with prosthetic devices, but the shoulder, elbow, ankle, and finger joints can also be replaced.

PCPs may choose to inject medications directly into a joint, muscle, or tendon for treatment. The injection may be an anesthetic for pain, a corticosteroid to reduce inflammation, or a substance that improves joint mobility.

Complementary Therapy

Proper diet, nutrition, and reduction of stress are beneficial. The amount of fatty meats, eggs, margarine, and dairy products is to be reduced. Caffeine, alcohol, tobacco, and sugar should be eliminated from the diet. Clients are advised to avoid carbonated soft drinks. Vitamins C, A, B, and E have proved to be helpful. Medications and biofeedback can reduce stress. Some people are finding benefits from over-the-counter remedies such as glucosamine for reducing pain, although they do not appear to grow new cartilage. Glucosamine is contraindicated for anyone with an allergy to sulfa drugs or shellfish. Acupuncture may reduce the pain of osteoarthritis, increase joint mobility, and reduce inflammation. Low-intensity exercise, such as walking, yoga, and tai chi, is beneficial for joint flexibility.

 CLIENT COMMUNICATION

Promote personal care, including adequate rest and appropriate exercise. For many, water exercise in a therapy pool is beneficial. Instruct clients on how and when to take prescribed medications and how to avoid overexertion. Regular physical therapy is often beneficial.

Prognosis

Prognosis of osteoarthritis depends on the site affected and the severity of the disease. Disability can range from minor to severe. The progression of osteoarthritis varies.

Prevention

There is no known prevention for osteoarthritis.

RHEUMATOID ARTHRITIS

ICD-10: M06.9

Description

Rheumatoid arthritis (RA) is a chronic, systemic, inflammatory disease affecting the synovial membranes of multiple joints. The disease has the capacity to destroy cartilage, erode bone, and deform joints. The course of the disease is characterized by spontaneous remissions and unpredictable exacerbations. RA affects 1.5 million Americans, mostly women, with the prevalence of the disease occurring in those ages 30 to 60.

As the disease develops, there is congestion and edema of the synovial membrane and joint. This causes formation of a thick layer of granulation tissue that invades the cartilage, destroying the joint and bone (Fig. 9.8). Finally, a fibrous immobility of joints, or **ankylosis,** occurs, causing visible deformities and total immobility.

Etiology

RA is a known autoimmune disease. The abnormal immune response causes inflammation that can damage joints and organs. Research suggests that some individuals may be genetically predisposed to acquiring the disease. Infections and endocrine factors also may be considered.

Signs and Symptoms

RA develops insidiously among most affected individuals. The earliest signs and symptoms may include malaise, persistent low-grade fever, fatigue, and weight loss. Joint pain and stiffness gradually emerge as the principal symptoms, usually affecting the joints of the fingers, wrists, knees, ankles, and toes in a symmetric pattern. The pain is characteristically aggravated by

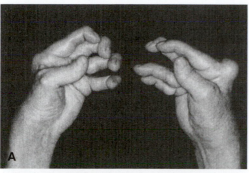
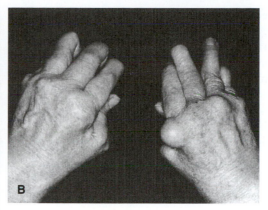
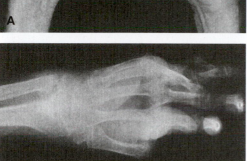

Figure 9.8 Severe rheumatoid arthritis can result in serious joint deformity (A and B) caused by the destruction of the joint tissues, as shown in the x-ray (C). *(From Stanley, BG, and Tribuzi, SM:* Concepts in Hand Rehabilitation. *Philadelphia: F.A. Davis, 1992, p 405, with permission.)*

movement of the affected joints. In advanced cases of RA affecting the hands, the interphalangeal joints are swollen and edematous and have a characteristic tapered appearance. Symptoms of RA may decrease or go into remission without treatment but will flare up, or become active, after weeks or months of a client being pain-free.

Diagnostic Procedures

A positive rheumatoid factor blood test is diagnostic in most cases. Other useful laboratory tests include serum protein electrophoresis, erythrocyte sedimentation rate (ESR), complete blood count (CBC), and synovial fluid analysis. X-rays are also useful. MRI and CT scan can show the extent of abnormality and track the progression of the disease.

Treatment

The primary objectives of treatment are to reduce inflammation and pain, preserve joint function, and prevent joint deformity. There are two groups of drugs for treatment: (1) NSAIDs, such as aspirin and ibuprofen, which help reduce joint pain, stiffness, and swelling, and (2) disease-modifying antirheumatic drugs (DMARDs), which slow joint degeneration. Hydroxychloroquine (Plaquenil) and methotrexate are oral DMARDs such as etanercept and adalimumab (Humira) that provide more rapid relief of symptoms. These tumor necrosis factor (TNF)–alpha inhibitors can help with morning stiffness and tender joints. Injections of corticosteroids into the joints can provide temporary relief of acute

inflammation. Advanced RA may require surgical repair of the hip, knee, or hand joints.

Complementary Therapy

See "Osteoarthritis." Also, 8 to 10 hours of sleep every night with frequent rest periods between daily activities is suggested. Moist heat application is often beneficial. Learning to relax and reducing stress as much as possible is helpful.

⊙ CLIENT COMMUNICATION

Make certain clients and family members understand RA is a serious chronic illness that is apt to require major changes in lifestyle. Provide emotional support. Physical and occupational therapists are helpful with activities of daily living. Staying active is key to treatment.

Prognosis

The course of RA is generally unpredictable. Permanent spontaneous remission may occur with return to normal function or less disability than previously; however, the disease generally is progressive, with some degree of consequent deformity. Only a small percentage of clients sustain total disability. RA usually requires lifelong treatment.

Prevention

There is no known prevention for RA.

Ankylosing Spondylitis

Ankylosing spondylitis, almost as common as RA, affects men three times more than women and usually begins between the ages of 15 and 30. It is a form of chronic inflammatory arthritis affecting mostly the spine. Back pain and stiffness result. Gradually the spinal bones fuse; other joints such as shoulders and hips may be involved. About 40% of cases affect the eyes, causing acute iritis and pain. Ankylosing spondylitis is likely genetic in origin. Pain and stiffness can be lessened by the use of new biological medications or TNF blockers such as Enbrel, Remicade, and Humira. Physical therapy is often prescribed to create a daily exercise protocol. The application of both cold and heat additionally provide relief.

CHAPTER EPISODE—PART II

Janet's internist performed an examination, asked her to identify the areas where she was having pain, and ordered comprehensive blood work for her. The internist suggested that because ulcerative colitis is an autoimmune disorder, there may be some relationship to her current symptoms. The internist asked about Janet's stress level. Janet revealed that she hated her job, but the pay was good and she could not leave. Her teenage son is going through a rebellious stage, is having problems in school, and doesn't always go to his classes. Her husband is supportive but doesn't really understand what is happening or why Janet often does not even have the energy to prepare dinner, let alone share any moments of intimacy. Sometimes Janet does not even want to be hugged.

- What do these additional symptoms and pieces of information suggest to you now about a possible diagnosis?
- Until a diagnosis is known, what might the internist suggest now? You may have to do a little Internet research.

GOUT

ICD-10: M10.9

Description

Gout, also called *gouty arthritis,* is a chronic disorder of uric acid metabolism. It is manifested as acute, episodic attacks of a form of arthritis in which crystals of uric acid compounds appear in the synovial fluid of joints (Fig. 9.9). The disease also is marked by **tophi,** which are deposits of urate compounds in and around the joints of the extremities; these frequently lead to joint deformity and disability. Gout is also characterized by hyperuricemia (increased urea in the blood), renal dysfunction, and kidney stones. Approximately 5 million Americans are treated for gout each year. The disease affects more men than women, usually appearing after age 30. Among women, gout usually appears after menopause.

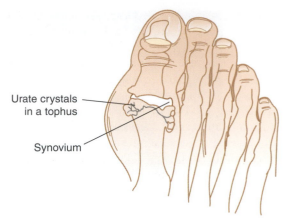

Figure 9.9   Gout of the big toe.

Etiology

The cause of gout may be metabolic, renal, or both. Metabolic gout is inherited, and several genetic factors have the potential to produce the condition. In metabolic gout, the body produces more uric acid than can be cleared by the kidneys into the urine. Renal gout is caused by one of many possible renal dysfunctions. In renal gout, the body may produce normal levels of uric acid, but the action of the kidneys is insufficient to clear the compound from the blood. Other risk factors for developing gout include obesity, moderate to high alcohol use, intake of aspirin, and low thyroid function.

Signs and Symptoms

The classic manifestation of gout is the sudden onset of excruciating joint pain, usually affecting the joints of the big toes. Other joints may be involved as well, especially those of the feet, ankles, and knees. The pain generally reaches a peak after several hours and then gradually subsides over 5 to 10 days. An acute attack also may be accompanied by mild fever and chills. The individual is characteristically free of any symptoms between attacks. As the disease progresses, the interval between acute attacks diminishes, and tophi may appear around the affected joints or at other points of the body.

Diagnostic Procedures

Identification of urate crystals in joint fluid or the presence of tophi in and around joints is indicative of gout. Urinalysis results will almost always reveal hyperuricemia. Other laboratory tests include ESR and differential count (white blood cell count), though symptoms of gout can be present even if blood uric acid levels are low. Skeletal x-rays may be used to assess the degree of damage to the affected joints.

Treatment

Treatment of an acute attack of gout may involve bed rest, immobilization of the affected part, local applications of heat or cold, and analgesics. NSAIDs usually provide excellent relief for clients who can tolerate them. Older clients are at risk for gastrointestinal bleeding when taking maximum doses of NSAIDs. Corticosteroids may be prescribed orally or by injection into the joint. Colchicine is an effective oral medication if NSAIDs or corticosteroids cannot be used, though it may cause nausea, vomiting, and diarrhea. Management of gout also may involve attempts to control the rate of uric acid formation by having the individual follow a low-purine diet. (Purines are end products of protein metabolism and are broken down to form uric acid.) Such a diet excludes sweetbreads, liver, kidney, poultry, fish, alcohol, rich pastries, and fried foods. To promote uric acid clearance by the kidneys, individuals with gout are usually encouraged to drink fluids frequently and may have to take various antihyperuricemic agents.

Complementary Therapy

Alcohol should be totally eliminated. A diet high in fiber and low in fat is suggested. Bioflavinoids found in cherries, grapes, and other dark fruits have been found to reduce uric acid levels. Fluid intake should be increased.

CLIENT COMMUNICATION

Remind clients to take NSAIDs with meals and to watch for any occult blood in the stool. Encourage increased fluids to prevent kidney stone formation.

Prognosis

Because of modern treatment procedures, gout is seldom as permanently disabling as it once was. Treatment measures may need to be maintained indefinitely. Complications include hypertension, kidney stones, and renal damage.

Prevention

There are no specific preventative measures for gout, but a low-purine diet and adequate hydration may lessen the chance of the disease occurring among those known to be at risk.

Muscles and Connective Tissue

SPRAINS AND STRAINS

ICD-10: T14.90

Description

A sprain is the tearing or stretching of a ligament surrounding a joint that usually follows a sharp twist. A strain is a tearing or overstretching of a tendon or a muscle. Both usually heal without surgery.

Etiology

Sprains and strains may be caused by trauma or result from excessive use of a body part. They are more common among athletes.

REALITY EPISODE

Schools were canceled due to a 6-inch snowfall. Keenan decided to use his day off to make some money shoveling the neighbors' driveways. After doing six driveways, Keenan was cold and tired and decided he had had enough of shoveling. Later that evening, when he reached for a glass from the top kitchen shelf, he felt a sharp pain across his right shoulder blade that extended into his upper arm. The area was tender and painful when he touched it. He told his mother about the shoulder pain, and she gave him some acetaminophen. Then she made Keenan an ice pack and applied it to his shoulder. She advised him to rest his arm and leave the ice pack on for 15 minutes.

What did Keenan's mother do correctly in this situation? How long might Keenan's pain last?

Signs and Symptoms

Symptoms are localized pain and inflammation, black-and-blue discoloration at the site of the injury, and loss of mobility. Sprains and strains caused by chronic overuse of a ligament, muscle, or tendon typically cause stiffness, soreness, and tenderness, whereas a sharp, transient pain may result when either condition is acute.

Diagnostic Procedures

A medical history revealing recent physical activities with the potential for causing sprains or strains may suggest the diagnosis. X-rays may be necessary to rule out the possibility of a fracture. An MRI may be necessary to determine the extent of the injury.

Treatment

Sprains and strains usually require immediate elevation and rest of the injured part. Cold compresses may be applied intermittently to the affected site for 12 to 48 hours to lessen swelling. Depending on the severity of the injury, immobilization of the affected part may be attempted by applying an elastic wrap or soft cast. Analgesics and NSAIDs may be necessary to control pain or discomfort. Surgical repair may be "indicated if the injury heals improperly or if a rupture results.

Complementary Therapy

Complementary therapy parallels traditional treatment. Proteolytic enzymes, which help digest proteins in food, may be given. A cold compress of camphor, lavender, chamomile, eucalyptus, and rosemary may be used on the joint.

CLIENT COMMUNICATION

Remind clients that the best repair and recovery will occur when the injured area has total rest. It may be necessary to teach crutch walking or performing daily tasks with limited mobility.

Prognosis

With proper treatment, healing of a strain or sprain generally occurs within 2 to 4 weeks.

Prevention

Prevention of these injuries includes warming up when preparing for exercise or physical activity, following safety precautions, and recognizing physical limitations.

BURSITIS AND TENDONITIS

ICD-10: M70.X, M71.X, or M75.X

Description

Bursitis is inflammation of a bursa, a thin-walled sac lined with synovial tissue and filled with a viscous fluid called *synovial fluid*. The bursae act as cushions that prevent friction between the bones at a joint and facilitate movement of tendons and muscles around the joints. Common forms of bursitis include subacromial (shoulder); subdeltoid (arm); olecranon (elbow), which is commonly referred to as *miner's* or *tennis elbow;* prepatellar (knee), which is referred to as *housemaid's knee;* and ischial (pelvis), which is commonly referred to as *weaver's bottom.*

Tendonitis is inflammation of a tendon or the fibrous band of tissue that connects a muscle to a bone, usually in the shoulder rotator cuff, hip, Achilles tendon, or hamstring. The condition is characterized by inflammation, fibrosis, and tears in the tendon.

Etiology

Bursitis may be caused by excessive frictional forces, trauma, and systemic diseases (such as gout or RA) or infection. Tendonitis generally results from overuse, another musculoskeletal disease such as RA, postural misalignment, or hypermobility.

Signs and Symptoms

The classic symptom is tenderness or pain, especially on movement of the affected part. Restricted movement and edema at the site are common. Fluid accumulation in the bursae causes irritation, inflammation, and sudden or gradual pain. Symptoms usually include dull aching in the affected tendon area and severe pain when the area is moved. At night, the pain often interferes with sleep.

Diagnostic Procedures

The client's clinical picture and a medical history may be all that are necessary for diagnosis. X-rays occasionally may show calcific deposits at the affected site, but CT scanning and an MRI may replace x-rays in the diagnosis.

Treatment

Treatment may include application of cold or heat, immobilization of the affected part, analgesics, NSAIDs, and local steroid injections. Active mobilization to prevent adhesions will prove helpful after the acute pain subsides. Physical therapy or hydrotherapy helps maintain range of motion.

Complementary Therapy

It is recommended that clients identify and cease the offending activity. Immobilization and rest of the affected area to prevent further irritation may be necessary. Acupuncture can provide symptomatic relief of the pain.

 CLIENT COMMUNICATION

See "Sprains and Strains." Clients who learn what caused the tendonitis or bursitis and are able to avoid that action will heal faster and have less chance of recurrence. Reinforce the importance of treatment.

Prognosis

The prognosis is good if the bursitis is treated as soon as possible. Bursitis may become chronic, in which case activity restrictions may be required or surgical intervention may be attempted to remove calcification. If infection results, surgical drainage or aspiration may be necessary followed by antibiotic therapy. Tendonitis usually responds to medical treatment and a change in physical activities. If untreated, it can become disabling. Chronic tendonitis may require surgical intervention to remove calcium deposits.

Prevention

Prevention of bursitis and tendonitis includes avoiding trauma, strenuous exercise, and overuse that might stress or cause pressure on a joint.

CARPAL TUNNEL SYNDROME

ICD-10: G56.00

Description

Carpal tunnel syndrome is a common condition that compresses the median nerve in the wrist found within the carpal tunnel (Fig. 9.10). This compression causes sensory and motor changes in the hand. It is most commonly seen in individuals who use their hands and wrists repetitively, such as computer users, assembly-line workers, packers, data-entry clerks, dental hygienists, and any others who make strenuous use of their hands.

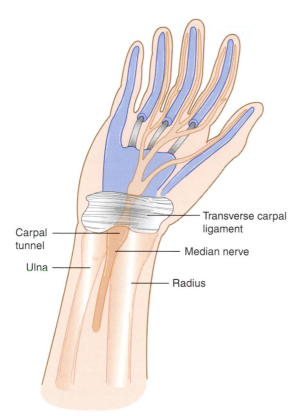

Carpal tunnel

Ulna

Transverse carpal ligament

Median nerve

Radius

Figure 9.10   Carpal tunnel.

Etiology

Overuse and incorrect use of the hands and fingers cause inflammation or fibrosis of the tendon sheaths that pass through the carpal tunnel. There is also the belief that some individuals' hands and wrists are particularly susceptible to the problem. Edema and compression of the median nerve result.

Signs and Symptoms

Pain, burning, weakness, numbness, or tingling in one or both hands are the classic symptoms. An individual with carpal tunnel syndrome is unable to clench the fist or demonstrate a strong grip. Discomfort is usually worse at night and in the morning.

Diagnostic Procedures

The medical history usually indicates a tendency for the syndrome. There will be decreased sensation to light touch or pinpricks of the fingers and a positive **Tinel sign,** tingling over the median nerve on light tapping. An electromyogram or a nerve conduction study may also be performed for diagnosis.

Treatment

Resting the wrist and supporting it with a splint represent the first treatment. If a client's occupation is the cause, ergonomic modifications of the workplace may be implemented. NSAIDs may be recommended. If the pain or numbness persists, surgery may be the best option.

Surgical decompression of the nerve through resection of the carpal tunnel ligament may be necessary.

Complementary Therapy

Yoga and other relaxation techniques may alleviate the pain. Acupuncture may be useful for easing the symptoms. However, magnet therapy, laser acupuncture, and chiropractic care have not provided much benefit.

⊖ CLIENT COMMUNICATION

Many clients benefit from reading material that educates them on relieving wrist and hand stress. Information on posture; wrist rests at computer keyboards; and proper holding, carrying, and lifting can be very helpful.

Prognosis

The prognosis for carpal tunnel syndrome is good, especially if the client responds to rest and a wrist splint. Surgical techniques are quite effective, but a change of occupation may be necessary if ergonomic alterations are not effective or possible.

Prevention

Proper workplace ergonomics, such as adjusting the keyboard so the wrists do not bend sharply and sitting in a chair positioned so both feet are flat on the floor can prevent injury. Instruct clients to avoid repetitive movements of the wrist or hand and use wrist rests at computer keyboards and mouse pads.

PLANTAR FASCIITIS

ICD-10: M72.2

Description

Plantar fasciitis is a common condition that results from irritation of the ligament on the bottom of the foot that connects the heel to the toes. This ligament is called the *plantar fascia* and supports the arch of the foot. Straining of the ligament leads to inflammation, swelling, and pain when standing or walking. This condition is more common in middle age but can occur in anyone at any age who stands or walks often.

Etiology

This condition occurs from small tears that appear after straining the ligament. Repetitive straining and tearing of the fascia results in pain and swelling of the heel (Fig. 9.11). Causes of strain can be due to several factors, such as having high arches; obesity; pregnancy; and walking, standing, or running for long periods of time, especially on hard surfaces. Poorly fitting shoes, feet that roll inward when walking (excessive pronation), and tight Achilles tendons are also contributing factors.

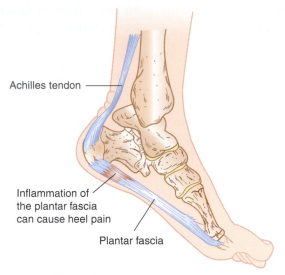

Figure 9.11 Plantar fasciitis.

Signs and Symptoms

Plantar fasciitis begins as pain or stiffness of the feet when getting out of bed or after sitting for long periods. Pain usually decreases as the day goes on but may return and be excessive after longs periods of standing, sitting in one position, or climbing stairs.

Diagnostic Procedures

Physical examination revealing pain, tenderness, or swelling on the bottom of the heel is sufficient for diagnosis. X-rays may be ordered to rule out other injuries or fractures.

Treatment

NSAIDs, ice, and rest are the first method of treatment. Flexibility exercises for the feet and legs and night splints may be recommended. If other treatments are not helpful, orthopedic shoe inserts may be prescribed. Injections of corticosteroids may bring relief, but multiple injections are not recommended and may weaken the fascia. For chronic discomfort, extracorporeal shock wave therapy can be used. This treatment uses sound waves directed at the heel to promote healing. Surgery to release the fascia is done if other treatments fail.

Complementary Therapy

It is suggested that clients stretch or massage their feet prior to getting out of bed in the morning. Flexing the foot up and down about 10 times can reduce pain. Using a towel stretched across the bottom of the foot when doing stretching is helpful. Shoes should have good arch support. Going barefoot is not advised. Another simple procedure is to freeze a small bottle of water, place it beneath the foot, and roll the bottle from the toes to the heel and back again. This stretches the tendon and ices the inflammation at the same time.

 CLIENT COMMUNICATION

Orthopedic shoe inserts should be worn in both shoes even if only one foot is painful.

Prognosis

With treatment and physical therapy, the prognosis for plantar fasciitis is good, and most patients improve within 1 year with nonsurgical treatment.

Prevention

Maintaining flexibility of the heel and Achilles tendon is the best prevention. Wearing supportive shoes on hard surfaces and replacing worn athletic shoes often can also prevent plantar fasciitis.

MYASTHENIA GRAVIS

ICD-910: G70.00

Description

Myasthenia gravis is a chronic, progressive neuromuscular disease that produces increasingly sporadic weakness and exhaustion of skeletal muscles. Curiously enough, neither the motor nerves nor the muscles themselves are directly affected by this disease. Rather, myasthenia gravis may be an autoimmune response resulting in the disappearance of receptors for the neurotransmitter acetylcholine, the substance that transfers a nerve impulse from the nerve ending across to the muscle fiber. The condition occurs more frequently in women than in men and has its highest incidence between ages 20 and 40. Thymomas (tumors of the thymus gland) accompany myasthenia gravis in approximately 15% of cases.

Etiology

The cause of this disease is not known, but it appears to be an acquired autoimmune disorder in which antibodies that are produced by the thymus gland destroy the acetylcholine receptors.

Signs and Symptoms

Skeletal muscle weakness and fatigability occur. Onset may be sudden, and most affected individuals will notice drooping eyelids and double vision as the first signs that something is wrong. Because the muscles most affected are usually those innervated by the cranial nerves (face, lips, tongue, neck, and throat), a blank expression, nasal regurgitation of fluids, **dysphagia** (difficulty swallowing), **blepharoptosis** (drooping eyelid), **dysphasia** (difficulty speaking), and a bobbing head may result (Fig. 9.12).

Muscle weakness typically occurs later in the day or after strenuous exercise. Although short rest periods characteristically restore muscle function, the muscle weakness is progressive in myasthenia gravis, and most muscles will be affected until paralysis occurs. Menses, emotional stress, prolonged exposure to sunlight or cold,

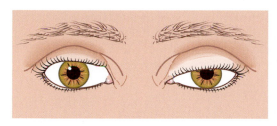

Ptosis
(drooping of the eyelid)

Figure 9.12 Ptosis. *(From Eagle, SE:* Diseases in a Flash: An Interactive Approach, *Flash-Card Approach, ed. 1. Philadelphia: F.A. Davis, 2012, Figure 14-25, p 479.)*

and infections heighten the symptoms. Respiratory muscle weakness or myasthenic crisis (the sudden inability to swallow and respiratory distress) may be severe enough to require mechanical ventilation.

Diagnostic Procedures

The improvement of muscle strength after resting or following injection of anticholinesterase drugs strongly suggests the diagnosis. The PCP will perform a neurological examination. Electromyography with repeated neural stimulation may assist in the diagnosis. The confirming diagnosis of myasthenia gravis is improved muscle function after an IV injection of edrophonium or neostigmine. An MRI or CT scan may be ordered to verify the presence of a thymus gland abnormality. When a drooping eyelid is present, the PCP may place a cool pack over the closed eyelid for a short period of time to determine if the eyelid function is then improved.

Treatment

Treatment is symptomatic and supportive. Anticholinesterase drugs are effective against fatigue and muscle weakness, but they become less effective as the disease progresses. Thymectomy is being used with success, bringing marked relief to more than half of those with severe myasthenia gravis. Corticosteroids may be beneficial. It is important to guard against myasthenic crisis and to treat it with emergency measures should it occur. Antibody therapies such as plasmapheresis that filter antibodies from the blood or injections of healthy immunoglobulins can alter the body's immune response against the acetylcholine receptors. Unfortunately, both of these therapies provide only short-term benefit.

Complementary Therapy

No significant complementary therapy is indicated.

> ⊕ **CLIENT COMMUNICATION**
>
> Help clients understand how to make the most of the periodic energy peaks throughout the day. Stress the need for frequent rest periods. Remind clients to avoid strenuous exercise, stress, infection, and unnecessary exposure to sun or cold.

Prognosis

Unexplained, spontaneous remissions may occur, but usually the disease is a lifelong condition with periodic remissions, exacerbations, and day-to-day fluctuations. There is no known cure for myasthenia gravis.

Prevention

There is no known prevention for myasthenia gravis.

POLYMYOSITIS

ICD-10: M33.20

Description

Polymyositis is a rare but chronic, progressive disease of connective tissue characterized by edema, inflammation, and degeneration of skeletal muscles. When the disease occurs with skin involvement, it is called *dermatomyositis.* Polymyositis and dermatomyositis develop slowly and have frequent exacerbations and remissions. Adults between ages 50 and 70 are most often affected. Women develop this condition twice as often as men, and it is much more common in African Americans.

Etiology

Polymyositis is an idiopathic disease. Viral, parasitic, and bacterial infections are rarely found, so an autoimmune etiology is suspected. Nearly one-third of cases are associated with other connective-tissue disorders, such as RA and systemic lupus erythematosus. Other cases, particularly among older adults are associated with malignancies, especially of the lung and breast.

Signs and Symptoms

Polymyositis usually develops insidiously over a period of a few months to a few years. The most frequent initial manifestation of the disease is muscle weakness in the hips and thighs. Consequently, the affected individual often reports difficulty in ascending or descending stairs or difficulty in rising from a sitting or kneeling position. Occasionally, the disease localizes in specific muscle groups, weakening only the neck, shoulder, or quadriceps muscles. Later symptoms include dysphagia and respiratory difficulties. In rare instances, the disease may appear as an acute condition, with the rapid onset and development of the symptoms noted.

When the disease develops as dermatomyositis, the previously mentioned symptoms may be preceded or accompanied by the appearance of a telltale lilac-colored rash on the eyelids, bridge of the nose, the cheeks, forehead, chest, elbows, and knees. The rash-covered portions of the body may itch severely. Dermatomyositis also may be accompanied by edema around the eye sockets.

Diagnostic Procedures

A muscle biopsy may reveal tissue changes characteristic of polymyositis, such as muscle fiber necrosis, infiltration of the muscle tissue with inflammatory cells (leukocytes), and patterns of tissue degeneration and regeneration. Blood testing typically indicates increased serum levels of creatine kinase, an enzyme normally present in skeletal muscles. The ESR also is usually elevated.

Treatment

High doses of corticosteroid drugs are often administered to bring the disease under control, followed by lower maintenance doses over a period of years. Cytotoxic drugs also may be used to lower the number of inflammatory cells affecting the muscles, especially if the response to corticosteroids is poor. Injections of immunoglobulins may inhibit the attack of muscle tissue by antibodies. Bed rest during an acute attack is beneficial. Physiotherapy and physical rehabilitation to regain muscle function are important components of the treatment process.

Complementary Therapy

Drug therapy using the biological injectable rituximab has been tested in small groups of clients. It has been found to improve muscle strength and skin rash. The U.S. Food and Drug Administration has not approved this drug for treatment of polymyositis, so it would need to be prescribed as an off-label usage. No other significant complementary therapy is indicated.

⊕► CLIENT COMMUNICATION

Encourage clients to pace activities to counteract muscle weakness. Explain the disease and its complications to clients and family members. Advise a low-sodium diet to prevent fluid retention. Discuss the side effects of corticosteroid therapy (weight gain, hypertension, edema, acne, and easy bruising), and remind clients that side effects are diminished after drugs are discontinued.

Prognosis

The prognosis is variable. Roughly half of those affected by polymyositis recover within 5 years and can discontinue therapy. Some individuals must remain on drug therapy indefinitely; others die from acute cardiac, pulmonary, or renal complications. Generally, the prognosis worsens with age. Individuals with polymyositis are monitored carefully for any sign of cancer.

Prevention

There is no specific prevention for polymyositis.

SYSTEMIC LUPUS ERYTHEMATOSUS

ICD-10: M32.10

Description

Systemic lupus erythematosus (SLE) is a chronic, inflammatory connective-tissue disorder in which cells and tissues throughout the body are damaged by a variety of autoantibodies and immune complexes. The disease affects women eight times more often than men. It is most often diagnosed between ages 15 and 45.

Etiology

The cause of the autoimmune response that characterizes SLE is not known. Genetic factors, as well as environmental and hormonal factors, may predispose an individual to the disease. Stress, overexposure to ultraviolet light, immunization reactions, and pregnancy are events that may precipitate the condition. Certain drugs also have the capacity to induce an SLE-like syndrome.

Signs and Symptoms

Because SLE can affect any part of the body, a host of symptoms are possible, including weight loss, fatigue, and fever. One manifestation of the disease is the "butterfly rash" (Fig. 9.13), which is found on the face, neck, and scalp of about 50% of clients with SLE. Similar rashes may appear on other body surfaces, especially on exposed areas. There also may be photosensitivity of the skin, joint and muscle pain, joint deformities, nausea, vomiting, and diarrhea. Other signs and symptoms include oral or nasopharyngeal ulcerations, patchy alopecia, pleuritis or pericarditis, and

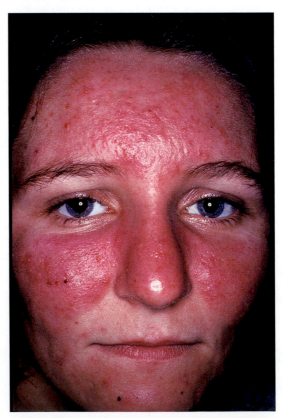

Figure 9.13 Butterfly rash of systemic lupus erythematosus. *(From Lazarus, GS, and Goldsmith, LA: Diagnosis of Skin Disease. Philadelphia: F.A. Davis, 1997, p 230, with permission.)*

Raynaud phenomenon. This disorder is exhibited by intermittent interruptions of blood supply to the fingers and toes, marked by severe pallor and accompanied by numbness, tingling, or severe pain.

Diagnostic Procedures

CBC with differential, ESR, serum electrophoresis, antinuclear antibody, anti-DNA, and lupus erythematosus (LE) tests are likely performed. LE cells (polymorphonuclear leukocytes) often are found in the bone marrow. The anti-DNA test, which detects a particular autoantibody, is the most specific test for diagnosing SLE, but it must be performed while the disease is in its active stage.

Treatment

The mild stage of the disease requires only anti-inflammatory agents, including aspirin. Skin lesions require topical treatment such as corticosteroid creams. Corticosteroid drugs remain the treatment of choice to control SLE, both for acute generalized exacerbations and for exacerbations of the disease localized to vital organ systems. It is recommended that clients with photosensitivity wear protective clothing when in the sun and use an effective sunscreen agent.

Complementary Therapy

A whole-foods diet that avoids cow's milk and beef products is recommended. Increasing intake of green, yellow, and orange vegetables and fish oil and flaxseed oil is recommended. Supplementation with vitamins B_{12}, B_5, and C may be helpful.

⊙ CLIENT COMMUNICATION

Urge clients to get plenty of rest and to consider a low-sodium, low-protein diet. Heat packs may be used to relieve joint pain and stiffness. Teach clients how to observe for multiple organ involvement.

Prognosis

The prognosis for SLE improves with early detection and careful treatment, but it remains poor for those who develop cardiovascular, renal, or neurological complications or serious bacterial infections.

Prevention

There is no specific prevention for SLE.

FIBROMYALGIA

ICD-10: M79.1, 60.9, or M79.7

Description

Fibromyalgia is a chronic condition characterized by pain in the muscles, ligaments, and tendons; constant fatigue; and muscle tenderness. Women are 80% more likely than men to develop this condition. It is most common in those of middle age, affecting 2% of the adult population in the United States.

Etiology

The exact cause of fibromyalgia is unknown, but a variety of factors seem to be involved. Genetics may be a key factor, as clients with the condition tend to have family members with fibromyalgia. Clients with fibromyalgia may have a lower pain threshold because of increased pain signals to the brain. Nerve stimulation causes an increase in neurotransmitters, and because the pain receptors are more sensitive, they become overreactive to the neurotransmitters. Other factors, such as emotional distress, trauma, and illness, may trigger or exacerbate the condition.

Signs and Symptoms

Pain begins as a constant, dull muscle ache. Additionally, pain comes from tender points or sites where firm pressure causes an increase in pain. These spots include the back of the head, tops of shoulders, outer elbows, upper hips, and inner knees. Exhaustion is also common because of the inability to enter into the restorative phase of sleep. Cognitive difficulties, commonly referred to as *fibro fog*, often occur. Coexisting conditions with fibromyalgia include chronic fatigue syndrome, SLE, osteoarthritis, post-traumatic stress disorder, restless leg syndrome, and depression.

Diagnostic Procedures

Fibromyalgia is difficult to diagnose and is often misdiagnosed. A physical examination showing widespread pain (both sides of the body and above and below the waist) lasting at least 3 months with no underlying cause is sufficient for diagnosis. Blood work that includes a CBC, an ESR, and thyroid function may be ordered to rule out other conditions.

Treatment

Reduction of pain is the first goal of treatment; the second is to improve sleep. Several different medications can be prescribed: analgesics, antidepressants such as duloxetine (Cymbalta), and antiseizure drugs can reduce pain and improve sleep. Recently, the drug milnacipran (Savella) was approved specifically for the treatment of fibromyalgia. Stress management and physical therapy are also recommended.

Complementary Therapy

Massage, acupuncture, and chiropractic care can help alleviate pain. Low-impact exercise, yoga, and meditation can reduce stress and alleviate symptoms. Physical therapy in a warm-water pool is beneficial.

CLIENT COMMUNICATION

Clients must understand that reducing stress and getting adequate sleep along with exercise and a healthy diet can help alleviate symptoms and exacerbation of the condition.

Prognosis

Fibromyalgia is a chronic condition, so prognosis depends on how the client responds to treatment. Even with treatment, symptoms may worsen and last for months or years.

Prevention

There is no known prevention for fibromyalgia.

CHAPTER EPISODE—PART III

Janet gets the test results the next week when she sees her internist a second time. Her spouse accompanies her on the visit. She begins to cry when she is told she has fibromyalgia, that there is no cure, and that the goal of treatment is to help her live as active a life as possible. It is much like the ulcerative colitis—she will have both the rest of her life. Her spouse asks, "What do we do now?"

- What might the internist suggest?
- What lifestyle changes might Janet and her spouse make?
- What is the possible prognosis for Janet?

CANCER

ICD-10: C41.9

Primary neoplasms of the musculoskeletal system are rare, but when they do occur, the prognosis usually is poor. Primary malignancy may arise from osseous tissue. These tumors include the following:

1. *Osteogenic sarcoma,* which primarily affects the long bones of the body
2. *Chondrosarcoma,* which also affects the long bones but tends to metastasize more slowly than osteogenic sarcoma
3. *Malignant giant-cell tumor,* which is common at the ends of long bones, especially near the knee and lower radius

Nonosseous tumors include fibrosarcoma, chondroma, and Ewing sarcoma, which is a malignant tumor originating from bone marrow, usually in the long bones or pelvis. The cause is unknown.

The classic symptom of nonosseous tumors is bone pain. It is dull and localized and may be more intense at night. A bone biopsy, bone x-ray, and radioisotope bone and CT scan may be necessary for diagnosis. The treatments of choice are radiation and surgery, which may involve amputation if surgical resection of the tumor is not effective. With any amputation, rehabilitation is necessary.

COMMON SYMPTOMS OF MUSCULOSKELETAL DISEASES AND DISORDERS

Individuals may present with the following common symptoms, which deserve attention from health-care professionals:

- Pain
- Tenderness and swelling
- Malaise, weakness, and fatigue
- Fever
- Obvious bone deformation, including spontaneous fractures
- Inflammation
- Stiffness
- Weight and height loss

SUMMARY

Musculoskeletal diseases and disorders can occur at any age. Most respond well to treatment; a few do not. All can affect body structure, function, or movement. If treatment protocols are followed, most clients will experience relief or remission of the disease or disorder, or they will learn to live more comfortably with it. Some require lifestyle changes. Fortunately, new treatment modalities, including alternative therapies, are being researched and tried. Many are successful.

 | For more resources and to sharpen your skills with interactive exercises, visit Davis*Plus* at http://davisplus.fadavis.com. Keyword *Tamparo.*

ONLINE RESOURCES

Arthritis
http://www.arthritis.org

Fibromyalgia
http://www.fmaware.org

https://www.rheumatology.org/Practice/Clinical/Patients/Diseases_And_Conditions/Fibromyalgia/

Myasthenia gravis
http://www.myasthenia.org

Osteomyelitis
http://www.nlm.nih.gov/medlineplus/ency/article/000437.htm

Systemic lupus erythematosus
http://www.lupus.org

CASE STUDIES

Case Study 1

Leon Best, a mail carrier in the middle of his daily 5-mile delivery route, suddenly experiences excruciating pain in his great left toe. As soon as his route is done, he calls his PCP.

Case Study Questions

1. What are some possible diagnoses?
2. What additional information might the PCP look for in making a diagnosis?
3. Is Leon's profession connected with his complaint? Explain.

Case Study 2

Thirty-five-year-old Donna Duckworth is learning how to care for her 5-week-old newborn, when she bends over the baby's crib and feels something give in her back. The next day and the following week, the pain becomes unbearable in her back. She is breast-feeding and does not want to take any medication, so she lives with the intense and continuing pain. Within a few weeks, she can no longer stand it, so she goes to see her primary care provider, who orders blood work and does a complete physical. As a result, he sends her to an orthopedist who takes x-rays and does a bone density test. The diagnosis comes back as "severe idiopathic osteoporosis." She has fractured three of her lumbar and four of her cervical vertebrae.

Case Study Questions

1. What is unusual about this diagnosis at this time?
2. What will Donna's future hold? What is the prognosis?
3. As a health-care practitioner, what teaching tips would you offer Donna?

REVIEW QUESTIONS

Matching

Match each of the following definitions with its correct term.

_____ 1. Outward curvature angulation of spine; round back

_____ 2. Bones become brittle and porous; fracture easily

_____ 3. Sideward curvature of the spine

_____ 4. Inward curvature of the spine; swayback

_____ 5. Ruptured or slipped disk

a. Lordosis

b. Osteoporosis

c. Kyphosis

d. Scoliosis

e. Herniated intervertebral disk

Short Answer

1. What are the names and descriptions of five major types of fractures?

   a._____

   b._____

   c._____

   d._____

   e._____

2. What is the difference between a sprain and a strain?

   _____

   _____

Multiple Choice

Place a checkmark next to the correct answer.

1. How might fibromyalgia be described?

   _____ a. An acute condition common in men

   _____ b. Progressive bilateral wasting of skeletal muscles

   _____ c. Condition accompanied by pain, fatigue, and inability to sleep well

   _____ d. Diagnosed by muscle biopsy

2. What is myasthenia gravis?

   _____ a. A chronic, progressive neuromuscular disease

   _____ b. A condition in which there is too much acetylcholine released at the junction

   _____ c. Diagnosed by muscle biopsy

   _____ d. Easily cured and prevented

3. What is carpal tunnel syndrome?

   _____ a. A syndrome that compresses the median nerve in the wrist

   _____ b. Inflammation of the tendon sheaths passing through the carpal tunnel

   _____ c. An ailment caused by excess viscous fluid in the carpal tunnel of the wrist

   _____ d. A problem that occurs by straining the ligament on the palm of the hand

4. Can you name the chronic disease of connective tissue characterized by edema, inflammation, and degeneration of skeletal muscles?

   _____ a. Systemic lupus erythematosus

   _____ b. Myasthenia gravis

   _____ c. Rheumatoid arthritis

   _____ d. Polymyositis

5. What is the treatment of choice to control systemic lupus erythematous symptoms?

   _____ a. Antidepressants such as Cymbalta

   _____ b. Thymectomy

   _____ c. Corticosteroid drugs

   _____ d. Physical therapy to minimize disability

6. What kind of therapy might be beneficial for those afflicted with rheumatoid arthritis?

   _____ a. Use of cold compresses on finger deformities

   _____ b. Applications of dry heat to inflamed joints

   _____ c. Occupational therapy to help with daily activities

   _____ d. Acupuncture to relieve stress

7. A tear or stress on the tendon or fibrous tissue connecting posterior thigh muscles to bone is likely called what?

_____ a. Weaver's bottom

_____ b. Achilles tendon strain

_____ c. Housemaid's knee

_____ d. Hamstring pull or strain

8. With proper treatment, what is the approximate healing time for a strain or a sprain?

_____ a. 2 to 4 weeks

_____ b. 6 weeks

_____ c. 2 months

_____ d. 7 to 10 days

9. The *terms tennis elbow, housemaid's knee,* and *weaver's bottom* refer to what kind of ailment?

_____ a. Tendonitis

_____ b. Plantar fascitis

_____ c. Bursitis

_____ d. Gout

10. What disease is identified with uric acid metabolism and tophi?

_____ a. Gout

_____ b. Bursitis

_____ c. Osteoarthritis

_____ d. Carpal tunnel syndrome

Discussion Questions/Personal Reflection

1. A postmenopausal woman slips while stepping off a curb, falls, and cracks her pelvic bone. During diagnosis, the primary care provider begins to consider the possibility of osteoporosis.

_____ a. What are the symptoms of osteoporosis?

_____ b. What diagnostic procedures would the primary care provider order to verify the diagnosis of osteoporosis?

_____ c. If the diagnosis is verified, what treatment will be initiated?

_____

_____

_____

_____

_____

_____

_____

_____

_____

_____

_____

_____

2. Compare and contrast bursitis and tendonitis.

_____

_____

_____

_____

_____

_____

_____

_____

_____

_____

_____

It is not enough to have a good mind. The main thing is to use it well.
—RENÉ DESCARTES, 1637

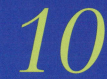

Nervous System Diseases and Disorders

● *chapter outline*

key words

Agnosia (ăg•nō'zē•ă)
Agraphia (ă•grăf'ē•ă)
Alexia (ă•lĕk'sē•ă)
Anticholinergic
(ăn"tī•kō"lĭn•ĕr'jĭk)
Aphasia (ă•fā′zē•ă)
Bradykinesia (brăd"ē•kĭ•nē'sē•ă)
Cerebrospinal fluid (CSF)
(sĕr"ĕ•brō•spī'nal flū'ĭd)
Cheyne-Stokes respiration
(chān'stōks' rĕs•pĭr•ā'shŭn)

Contracture (kŏn•trăk'chūr)
Craniotomy (krā"nē•ŏt'ŏ•mē)
Deoxyribonucleic acid (DNA)
(dē•ŏk"sē•rī"bō•nū'klē•ĭk ă'sĭd)
Diplopia (dĭp•lō'pē•ă)
Dysphasia (dĭs•fā'zē•ă)
Endoplasmic reticulum
(ĕn'dō•plăz"mĭk rē•tĭk'ū•lŭm)
Foramen magnum (for•ā'mĕn
măg'nŭm)
Hemiparesis (hĕm"ē•păr'ĕ•sĭs)

Meninges (mĕn•ĭn'jēz)
Mitochondria (mīt″ō•kŏn'drē•ă)
Neuropeptide (noor"ō•pĕp'tĭd)
Nuchal rigidity (nū'kăl rĭ•jĭ'dĭ•tē)
Photophobia (fō"tō•fō'bē•ă)
Ribosome (rī'bō•sōm)
Serotonin (sĕr"ō•tōn'ĭn)
Somatic (sō•măt'ĭk)
Stupor (stū'pŏr)
Tinnitus (tĭn•ī'tŭs)
Visceral (vĭs'ĕr•ăl)

learning outcomes

Upon successful completion of this chapter, you will be able to:

- Interpret key terms.
- Recall anatomy and physiology of the nervous system.
- Identify the main divisions of the nervous system.
- Describe the basic unit of the nervous system and how it functions.
- List the concerns in using over-the-counter medications for headache.
- Recall the etiology for migraine headaches.
- Compare the prognoses for migraine and tension headaches.
- Describe traumatic brain injury.
- Contrast concussion with contusion.
- Recall possible treatment for acute subdural hematomas.
- Discuss the signs and symptoms of abusive head trauma.
- Recall four courses of treatment for spinal cord injuries.
- Distinguish the signs and symptoms of paraplegia and quadriplegia.
- Restate the cause of hemiplegia.
- Identify the classifications of meningitis.
- Describe acute bacterial meningitis.

- Describe complementary therapies for peripheral neuropathy.
- Explain the characteristic symptoms of Bell palsy.
- Discuss cerebrovascular accident.
- Restate the relationship between cerebrovascular accident and transient ischemic attack.
- Recall the less invasive treatment for cerebral aneurysm.
- Identify at least three diagnostic procedures for epilepsy.
- Recall the etiology and the 10 warning signs for Alzheimer disease.
- Recognize the signs and symptoms of Parkinson disease.
- Recall the etiology of multiple sclerosis.
- Discuss the appropriate treatment protocol for amyotrophic lateral sclerosis.
- Summarize the diagnostic tools for narcolepsy.
- Discuss the prognosis of restless leg syndrome.
- Describe the progression of brain tumors.
- List at least four symptoms characteristic of nervous system diseases and disorders.
- Recall the diseases/disorders in the nervous system that are a medical emergency.

CHAPTER EPISODE—PART I

Breyona, now 26, faced a very difficult challenge when an automobile crash left her paralyzed from the waist down 6 years ago in her home state of Florida. She was a skilled volleyball player attending a community college in a nearby state on a volleyball scholarship. She fought for her life during her several months' stay in a teaching hospital near her home. She wondered if she would ever play volleyball again.

- What type of paralysis does Breyona have?
- What chances does she have of playing volleyball again?
- What might her life look like this many years from her accident?

NERVOUS SYSTEM ANATOMY AND PHYSIOLOGY REVIEW

The body's nervous system is an elaborate, interlaced network of nerve cells of astonishing complexity and sophistication. This network includes the brain, spinal cord, and nerves. The entire system functions to regulate and coordinate body activities and bring about responses by which the body adjusts to changes in its internal and external environments.

The nervous system consists of two divisions: the central nervous system (CNS) and the peripheral nervous system (PNS). The CNS consists of the brain and spinal cord. It processes and stores sensory information and includes the parts of the brain governing consciousness. The PNS is composed of all other nervous tissue outside the CNS and includes 12 pairs of cranial nerves, 31 pairs of spinal nerves, all sensory nerves, and the sympathetic and parasympathetic nerves. The sympathetic and parasympathetic nerves comprise the autonomic nervous system (ANS), which regulates involuntary muscle movements and the action of glands.

The PNS is the conduit for information both to and from the CNS. The brain is the control center for this information; it receives the information, processes it, and initiates the appropriate responses.

Neurons

The nervous system contains billions of neurons, or nerve cells, that make up nerves. Neurons are specialized cells that initiate or conduct electrochemical impulses and react to physical and chemical changes in their surroundings. The cell body of each neuron contains **deoxyribonucleic acid (DNA)** in its nucleus, **endoplasmic reticulum** and **ribosomes** for building proteins, and mitochondria for making energy.

Each neuron has a long axon that may be sheathed in myelin and many tiny branches called *dendrites*. The dendrites carry messages *to* the cell body coming from other neurons; the axon of the neuron carries impulses *away from* the cell body to other neurons, sometimes at a great distance. For example, the neurons making up the nerves going from the spinal cord to the toes may be as long as 3 feet (Fig. 10.1). The neuron cell bodies and all their dendrites appear gray to the naked eye—thus the reference to gray matter. The neuron axons and their myelin sheaths appear white in color—thus the reference to white matter.

There are three types of neurons: sensory, motor, and interneuron. Sensory neurons, also called *afferent neurons*, transmit impulses to the central nervous system, where they are interpreted as a sensation. The sensory neurons coming from the skin, skeletal muscles, and joints are called **somatic.** The sensory neurons coming from internal organs are called **visceral.**

Motor neurons, also called *efferent neurons*, transmit impulses *from* the central nervous system to muscles and glands. Similar to sensory neurons, somatic motor neurons relate to skeletal muscle and the visceral neurons to smooth muscle, cardiac muscle, and glands.

Interneurons provide connections between sensory and motor neurons and between themselves. The neurons of the CNS are all interneurons.

Neurons transmitting impulses do not actually touch each other. There is a small space, called a *synapse,* between the axon of one neuron and the dendrite of another neuron. When a nerve impulse arrives at the synapse, it releases chemicals called *neurotransmitters* that sail across the gap to the next neuron to influence another neuron either in an inhibitory or excitatory way.

Central Nervous System

Brain

The brain, an organ about the size of a small head of cauliflower, coordinates, controls, and regulates a number of life-sustaining tasks (Fig. 10.2):

- Controls heart rate and respirations, blood pressure, and body temperature
- Processes all the information obtained from seeing, hearing, smelling, tasting, and touching
- Produces and releases a number of hormones for body functioning
- Coordinates physical movement
- Enables thought, learning, speech, emotions, and social behavior

The major sections of the brain and their function are summarized in Table 10.1. Refer to Figure 10.2 as you read the table.

Spinal Cord

The spinal cord transmits electrochemical messages to and from the brain and processes spinal cord reflexes. The spinal cord runs from an opening in the occipital

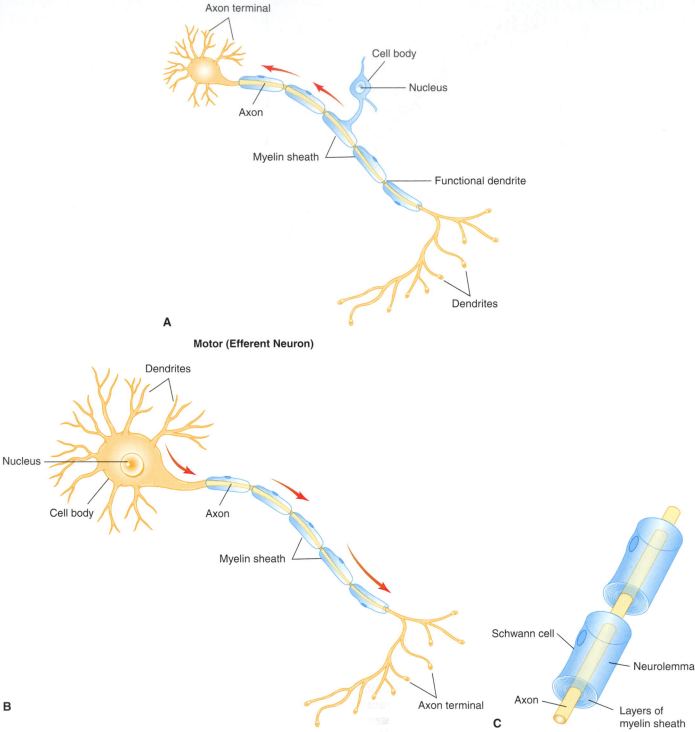

Figure 10.1 Neuron structure. (A) Afferent (sensory) neuron. (B) Motor (efferent) neuron. Arrows indicate the direction of impulse transmission. (C) Close-up of the myelin sheath and neurolemma formed by Schwann cells.

bone called the **foramen magnum** to the area between the first and second lumbar vertebrae.

Peripheral Nervous System

Together the CNS and the PNS provide three general functions: sensory, integrative, and motor. The sensory function consists of receptors that monitor the body both externally and internally. The sensory receptors convert their information into nerve impulses, which are then transmitted via the PNS to the CNS, and the signals are integrated. They are brought together, creating sensations and helping to produce thoughts and

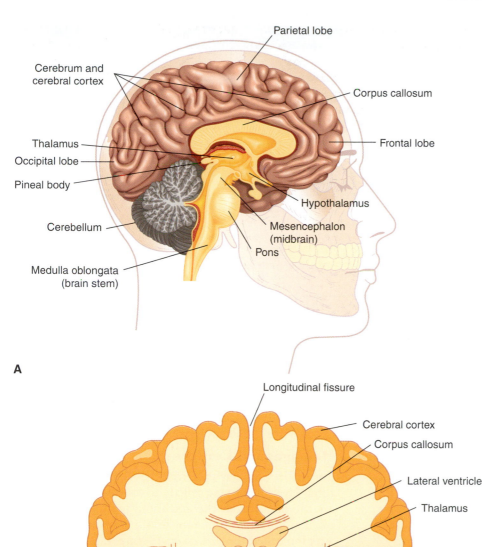

A

B

Figure 10.2 (A) Midsagittal section of the brain as seen from the right side. This medial plane shows internal anatomy and the lobes of the cerebrum. (B) Frontal section of the brain in anterior view.

perceptions. As a result, we make decisions and use motor functions to act on them. The PNS includes the cranial and spinal nerves as well as the ANS.

Cranial Nerves

Twelve pairs of cranial nerves come from the brain. They are named by Roman numeral and name (e.g., "I olfactory"). The Roman numeral partially identifies the cranial nerves' location in the brain. Refer to Table 10.2 for a summary of the cranial nerves and their function.

Spinal Nerves

Thirty-one pairs of spinal nerves branch from the spinal cord. There are eight pairs of cervical nerves (C1–C8),

twelve pairs of thoracic nerves (T1–T12), five pairs of lumbar nerves (L1–L5), five pairs of sacral nerves (S1–S5), and one pair of coccygeal nerves. Each set of nerves has a specialized task (Fig. 10.3).

Autonomic Nervous System

The ANS is actually part of the PNS. It helps individuals adapt to changes in the environment. There are two parts to the ANS: the sympathetic and the parasympathetic systems.

Sympathetic System

Neuron cell bodies of the sympathetic system are located in the thoracic and lumbar areas of the spinal cord. They

Table 10.1 Structure and Function of Major Brain Areas

STRUCTURE	FUNCTION
Cerebrum: the largest part of the brain; splits vertically into right and left hemispheres; identified in four lobes: frontal, parietal, temporal, and occipital; surface is called *cerebral cortex;* consists of gray matter.	Each lobe is specific in function, but the cerebrum is important for its coordination of motor control, behavior, skin sensations, smell, meaning of words, speech, interpreting what is seen, and spatial ability. The right hemisphere controls the left side of the body; the left hemisphere controls the right side of the body.
Cerebellum: located at the base of the brain under the occipital lobes of the cerebrum.	Controls involuntary movements of muscles, posture, balance and equilibrium, and some memory for reflex motor acts. It contains more neurons than all other brain areas combined.
Thalamus: lies beneath the cerebrum and above the hypothalamus.	Processes and relays information to the cerebral cortex; important in sleep, consciousness, and activity.
Hypothalamus: is below the thalamus; a small area of the brain sitting on either side of the third ventricle. Shaped like two eggs side by side.	Responsible for many functions, including producing hormones, regulating body temperature, regulating the food we eat, assisting with the autonomic nervous system, and causing visceral responses in emotional situations.
Medulla oblongata: is behind the cerebellum; extends from the spinal column to the pons.	Regulates heartbeat, blood pressure, and respiration; reflex center for coughing, sneezing, swallowing, and vomiting.
Pons: means "bridge"; connects medulla to other brain parts. Serves as the pathway for signals to and from different parts of the brain.	With the medulla, creates a normal breathing pattern.

are responsible, in part, for the fight-or-flight response during times of stress, anger, or fear, and they operate through a series of interconnected neurons. This response enables the body to perform at its peak in stressful circumstances.

Table 10.2 Cranial Nerves

NUMBER AND NAME	FUNCTION
I Olfactory	• Sense of smell
II Optic	• Sense of sight
III Oculomotor	• Movement of the eyeball • Constriction of pupil in bright light or for near vision
IV Trochlear	• Movement of eyeball
V Trigeminal	• Sensation in face, scalp, and teeth • Contraction of chewing muscles
VI Abducens	• Movement in the eyeball
VII Facial	• Sense of taste • Contraction of facial muscles • Secretion of saliva
VIII Acoustic (vestibulocochlear)	• Sense of hearing • Sense of equilibrium
IX Glossopharyngeal	• Sense of taste • Sensory for cardiac, respiratory, and blood pressure reflexes • Contraction of pharynx • Secretion of saliva
X Vagus	• Sensory in cardiac, respiratory, and blood pressure reflexes • Sensory and motor to larynx (speaking) • Decreases heart rate • Contraction of alimentary tube (peristalsis) • Increases digestive secretions
XI Accessory	• Contraction of neck and shoulder muscles • Motor to larynx (speaking)
XII Hypoglossal	• Movement of the tongue

From Scanlon, VC, and Sanders, T: Essentials of Anatomy and Physiology, ed. 6. Philadelphia: F.A. Davis, 2011, p 201, with permission.

Parasympathetic System

The parasympathetic system's neuron cell bodies are found in the brain stem and the sacral region of the spinal cord. This system complements the sympathetic system in that it calms and relaxes the body in nonstress situations. It helps to regulate heart rate and respirations appropriate to the circumstances.

Meninges and Cerebrospinal Fluid

The entire nervous system is covered in a protective three-layer membrane called the **meninges.** The layers are the dura mater, the arachnoid membrane, and the pia mater. Between the arachnoid and the pia mater is a region called the *subarachnoid space.* It is in this space that **cerebrospinal fluid (CSF)** is found. The CSF bathes the brain and spinal cord, carrying nutrients to the neurons, acting as a cushion of protection, and moving waste products to the blood for absorption.

Reviewing the anatomy and physiology of the nervous system enables a clearer understanding of the numerous diseases and disorders of the brain and spinal cord.

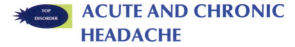

Headache

ACUTE AND CHRONIC HEADACHE

ICD-10: G44.1 or R51

Description

A headache is any diffuse pain occurring in any portion of the head. The condition may be acute or chronic. Headache is one of the most common maladies afflicting humans. The International Headache Society classifies headaches into three major categories:

• Primary headaches, which include tension, migraine, and cluster headaches

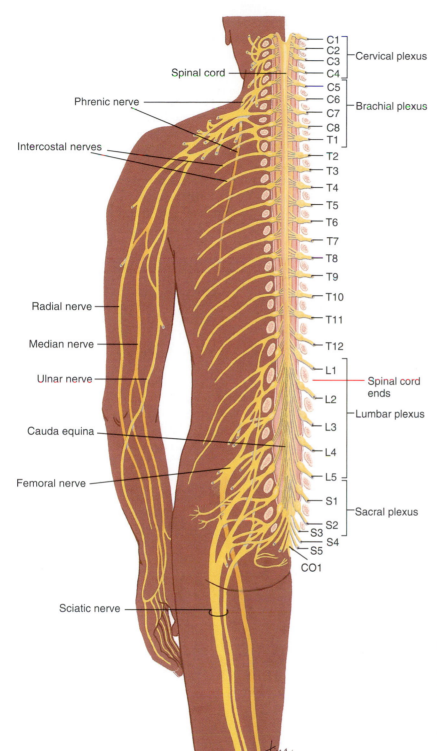

Labels on figure:
Spinal cord
Phrenic nerve
Intercostal nerves
Radial nerve
Median nerve
Ulnar nerve
Cauda equina
Femoral nerve
Sciatic nerve

C1
C2
C3
C4 — Cervical plexus
C5
C6
C7 — Brachial plexus
C8
T1
T2
T3
T4
T5
T6
T7
T8
T9
T10
T11
T12
L1 — Spinal cord ends
L2
L3 — Lumbar plexus
L4
L5
S1
S2 — Sacral plexus
S3
S4
S5
CO1

Figure 10.3 The spinal cord and spinal nerves. The distribution of spinal nerves is shown only on the left side. The nerve plexuses are labeled on the right side. A nerve plexus is a network of neurons from several segments of the spinal cord that combine to form nerves to specific parts of the body. For example, the radial and ulnar nerves to the arm emerge from the brachial plexus. *(From Scanlon, VC, and Sanders, T:* Essentials of Anatomy and Physiology, *ed. 6. Philadelphia: F.A. Davis, 2011, p 184, with permission.)*

- Secondary headaches, which occur because of some underlying structural problem
- Cranial neuralgias, facial pain, and other headaches

Tension headaches are the most common, followed by migraines. Cluster headaches are rare. Tension headaches are the basis for this content; migraine headache information follows. In most cases, headache signals nothing more serious than fatigue or tension. Less frequently, headache may be the manifestation of an underlying disorder or may be secondary in nature. For this reason, an individual's complaint of headache should not be minimized or unthinkingly treated with analgesics before the underlying cause has been determined.

Etiology

The cause of tension headaches is essentially unknown. Generally, however, when contracting muscles that cover the skull become stressed, they spasm and cause pain. Common sites include the forehead, the base of the skull, and the temple area. Tension headaches may result from physical or emotional stress.

Signs and Symptoms

The character of headache pain varies markedly among individuals. (Recall from Chapter 3 that pain is exactly what an individual says it is.) The pain may be dull and aching or acute and pounding. The pain may be intermittent and sometimes seem intense. It may focus in the front, sides, or back of the head and is usually not disabling. Pain also may be intense over one or both eyes.

Diagnostic Procedures

If a medical history reveals a pattern of recurrent or unusually severe headaches, further medical testing is usually undertaken to try to detect an underlying secondary cause. This may include neurological testing. The medical history is essential for diagnosis of the tension headache, as it will reveal specific information about the headache—its quantity, quality, and duration, as well as any other symptoms. There will be no nausea, vomiting, or light sensitivity with a tension headache.

Treatment

Analgesics are generally effective in providing temporary, symptomatic relief of headache pain. These are often over-the-counter (OTC) medications, such as ibuprofen (e.g., Advil, Motrin), acetaminophen (e.g., Tylenol), and naproxen (e.g., Aleve). Sometimes muscle relaxants and minor tranquilizers may be prescribed.

Complementary Therapy

Food allergies can be a major source of headache pain. Common offenders include refined sugars, chocolate, caffeine, sodas, alcohol, nuts, and dried fruit (due to molds or sulfites); these should be omitted from the diet if they are suspected of causing pain.

Massage and acupressure are beneficial in releasing muscle tension, thereby reducing headaches. Many bodywork therapies require a professional, but acupressure self-help techniques can be practiced by anyone. Acupressure involves placing pressure with the thumbs and the index fingers on various points on the back of the neck and near the bridge of the nose. Pressing fingertips into any area of the neck that is sore and tender can be helpful. Moving shoulders in a gentle rhythmic motion encourages relaxation and tension release.

Techniques for relaxation include meditation, biofeedback, and yoga. Deep breathing for 5 minutes is relaxing, and progressive muscle relaxation exercises can help prevent some headaches. Another method of treating headaches without drugs is hydrotherapy. Hot baths, saunas, heat lamps, and steam baths reduce tension, increase circulation, and remove metabolic wastes from the body. Sometimes the addition of peppermint or menthol aromatherapy is beneficial.

⊙ CLIENT COMMUNICATION

Remind clients to prevent complacency when using OTC medications for pain. The Food and Drug Administration (FDA) now requires pharmaceutical companies to place stricter warnings on their pain medications. Acetaminophen products such as Tylenol must now warn users of the danger of liver damage. NSAIDs, such as aspirin, ibuprofen, and naproxen, must carry warnings of stomach bleeding. The use of alcohol, taking more than the recommended dosage, and using the medication longer than suggested can cause severe side effects.

Prognosis

The prognosis for most tension headaches is good. Recurring headaches are a signal that further medical attention may be necessary.

Prevention

Recognizing and practicing methods of reducing stress and tension can be beneficial in reducing the number of tension headaches.

MIGRAINE HEADACHE

ICD-10: G43.XX*

Description

A migraine is a recurrent, frequently incapacitating type of headache characterized by intense, throbbing pain often accompanied by nausea and vomiting. Migraine headaches usually begin in adolescence or early adulthood and diminish slowly in frequency and intensity with advancing age. Women are affected more than twice as frequently as men. Migraine headaches are often familial.

---

*The X represents the fourth and fifth digits that are often required and supplied once more detailed information about the disease or disorder is made known to the provider.

Etiology

Migraines are not psychogenic. They are occasioned by changes in the cerebral blood flow, presumably due to vasoconstriction and subsequent vasodilation of cerebrocranial arterioles. It is likely that the trigeminal cranial nerve releases substances called **neuropeptides** when **serotonin** levels fall, usually the result of a chemical imbalance. What initiates this process is not known. Susceptibility to migraine headaches may be hereditary. There are some known migraine triggers:

- Certain foods, such as chocolate, aged cheese, red wine, caffeine, and the ingredient monosodium glutamate
- Hormonal changes in women near or during their menstrual cycle when there is a major drop in estrogen
- Sensory stimuli, such as sun glare, bright lights, and loud sounds
- Some odors such as paint thinner, perfumes, and smoke
- Changes in weather or barometric pressure
- Some medications

Signs and Symptoms

Before the onset of pain, many migraine sufferers report symptoms such as flashing lights before their eyes, **photophobia,** or **tinnitus** (a ringing or buzzing sound in the ears). Other symptoms occurring before the migraine attack, called *premonitory symptoms* or *aura,* may include unusual thirst, craving for sweet foods, unusual energy peaks, and alterations in mood or mental clarity. Once the pain of the attack begins, it is typically accompanied by nausea, vomiting, and photophobia. During attacks, some clients develop stroke-like symptoms with numbness and/or loss of muscle strength on one side of the body. In these cases, clients need to be evaluated for stroke.

Diagnostic Procedures

The diagnosis depends almost totally on the medical history. A recurrent pattern of severe headaches preceded by any of the classic premonitory symptoms noted previously suggests the diagnosis of migraine headache. To rule out organic causes, a computed tomography (CT) scan or magnetic resonance imaging (MRI) scan may be ordered.

Treatment

Drug therapy may include the use of NSAIDs, such as ibuprofen or aspirin, triptans (Imitrex), ergot preparations, antinausea medications, combination medications, and opiates. A number of medications have been effective in preventing migraines, such as those used as cardiovascular drugs, antiseizure medications, antidepressants, and botulinum toxin type A. Sometimes no treatment is chosen other than bed rest in a quiet, darkened room for the duration of the attack.

Complementary Therapy

See "Headaches." Acupuncture has shown success in migraine treatment. Massage may help reduce the frequency of migraines and improve sleep. There is some evidence that the herbs feverfew and butterbur may reduce the severity of migraines, but these should not be taken by pregnant women or without consultation with the primary care provider (PCP).

⊕ CLIENT COMMUNICATION

Avoidance of anything that provokes an attack is essential. Once premonitory symptoms are experienced, it is necessary to begin treating immediately. Decrease stimuli once the migraine pain begins.

Prognosis

The prognosis varies. No form of therapy has proved successful in permanently disrupting the cycle of migraine attacks. As noted earlier, migraine headaches tend to become less frequent and less severe with age.

Prevention

There is no specific prevention for migraine headaches unless the actual cause is known and can be avoided. Keeping a headache diary can help determine what triggers, if any, might be the cause of the migraines.

Head Trauma

Head trauma usually results from an accident, a blow to the head, or a serious fall. Recovery may be rapid or extended, depending on the severity of the trauma. It is important to watch an individual who has suffered head trauma for any signs of dizziness, nausea, severe headache, and loss of consciousness. Diagnosis of head trauma likely includes a neurological workup using the Glasgow Coma Scale. The examination will include assessment of hearing, vision, balance and strength, coordination, and reflexes. For an explanation of the Glasgow Coma Scale, see http://www.brainline.org/content/2010/10/what-is-the-glasgow-coma-scale.html. Keep in mind, however, that while the Glasgow Coma Scale is very helpful in diagnosis, it gives no indication on the long-term issues caused by head trauma. Head traumas considered here are all identified as a form of traumatic brain injury (TBI) and include concussions, contusions, and hematomas.

TRAUMATIC BRAIN INJURY

ICD-10: S06.89X

Description

Today, the majority of head injuries fall under the general classification of traumatic brain injuries. They occur when the brain collides with the inside of the skull, sometimes bruising the brain, tearing nerve fibers, and causing bleeding. The TBIs discussed here include concussion, subdural hematoma, and abusive head trauma. Many veterans return from military conflicts with TBIs that are the result of explosions or bullets shattering the skull and piercing brain tissue.

Etiology

The most serious TBIs are caused by sudden, violent blows to the head that bruise the brain. Military conflicts, serious assaults, bullet wounds, serious vehicular crashes, catastrophic events (e.g., earthquake, building/bridge collapse), and severe sports injuries are major causes of TBIs.

Signs and Symptoms

The signs and symptoms may be mild or severe. Mild symptoms include brief unconsciousness, amnesia, headache, confusion and problems concentrating, balance problems, blurred vision, ringing in the ears, bad taste in the mouth, and mood changes. Serious symptoms include persistent headache, vomiting or nausea, convulsions or seizures, slurred speech, numbness in extremities, agitation and combativeness, and the inability to be awakened from sleep. Children with TBI may complain of headache, refuse to eat, be cranky, have unusual sleep patterns, and lose interest in their favorite activities.

Diagnostic Procedures

TBIs pose an emergency. Prompt diagnosis is important and includes CT scans and MRIs. A 15-point test called the Glasgow Coma Scale is used to test the severity of the brain injury. This test checks for mental alertness, ability to blink eyes and move extremities, and speech coherence. It may be necessary to insert a probe into the skull to monitor increased pressure from the trauma. Excess fluid may be drained in the same way.

Treatment

Mild TBIs may necessitate only bed rest and mild analgesics. Severe TBIs, however, require hospitalization, perhaps intensive care. Diuretics administered via IV to reduce the amount of fluid in tissues and antiseizure and coma-inducing medications may be ordered. Individuals may deliberately be placed into a temporary coma to reduce the need for oxygen, especially if the damaged vessels are unable to deliver the normal amount of oxygen to the brain cells. Surgery may be necessary to remove clotted blood, repair skull fractures, or create an opening for drainage and additional space as the brain continues to swell.

Complementary Therapy

No significant complementary therapy is indicated.

 CLIENT COMMUNICATION

The individual with the TBI and the person's family members need support in coping with rehabilitation and recovery. A fair amount of memory may be erased, and it is difficult to learn new tasks. Help individuals learn to slow down, stop and think, break a task into smaller components, ask questions, pay attention to details, and be patient.

Prognosis

Rehabilitation is usually required to relearn basic skills, such as walking and talking. The goal is to enable individuals to return to as many of their regular activities of daily living as possible.

Prevention

Teach clients to wear seat belts, never drive under the influence of drugs or alcohol, separate firearms from their bullets and store all in a locked cabinet, wear protective gear such as helmets and hard hats, and take precautions to avoid falls.

CEREBRAL CONCUSSION

ICD-10: S06.0XX

Description

A cerebral concussion is the mildest form of TBI that changes brain function. It may or may not be immediately apparent. Cerebral concussion may result in a temporary loss of consciousness, typically lasting from a few seconds to a few minutes, followed by a short period of amnesia. The reaction of a boxer who has just been "knocked out" is a classic example of cerebral concussion. It is the most common head injury in sports.

Etiology

This condition is usually caused by a blunt impact to the head of sufficient force to cause the brain to strike and rebound from the skull. The loss of consciousness, subsequent amnesia, and other bodily symptoms of cerebral concussion are due to disruption of normal electrical activity in the brain. The brain tissue itself is usually not injured.

Signs and Symptoms

Primary symptoms are dizziness, temporary loss of consciousness with shallow respirations, depressed pulse rate, and flaccid muscle tone. After the individual regains consciousness, there is usually a variable period of amnesia that may be accompanied by bradycardia, faintness, pallor, hypotension, and photophobia. Delayed symptoms may include headache, nausea, vomiting, tinnitus (ringing in the ears), and blurred vision.

Diagnostic Procedures

A careful physical and neurological assessment are typically performed. Cranial CT scans usually reveal no evidence of brain tissue damage (compare with cerebral contusion). MRI may prove helpful as well.

Treatment

Treatment usually involves nothing more than quiet bed rest. The affected individual should be closely watched for any behavioral changes that may indicate progressive brain injury. If pain exists, a mild analgesic may be ordered. A gradual return to daily activities at a pace that does not worsen symptoms is allowed.

Complementary Therapy

No significant complementary therapy is indicated.

CLIENT COMMUNICATION

Immediate medical attention should be sought if any of the following signs and symptoms occur: difficulty in walking, difficulty in speaking, confusion, severe headache, and vomiting.

Prognosis

If the individual remains alert with only one or two symptoms, such as headache, nausea, a brief episode of vomiting, impaired concentration, or slightly blurred vision, the prognosis is usually good, with a low risk of subsequent complications. Brain edema is a life-threatening complication most often seen in children and adolescents with a concussion. Most clients recover in 24 to 48 hours. Having a concussion doubles the risk of developing epilepsy within 5 years of the concussion.

Prevention

Prevention of concussions includes following work and play safety measures that minimize the risk of head injury, such as the use of approved head protection when playing sports, riding bikes, skiing, and skating. Hard hats are to be worn in construction areas, and seat belts must be used while driving or riding in motor vehicles.

REALITY EPISODE

Brian plays varsity football. He loves the game and plays with abandon. On Friday night, the game was close and his team was behind by 3 points. While completing a running catch close to the end zone, Brian was tackled and dropped to the field. Several players from the opposing team immediately piled on top of him. When the referee pulled everyone off the pile, Brian had difficulty getting up. In fact, he fell back down. The coach and the team's doctor immediately ran to Brian. After just a few moments, Brian was helped up and walked off the field. He sat on the bench for the next few plays and begged to go back into the game, but his coach refused.

Brian's team lost the game; he and his teammates were pretty upset about Brian not being able to play.

Identify the positive action of this scenario. What might have occurred had Brian been permitted to return to the game?

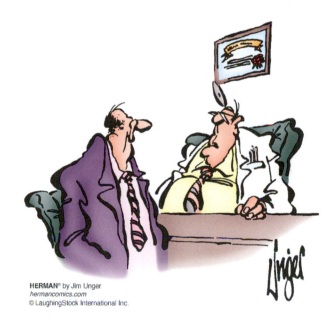

HERMAN® by Jim Unger
hermancomics.com
© LaughingStock International Inc.

"If I don't cure your amnesia, you get ten times your money back."

HERMAN© is reprinted with permission from LaughingStock Licensing Inc., Ottawa, Canada. All rights reserved.

CEREBRAL CONTUSION

ICD-10: S06.33

Description

A cerebral contusion is a type of TBI in which the tissue along or just beneath the surface of the brain is bruised. Blood from broken vessels usually accumulates in the surrounding brain tissue. It is far more serious than a concussion.

Etiology

Cerebral contusions are produced by a blow to the head or after the head impacts a surface, causing the hemispheres of the brain to twist against or slide along the inner surface of the skull. The twisting or shearing force may be sufficient to damage deep structures in the brain as well.

Signs and Symptoms

The signs and symptoms of cerebral contusions vary according to the location and extent of the tissue injury to the brain. Symptoms may range from transient loss of consciousness to coma. When conscious, an individual may exhibit hemiparesis; severe headache; nausea; vomiting; and a variety of behavioral disturbances ranging from lethargy, apathy, and drowsiness to hostility and combativeness. Blood pressure and temperature are subnormal.

Diagnostic Procedures

A thorough neurological assessment is required. Cranial CT scans and MRI typically reveal the location and extent of tissue damage produced by a cerebral contusion.

Treatment

The condition is acute and considered a medical emergency. The treatment varies according to the location and severity of the contusion. Individuals with contusions are hospitalized so their vital signs can be monitored and rapid medical intervention can take place should it be required. Surgery may be necessary to control bleeding.

Complementary Therapy

No significant complementary therapy is indicated.

> ### ⊕ CLIENT COMMUNICATION
>
> When a client is hospitalized and unconscious or in a coma, attention must be given to family members, who will have many questions. Teach them what they can do to be helpful to their loved one.

Prognosis

The prognosis for cerebral contusion ultimately depends on the extent of the brain injury. Sudden, progressive edema of the brain with a consequent escalation of intracranial pressure is a serious, life-threatening complication. Other complications include cerebral hemorrhage and epidural or subdural hematoma. Permanent neurological deficits, including epilepsy caused by scar tissue formation at the site of the contusion, may result.

Prevention

See preventive measures for cerebral concussion.

SUBDURAL HEMATOMA (ACUTE)

ICD-10: S06.36X

Description

After a severe blow to the head, a subdural hematoma may form, where blood collects between the dura mater and the arachnoid membrane (the second membrane covering the brain) (Fig. 10.4). Pressure from the mass of blood can be sufficient to impair brain function. Acute subdural hematomas are one of the deadliest types of head injuries.

Etiology

Acute subdural hematomas are caused by blood seeping from ruptured vessels below the dural membrane and are almost always the result of severe head injury. Chronic subdural hematomas may occur spontaneously or follow only a minor head injury, especially in elderly clients.

Signs and Symptoms

The symptoms of subdural hematoma typically include difficulty walking, headache, confusion, confused or slurred speech, visual problems, and an initial loss of consciousness. As the condition worsens, there may be

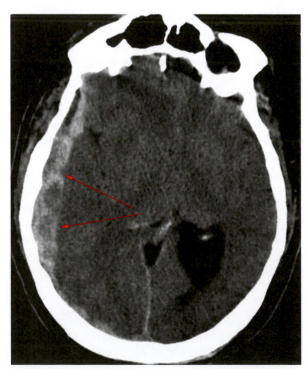

Figure 10.4 Axial CT demonstrating an acute subdural hematoma (arrows). Deep to the hematoma there is severe cerebral edema with positive mass effect. *(From Weber, EC, Vilensky, JA, and Fog, AM: Practical Radiology: A Symptom-Based Approach, ed. 1. Philadelphia: F.A. Davis, 2013, p 86, with permission.)*

paralysis of half the body **(hemiparesis)**, severe headache, and dilated pupils. These symptoms may appear within a short period of time or over a period of days, depending on the rate at which blood accumulates.

Diagnostic Procedures

The individual's clinical picture and a medical history revealing head trauma should suggest a potential diagnosis of subdural hematoma. CT scans or MRI are likely ordered to pinpoint the position of the hematoma.

Treatment

A subdural hematoma is a medical emergency. It may be necessary to perform a **craniotomy,** an incision into the cranium to aspirate the accumulated blood and control further bleeding.

Surgery may be performed on an emergency basis if rising intracranial pressure proves to be life-threatening. There are medications to help reduce the swelling and to control seizures.

Complementary Therapy

No significant complementary therapy is indicated.

 CLIENT COMMUNICATION

Remember that the risk of a subdural hematoma increases with anticoagulant medication use, such as blood thinners and aspirin, abuse of alcohol, recurrent falls, and in the very young and in older people.

Prognosis

The prognosis for acute subdural hematomas is always guarded. Barring any complications, a person can recover with few, if any, residual effects. Seizures that often follow a subdural hematoma can be controlled with medications. In the most serious cases of subdural hematoma, however, irreversible brain damage, coma, or death may result.

Prevention

The best prevention is to minimize the risk of head trauma. Front and side air bags in automobiles are helpful. It is important to properly restrain children in car seats. Helmets should be worn when playing contact sports, riding bicycles or motorcycles, skiing or snowboarding, skating, and skateboarding.

ABUSIVE HEAD TRAUMA (SHAKEN BABY SYNDROME)

ICD-10: T74.4

Description

Shaken baby syndrome (SBS) was renamed *abusive head trauma* by the American Academy of Pediatrics in April 2009; however, the term *shaken baby syndrome* is still commonly used in many circles. The syndrome is a TBI in children caused by abuse. Because there is legal debate about whether an infant can be shaken hard enough to cause serious damage, the new term avoids that debate and more clearly directs attention to the more important consideration of whether abuse occurred. Abusive head trauma in children is manual vigorous shaking of an infant or young child by the arms, legs, chest, or shoulders that results in subdural hematoma of the brain, occult bone fractures, and retinal hemorrhages. Brain damage, decreased mental capacity, paralysis, seizures, hearing loss, and even death can result. Generally, the infant is under age 3. SBS was first described in 1946 and affects 1,500 infants per year. However, some resources have estimated that there are more than 50,000 cases each year. The abuse is generally triggered by anger that results when a baby will not stop crying. The father, the mother's boyfriend, the babysitter, or the mother are usually the perpetrators.

Etiology

Abusive head trauma is the result of violent shaking of an infant or a child. Babies have very weak neck muscles, and violent shaking can cause any or all of the following:

- Subdural hematoma when the veins from the brain to the dura are torn and bleed.
- Subarachnoid hemorrhage.
- Brain trauma when the brain hits the inner surface of the skull.
- Breaking off of nerve cell axons.
- Lack of oxygen when the infant stops breathing during the shaking.
- Retinal hemorrhage.
- Skull fractures if the infant's head hits a wall or hard object.

Signs and Symptoms

The condition may go unnoticed and unreported because there are no outward symptoms. Often the infant is not brought in for medical treatment until some time after the initial injury. Some cases may be mild and the infant's condition attributed to a mild viral infection or colic. Other symptoms may include difficulty feeding, vomiting, listlessness, lethargy, apnea, seizures or convulsions, irritability, and dilated pupils that do not respond to light.

Diagnostic Procedures

Abusive head trauma is not always easily diagnosed. A careful history and physical examination, including a neurological assessment, are performed. Primary care providers look for retinal hemorrhages, blood in the brain (subdural hematoma), and increased head size, indicating the increased fluid and pressure in the brain. Ophthalmologic examination may reveal any retinal hemorrhage. Ultrasound and radiology as well as CT scans and MRI may be ordered. Other diseases and disorders, such as birth trauma, meningitis, infection, and seizure disorders, must be ruled out. Interviewing parents can be helpful, but not everyone is willing to acknowledge responsibility for the abuse. Some say the injuries occurred because the infant stopped breathing and they were trying to resuscitate him or her.

Treatment

Abusive head trauma is a medical emergency, and treatment is essential to save the infant. Immediate treatment is important to prevent further damage and may require that the infant or child be hospitalized, especially if there is a head injury. Observation is important to note any neurological changes needing treatment. Safety of the infant is essential and may necessitate removal from his or her environment.

Complementary Therapy

No significant complementary therapy is indicated.

 CLIENT COMMUNICATION

Instruct parents and caregivers how to calm a crying and upset baby or child and how shaking can lead to permanent injury. Provide education about normal human growth and development. If caregivers are high risk, refer to the appropriate resources for support and education.

Prognosis

One-third of the infants with abusive head trauma die from these injuries, and one-third more have permanent injuries, such as diminished mental ability, seizures, epilepsy, and paralysis.

Prevention

Abusive head trauma is completely preventable. Education is paramount for caregivers and family members to ensure the safety of children. Encourage parents and caregivers to bring in their children for well-baby checks as directed by pediatricians and primary care providers. Refer parents and caregivers to appropriate community resources if they have stressful events in their lives.

Cumulative Effects of Multiple Brain Injuries

Before leaving this section, it should be noted that subsequent head injuries identified must also be considered. The effect of multiple traumatic brain injuries is significant and can result in long-term neurological and functional deficits.

Preventing Abusive Head Trauma (Shaken Baby Syndrome)

These tips may be given to parents and caregivers to help prevent abuse:

- Count to 10 and take several deep breaths.
- Go to another room and allow the infant to cry for a time.
- Call someone close for emotional support.
- Call a primary care provider; there may be a reason the infant is crying.
- Never leave the infant with anyone not trusted completely.
- Carefully check references before leaving an infant with a caregiver or day-care facility.

Paralysis

HEMIPLEGIA

ICD-10: G81.90

Description

Hemiplegia is the loss of voluntary muscular control and sensation on one side of the body.

Etiology

Hemiplegia is most frequently caused by disease processes such as cerebrovascular accident (CVA, or stroke) that disrupt the blood supply to the brain and brain stem. The condition also may result from cerebral contusion, subdural hematoma, or TBI. A brain tumor or brain infection may also cause hemiplegia. Damage to the right side of the brain causes left-sided paralysis, and vice versa.

Signs and Symptoms

Symptoms of hemiplegia include one-sided paralysis or weakness of the arm, leg, and (usually) face. The condition often is accompanied by communication disorders, such as **aphasia,** an inability to communicate through speech or writing; **agnosia,** an inability to understand auditory or visual information; **agraphia,** an inability to convert thought into writing; and **alexia,** an inability to understand the written language. Individuals have difficulty with balance and walking and most likely are incontinent. The onset of these symptoms is usually sudden, as in the case of CVA or injury, but may occur more gradually, as in the case of a tumor.

Diagnostic Procedures

A thorough physical and neurological assessment is necessary. Cranial CT scans, MRI, and a complete blood analysis may be performed as well.

Treatment

Treatment is directed at the cause of the hemiplegia and usually takes place in an acute care hospital. Otherwise, treatment measures are largely supportive. Physical rehabilitation should begin as soon as possible, no later than 24 to 48 hours following the CVA. In January 2009, research began on the use of injecting embryonic stem cells into individuals who are paralyzed. It is believed that the stem cells can insulate and stimulate nerve fibers that may restore some of the lost function caused by paralysis. To date, the therapy has only been used on rats and mice and is still in the developmental stage.

Complementary Therapy

No significant complementary therapy is indicated.

CLIENT COMMUNICATION

Depending on the resulting paralysis, the following factors must be taken into consideration. It is most beneficial if both the client and family are actively involved in teaching to increase mobility, promote good skin care, improve bladder and bowel control and management, encourage the client's coping mechanisms, prevent any possible complications, and focus on community-based care versus hospitalization. It is helpful to remember that clients and family are often filled with anxiety, fear, frustration, anger, and depression.

Prognosis

The extent of neurological damage determines, in part, the prognosis. Physical rehabilitation, always an arduous process, is the best hope for recovering any lost motor and sensory function. Rehabilitation does not reverse brain damage.

Prevention

The only preventive measures refer to the causes of hemiplegia. Follow the best care to avoid strokes, accidents, and traumatic injuries.

PARAPLEGIA AND QUADRIPLEGIA

ICD-10: G82.XX

Description

Paraplegia and quadriplegia are caused by spinal cord injuries. They are often characterized by the degree of motor and sensory disability they occasion. Paraplegia is the loss of voluntary motion or sensation (paralysis) of the trunk and lower extremities. Quadriplegia is paralysis of all four extremities and, usually, the trunk. Paralysis may not be instant but likely increases over a period of time, usually within 6 months.

Spinal cord injuries occur much more frequently in males than females, especially between ages 16 and 30. Motor vehicle crashes account for 46%; falls, 22%; acts of violence, 16%; sports, 12% (mostly diving); and other, 4%. After age 45, falls become more prevalent than motor vehicle crashes. Alcohol was found to be a factor in 25% of cases.

Etiology

In general, spinal cord injury resulting in paraplegia or quadriplegia is a consequence of fracture, dislocation, or both of the vertebral column. The location of the spinal cord injury, the type of trauma inflicted on the cord, and the severity of that trauma determine whether paraplegia or quadriplegia may result. Refer to Figure 10.3 during this discussion for a better understanding of the location of spinal cord injuries resulting in paraplegia or quadriplegia.

Spinal cord injury resulting in paraplegia is usually due to trauma to the thoracic and lumbar portions of the vertebral column (T1 or lower). Trauma that produces vertical compression and twisting (flexion) of this portion of the spinal cord is the usual mechanism of injury.

Spinal cord trauma at or above C5 in the cervical portion of the vertebral column may result in quadriplegia. Injuries between C5 and C7 may result in varying degrees of motor and sensory weakness in the arms and shoulders. Injuries above C3 usually result in death. Trauma that produces stretching, hyperextension, or flexion of this portion of the spinal cord is the usual mechanism of injury.

Signs and Symptoms

Loss of motor and sensory functions in the legs and trunk are the symptoms of paraplegia. Bowel, bladder, and sexual function are likely lost.

The symptoms of quadriplegia are those of paraplegia plus total or partial loss of motor and sensory functions in the upper limbs and trunk. These symptoms also may be accompanied by falling blood pressure and body temperature, bradycardia, and respiratory difficulties. In some cases, unassisted respiration may cease, causing death.

Diagnostic Procedures

A thorough neurological assessment is necessary. Spinal x-rays, spinal CT scanning, and MRI are typically performed to gauge the nature of the spinal cord injury as well as to detect possible spinal ischemia, edema, or blockage of the flow of CSF.

Treatment

All the spinal cord injuries are a medical emergency, because immediate treatment is important in order to control the paralysis as much as possible. The treatment for all spinal cord injuries includes (1) restoration of spinal alignment, (2) stabilization of the injured spinal area, (3) decompression of neurological structures, and (4) early rehabilitation to minimize long-term paralysis. Much of the early treatment effort is directed at preventing progressive spinal cord tissue damage that may occur following the initial trauma. This may involve surgery to restore spinal alignment, specialized drugs to lessen cell damage, or cooling the affected portion of the spine. As in hemiplegia, stem cell research still offers hope for restoration of some nerve function.

Complementary Therapy

No significant complementary therapy is indicated.

 CLIENT COMMUNICATION

See "Hemiplegia."

Prognosis

The prognosis for individuals with spinal cord injuries is always guarded. It may take several months to adequately assess the extent of the paralysis. If the damage to the spinal cord is complete, there is little hope of regaining lost motor and sensory functions. In general, though, the sooner treatment procedures are begun following spinal cord trauma, the better is the prognosis. Nearly 85% of spinal cord injury clients who survive the first 24 hours are still alive 10 years later. The most common cause of death is a respiratory ailment, such as pneumonia, pulmonary emboli, and septicemia.

Prevention

Preventing paraplegia and quadriplegia involves teaching clients to follow safety measures that minimize the risk of spinal cord injury. Such measures include wearing seat belts while driving or riding in motor vehicles, checking the water depth before diving into any body of water, and wearing protective gear when participating in contact sports.

CHAPTER EPISODE—PART II

Breyona and her dedicated parents grew weary of the attitude of many professionals whose primary goal seemed to be to make Breyona comfortable living her life in a wheelchair. They gave little hope for anything else, and she was taking 14 different medications daily. The family sought assistance from nontraditional practitioners, namely homeopathic and naturopathic therapy when they felt that the traditional specialists had given up hope on Breyona.

Breyona was determined to accomplish her goals. She struggled but was able to finish her schooling and

get her bachelor's degree by attending an accredited, nontraditional program in her state. In the meantime, she started an extensive and rigorous therapy schedule. She has a specially designed treadmill built by a neighbor that allows her to move while being held in place with a harness. She is thrilled at being upright during this time.

- Can you identify one or more positive aspects of this episode?
- Are homeopaths and naturopaths licensed health-care providers in Florida? (See Chapter 2.)
- What is likely the attitude of the traditional health-care practitioners regarding homeopaths and naturopaths?

Infections of the Central Nervous System

MENINGITIS

ICD-10: G00.X (ACUTE BACTERIAL)
ICD-10: A87.X (VIRAL)

Description

Meningitis is inflammation of the three-layer membrane called the *meninges* that surrounds the brain and spinal cord (Fig. 10.5). It can be classified as acute or chronic, bacterial or viral. The majority of cases are viral in origin, but bacterial and fungal infections can also cause meningitis. **Acute bacterial meningitis is a medical emergency.** Depending upon the cause, some cases will improve in 2 to 3 weeks, or it can become life-threatening. The disease can occur at any age, but those at the highest risk include infants, older adults, and individuals whose immune systems are compromised.

Etiology

Meningitis occurs when the offending agent enters the bloodstream and navigates to the brain and spinal cord or invades the meninges directly as a result of ear or sinus infection or skull fracture. Enteroviruses are the leading cause of the viral form of the disease. These viruses include herpes simplex virus, HIV, mumps, and West Nile virus. This form of meningitis is mild and often clears on its own. Acute bacterial meningitis stems from *Streptococcus pneumoniae* (commonly causes ear and throat infections, especially in children), *Neisseria meningitides* (upper respiratory infections, mostly in teenagers and young adults), *Haemophilus influenzae* type b (mostly seen in children), or *Listeria monocytogenes*

Structure of the Meninges

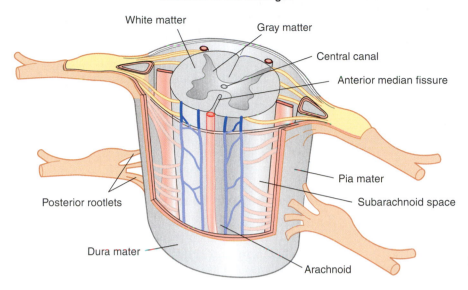

White matter

Gray matter

Central canal

Anterior median fissure

Posterior rootlets

Pia mater

Subarachnoid space

Dura mater

Arachnoid

Figure 10.5 The structure of the meninges.

(a threat to children, older adults, and the immuno-compromised).

Signs and Symptoms

Early signs of the disease are often difficult to distinguish from influenza symptoms. However, within a few hours symptoms likely include severe headache, fever, vomiting, **nuchal rigidity,** initial drowsiness or **stupor,** and seizures. Very young children may have difficulty feeding, show irritability, and have high-pitched crying. A red and purple rash may appear on the trunk and lower extremities in meningococcal meningitis.

Diagnostic Procedures

A thorough medical history and physical examination are essential. Blood, urine, and throat cultures may be useful in isolating the infectious agent. Chest, skull, sinus x-rays, CT scan, and MRI may be ordered. A biopsy of the skin rash may be obtained. The diagnosis is usually established by performing a lumbar puncture to confirm elevated CSF pressure and to analyze the CSF for the presence of bacteria and elevated levels of proteins and leukocytes.

Treatment

If the cause is bacterial, the client is hospitalized, and an aggressive, sustained course of antibiotic therapy begins as soon as possible. Corticosteroids are usually given at the time of the first antibiotic dose to ward off the inflammation that causes swelling in the brain and prevent blockage in the movement of CSF. Isolation may be required. Good nutrition and adequate fluid intake are important to replace fluids lost because of the fever, sweating, and vomiting. If the cause is viral, bed rest, plenty of fluids, and over-the-counter medications to reduce aches and fever is usually all that is necessary. In certain cases, an antiviral medication will be prescribed.

Complementary Therapy

No significant complementary therapy is indicated.

CLIENT COMMUNICATION

In the case of elderly individuals, infants, or children, follow-up care is vital. If older clients have existing medical problems, they are more likely to have complications, whereas infants need to be checked for long-term complications, such as neurological impairment, hearing loss, and paralysis.

Prognosis

Acute bacterial meningitis can prove fatal, especially among infants and older persons. The prognosis is good, however, in the event of prompt treatment and diagnosis accompanied by effective treatment. Meningitis can cause lasting neurological damage in children, particularly hearing loss, decreased mental ability, and epilepsy.

Prevention

The best prevention comes from available vaccinations, but careful handling of excretions and proper hand-washing techniques help prevent the spread of the infection. Vaccines are available for several forms of meningitis. The meningococcal meningitis vaccine is given to adolescents, students living in dormitories, military personnel, and individuals who are repeatedly exposed to bacterial infections. Hib vaccines are available and are a part of the routine childhood immunization schedule in the United States.

Peripheral Nervous System Diseases and Disorders

PERIPHERAL NEUROPATHY

ICD-10: G60.0

Description

Peripheral neuropathy, also called *multiple neuritis, polyneuritis,* and *peripheral neuritis,* is a degeneration of the nerves carrying impulses to and from the brain and spinal cord. One set of peripheral nerves supplies the distal muscles of the extremities; another set relays information from the skin, joints, and other organs. The syndrome causes loss of sensation and pain as well as the inability to control muscles. It is very common.

Etiology

There are several causes of peripheral neuropathy, but in many instances, no cause is determined. Causes include diabetes, deficiencies in vitamin B_{12}, chronic alcohol intoxication, uremia from kidney failure, and cancer. Toxicity from poisons, drugs, or heavy metals such as lead and arsenic is also a known cause. Infections, such as hepatitis, HIV, and rheumatoid arthritis, may induce peripheral neuropathy, as may metabolic disorders such as lupus erythematosus. Peripheral neuropathy may be the result of some chemotherapeutic agents used in treating cancer. Diabetic neuropathy is the most common of all forms.

Signs and Symptoms

The symptoms depend on the nerve(s) affected. The most common locations for pain and loss of sensation are in the extremities. The pain is often described as tingling, prickling, burning, or freezing, with extreme sensitivity to touch. The onset is slow in most cases and may be marked by progressive muscular weakness, loss of dexterity, tenderness, and pain. Physical wasting, loss of reflexes, and clumsiness may result. When the autonomic nerves are affected, a number of symptoms result. They can include blurred vision, dizziness, abdominal bloating, constipation or diarrhea, urinary hesitancy or incontinence, and heat intolerance.

Diagnostic Procedures

A thorough history and physical examination, including a neurological workup, to determine motor and sensory deficits are necessary. Electromyography may be ordered to record the muscles' electrical activity. Blood tests, CT scan and MRI, and nerve conduction tests are helpful. A lumbar puncture may be ordered to determine the cause.

Treatment

The treatment depends on identifying the underlying cause and treating or curing it. Toxins must be neutralized, infections and metabolic diseases treated, and nutritional deficiencies corrected. Analgesics and bed rest, especially of the affected limbs, are essential. Low doses of anticonvulsants or antidepressants may help in controlling the discomfort. A Lidocaine patch applied to the area of greatest pain is often prescribed. Physical therapy, occupational therapy, and orthopedic interventions may be recommended. Elastic support stockings, sleeping with the head elevated, and adjusting positions is useful.

Complementary Therapy

There are a number of therapies to consider that may provide relief. They include biofeedback accompanied by visualization and relaxation, acupuncture, lower stress exercise such as water therapy or tai chi, and the use of a transcutaneous electrical nerve stimulation unit (see Chapter 3). A rich diet in omega-3 fatty acids should be encouraged. Studies have shown that wearing static magnetic shoe soles for a few months does not reduce peripheral neuropathy in the feet.

⊙ CLIENT COMMUNICATION

Depending on the cause of the neuropathy, individuals may have to alter their lifestyle. Exercise in moderation may be recommended. Supportive measures are tried to control the pain or loss of motion.

Prognosis

The prognosis depends on how successfully the underlying cause can be treated and the extent of existing nerve damage. Peripheral neuropathy is problematic for clients, especially when it seems that the problem will be chronic. Loss of function and mobility is difficult. The inability to feel or to notice injuries can lead to infections and further structural damage. When the autonomic nerves are affected, rapid heartbeat, loss of consciousness for even a few minutes, and difficulty breathing or swallowing constitutes an emergency.

Prevention

Prevention includes prompt treatment of nutritional deficiencies, infections, and metabolic diseases. Avoidance of toxins is also essential for prevention. It is important not to smoke.

BELL PALSY

ICD-10: G51.0

Description

Bell palsy is a disruption of the seventh cranial facial nerve's message sent from the brain to facial muscles, causing paralysis of the muscles on one side of the face. It may be transient or permanent and is more common in persons between ages 20 and 60, especially those with diabetes or upper respiratory infections.

Etiology

Bell palsy is mostly idiopathic, although possible causes include viral infections, tumors, vascular ischemia, autoimmune disease, Lyme disease, trauma to the seventh cranial nerve, high blood pressure, diabetes, viral diseases such as viral meningitis, and the common cold sore caused by the herpes simplex virus (HSV-1).

Signs and Symptoms

Signs and symptoms vary greatly from person to person but include facial weakness and the characteristic drooping mouth with drooling saliva. The sense of taste may be disrupted. Pain in the jaw or behind the ear and headache may precede or accompany the paralysis. Another sign is Bell phenomenon, in which the eye cannot close completely. When the person attempts to close the eye, the eyeball rolls upward and the eye may tear excessively.

Diagnostic Procedures

The clinical picture of the sudden, unexplained onset of facial paralysis suggests the diagnosis. Physical and neurological examinations are necessary to check for nerve function. Bell palsy must be differentiated from CVA or an autoimmune disease. An electromyography can determine the severity and extent of the nerve involvement.

Treatment

Antiviral medications and anti-inflammatory drugs may be prescribed if the etiology is found to be viral. The affected portion of the face, particularly the eye, must be protected from trauma, wind, or temperature extremes. Electrical stimulation, warm moist heat, and analgesia may be prescribed. Corticosteroid drugs may be prescribed to reduce edema in some instances.

Complementary Therapy

Facial exercises and massage are recommended to prevent contractures. Relaxation and acupuncture have promising benefits as well.

CLIENT COMMUNICATION

It is important to teach clients to keep the affected eye moist through the use of either artificial tears or an eye patch. Smoking should be avoided.

Prognosis

The prognosis is good in the majority of cases. The palsy usually disappears spontaneously within 1 to 8 weeks, but it can recur. If the palsy remains, facial **contractures,** a permanent shortening of facial muscles, may develop.

Prevention

There is no known prevention for Bell palsy.

Cerebral Diseases and Disorders

CEREBROVASCULAR ACCIDENT (STROKE OR BRAIN ATTACK)

ICD-10: I63.50

Description

Cerebrovascular accident (CVA) is a clinical syndrome marked by the sudden impairment of consciousness and subsequent paralysis. It is caused by occlusion or hemorrhaging of blood vessels supplying a portion of the brain. Deprived of adequate blood supply, the tissue in the affected area becomes necrotic. The condition is commonly known as a *stroke* or *brain attack*. The latter term is more current and used to denote its need for emergency treatment and its neurological deficits, similar to a heart attack in timelines.

There are two types of brain attack: (1) ischemic stroke, in which there is an interruption of the blood flow in a cerebral vessel, such as a thrombosis or emboli (this type accounts for 70% to 80% of brain attacks), and (2) hemorrhagic stroke, when a blood vessel on the brain's surface ruptures and bleeds into just the subarachnoid space or when the blood floods the brain itself. In hemorrhagic stroke, the cause can be hypertension, aneurysm, head injury, arteriovenous malfunction, or blood disease. The fatality rate is higher for hemorrhagic stroke.

Etiology

Contributing factors include a family history of atherosclerotic disease, hypertension, smoking, lack of exercise, a poor or high-fat diet, obesity, the use of oral contraceptives, high cholesterol, and diabetes mellitus. Other risk factors include prior stroke, illicit drug use, and heart disease.

Signs and Symptoms

The National Stroke Association has identified four simple signs of stroke that every person should recognize. If there is any hint that an individual shows signs of a CVA, follow the four guidelines indicated in Figure 10.6. The signs and symptoms of CVA will

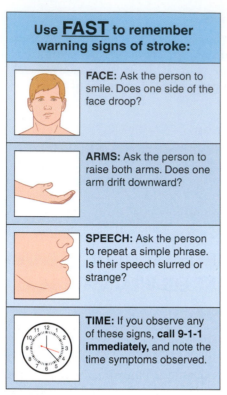

Use FAST to remember warning signs of stroke:

FACE: Ask the person to smile. Does one side of the face droop?

ARMS: Ask the person to raise both arms. Does one arm drift downward?

SPEECH: Ask the person to repeat a simple phrase. Is their speech slurred or strange?

TIME: If you observe any of these signs, **call 9-1-1 immediately,** and note the time symptoms observed.

Figure 10.6 Warning signs of stroke—FAST (**f**ace, **a**rms, **s**peech, **t**ime).

reflect the portion of the brain involved in the attack and whether the attack is caused by a thrombus, an embolus, or a hemorrhage. The symptoms of strokes caused by an embolus or a hemorrhage are often sudden in onset, whereas those caused by a thrombus may appear more gradually. Common symptoms include impaired consciousness, ranging from stupor to coma, full and slow pulse, hemiparesis, and **Cheyne-Stokes respiration.** With this type of respiration, there is a period of apnea lasting 10 to 60 seconds, followed by gradually increasing depth and frequency of respirations. Other symptoms include loss of balance and coordination, speech impairment **(dysphasia)**, numbness, sensory disturbances, double vision **(diplopia)**, poor coordination, confusion, severe headache, and dizziness.

Diagnostic Procedures

A comprehensive history, physical examination, and neurological workup may reveal the diagnosis. Cerebral angiogram, computed tomography angiogram (CTA, MRI, and magnetic resonance angiography (MRA) are useful in diagnosis. Carotid ultrasonography, which is an ultrasound of the neck, may be used. A transcranial Doppler (TCD) test shows the blood flow through the cerebral vessels.

Treatment

Stroke or brain attack is a medical emergency. Treatment of CVA depends on the severity of the event and whether it was hemorrhagic or ischemic in origin. The goal of treatment is to salvage damaged brain tissue and to minimize permanent disability. General treatment protocols may include drug therapy, anticoagulant or antiplatelet agents, and surgery (carotid endarterectomy or cerebral angioplasty) to improve cerebral circulation or to remove clots. Other therapeutic procedures may include measures to guard against or to control brain edema. Physical rehabilitation is necessary for most stroke clients; it needs to be started early and continued until the client can perform as many basic and instrumental activities of daily living as possible.

Complementary Therapy

Treatment and prevention of CVA suggests eating a diet that includes lots of fruit, vegetables, whole grains, and fish. Eliminating foods containing trans fats is recommended. Teach clients the advantages of replacing coffee with a cup of green tea. In addition, encourage daily aerobic exercise, which helps reduce hypertension and enhances elasticity of the brain's arteries.

⊙ CLIENT COMMUNICATION

It is essential to prevent complications and to promote the fullest recovery possible. Focus on improving any motor deficits and language and speech problems. Care for clients is a long-term concern. Support and encouragement from caregivers and family are essential.

Prognosis

The prognosis for an individual experiencing a CVA is determined by the extent of damage to the affected portion of the brain. In general, the greater the delay in recovery following the event, the poorer is the ultimate prognosis. Early diagnosis and treatment are necessary. Some individuals may remain permanently disabled or have a recurrence.

Prevention

Prevention includes prompt treatment of cardiac and circulatory problems. Encourage clients to seek methods to lower hypertension, stop smoking, improve dietary habits, and control weight—all are essential in preventing a CVA.

TRANSIENT ISCHEMIC ATTACKS

ICD-10: G45.9 or I67.848

Description

Transient ischemic attacks (TIAs) are temporary, often recurrent episodes of impaired neurological activity resulting from insufficient blood flow to a part of the brain. These "little strokes" or little brain attacks may last for seconds or hours, after which the symptoms gradually subside. TIAs share a common pathophysiology with brain attacks and may serve as a warning of an impending CVA. Ten percent of individuals who have TIAs suffer a stroke within 3 months.

Etiology

TIAs are caused by the temporary obstruction of cerebral arterioles by very small emboli or by ischemia of a small portion of brain tissue due to arterial narrowing in that region. These processes are usually the result of atherosclerotic disease. (See "Cerebrovascular Accident" for other potential causes and risk factors.)

Signs and Symptoms

The particular combination of symptoms during a TIA, like those for a CVA, depend on which portion of the brain is affected. Symptoms may include the sudden onset of muscle weakness in the arm, leg, or foot on one side of the body. Other symptoms may include diplopia, speech deficits, dizziness, and staggering or uncoordinated gait. TIAs generally do not result in unconsciousness.

Diagnostic Procedures

A full physical and neurological examination is conducted. Carotid ultrasound, cranial CT scans, and cranial MRI are helpful in isolating the area of ischemia within the brain.

Treatment

Prompt treatment is important to prevent a future brain attack. The course of treatment selected depends on locating the area of ischemia and finding the underlying cause. Antiplatelet agents and aspirin or anticoagulant drugs are typically used to treat an ongoing attack and minimize the chance of another. Surgery to promote blood flow to the affected area may be attempted in certain cases.

Complementary Therapy

See "Cerebrovascular Accident."

> ### ⊕ CLIENT COMMUNICATION
>
> It is important to keep clients hydrated. Provide instruction about the desired effects and adverse reactions of medication. Helping clients understand the risk of a more serious brain attack can be helpful.

Prognosis

The prognosis for an individual experiencing a TIA is dependent on the underlying cause. Although the symptoms subside, TIAs tend to be recurrent and may signal an impending CVA.

Prevention

See preventive measures for cerebrovascular accident, which include eliminating risks for a brain attack.

CEREBRAL ANEURYSM

ICD-10: I67.1

Description

A brain or cerebral aneurysm occurs when there is a bulging outward of an artery in the brain. The Brain Aneurysm Foundation reports that there is a brain aneurysm rupturing every 18 minutes in the United States. Cerebral aneurysms are not often discovered until they rupture, causing a subarachnoid hemorrhage in the brain. They are more common in women than in men over the age of 40.

Etiology

When the artery walls become thin and deteriorate, the vessel can balloon. This more likely occurs at branches of the arteries because the walls are thinner and weaker at those junctions. Aneurysms develop over a period of time due to an unknown cause. Risk factors, however, include some congenital diseases and disorders, such as having a close relative with brain aneurysms, smoking, hypertension, high cholesterol, alcohol consumption, and cocaine use.

Signs and Symptoms

Severe headache, dilated pupils, blurred or double vision, neck pain, nausea, sensitivity to light, and loss of sensation are the usual symptoms of a ruptured cerebral aneurysm. Before the rupture occurs, clients may report speech problems, diminished thought processes, loss of balance and coordination, and vision deficits.

Diagnostic Procedures

When the aneurysm ruptures, it will show on a CT scan. A lumbar puncture will reveal blood in the CSF. Cerebral angiography is necessary to identify the exact location and size of the aneurysm. An electroencephalogram (EEG) or an MRI may be ordered as well.

Treatment

A neurosurgeon is usually consulted to determine appropriate treatment, which is most often surgery or a less-invasive technique known as *endovascular coiling.* This procedure is performed through the blood vessel, where a catheter in the femoral artery is navigated toward the aneurysm. Tiny platinum flexible coils threaded through the catheter are directed into the aneurysm where they are used to fill the aneurysm, thus stopping blood flow and preventing rupture. If surgery is used, the blood flow to the aneurysm must first be stopped, and then the aneurysm is snipped off.

A craniotomy must be performed for this surgery to take place.

Complementary Therapy

There is no significant complementary therapy identified.

 CLIENT COMMUNICATION

Carefully explain to clients any procedures to be performed. Recognize their fears upon learning of the diagnosis.

Prognosis

The prognosis is guarded, and much depends on a client's well-being at the time of the diagnosis. If rupture occurs, the goal is to stop the bleeding and prevent complications. Surgical procedures require significant recovery periods. The goal then becomes the prevention of other aneurysms. A cerebral aneurysm is fatal in about 40% of cases, and for those who survive, nearly 66% will have some neurological deficit.

Prevention

Recognition of the risk of aneurysm is helpful. Family history of a ruptured aneurysm is an important consideration in prevention. Encourage clients to stop smoking, reduce stress, control hypertension, limit alcohol intake, and do not use cocaine.

EPILEPSY

ICD-10: G40.XX

Description

Epilepsy is a chronic brain disorder characterized by recurring attacks of abnormal sensory, motor, and psychological activity. During these attacks, the individual may or may not lose consciousness. Each epileptic episode is called a *seizure,* although not all seizures indicate epilepsy. Epileptic seizures exhibit a chronic pattern, with similar characteristics at each recurrence. Epilepsy represents a disruption of the normal pattern of electrical activity within the brain. During an epileptic seizure, neurons within the brain discharge in a random, intense manner. This hyperactivity may be focused within a small section of the brain or may involve several areas of the brain at once. Epilepsy can begin at any time of life.

Seizures generally are categorized as partial or generalized. Partial seizures are focal in origin—that is, they affect only one part of the brain and cause specific symptoms. Generalized seizures are nonfocal in origin and may affect the entire brain.

Etiology

Most cases of epilepsy are idiopathic. Epilepsies may follow birth trauma, congenital malformations of the brain, head trauma, fever, metabolic and nutritional disorders, CVA, CNS infections such as meningitis, or neoplasms. Other causes may include brain tissue damage produced by chemicals, drugs, and toxins or degenerative brain disorders and structural defects of the brain.

Signs and Symptoms

Individuals may experience a warning or "aura" of the impending seizure or no warning at all. Symptoms of the seizure may be a simple uncontrollable twitch of the finger, hand, or mouth. The person may be dizzy and experience unusual or unpleasant sights, sounds, or odors, all without losing consciousness. Some individuals experience sudden loss of consciousness and intense rigidity of the body, with alternating relaxation and contraction of muscles. A characteristic cry may be uttered. Cyanosis, inhibited respiration, incontinence, and chewing of the tongue may occur. After the seizure has passed, amnesia, headache, and drowsiness are common. Some individuals may sleep for hours following a seizure; others may not feel quite like themselves for days.

Diagnostic Procedures

A thorough physical examination and medical history, focusing on the person's developmental history and any head trauma or illness, are essential, followed by a neurological examination. Recurrent seizures or a family history of epilepsy should help to suggest the diagnosis. Epilepsy is also indicated in the presence of seizures following head trauma, CNS infections, or CVA. Because many individuals with epilepsy exhibit abnormalities in brain-wave patterns, even between seizures, electroencephalograms are very helpful in diagnosis. Cranial CT scans also are useful in pinpointing brain lesions that may be triggering seizures. MRI provides clear images of the brain, shows structural changes resulting from disorders, and helps to diagnose epilepsy.

Treatment

An array of anticonvulsant drugs exists that have proved effective in controlling epileptic seizures. Because certain drugs are more effective in controlling specific forms of seizures, the client and the PCP may have to engage in a process of trial and error before settling on one drug that best controls the individual's seizures with the fewest side effects. Neurosurgery may be attempted in some cases when a severe case of epilepsy can be traced to the presence of a specific, accessible brain lesion. Education about the nature of the disease and counseling the person with epilepsy are essential parts of the treatment process.

Complementary Therapy

Teach clients to avoid common triggers for epilepsy, such as poor sleep patterns, heavy use of alcohol, skipping meals, and inadequate diet. Encourage them to get plenty of rest and reduce stress with yoga, acupuncture, and aromatherapy. Suggest biofeedback. Stress how important it is to take prescribed medications regularly.

 CLIENT COMMUNICATION

> The incidence of new-onset epilepsy is high among older individuals. Hence, it is important to know what medications they are taking for other diseases, because drug interactions can be dangerous. Also, the complete removal of certain medications may precipitate a seizure in some. Older clients may absorb, metabolize, and excrete medications differently, so they must be closely monitored. Teach clients how to create a safe environment and to understand what might trigger a seizure.

Prognosis

The prognosis varies from case to case. The prognosis is good if a drug therapy can be found that effectively suppresses the seizures. An individual in these circumstances can generally expect to live a normal life. The prognosis is not so favorable if seizures cannot be controlled. Such individuals may have restrictions on their independence. Some states refuse drivers' licenses to people with epilepsy.

Prevention

Only certain forms of epilepsy are preventable. Preventive measures involve avoiding head injuries, seeking prompt treatment of brain infections, and avoiding the abuse of drugs and alcohol.

Degenerative Neural Diseases and Disorders

 ## ALZHEIMER DISEASE

ICD-10: G30.9

Description

Alzheimer disease, the most common form of dementia, is a type of progressive, chronic, ultimately fatal, organic brain syndrome characterized by the death of neurons in the cerebral cortex. The result is neurofibrillary tangles, a tangled mass of nonfunctioning neurons, and their replacement by microscopic senile or neurotic "plaques." Biochemically, acetylcholine production, used for memory processing, is reduced, resulting in progressive memory impairment followed by gradual deterioration of judgment, reasoning ability, verbal fluency, and other cognitive skills. This impairment and deterioration is accompanied by disturbances in behavior and affect. The disease affects mainly older persons, with one in eight having Alzheimer disease after age 65. In a few families with a genetic predisposition for the disease, symptoms occur as early as age 30 or 40.

Facts About Alzheimer Disease

Alzheimer disease is named for the German physician who first described the disorder in 1906. Today, it is the sixth leading cause of death in the United States. Close to 5.2 million Americans have Alzheimer disease, the majority who are 65 and older. Costs of care for persons with Alzheimer disease and other forms of dementia is projected to be $1.2 trillion per year by 2050.*

Etiology

The cause of Alzheimer disease is unknown, but hereditary factors, autoimmune reactions, and cellular changes of viral origin have all been proposed. Risk factors include a family history of Alzheimer disease, advancing age, and history of head trauma.

Signs and Symptoms

In the early stages, the person with Alzheimer disease has small difficulties at work or in social settings with memory loss but generally can hide the loss and function independently. Depression may occur. As the disease progresses, the person exhibits mild mental impairment. This impairment includes loss of short-term memory, inability to learn new tasks, and subtle changes in personality. Then increased forgetfulness, agitation, irritability, and extreme restlessness occur. The person may retell the same stories, and others can no longer reason with him or her, which may further increase the person's anxiety. Conversations become difficult. Eventually, the individual is unable to perform self-care, becomes incontinent, and is unable to communicate. The person becomes emotionally detached and may show sleep disturbances, restlessness, and hostility. In the terminal stage, the person usually requires total care. The rate at which an individual progresses through the disease varies; within 5 to 10 years, there is profound deterioration of intellectual and physical ability.

Diagnostic Procedures

The goal of diagnosis is to rule out other degenerative brain diseases that produce similar symptoms. A comprehensive history and physical examination that

*From 2013 Alzheimer's Disease Facts and Figures http://www.alz.org/downloads/facts_figures_2013.pdf

The 10 Warning Signs of Alzheimer Disease

1. Memory changes that disrupt daily living
2. Difficulty in planning or solving problems
3. Problems completing familiar tasks at home, at work, or in leisure
4. Confusion with time and place
5. Trouble understanding visual images and spatial relationships
6. Difficulty with words in speaking or in writing
7. Misplacing items, losing ability to retrace steps
8. Decreased or poor judgment
9. Withdrawal from work or social activities
10. Changes in mood or personality

includes mental and functional health status examinations are essential. A cranial CT and MRI are performed. A positron emission tomography (PET) scan is sometimes used and appears to be quite accurate in identifying the tangles and plaques in the brain. A depression scale and cognitive functioning test should be administered. Laboratory testing of urine and blood may help in the diagnosis, although they do not confirm it.

Treatment

There is no cure; however, there are two types of medication used to treat the cognitive symptoms of Alzheimer disease: (1) cholinesterase inhibitors, which prevent the breakdown of acetylcholine and support communication between neurons, and (2) memantine, which works by regulating the activity of glutamate, one of the chemical messengers involved in learning and memory. Both drugs may delay worsening of symptoms for a period of time. Some medications may lessen behavioral changes, but they also have side effects. It may be more helpful to seek nondrug approaches when treating this disease. Another focus of treatment is to maintain client safety, reduce anxiety and agitation, promote independence, improve communication, and provide socialization for as long as possible. Treatment is merely palliative and directed toward maintaining nutrition, hydration, and safety. Emotional support and education of family members are important.

Complementary Therapy

There is some indication that a quiet environment, with soft lights and soft music, may benefit some clients. Also, aromatherapy has shown possibilities. Persons with Alzheimer disease seem to respond favorably to the smell of baking bread or brewing coffee, which can help to calm them. Integrative medical practitioners recommend daily exercise and a diet low in fat and high

in omega 3-rich foods as preventive measures. Vitamin E and ginkgo biloba have not shown to be of any help.

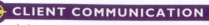

CLIENT COMMUNICATION

Adequate nutrition and hydration are important, as are sleep and exercise. More frequent meals with liquids may provide the necessary nourishment. If sleep is elusive, warm milk and back rubs may help. Physical clues become especially important when clients lose their ability to speak. The families are equally important in the treatment of Alzheimer disease because they will need support and education. Referrals to local support systems and advocacy groups are beneficial. Respite care is available to caregivers. Being sensitive to the emotional needs of the family, caregivers, and clients is paramount.

Prognosis

The prognosis is poor, with the disease progressing over a period of 5 to 10 years. Death may occur from secondary causes, such as pneumonia, malnutrition, dehydration, or infection.

Prevention

There is no known prevention for the disease. Research currently points increasingly to a genetic marker abnormality, which if identified and corrected may prevent Alzheimer disease. Those at risk should undertake activities that require focus and concentration. They can plan and carry out projects to keep their mental state alert.

PARKINSON DISEASE

ICD-10: G20

Description

Parkinson disease is a chronic brain disease characterized by progressive muscle rigidity and involuntary tremors (Fig. 10.7). Parkinson is a common crippling disease in the United States, affecting more men than women, usually over age 50.

Etiology

The cause is unknown, but the condition is related to a loss of brain cells that make the neurotransmitter chemical dopamine. Dopamine is necessary for brain cell functioning. Other suggested causes include genetic mutations or environmental toxins.

Signs and Symptoms

The onset of Parkinson disease is slow and insidious. Symptoms eventually may include **bradykinesia,** or abnormally slow movements; progressively rigid extremities; and "pill-rolling" tremors beginning in the

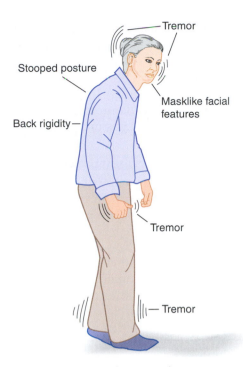

Tremor

Stooped posture

Masklike facial features

Back rigidity

Tremor

Tremor

Figure 10.7 Woman with Parkinson disease.

fingers. There often is difficulty with balance, a shuffling walk, and muffled speech. The individual's facial expression may appear fixed. Stress, fatigue, and anxiety tend to aggravate the tremors, whereas purposeful movement and sleep decrease the tremors. Symptoms of parkinsonism (but not the disease itself) can be attributed to other diseases or difficulties, such as increase of fluid on the brain, other neurological disorders, certain medications, and environmental toxins. In these cases, when the underlying cause is removed or stops, the parkinsonian symptoms also subside.

Diagnostic Procedures

Diagnosis is made on the basis of the unique set of physical symptoms and a neurological examination characteristic of Parkinson disease. The tremors, bradykinesia, and rigidity must be differentiated from the symptoms of other diseases. Blood tests and MRI can rule out other conditions with similar symptoms.

Treatment

The disease progression cannot be controlled; therefore, the goals are to control the symptoms and to promote independence. Levodopa, a dopamine replacement, is the most effective treatment. Because of levodopa's side effects, other drugs are sometimes given at the same time. Some drugs that mimic the effects of dopamine in the brain are useful. Drugs that help prevent the breakdown of levodopa are often given. **Anticholinergics** can help control the tremors, and some antivirals may be given in the early stages of the disease to provide some relief. Physical therapy and psychological support

and reassurance are also necessary. If drug therapy is unsuccessful, certain surgical techniques may be attempted. Deep brain stimulation is the surgery most often used. A thin wire lead with four electrodes at its tip is implanted in the affected area of the brain; the lead runs under the skin to a pulse generator, which is placed underneath the chest skin, close to the clavicle. The battery-operated pulse generator emits electrical pulses to interfere with neural activity. It can be calibrated by the neurologist or other trained professional and can also be turned off (e.g., for sleeping) and on by the client.

Complementary Therapy

A diet with lots of fruits, vegetables, and whole grains is beneficial. Massage therapy can reduce muscle tension, increase strength, and promote relaxation. Tai chi, especially in classes designed specifically for individuals with Parkinson disease, can help in balance and improve flexibility.

➔ CLIENT COMMUNICATION

Teach clients to walk carefully, to not move too quickly, and to take steps to prevent falls. Helping individuals maintain their center of gravity right over their feet is helpful. Clothing that is easy to fasten (e.g., with elastic waistbands and without buttons, zippers, and belts) will be less frustrating for clients as the disease progresses. Support systems prove helpful for some clients and their families.

Prognosis

Although the disease is slowly progressive and debilitating, because of effective treatment strategies, many individuals with Parkinson disease can live comparatively normal lives for many years. Complications can include sleep difficulties, urinary incontinence or retention, constipation, depression, and sexual dysfunction. Clients are at risk for respiratory and urinary infection, skin breakdown, and injury due to falls. Parkinson disease is not usually a direct cause of death; rather, complications from the disease are more likely the cause.

Prevention

There is no known prevention for Parkinson disease.

MULTIPLE SCLEROSIS

ICD10: G35

Description

Multiple sclerosis (MS) is a chronic, progressive, and irreversible autoimmune disease characterized by the destruction of the myelin sheath—the lipid and protein layer that insulates and protects the axons of certain nerve cells. The demyelination process occurs at scattered sites throughout the CNS and results in progressive physical disability. The onset of MS usually occurs during early adulthood and rarely after age 60. It occurs twice as often in women than in men. The disease is a common cause of chronic disability.

Etiology

The cause of MS is believed to be immunologic; the body's immune system attacks its own tissues. The reasons are not fully understood, but genetics have been proposed. Recent research reveals that the incidence of MS is higher farther from the equator. This causes some to believe that vitamin D plays a role, because closer to the equator, individuals receive much higher doses of vitamin D than those who live farther away. It is believed that naturally produced vitamin D supports the immune function and protects against immune-related diseases like MS.

Signs and Symptoms

Symptoms vary widely among individuals because of the scattered sites of demyelination throughout the CNS. A change in vision may be the first symptom. Others may include sudden and transient motor and sensory disturbances, muscle weakness, paralysis, incontinence, fatigue, balance problems, numbness, and mood swings. The initial onset of symptoms, and later relapses, may occur following acute infection, trauma, serum injections, pregnancy, or stress. The symptoms usually come and go with no pattern or warning but are often triggered by a rise in body temperature. They may last hours or weeks. Most individuals have an episodic pattern of attacks and remissions throughout the disease.

Diagnostic Procedures

There is no one definitive test for MS; the diagnostic process includes ruling out other possibilities. A neurological examination, eye examination by an ophthalmologist, CSF analysis, cranial CT scans, and MRI may be useful in diagnosing MS. The disease is difficult to diagnose, however, because the onset may be mild and symptoms may take years to progress. Periodic testing and observation are usually necessary.

Treatment

Early treatment is essential and is directed at relieving symptoms and forestalling future attacks. There is no cure. Medications include interferon-beta products, which can reduce the number of exacerbations of the disease and slow the progression of physical disability. In some cases, corticosteroids can be used for acute attacks. Symptomatic treatment and medical, rehabilitative, and psychological approaches are also needed.

Complementary Therapy

Complementary therapy embraces the use of pharmaceuticals to reduce the number of MS attacks. It is also suggested that aquatic or water therapy, physical therapy, and yoga may be helpful. A healthy diet, adequate rest and relaxation, and meditation to reduce stress can boost an immune system that is under attack.

⊙ CLIENT COMMUNICATION

Although diet cannot suppress or cause exacerbation, a well-balanced diet can help prevent complications, such as bladder and bowel disorders. Medication must be carefully monitored, because some may become less effective after 5 to 10 years. Sometimes medication may be discontinued for a time and then restarted. Exercise is important, as is the prevention of any injury. Sexual problems are common and require attention as well. An experienced sexual counselor may prove helpful to clients and their partners.

Prognosis

Because the course of the disease is varied, the prognosis varies, too. Individuals with MS experience remissions and exacerbations of symptoms and generally have a life expectancy of 50 years after onset. Secondary complications include bowel and bladder problems, pressure ulcers, contracture deformities, pneumonia, and depression.

Prevention

There is no known prevention for MS.

AMYOTROPHIC LATERAL SCLEROSIS

ICD-10: G12.21

Description

Amyotrophic lateral sclerosis (ALS), commonly known as *Lou Gehrig disease*, is a disease of motor neurons that results in progressive muscular atrophy and weakness. The neurodegeneration affects the nerve cells in the brain and spinal cord, resulting in the death of nerve cells. Lou Gehrig was a famous baseball player who died of the disease in 1941. The disease generally occurs between ages 50 and 60 and slightly more often in men than in women.

Etiology

The cause is unknown, although some cases may be due to autosomal inherited traits.

Signs and Symptoms

Symptoms of ALS include involuntary muscle contractions and muscular atrophy, weakness, and twitching, especially in the muscles of the extremities. The individual may have problems with speech, chewing, swallowing, and even breathing if the brain stem is affected. There is no sensory nerve involvement. With all voluntary muscle action affected, the person in the later stages of the disease becomes totally paralyzed.

Diagnostic Procedures

The disease is difficult to diagnose and usually is diagnosed on the basis of the presenting signs and symptoms. Electromyography, a nerve conduction test, and muscle biopsy will help ascertain whether there is nerve rather than muscle disease. An MRI may be useful. It is necessary to rule out several other disorders that may produce similar symptoms, such as MS, spinal cord neoplasm, and myasthenia gravis.

Treatment

There is no effective treatment for ALS. Treatment is symptomatic and may include emotional and physical support. Persons afflicted with the disease are likely to become confined to a wheelchair or a bed, need to be taught to suction themselves to prevent choking, require assistance with personal hygiene, and need a great deal of emotional support. The antiglutamate drug riluzole (Rilutek) is the only medication approved by the FDA that appears to slow the progression of the disease and prolong the life of persons with ALS for at least a few months. Other drugs are undergoing clinical trials.

Complementary Therapy

A combination of the following therapies can be beneficial: physical therapy to maintain muscle strength as long as possible; occupational therapy to assist in the use of braces and walkers and to make the activities of daily living easier; and speech therapy to ease the difficulty in communicating as the disease progresses.

⊖ CLIENT COMMUNICATION

Symptomatic treatment is given mostly to support the person and improve quality of life. Drugs for muscle cramps, constipation, depression, and fatigue may be prescribed. Mechanical ventilation and artificial feeding may be required for the client, and caregivers will need information and training on proper use and care.

Prognosis

The prognosis is dependent on the speed at which the disease progresses. ALS is usually fatal 3 to 10 years after onset. Death most often results from respiratory failure or aspiration pneumonia. Research is ongoing, and there is hope that stem cell research may open doors to ALS treatment.

Prevention

There is no known prevention of ALS.

Chronic Neurological Diseases and Disorders

NARCOLEPSY

ICD-10: G47.419

Description

Narcolepsy causes individuals to want to sleep during the day; they often are overwhelmed by the need to sleep, even for just a few seconds. They may fall asleep while in a conversation, while working, even while driving. It is most common between ages 40 and 50 and may decline after age 60.

Etiology

The cause is essentially unknown. However, a number of factors may contribute to the neurological dysfunction that occurs when the brain in unable to regulate sleep-wake cycles. Scientists have discovered that people with narcolepsy lack a chemical in the brain called hypocretin (orexin), which activates arousal and regulates sleep. Heredity may also play a role.

Signs and Symptoms

Excessive daytime sleepiness and abnormal rapid eye movement (REM) sleep are the classic symptoms. There are three additional symptoms that may accompany narcolepsy: (1) cataplexy, or the sudden loss of voluntary muscle tone; (2) hallucinations during sleep or upon awakening; and (3) brief but total paralysis at the start or the end of sleep. Other symptoms may be nighttime wakefulness, rapid entry into REM sleep, and microsleep. Microsleep is a period of very brief sleep when individuals continue to function but have no recollection of their actions.

Diagnostic Procedures

Narcolepsy is often misdiagnosed or undiagnosed. Diagnosis of narcolepsy can take a long time. Sleep specialists may have clients complete a general sleep questionnaire called the Epworth Sleepiness Scale. A sleep study or nocturnal polysomnography may be conducted showing electrical activity of the brain and heart as well as muscle and eye movements. A multiple sleep latency test (MSLT) can measure how long it takes to fall asleep during the day. More recently, examining spinal fluid to determine if hypocretin is absent is being used for diagnosis.

Treatment

There is no cure for narcolepsy, so the goal is to control the symptoms. Some medications may be useful. They include antidepressants and stimulants, but their use varies according to individual needs.

Complementary Therapy

Integrative practitioners agree on a number of steps that include:

- Avoiding caffeine, alcohol, and nicotine
- Scheduling sleep periods and naps
- Telling friends, family, and coworkers of your diagnosis
- Avoiding activities that would be dangerous in a sudden sleep episode
- Avoiding large or heavy meals at bedtime

⊕ CLIENT COMMUNICATION

Encourage clients to wear an alert bracelet. A support group may be recommended for some individuals.

Prognosis

There is no cure for narcolepsy. It is a lifelong condition, and narcolepsy can be frustrating for all involved. With patience, proper medications, and some lifestyle changes, however, it can be managed.

Prevention

There is no known prevention for narcolepsy.

RESTLESS LEG SYNDROME

ICD-10: G25.81

Description

Restless leg syndrome (RLS) is a neurological disorder in which sensations in the leg create an uncontrollable urge to move the leg when at rest. Trying to relax the leg only makes it worse. The only relief is to get up and move around. This action creates poor sleep patterns and exhaustion during the next day. It is believed that as many as 12 million individuals in the United States have RLS and many more are undiagnosed.

Etiology

The cause is essentially unknown; however, risk factors include heredity, pregnancy, stress, and related disorders. Peripheral neuropathy and/or an iron deficiency, diabetes, and Parkinson disease can cause or worsen RLS.

Signs and Symptoms

Individuals describe a restless or unpleasant sensation in their legs. The terms *creeping, tingling, burning,* and *crawling* are often used to describe the feeling. RLS begins when an individual is inactive, is relieved by moving, and worsens at night.

Diagnostic Procedures

RLS, much like narcolepsy, is often undiagnosed. A physical examination and medical history review are conducted. A diagnosis involves ruling out any other disorders that might cause the syndrome. A sleep study or nocturnal polysomnography may be conducted showing electrical activity of the muscle movements. Blood tests can rule out iron and vitamin deficiency.

Treatment

Treating any underlying cause can relieve symptoms. Otherwise, controlling RLS is the goal. Taking an OTC pain reliever may help. Warm baths, relaxation techniques, and yoga are beneficial for some. A regular exercise regimen is recommended. Some medications may be prescribed, including muscle relaxants, sleep medications, and medications for parkinsonian symptoms.

Complementary Therapy

Integrative practitioners agree on a number of steps, including:

- Avoiding caffeine, alcohol, and nicotine
- Sharing the diagnosis with friends and family
- Not suppressing the urge to move, get out of bed, or stop when traveling
- Keeping a sleep diary
- Reducing stress and anxiety

⊕ CLIENT COMMUNICATION

Listening to clients is helpful. Many do not seek treatment because they believe their complaint is insignificant or foolish. Assure them this is not the case.

Prognosis

Older adults experience symptoms more frequently than others. RLS is a lifelong condition with no cure. Symptoms may decrease for a time but later return. About 80% of individuals with RLS also have a condition known as *periodic limb movement disorder*. This disorder occurs during sleep and causes leg twitching or jerking movements every 10 to 60 seconds, often disrupting sleep patterns.

Prevention

There is no known prevention for RLS.

Cancer

TUMORS OF THE BRAIN

ICD-10: C71.9 (PRIMARY)

Description

Primary brain tumors are benign or malignant neoplasms originating within the brain. In children, most brain tumors are primary tumors. Secondary brain tumors are the result of metastasis of neoplasms from elsewhere in the body and account for the majority of cases. In adults, most tumors in the brain have spread there from the lung, breast, or other parts of the body. The condition is not a brain tumor; rather the tumor is named for the organ or tissue in which it began. Tumors in the brain cause neurological deterioration by replacing healthy brain tissue, by compressing brain tissue, or by blocking the blood supply or the flow of CSF to a portion of the brain. Benign tumors of the brain can be life-threatening because of their location; however, most benign tumors can be removed and seldom grow back. Malignant tumors are more serious and often are life-threatening. They generally grow rapidly.

Etiology

The cause is unknown. Risk factors include a family history of brain tumor and exposure to radiation, especially nuclear; formaldehyde; vinyl chloride; or acrylonitrile (textile and plastics). Most tumors occur after age 70 and are more common in white males; however, brain tumors are the second most common cancer in children.

Signs and Symptoms

Brain tumors may be difficult to diagnose because of vague symptoms and their slow onset. The location of the growth in the brain partially dictates the symptoms. Headache, vomiting, defective memory, mood changes, seizures, visual disturbances, motor impairment, and personality changes may occur.

Diagnostic Procedures

A complete history and physical examination, including neurological assessment, are essential. Skull x-rays, lumbar puncture for CSF, cranial CT scans and MRI, or biopsy of the lesion will confirm the diagnosis. Further studies may be done to locate the primary site of a metastatic brain tumor.

Treatment

Treatment is dependent on the stage and type of brain tumor. Surgery, radiation therapy, or chemotherapy—individually or in combination—may be used to treat the tumor. Medications may be ordered for symptomatic treatment of seizures, edema, and headache.

Complementary Therapy

Speech, occupational, and physical therapy may be indicated. Some complementary therapies that make conventional treatment easier include acupuncture to decrease pain and nausea, and visualization, meditation, and prayer to decrease anxiety.

↪ CLIENT COMMUNICATION

Because the shock of hearing the diagnosis remains with clients for some time, it is important to include family members when treatment options are being determined. It is important for some clients and their families to be referred to support systems. The Cancer Information Service (National Cancer Institute) is a nationwide telephone service for cancer patients, their families and friends, and health-care professionals. The staff can answer questions in English and Spanish and can send booklets about cancer. The toll-free number, 1-800-4-CANCER (1-800-422-6237), connects callers with the office that serves their area.

Prognosis

The prognosis is dependent on the size, location, and type of tumor.

Prevention

There is no known prevention for brain tumors.

CHAPTER EPISODE—PART III

The nontraditional therapy seemed to be helping. Breyona still maintained her primary care provider, who was astonished at the progress she was making. It wasn't long before she was able to quit taking some of the medications. She is beginning to have some sensations in her feet and can do modified situps from her wheelchair. The new therapy has helped to regulate her temperature better—a common problem in spinal cord injuries. Breyona was determined to be as independent as possible. When she saw an ad in the newspaper that her local high school (where she had played volleyball) was looking for a part-time volleyball coach, she applied. She got the job. To date, she is doing well with the position and her players. They admire her ability to not let the tragedies of life get her down. While Breyona misses the play of volleyball, she is able to move herself around the gym floor in her wheelchair and coach the players quite well.

- Would you classify Breyona's medical care as alternative, complementary, or integrative? (See Chapter 2.)
- What does Breyona's story say for others who might have similar circumstances?

COMMON SYMPTOMS OF NERVOUS SYSTEM DISEASES AND DISORDERS

Individuals may present with the following common symptoms, which deserve attention from health-care professionals:

- Headache
- Weakness
- Nausea and vomiting
- Motor disturbances, such as stiff neck or back, rigid muscles, seizures, convulsions, or paralysis
- Sensory disturbances of any kind, especially vision or speech
- Drowsiness, stupor, unconsciousness, or coma
- Mood swings
- Fever
- Pain

SUMMARY

The nervous system provides a major control center for the body. Its complexity and sophistication are sometimes baffling to health-care providers. New discoveries are made almost daily that provide important information related to diseases and disorders of the nervous system. These new discoveries offer hope to those who suffer from the devastation of any dysfunction in the nervous system.

 DavisPlus | For more resources and to sharpen your skills with interactive exercises, visit Davis*Plus* at http://davisplus.fadavis.com. Keyword *Tamparo*.

ONLINE RESOURCES

ALS Association
http://www.alsa.org

Alzheimer's Association
http://www.alz.org/index.asp

American Brain Tumor Association
http://www.abta.org

Cerebral aneurysm
http://www.brainaneurysm.com

Epilepsy Foundation
http://www.epilepsyfoundation.org

Hemiplegia
http://www.nlm.nih.gov/medlineplus/paralysis.html

Meningitis
http://www.cdc.gov/meningitis/about/faq.html

Neuropathy Association
http://www.neuropathy.org

Paralysis
http://www.nlm.nih.gov/medlineplus/paralysis.html

Transient ischemic attack
http://www.americanheart.org/presenter.jhtml?identifier=4781

Traumatic brain injury
http://www.dvbic.org

http://www.aans.org/Patient%20Information.aspx

CASE STUDIES

Case Study 1

Will calls the clinic of his PCP about his 45-year-old wife, Rene, to make an appointment. Rene is exhibiting progressive muscular atrophy and weakness in all her extremities. She has difficulty talking, chewing, and swallowing.

Case Study Questions

1. What diagnostic procedures might the primary care provider order?
2. What disease or disorder might be causing such symptoms?
3. What support services might Rene and Will need?

Case Study 2

The first sign family members had that something was not quite right was Julie getting lost while driving to church. Although she was fairly new to the community, she had been to the church many times. She never did find the church that Sunday morning, but she eventually found her way home. Julie's speech and her writing became very disconnected and disjointed. Her husband, Phil, was taking over more and more of the household activities. After an extensive history and physical examination that included a CT scan, a mental health assessment was performed. The diagnosis was Alzheimer disease.

Case Study Questions

1. What steps must Julie and her husband take at this point?
2. Describe any treatment for this disorder.
3. Julie has a sister who also has Alzheimer disease. Does this have any significance for Julie's only child, a daughter? Explain your response.

Case Study 3

Jed was just 18 when the terrible crash happened. While Jed was returning home from work one evening, a driver in a sports utility vehicle sped through a red light and smashed into the driver's side of Jed's car. He was unconscious when he arrived at the hospital. Swelling in the brain required removal of skull bone on both sides of his head. The family members, including grandparents who drove from another state, were determined to not leave Jed alone at the hospital. They talked with all the caregivers to decide what would be beneficial for Jed in his recovery. His friends took turns spending time with him. Friends came to tell him about his favorite baseball team. Individuals sang to him, read to him, recalled funny stories that included him, and kept Jed up on all their activities. Jed's 19th birthday was celebrated in a rehabilitation center. He was to be released to his home and in the care of his parents nearly 11 months later—still not fully conscious but responding to stimuli and eating and swallowing when fed.

Case Study Questions

1. Discuss the possible consequences of such an accident when and if Jed becomes fully conscious.
2. What kind of resources might be provided for family members?

REVIEW QUESTIONS

Matching

Match each of the following definitions with its correct term.

_____ 1. Sensory loss in lower extremities

_____ 2. Little brain attack

_____ 3. Sensory loss in all extremities

_____ 4. Unilateral sensory loss

_____ 5. Classic symptom for narcolepsy

a. Quadriplegia

b. Paraplegia

c. Hemiplegia

d. Transient ischemic attack

e. Acute bacterial meningitis

f. Excessive daytime sleepiness

Short Answer

1. List at least four common signs and symptoms of CNS infections:

   a. _____

   b. _____

   c. _____

   d. _____

2. Name and define the two classifications of seizures:

   a. _____

   b. _____

3. Recall complementary therapies for acute and chronic headache.

   _____

   _____

4. Compare and contrast cerebral concussion and cerebral contusion.

   _____

   _____

Multiple Choice

Place a checkmark next to the correct answer.

1. What is known about abusive head trauma?

   _____ a. It occurs most frequently after age 3.

   _____ b. It is not easily diagnosed.

   _____ c. It was renamed by the American Association of Physicians in 2009.

   _____ d. It is not considered a medical emergency.

2. What are contributing factors for cerebrovascular accident?

   _____ a. Smoking and high-fat diet

   _____ b. Hypotension

   _____ c. Viral infection

   _____ d. Stress and anxiety

3. What are possible risk factors for Alzheimer disease?

   _____ a. Down syndrome

   _____ b. High cholesterol and alcohol consumption

   _____ c. Autoimmune reactions and cellular changes of viral origin

   _____ d. Deficiency of brain cells that make dopamine

   _____ e. Autosomal inherited traits

4. What is known about Parkinson disease?

   _____ a. It is an acute progressive disease causing muscle rigidity.

   _____ b. It affects more men than women, usually after age 65.

   _____ c. It has an insidious and slow onset.

   _____ d. It is curable with appropriate drug therapy.

5. How might you describe multiple sclerosis?

   _____ a. It is a chronic, autoimmune, progressive, and irreversible disease.

   _____ b. It is the result of genetic mutations or environmental toxins.

   _____ c. It is commonly known as Lou Gehrig disease.

   _____ d. It does not respond to most treatment plans.

Discussion Questions/Personal Reflection

1. It has been said that Alzheimer disease is harder on the family members than on the person who has the disease. Discuss why or how this might be true. Talk with someone who has lived with a person who has Alzheimer disease. How can one remain connected to a person with Alzheimer disease?

_____

_____

_____

_____

_____

_____

_____

_____

_____

_____

_____

2. Identify training or education that might be helpful to stressed parents and caregivers to help prevent such tragedies as abusive head trauma.

_____

_____

_____

_____

_____

_____

_____

_____

_____

_____

_____

_____

_____

To keep a lamp burning, we have to keep putting oil in it.
—MOTHER TERESA

11

Endocrine System Diseases and Disorders

● *chapter outline*

ENDOCRINE SYSTEM ANATOMY AND PHYSIOLOGY REVIEW

PITUITARY GLAND DISEASES AND DISORDERS

Hyperpituitarism (Gigantism, Acromegaly)

Hypopituitarism

Diabetes Insipidus

THYROID GLAND DISEASES AND DISORDERS: HYPERTHYROIDISM

Simple Goiter

Graves Disease

THYROID GLAND DISEASES AND DISORDERS: HYPOTHYROIDISM

Hashimoto Thyroiditis (Chronic Thyroiditis)

Hypothyroidism (Cretinism, Myxedema)

Thyroid Cancer

PARATHYROID GLAND DISEASES AND DISORDERS

Hyperparathyroidism (Hypercalcemia)

Hypoparathyroidism (Hypocalcemia)

ADRENAL GLAND DISEASES AND DISORDERS

Cushing Syndrome

Addison Disease

PANCREAS AND THE ISLETS OF LANGERHANS DISEASES AND DISORDERS

Diabetes Mellitus

GONADAL DISEASES AND DISORDERS

Polycystic Ovary Syndrome

COMMON SYMPTOMS OF ENDOCRINE SYSTEM DISEASES AND DISORDERS

SUMMARY

ONLINE RESOURCES

CASE STUDIES

REVIEW QUESTIONS

● *key words*

Adenoma (ăd″ĕ•nō′mă)
Alopecia (al″ō•pē′shē•ă)
Exophthalmos (ĕks″ŏf•thăl′mōs)
Glycogen (glī′kŏ•jĕn)
Glycosuria (glī″kō•sū′rē•ă)
Goitrogens (goy′trō•jĕns)
Hemoglobin (hĕm″ō•glō′bĭn)
Hirsutism (hŭr′sūt•ĭzm)
Hyperglycemia (hī″pĕr•glī•sē′mē•ă)

(key words continued)

● learning outcomes

Upon successful completion of this chapter, you will be able to:

- Define key words.
- Recall endocrine system anatomy and physiology.
- Compare/contrast the endocrine and nervous systems.
- Recall where the nervous system and the endocrine system meet to communicate.
- Discuss the importance of the body's master gland—the pituitary.
- Describe the two forms of hyperpituitarism.
- Discuss the etiology and signs and symptoms of hypopituitarism.
- Describe diabetes insipidus and its classic symptoms.
- Recall the cause and diagnosis of simple goiter.
- Describe the possible complications of Graves disease.
- Explain the description and treatment for Hashimoto thyroiditis.
- Recognize the signs and symptoms of hypothyroidism.

- Compare cretinism with myxedema.
- Identify the treatment and prognosis criteria for thyroid cancer.
- Relate hypercalcemia to hyperparathyroidism and its signs and symptoms.
- Relate hypocalcemia to hypoparathyroidism.
- Review the classic symptoms of Cushing syndrome.
- Describe an Addisonian crisis.
- Recall the etiology and signs and symptoms of diabetes mellitus.
- Compare and contrast type 1 and type 2 diabetes mellitus.
- Describe the complications of diabetes mellitus.
- Recall the treatment of polycystic ovary syndrome.
- List common symptoms of endocrine diseases and disorders.

CHAPTER EPISODE—PART I

Susan is 17 years old and is ready to leave home for college in a neighboring state. She is spending a couple of days with her grandmother at the family beach house before she goes. Susan's mom told her grandmother that Susan will probably want to talk a little about PCOS, since she has just been diagnosed and knows her grandmother suffered from PCOS all her life.

- What is PCOS?
- Does the disease have a genetic connection?

ENDOCRINE SYSTEM ANATOMY AND PHYSIOLOGY REVIEW

In cooperation with the nervous system, the endocrine system regulates and integrates the body's metabolic activities. While the nervous system is the rapid response to stimuli, the endocrine system is the slower response. They do, however, complement each other to maintain the body's homeostasis.

The endocrine system consists of a group of ductless glands that act to regulate many of the body's physiological processes. Each type of endocrine gland produces one or more secretions that are discharged into the blood or lymph and circulated to target organs upon which they act. These secretions are called *hormones*, which are chemical substances that produce a specific effect on a particular type of tissue, organ, or the body as a whole. Many hormones work as antagonists to one another, having opposite effects on target organs. Hormonal regulation also relies on feedback from target organs or tissues to maintain balance and homeostasis. Hormones are classified by their structure as follows:

- Derivatives from tyrosine or tryptophan include norepinephrine, epinephrine, thyroxine, and melatonin.
- Polypeptide proteins and amino acid derivatives include antidiuretic hormone (ADH), growth hormone, insulin, oxytocin, glucagon, adrenocorticotrophic hormone (ACTH), and parathyroid hormone (PTH).
- Glycoproteins include luteinizing hormone (LH), follicle-stimulating hormone (FSH), and thyroid-stimulating hormone (TSH).
- Steroid hormones derived from cholesterol include testosterone, estrogen, progesterone, and cortisol.

Hormones work slowly to regulate much of the body's physiological functions:

- Body energy, metabolism
- Sexual function and reproduction
- Growth and development
- Homeostasis
- Response to surroundings, stress, and injury

The hypothalamus is where the nervous system and the endocrine system meet to communicate, control, and coordinate the body's work. The hypothalamus controls the function of endocrine glands through its neural and hormonal paths connected to the anterior pituitary gland.

The principal organs of the endocrine system are the pituitary gland, the thyroid gland, the parathyroid glands, the pancreas, the adrenal glands, the gonads (testes and ovaries), and the pineal body. The pineal body secretes melatonin that seems to encourage sleep; however, its function is not well understood. Additionally, the hypothalamus releases hormones that offset the production of some other hormones. The pancreas and the gonads serve as endocrine glands but also have other important roles in the body's functioning. Figure 11.1 shows the location of the endocrine glands within the body. Table 11.1 lists the hormones produced by the principal endocrine glands and summarizes their major effects on the body.

The secretion of hormones by the endocrine system is governed by an amazingly intricate interrelationship among the glands, the nervous system, and the levels of various substances in the blood. Dysfunction of an endocrine gland may result in either too little secretion of its hormone (hyposecretion) or too much secretion (hypersecretion) because of a problem in the gland itself, difficulties in the feedback system, or problems in the target cells' response. Dysfunction can also be

related to infection, disease, trauma, tumor, or genetics. Endocrine gland tumors are usually benign and quite small, and inherited conditions are rare. Because of the effect the endocrine system has on the entire body, many disease conditions result from or are associated with endocrine dysfunction. Also of note is the connectedness of hormone production and function. If one of a gland's hormones malfunctions, other glands' hormones are affected. Even a minor malfunction can cause serious problems in one or more body systems.

Pituitary Gland Diseases and Disorders

The pituitary gland, located at the base of the brain, is only pea size but is often called the *master gland*. That term denotes the function of the pituitary gland in its relationship to the hypothalamus and the number of important hormones they control (Fig. 11.2). Many are related to female menstruation, pregnancy, birth, lactation, and sex characteristics. These include the following:

- *Follicle-stimulating hormone (FSH)* stimulates the development and maturation of a follicle of a woman's ovaries and promotes sperm production in men.
- *Luteinizing hormone (LH)*, a gonadotropin, causes the follicle to burst and a corpus luteum to be formed; it also helps to regulate testosterone in men and estrogen in women.
- *Prolactin* (or *luteotropic hormone*) *(LTH)* and *oxytocin* control lactation and affect sex hormone levels in both the ovaries and the testes.

Other hormones include the following:

- *Antidiuretic hormone (ADH)* limits water excretion from the kidneys.
- *Human growth hormone (hGH)* stimulates growth and cell reproduction and maintains muscle and bone mass in adulthood.
- *Thyroid-stimulating hormone (TSH)* stimulates the thyroid and its hormones, which help to regulate body metabolism, growth, energy, and nervous system activity.
- *Adrenocorticotrophic hormone (ACTH)* stimulates cortisol in the adrenal cortex, which helps to maintain blood glucose levels and blood pressure.

HYPERPITUITARISM (GIGANTISM, ACROMEGALY)

ICD-10: E22.0

Description

Hyperpituitarism is the hypersecretion of human growth hormone (hGH) by the anterior pituitary or

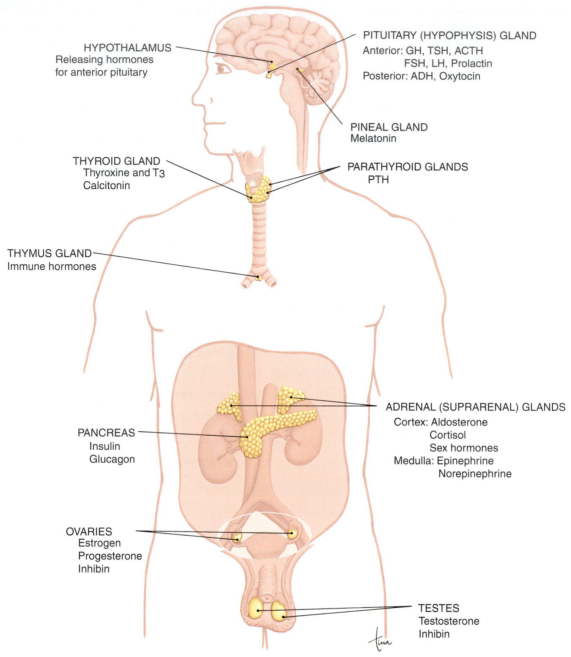

Figure 11.1   The endocrine system showing the location of many endocrine glands. Both male and female gonads (testes and ovaries) are shown. *(From Scanlon, VC, and Sanders, T:* Essentials of Anatomy and Physiology, *ed. 5. Philadelphia: F.A. Davis, 2007, p 224, with permission.)*

adenohypophysis gland. Two distinct conditions may result from hyperpituitarism, depending on the time of life at which this dysfunction begins. Gigantism results from the hypersecretion of hGH during an individual's growing years, especially before puberty. The person with gigantism grows abnormally tall, although the relative proportion of the body parts and sexual development remain unaffected. When hGH hypersecretion occurs during adulthood, acromegaly results. This is a chronic, disfiguring, life-shortening disease characterized by the overgrowth of bones and soft tissues and cardiac dysfunction.

Etiology

The hypersecretion of hGH that produces gigantism and acromegaly is typically due to benign, slow-growing glandular tumors, or **adenomas,** in the anterior pituitary. Not subject to normal control, these neoplastic cells release abnormally high levels of hGH. A genetic cause also has been suggested.

Signs and Symptoms

The principal symptom of gigantism is excessive growth of the long bones of the body. It develops abruptly and results in an abnormal increase in height.

Table 11.1 Principal Endocrine Glands

NAME AND POSITION	HORMONE	FUNCTION	ENDOCRINE DISORDER
Adrenal gland; adrenal cortex	Aldosterone	Balances sodium/potassium levels in blood	*Hypofunction:* Addison disease
Outer portion of gland on top of each kidney	Cortisol	Releases glucose to brain	*Hyperfunction:* adrenogenital syndrome; Cushing syndrome
Gonads (ovaries)	Androgen	Produces or stimulates male sex characteristics	
Adrenal medulla	Epinephrine	Mimics sympathetic nervous system	*Hypofunction:* almost unknown
Inner portion of adrenal gland; surrounded by adrenal cortex	Norepinephrine	Increases carbohydrate use of energy	*Hyperfunction:* pheochromocytoma
Pancreas (islets of Langerhans)	Glucagon (alpha cells)	Increases blood glucose level to produce energy	*Hypofunction:* diabetes mellitus
Head adjacent to duodenum; tail close to spleen and kidney	Insulin (beta cells)	Decreases blood glucose level	*Hyperfunction:* if a tumor produces excess insulin, hypoglycemia
Parathyroid Four or more small glands on back of thyroid	Parathyroid hormone	Regulates calcium and phosphates in blood; targets bones, small intestine, and kidneys	*Hypofunction:* tetany *Hyperfunction:* resorption of bone; renal calculi
Pituitary, anterior (adenohypophysis) Front portion of small gland below hypothalamus	Growth hormone Thyroid-stimulating hormone Adrenocorticotropic hormone Prolactin Follicle-stimulating hormone Luteinizing hormone	Influences growth, cell reproduction Stimulates thyroid function Stimulates cortisol in adrenal cortex Stimulates lactation Stimulates maturation of ovarian follicles With FSH promotes spermatogenesis (in men) and ovulation (in women)	*Hypofunction:* dwarfism in child; decrease in all other endocrine gland functions except parathyroids *Hyperfunction:* acromegaly in adult; gigantism in child
Pituitary, posterior (neurohypophysis)	Oxytocin	Stimulates uterine contraction and lactation	*Hyperfunction:* unknown
Back portion of small gland below hypothalamus	Antidiuretic hormone	Increases absorption of water by kidney tubule	*Hypofunction:* Diabetes insipidus
Gonads (testes) In scrotum	Testosterone Inhibin	Influences sperm maturation and secondary sex characteristics Works with anterior pituitary; maintains spermatogenesis	*Hypofunction:* Lack of sex development or regression in adult *Hyperfunction:* Abnormal sex development
Gonads (Ovaries) In pelvic cavity	Estrogen Progesterone Inhibin	Induces ovum maturation; prepares for fertilized egg; induces development of secondary sex characteristics Stores glycogen; secretes through mammary glands Works with anterior pituitary to decrease FSH	
Thyroid	Thyroxine (T$_4$)	Controls metabolic processes	*Hypofunction:* cretinism in young; myxedema in adult; goiter
Two lobes in anterior portion of neck	Triiodothyronine (T$_3$) Calcitonin	Affects heart rate, body temperature; indirectly influences growth and nutrition Helps maintain calcium levels in blood	*Hyperfunction:* goiter; thyrotoxicosis

Source: Venes, D (ed): Taber's Cyclopedic Medical Dictionary, ed. 22. Philadelphia: F.A. Davis, 2013, pp 1141–1143, with permission. (Adapted from Taber's by Carol D. Tamparo.)

Other symptoms include obesity; macrocephaly; headaches; an exaggerated growth of hands and feet; vision disorders; and **paresthesia,** a sensation of numbness, prickling, or tingling. The symptoms of acromegaly generally appear very gradually, causing the deformation of and doughy-feeling facial skin, thick and hard nails, oily skin, and thick eyelids. Serious physiological symptoms also may appear, such as increased sweating, hypertension, and chronic sinus congestion.

Diagnostic Procedures

The clinical picture of symptoms suggests the diagnosis. A glucose tolerance test is the standard method for confirming elevated hGH levels. Magnetic resonance imaging (MRI) and computed tomography (CT) scans are useful in pinpointing the location and estimating the extent of any pituitary tumor or lesion. Bone x-rays may exhibit bone thickening, especially of the cranium and long bones.

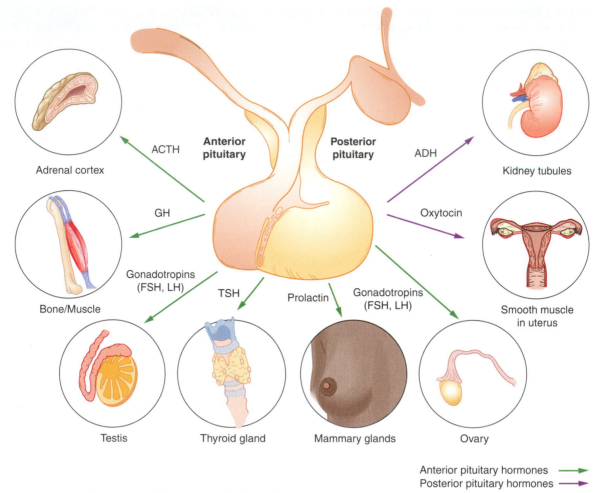

Figure 11.2 Hormones of the pituitary gland and their target organs.

Treatment

Treatment goals involve lowering hGH levels to normal and stabilizing or removing the underlying tumor while minimizing damage to the pituitary gland. Depending on the size and location of the tumor, a **transsphenoidal** (incision through the nose to remove the tumor) surgery may be performed. Otherwise, radiation therapy to reduce or destroy the tumor or medication therapy to shut off hGH hormone production may be used.

Complementary Therapy

No significant complementary therapy is indicated.

⊖ CLIENT COMMUNICATION

Clients will be concerned about body changes; therefore, emotional support is very helpful. Remind clients and family members what can happen with this disease, and prepare them for surgery as needed. Hormone replacement therapy following surgery or radiation is necessary and should be regularly monitored by a primary care provider. Refer to Hormone Health Network at www.hormone.org.

Prognosis

The prognosis for an individual with either gigantism or acromegaly depends on how far the condition has advanced before successful treatment. Gigantism is generally not life-threatening, and the prognosis is usually good. An individual with advanced acromegaly, however, may suffer serious complications, such as congestive heart failure, type 2 diabetes mellitus, respiratory disease, or cerebrovascular disease. For acromegaly, the mortality rate is two to three times that of the general population.

Prevention

There is no specific prevention for hyperpituitarism. Early treatment helps to prevent complications.

HYPOPITUITARISM

ICD-10: E23.0

Description

Hypopituitarism is an endocrine deficiency in which any of the hormones produced by the anterior portion of the pituitary gland (adenohypophysis) are secreted at insufficient levels or are absent. Gonadotropin and hGH are the most commonly deficient hormones in hypopituitarism. This is a complex disorder causing metabolic dysfunction, sexual immaturity, and growth retardation in childhood. Less frequently, ACTH and TSH are deficient. When all the anterior pituitary hormones are affected, the condition is called *panhypopituitarism*. As Table 11.1 indicates, the major effect of some anterior pituitary hormones is the stimulation of hormone production by other endocrine glands. For this reason, hypopituitarism has a cascading effect, resulting in hyposecretion of essential hormones by the "target" glands and producing symptoms that may mimic disorders of these glands.

Etiology

Hypopituitarism is often caused by a pituitary tumor or a tumor of the hypothalamus. It may result from a genetic mutation; other significant causes include pituitary vascular diseases, especially postpartum hemorrhage of the pituitary gland, which occurs because the enlarged pituitary gland of pregnancy becomes vulnerable to ischemia. Head injuries and **iatrogenic** damage—the result of surgery, chemotherapy, and radiation therapy—also may result in hypopituitarism. Less frequently, infection and inflammation of these structures are causes.

Signs and Symptoms

The symptoms usually develop over a period of time and may be vague and easily overlooked. Symptoms depend on the age and sex of the affected individual and on the specific hormones that are deficient. In children, hGH deficiency produces dwarfism, a condition of being abnormally small, whereas gonadotropin deficiency may interfere with the emergence of secondary sexual characteristics. Gonadotropin deficiency in adult women may cause amenorrhea and infertility. In men, the deficiency can result in lowered testosterone levels, decreased libido, and loss of body and facial hair. ACTH and TSH deficiencies may produce generalized symptoms, such as fatigue, anorexia, weight gain or loss, loss of skin pigmentation, low tolerance to cold, muscle weakness, stiff joints, and a poor response to stress. Naturally enough, panhypopituitarism may result in all of the preceding symptoms as well as mental and physiological abnormalities.

Diagnostic Procedures

The individual's clinical history of symptoms will suggest the diagnosis. A battery of laboratory tests to measure the levels of each of the principal pituitary hormones is typically run to confirm the diagnosis. It is essential that laboratory tests also be run to measure the normal output of "target" glands (e.g., cortisol production by the adrenal glands), because deficiencies of these secretions may prove life-threatening. A vision test may be given to check for impaired sight. MRI and cranial CT scans are useful in pinpointing pituitary tumors or lesions.

Treatment

Hormone replacement therapy, both of pituitary hormones and of hormones secreted by the target glands, is the typical course of treatment. Because hormonal balances normally change during growth and development, serious illness, or major physical stress, constant monitoring is necessary during hormone replacement therapy to make certain that appropriate hormonal levels are maintained. Surgical removal of pituitary tumors may be required. (Refer to the "Treatment" section under "Hyperpituitarism.")

Complementary Therapy

It can be helpful to manage chronic stress, maintain appropriate weight, eat healthy foods, limit fat intake, and avoid sugar and simple carbohydrates.

 CLIENT COMMUNICATION

Help clients and family members understand the effects of deficient hormones on the body. Monitor hormone replacement therapy carefully throughout a client's lifetime. Recommend the client wear a medical alert bracelet or pendant to provide information about the condition in an emergency.

Prognosis

Even though lost pituitary function generally cannot be restored, the prognosis can be good with adequate hormone replacement therapy. Total loss of all hormonal secretions from the anterior pituitary may result in fatal complications.

Prevention

There is no specific prevention for hypopituitarism. Because of the impact hypopituitarism has on multiple target organs, it is fortunate that this disorder is rare.

DIABETES INSIPIDUS

ICD-10: E23.2

Description

Diabetes insipidus, sometimes called *pituitary diabetes insipidus*, occurs when the kidneys are unable to conserve water. When the problem is the result of insufficient secretion of **vasopressin** by the posterior portion of the pituitary gland, or neurohypophysis, the term *central diabetes insipidus* is used. When the problem is caused by a failure of the kidneys to respond to vasopressin, the term *nephrogenic diabetes insipidus* is used. Vasopressin, or *antidiuretic hormone (ADH)*, helps regulate the amount of fluid the kidneys release as urine. Other things being equal, the higher the level of vasopressin, the greater is the fluid reabsorption by the kidneys. In diabetes insipidus, the decreased vasopressin allows the filtered water to be excreted, which means that large quantities of diluted water must pass through the body as urine. Diabetes insipidus usually starts in childhood or early adulthood and affects men more commonly than women.

Etiology

Central diabetes insipidus results from tumors, hypophysectomy, skull fracture, or head trauma. It can also result from infection, or it may be idiopathic. Nephrogenic diabetes insipidus is less common than central diabetes insipidus. It can be inherited or caused by kidney dysfunction, higher than normal levels of calcium in the blood (hypercalcemia), or certain drugs such as lithium.

Signs and Symptoms

The classic symptoms are polyuria and polydipsia. As much as 4 to 16 liters of dilute urine may be produced in 24 hours. This makes the person extremely thirsty because of the need to replace the fluids lost from the body. Consequently, there may be signs of dehydration, such as dry skin, weakness, fever, mental confusion, and prostration.

Diagnostic Procedures

Urinalysis reveals a colorless urine with low osmolality (i.e., containing low levels of dissolved wastes). A "dehydration test" is often done to differentiate diabetes insipidus from other diseases causing polyuria. In this test, the person is denied fluids while hourly measurements are made of urine osmolality, body weight, and blood pressure. After a period of several hours, the individual is given a vasopressin medication. If the person has diabetes insipidus, the vasopressin will decrease the urine output and increase the osmolality of the urine. An MRI may be necessary to determine any pituitary tumor.

Treatment

Treat the underlying cause if possible. Mild cases may require only increased fluid intake. Hormone replacement therapy using various vasopressin medications is the most common treatment protocol for central diabetes insipidus. ADH is usually administered via tablet or nasal spray. For nephrogenic diabetes insipidus, stopping the offending medications may reverse the problem. Drugs may be used to treat the nephrogenic type; they include anti-inflammatory medications and diuretics.

Complementary Therapy

No significant complementary therapy is indicated.

 CLIENT COMMUNICATION

During treatment, monitor symptoms to ensure a proper maintenance of fluid balance. It is recommended that clients report any weight gain and recurrence of polyuria.

Prognosis

The prognosis of an individual with diabetes insipidus depends on the underlying cause of the condition. If the underlying cause is difficult to treat, such as cancer, the prognosis is guarded. In most cases, though, with effective vasopressin replacement therapy and administration of the appropriate medications, individuals should be able to lead a normal life. Complications, such as electrolyte imbalance and dehydration, occur when not enough fluids are consumed.

Prevention

There is no specific prevention for diabetes insipidus.

CHAPTER EPISODE—PART II

Susan's grandmother waits until Susan raises the issue of PCOS and shares her fears and concerns with her grandmother. In the past 3 to 4 years, Susan's menstrual cycle had grown less frequent and more irregular, often accompanied by serious cramping and excessive bleeding when it did occur. Susan begins to cry when she says she thought the worst thing about her irregular periods was that she could never count on when her excessive flow would interfere with her swim team activities. Now, however, she fears that she might not ever be able to have a child.

- How might Susan's grandmother respond?
- How is Susan's situation likely different from her grandmother's?

Thyroid Gland Diseases and Disorders: Hyperthyroidism

The thyroid gland is a butterfly-shaped endocrine gland in the neck. Diseases and disorders of the thyroid gland are far more common than those of the pituitary gland. Literally millions of individuals live with a thyroid disorder. The majority are women. The four main types of thyroid disease are (1) hyperthyroidism, (2) hypothyroidism (see next section), (3) benign thyroid neoplasms, and (4) thyroid cancer. The thyroid gland secretes the following hormones:

- *Thyroxine* (T_4) contains iodine and is responsible for cell metabolism and regulates growth.
- *Triiodothyronine* (T_3) is a powerful hormone affecting every part of the body, including body temperature, growth, heart rate.

SIMPLE GOITER

ICD-10: E04.0

Description

A goiter is an enlargement or hyperplasia of the thyroid gland. A simple goiter is any thyroid enlargement that is not caused by an infection or neoplasm and that does not result from another hypothyroid or hyperthyroid disorder. It is classified as endemic or sporadic. Endemic or colloid goiter is the result of insufficient dietary intake of iodine. Sporadic or nontoxic goiter follows ingestion of certain drugs or foods. Simple goiter is more common in women, especially during adolescence, pregnancy, and menopause. During these times, the body's demand for thyroid hormone is increased.

Etiology

The thyroid gland hyperplasia that characterizes a goiter occurs when the thyroid gland cannot secrete sufficient levels of the two iodine-rich hormones: thyroxine (T_4) and triiodothyronine (T_3). The thyroid gland tissue enlarges to compensate for the deficiency. In simple goiter, the inadequate secretion of these thyroid hormones may be caused by a dietary iodine deficiency, the ingestion of substances known to induce goiter (**goitrogens**), or some error in the hormone formation process within the thyroid gland. Risk factors include being female, being over age 40, and having a family history of goiter. In many cases, though, the condition is idiopathic.

Signs and Symptoms

The extent of thyroid enlargement varies from case to case. A simple goiter may appear as a small nodule, or it can be quite massive, presenting a conspicuous swollen mass at the front of the neck, just above the sternum (Fig. 11.3). The goiter shown in Figure 11.3 is more commonly seen in countries that, unlike the United States, do not put iodized salt in foods. The goiter may compress the esophagus or trachea, producing dysphagia, dyspnea, dizziness, and syncope.

Diagnostic Procedures

A thorough history and physical examination to rule out disorders with similar clinical effects, such as Graves disease and Hashimoto thyroiditis, is necessary. Diagnosis

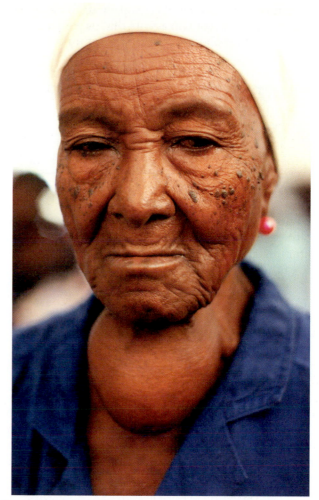

Figure 11.3 Haitian woman with nontoxic goiter. *(James Gray, MissionFoto, Gosport, Indiana.)*

of simple goiter is made on the basis of thyroid gland enlargement in the presence of normal levels of T_3 and T_4 hormones. A T_3 and T_4 radioimmunoassay test accurately measures the levels of these two hormones. If an ultrasound locates any nodules, a biopsy is necessary to check for thyroid cancer.

Treatment

The treatment goal is to reduce the size of the goiter. How this is accomplished depends in part on the underlying cause of the condition. Treatment procedures may include dietary supplements of iodine or T_3 and T_4 hormone replacement therapy. Sporadic goiter requires avoidance of known goitrogenic foods and drugs. A large goiter that is unresponsive to therapy may require excision, resulting in lifelong thyroid replacement therapy.

Complementary Therapy

Nutritional supplements may be helpful. A diet that includes iodized salt but avoids goitrogenic foods is recommended; those foods include rutabagas, cabbage, peas, spinach, radishes, soybeans, peanuts, peaches, and pears, all of which contain agents that decrease T_4 production. Shrimp and other shellfish are a good source of iodine.

 CLIENT COMMUNICATION

Iodized salt should be used to supply the daily 150 to 300 mg of iodine necessary to prevent goiters. Measuring the neck circumference to monitor for progressive thyroid enlargement may be beneficial.

Prognosis

The prognosis is generally good following effective treatment. Complications from severe cases of simple goiter include tachycardia, congestive heart failure, and atrial fibrillation.

Prevention

Prevention of simple goiter includes adequate dietary intake of iodine.

GRAVES DISEASE

ICD-10: E05.0X*

Description

Graves disease is a condition caused by the oversecretion of hormones by the thyroid gland. As Table 11.1 reveals, thyroid hormones such as T_4 and T_3 influence the metabolism of cells throughout the body. Consequently, when levels of these hormones are constantly elevated, as occurs in hyperthyroidism, profound changes can occur in the body's normal physiological processes. Graves disease is the most common form of hyperthyroidism and occurs more frequently in women than in men.

Etiology

Oversecretion of T_3 and T_4 influences the speed at which the body converts food into energy. Graves disease may be genetic but is more likely immunologic in nature. The immune system attacks the thyroid gland, causing hypersecretion of its hormones.

Signs and Symptoms

The classic manifestations of Graves disease are goiter, nervousness, anxiety, loss of sleep, excessive perspiration, and heat intolerance. Wasting of muscle and decalcification of the skeleton may lead to persistent weight loss and fatigue. The disorder may cause a condition known as Graves ophthalmopathy. The ophthalmopathy characteristic of Graves disease is **exophthalmos,** which is when the eyeballs protrude, giving the affected individual a "frightened" appearance (Fig. 11.4). Inflammation

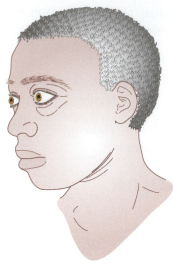

Figure 11.4 Exophthalmos caused by hyperthyroidism (Graves disease).

of the muscles surrounding the eye may interfere with normal eye movements, including blinking. A rare form of dermopathy associated with Graves disease is marked by thickened patches of skin, usually on the feet or legs, giving an "orange skin" texture and uneven pigmentation.

The symptoms of **thyrotoxicosis** include a host of cardiac manifestations, such as tachycardia, arrhythmias, heart murmurs, and cardiomegaly.

Diagnostic Procedures

Diagnosis is based largely on the characteristic physical manifestations of the disease. Primary care providers will do a physical examination and order blood tests to determine TSH levels, and a radioimmunoassay will confirm increased serum levels of T_4 and T_3. A nuclear thyroid scan reveals increased uptake of radioactive iodine (^{131}I). Blood tests indicating elevated levels of certain antithyroid immunoglobulins also strongly suggest a diagnosis of Graves disease.

Treatment

The course of treatment depends on the affected individual's age and the severity of the case. One approach involves the use of antithyroid agents (i.e., drugs that block hormone synthesis within the thyroid gland). Another approach involves altering the structure of the thyroid gland itself through either surgery or radioactive iodine therapy. Short-term control of the hyperthyroidism of Graves disease also may be obtained by administration of iodide compounds. Beta blockers can relieve some of the symptoms of Graves disease and are usually prescribed in combination with one of the other treatments. Because treatment causes thyroid activity to decline, most

The X represents the fourth and fifth digits that are often required and supplied once more detailed information about the disease or disorder is made known to the provider.

individuals require thyroxine treatment to supply the body with necessary amounts of thyroid hormones.

Complementary Therapy

See "Simple Goiter." Cool compresses and lubricating eyedrops may help relieve discomfort of exophthalmos. Over-the-counter hydrocortisone creams may help relieve symptoms of dermopathy.

 CLIENT COMMUNICATION

Drug and iodide compound therapy require careful monitoring and follow-up care. Remind clients to watch for any form of hypothyroidism. Clients may need help coping with anxiety and the physical discomforts of the disease.

Prognosis

The prognosis of Graves disease varies from case to case. If treatment results in the remission of symptoms and the disappearance of immunoglobulins associated with the disease, then the prognosis for a complete recovery without recurrence is good. Cardiovascular problems and osteoporosis are complications of untreated hyperthyroidism. A potentially fatal complication of untreated Graves disease is thyroid storm, a severe episode of thyrotoxicosis; it is marked by the rapid onset of fever, sweating, tachycardia, pulmonary edema, congestive heart failure, and death. **Thyroid storm requires emergency medical intervention.**

Prevention

There is no specific prevention for Graves disease.

Thyroid Gland Diseases and Disorders: Hypothyroidism

HASHIMOTO THYROIDITIS (CHRONIC THYROIDITIS)

ICD-10: E06.3

Description

Hashimoto thyroiditis was first described by Dr. Hakaru Hashimoto in 1912. It is the most common type of hypothyroidism. The swelling and inflammation of the thyroid gland is also known as *autoimmune thyroiditis*. The disease is chronic and more common in women than in men.

Etiology

Autoimmune thyroiditis, a long-term inflammatory disease, is due to antibodies to thyroid antigens in the blood. When the inflammation causes lymphocytic infiltration, it is called *Hashimoto thyroiditis*. Myxedema and Graves disease are both linked to autoimmune thyroiditis. While the cause is essentially unknown, it is probably familial and may appear with other diseases, such as celiac disease and type 1 diabetes.

Signs and Symptoms

There may be moderate thyroid enlargement accompanied by pain and tenderness. Dysphagia may occur. The signs and symptoms begin slowly, are often subtle, and mimic other disorders. They include fatigue and excessive sleepiness, difficulty concentrating, depression, cold intolerance, and dry skin and hair.

Diagnostic Procedures

Blood testing will reveal elevated immunoglobulin levels and the presence of antibodies that react with thyroid tissue. A thyroid scan and MRI may also be helpful. A thyroid biopsy may identify characteristic changes.

Treatment

Treatment includes lifelong hormone replacement therapy for hypothyroidism, analgesics, and anti-inflammatory drugs for acute inflammation. Without medication, the thyroid gland is unlikely to be able to carry out its hormonal function. Because there is no way to tell how long the autoimmune process will continue, consistent monitoring of thyroid hormone levels is necessary.

Complementary Therapy

Stress appears to affect the thyroid hormones. Therefore, measures to reduce stress can be attempted along with hormone replacement as necessary.

 CLIENT COMMUNICATION

Carefully explain treatment protocols to clients. It is recommended that clients understand symptoms of both hypothyroidism and hyperthyroidism, because treatment may cause either problem. Signs of hypothyroidism include lethargy, restlessness, sensitivity to cold, dry skin, and forgetfulness. Signs of hyperthyroidism include nervousness, tremors, and weakness.

Prognosis

The prognosis is good with proper diagnosis and treatment. Since permanent loss of thyroid function requires lifelong thyroid replacement therapy, medical monitoring should continue even after recovery.

Prevention

There is no known prevention for Hashimoto thyroiditis.

HYPOTHYROIDISM (CRETINISM, MYXEDEMA)

ICD-10: E03.9

Description

Hypothyroidism, the undersecretion of hormones by the thyroid gland, is called *cretinism* when it appears as a congenital condition, and it is called *myxedema* when it is acquired later in childhood or during adulthood. Hypothyroidism is a common condition seen more in women than men.

Etiology

Hypothyroidism may be caused by either an insufficient quantity of thyroid tissue or the loss of functional thyroid tissue. The former condition may be iatrogenic, resulting from thyroid surgery, radioactive iodine therapy performed to treat another thyroid disease, or a congenital thyroid abnormality. Inflammation and chronic autoimmune thyroiditis or Hashimoto disease are also common causes.

Other forms of hypothyroidism may be caused by dietary or metabolic iodine deficiencies or may be induced by certain drugs. Hypothyroidism also may arise secondarily from diseases of the anterior pituitary lobe that result in hyposecretion of TSH.

Signs and Symptoms

Because the thyroid hormones T_3 and T_4 influence the metabolism of cells throughout the body, persistently low levels of these hormones can result in a host of symptoms. The assortment of symptoms varies with the age of the affected individual.

Neonates with hypothyroidism may exhibit constipation and feeding problems, may sleep too much, and may have a hoarse cry. The brain and skeleton fail to develop properly without treatment. Children with the condition (either congenital or acquired) typically show retarded growth, a delayed emergence of secondary sexual characteristics, impaired intelligence, and one or more of the adult symptoms of hypothyroidism.

The onset of hypothyroidism during adulthood is often insidious. Initial symptoms may include fatigue, constipation, intolerance to cold, muscle cramps, and excessive sleepiness. Later symptoms may include mental clouding, diminished appetite, and weight gain. The skin may become dry, and the hair and nails may become brittle. In advanced forms of the disease, the affected individual may have an expressionless face and sparse hair.

Diagnostic Procedures

The presenting signs and symptoms may suggest the diagnosis. Radioimmunoassay typically shows depressed levels of T_3 and T_4. A similar test usually reveals elevated levels of TSH, except for hypothyroidism arising from pituitary gland dysfunction, in which case TSH levels may range from undetectable to near normal. Thyroid scan shows diminished levels of iodine uptake. There are likely to be higher-than-normal levels of serum cholesterol, alkaline phosphates, and triglycerides.

Treatment

Treatment for hypothyroidism usually requires lifelong hormone replacement therapy with synthetic or animal-derived thyroid hormones. In the case of infants and children, therapy should begin as soon as possible to avoid or minimize intellectual impairment.

Complementary Therapy

No significant complementary therapy is known.

 CLIENT COMMUNICATION

Continued monitoring of thyroid replacement hormone is necessary and should be checked every 6 weeks until the thyroid hormone level is stable, and then periodically throughout the client's life.

Prognosis

With effective thyroid hormone replacement therapy, the prognosis for an individual with hypothyroidism is good. A life-threatening complication of severe hypothyroidism is myxedema coma. This condition is marked by the onset of hypothermia and stupor and is considered a medical emergency.

Prevention

Only hypothyroidism due to dietary iodine deficiency, radiation or surgical removal of the thyroid, and drug-induced forms of the disease are preventable.

THYROID CANCER

ICD-10: C73

Description

According to the National Cancer Institute, cancer of the thyroid is becoming more common. There are four main types:

1. *Papillary thyroid cancer* accounts for about 80% of cases; seen mostly in individuals aged 30 to 50, it grows slowly but often spreads to lymph nodes.
2. *Follicular thyroid cancer* accounts for about 10% of cases, usually occurs in people over age 50, and more likely spreads to lungs or bones.
3. *Medullary thyroid cancer* is mostly sporadic and may be associated with tumors of other glands; it can run in families.
4. *Anaplastic thyroid cancer* is very aggressive and usually occurs in people over age 60. Fortunately, it is

very rare, because the chances for survival beyond 6 to 12 months is low.

Etiology

What causes thyroid cells to mutate, grow abnormally, and cause a tumor is unknown. Risk factors to consider include having a family history of goiter or thyroid cancer; being over age 40; and receiving radiation treatments to the head, neck, or chest in childhood.

Signs and Symptoms

There are only a few symptoms, and they include increasing hoarseness or voice changes, difficulty swallowing, and a lump that can be felt in the neck.

Diagnostic Procedures

A complete physical examination that includes palpation of the neck area to check for lumps or nodules and lymph node swelling is performed. Ultrasound to visualize lumps, aspiration needle biopsy to check for cancer cells, and a blood test to measure for TSH in the body are the best tools for diagnosis. The blood test, however, can evaluate the function of the thyroid but is rarely abnormal in individuals with thyroid cancer.

Treatment

Treatment depends on the type and stage of the cancer diagnosed. Most commonly, surgery is performed to remove all or part of the thyroid gland (thyroidectomy). Radioactive iodine therapy requires swallowing a small amount of radioactive iodine to destroy any thyroid tissue remaining after surgery or to destroy cancer cells that have spread. The radioactive iodine attaches to thyroid cells and is not harmful to other tissues. It is excreted from the body in urine within a few days; however, it is advised that close contact with children and pregnant women be avoided during that time. External radiation directs high-energy beams directly to the cancerous nodule a few moments a day for several weeks. Those with advanced cancer may benefit most from external radiation. Chemotherapy, typically given intravenously, is used mostly for those with anaplastic thyroid cancer.

Complementary Therapy

No significant complementary therapy is known.

⊖ CLIENT COMMUNICATION

Remind clients that when the thyroid is destroyed, replacement therapy will follow and should be monitored regularly until a proper dosage is determined and blood levels are sustained. The thyroid hormone level should be checked periodically throughout the client's life.

Prognosis

Despite successful treatment, thyroid cancer can return. It may return in the lymph nodes of the neck, in the lungs, or in the bones.

Prevention

There is no known prevention for thyroid cancer. Avoid radiation therapy of the neck if possible. Individuals who live within 10 miles of a nuclear power plant may qualify for the medication potassium iodide that blocks the effect of radiation on the thyroid gland. The medication would be taken in case of an emergency or accident at the power plant.

Parathyroid Gland Diseases and Disorders

The parathyroids are four small glands surrounding the thyroid in the neck. They are quite small—about the size of a grain of rice. These glands produce the parathyroid hormone (PTH), which maintains the balance of calcium and phosphorus in the bloodstream and serves as an antagonist to calcitonin secreted by the thyroid gland (Fig. 11.5). A dysfunction of the glands causes either hyperparathyroidism (too much calcium in the blood or hypercalcemia) or hypoparathyroidism (too little calcium in the blood or hypocalcemia). Both conditions can cause a number of complications.

HYPERPARATHYROIDISM (HYPERCALCEMIA)

ICD-10: E21.3

Description

Hyperparathyroidism is a general disorder of calcium and phosphorus metabolism caused by excessive secretion

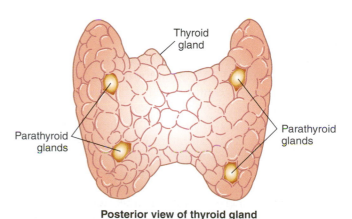

Posterior view of thyroid gland

Figure 11.5 Posterior view of thyroid gland.

of PTH by the parathyroid glands. The persistently high level of PTH typically depresses the concentration of phosphorus in the extracellular fluid and elevates the concentration of calcium (hypercalcemia). Most of the troubling effects associated with hyperparathyroidism result from hypercalcemia. Hyperparathyroidism is more common than once suspected, and it affects women twice as frequently as men.

Etiology

Hyperparathyroidism may have either a primary or a secondary etiology. The most common primary etiology is an adenoma on one of the parathyroid glands. Less commonly, two or more of the parathyroid glands may become enlarged, or a malignant tumor may cause hyperparathyroidism. Secondary hyperparathyroidism occurs when another condition lowers calcium levels, causing the parathyroids to overcompensate for the calcium loss. Factors that contribute to secondary hyperparathyroidism are severe calcium deficiency or vitamin D deficiency and chronic kidney failure. Hypercalcemia may also be the result of certain diseases, such as tuberculosis and sarcoidosis, which are inflammatory diseases of the lungs. Certain medications can cause hypercalcemia, such as lithium (used to treat bipolar disorder) and thiazide diuretics (used to treat high blood pressure).

Signs and Symptoms

The onset of hyperparathyroidism is usually very gradual, with more than half the affected individuals remaining asymptomatic for extended periods of time. Symptoms are usually related to hypercalcemia and may include weak, brittle bones; joint pain; or kidney stones. Polyuria is a common effect of hyperparathyroidism. Other hypercalcemic symptoms include central nervous system disturbances, such as depression or forgetfulness, or gastrointestinal disturbances, such as nausea, vomiting, and loss of appetite. Additional symptoms may include muscle weakness or atrophy, chronic fatigue, and cardiac disturbances.

Diagnostic Procedures

Radioimmunoassay typically reveals elevated concentrations of serum PTH. Blood testing usually shows abnormally high serum calcium levels in primary forms of the disease and diminished or nearly normal levels in secondary forms. Serum phosphorus levels are decreased. A 24-hour urine collection measures how much calcium is being excreted in urine. A bone mineral density test measures the amount of calcium and other minerals in bone. CT scans of bone may reveal evidence of demineralization or increased bone turnover (i.e., newly formed bone mass balancing the reabsorption of older bone mass).

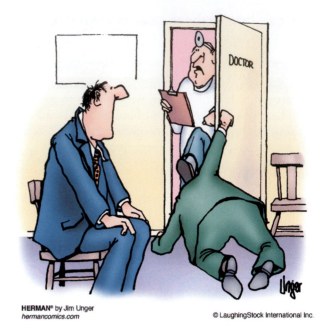

HERMAN® by Jim Unger
hermancomics.com

© LaughingStock International Inc.

"Okay, who's next?"

HERMAN© is reprinted with permission from LaughingStock Licensing Inc., Ottawa, Canada. All rights reserved

Treatment

The treatment of hyperparathyroidism varies with the etiology. In primary forms of the disease, the goal is to reduce the level of circulating calcium. This may be accomplished surgically by removing the neoplastic or hypertrophied parathyroid gland(s). All except half of one parathyroid gland can be removed in order to maintain normal PTH levels. Increased hydration and sodium intake also may be used to lower serum calcium levels. In some cases, drugs that increase the excretion of calcium by the kidneys or inhibit the reabsorption of calcium from bone may be used. Secondary forms of hyperparathyroidism can only be corrected by treating the underlying cause.

Outpatient Surgery

Surgical excision of the parathyroids can be done on an outpatient basis by making tiny incisions in the neck under a local anesthesia. Usually, a small portion of one parathyroid gland is left in order to maintain as much normal PTH as possible.

Complementary Therapy

Careful monitoring of calcium and vitamin D supplements is important and should be carried out only by a primary care provider. Drinking plenty of water and participating in daily exercise is helpful. Smoking, which can increase bone loss, should be avoided.

CLIENT COMMUNICATION

Instruct clients about the disease and its treatment. Prepare clients for surgery as needed and emphasize the importance of follow-up care.

Prognosis

The prognosis for an individual with hyperparathyroidism is generally good, given successful treatment. Without successful treatment, osteoporosis, kidney failure, and cardiac arrest may result. Severe hypercalcemia can also lead to confusion and dementia.

Prevention

There is no known prevention for hyperparathyroidism.

HYPOPARATHYROIDISM (HYPOCALCEMIA)

ICD-10: E20.9

Description

Hypoparathyroidism is undersecretion of PTH by the parathyroid glands. Consequently, circulating concentrations of calcium are reduced, resulting in hypocalcemia and an increased amount of phosphorus. There is excessive deposit of calcium into bone tissue.

Etiology

Some cases of hypoparathyroidism are caused by hereditary disorders in which parathyroids are absent or seriously underdeveloped. Far more frequently, however, hypoparathyroidism is iatrogenic, usually resulting from the deliberate or inadvertent removal of parathyroid tissue during surgery.

Signs and Symptoms

The signs and symptoms of hypoparathyroidism are generally dependent on the degree of hypocalcemia. Symptoms may include **tetany** and paresthesia of the extremities, neuromuscular irritability, and muscle cramps. Central nervous system symptoms may include general irritability, anxiety, memory problems, and depression. Women are likely to have painful menstruation, brittle fingernails, and suffer hair loss.

Diagnostic Procedures

Radioimmunoassay revealing decreased PTH and serum calcium levels will suggest the diagnosis. Serum phosphorus typically is increased and serum calcium decreased. There will also be a lower than normal parathyroid hormone level. Electrocardiograms (ECGs) may indicate increased QT and ST cardiac waveform abnormalities due to hypocalcemia. A 24-hour urine collection measures how much calcium is being excreted in urine. A bone mineral density test measures the amount of calcium and other minerals in bone.

Treatment

Treatment usually consists of lifelong vitamin D and calcium supplementation. Serum calcium levels should be tested regularly because of side effects that may occur. A diet high in calcium (dairy products, fortified orange juice, and green leafy vegetables) and low in phosphorus is encouraged.

Complementary Therapy

Other than following a diet high in calcium and low in phosphorus, no known significant complementary treatment is indicated. Following a low-phosphorus diet means avoiding all carbonated soft drinks, which are high in phosphorus.

 CLIENT COMMUNICATION

Emphasize the importance of checking serum calcium levels at least three times yearly. Teach clients how to watch for signs of tetany and paresthesia. As tetany worsens, muscle tension and spasms occur, and the client may have difficulty walking.

Prognosis

Although the condition is chronic, with successful treatment the individual with hypoparathyroidism can lead a relatively normal life.

Prevention

There is no known prevention for hypoparathyroidism.

Adrenal Gland Diseases and Disorders

The adrenal glands are located near the top of each kidney. The adrenal cortex (outer layer of the adrenal gland) produces the hormones aldosterone, cortisol, and androgen. Aldosterone maintains normal levels of sodium and potassium in the blood, cortisol responds to stress by releasing glucose to the brain, and androgen is partly responsible for male sex characteristics. The adrenal medulla (inner portion of the adrenal gland) secretes epinephrine and norepinephrine, which mimic the sympathetic response to fright or flight.

Adrenal disorders cause the adrenal glands to hyperfunction or hypofunction. In Cushing syndrome, there is hyperfunction and too much cortisol. In Addison disease, there is hypofunction and too little cortisol.

CUSHING SYNDROME

ICD-10: E24.X

Description

Cushing syndrome is hypersecretion of cortisol from the adrenal cortex. It is most common in females.

Etiology

One cause of Cushing syndrome is bilateral **hyperplasia** of the adrenal glands due to elevated serum levels of ACTH. Elevated concentrations of ACTH may result from overproduction of this hormone by a malfunctioning pituitary gland or from ACTH-secreting neoplasms elsewhere in the body. In either case, the result is overstimulation of the cortices of the adrenal gland and hypersecretion of cortisol. Another cause of Cushing syndrome is benign or malignant neoplasm of an adrenal cortex. Finally, the disease is frequently iatrogenic, produced as a side effect of the long-term administration of corticosteroid drugs used to treat other diseases, such as asthma, or repeated injectable corticosteroids for joint and back pain.

Signs and Symptoms

Like other endocrine disorders, Cushing syndrome causes changes in multiple body systems. The classic symptom of Cushing syndrome is a round "moon-shaped" face, a "buffalo" hump on the upper back, and purple striae or stretch marks on the skin. There may be impaired glucose tolerance that can lead to diabetes, muscle weakness, fragile skin that bruises easily, emotional changes, hypertension, and increased susceptibility to infection. The menstrual cycle may be irregular or absent in women, and men may have erectile dysfunction.

Diagnostic Procedures

The primary care provider performs a complete physical examination and will likely know if long-term corticosteroids have been administered for some other disorder or disease. The diagnostic procedures are chosen so as to establish the diagnosis and to pinpoint its etiology—frequently a difficult task. A 24-hour urine test typically exhibits elevated free cortisol levels. It is important to determine steroid levels in both serum and urine. A low-dose dexamethasone suppression test confirms the diagnosis. Brain MRI and abdominal CT scans may be helpful in locating any tumors.

Treatment

The treatment goal in each case is to restore the concentration of serum cortisol to normal levels. The approach chosen, however, necessarily varies according to the etiology. Reducing corticosteroid use may be the first step. In the case of adrenal hyperplasia due to elevated ACTH levels, surgery is usually performed to remove tumors on the pituitary gland or at ectopic sites. In some cases, drug therapy or radiation therapy may be attempted to suppress ACTH secretion. Occasionally, total adrenalectomy is the treatment of choice, but there is a subsequent lifelong requirement for cortisol replacement therapy.

Complementary Therapy

No significant complementary therapy is indicated.

 CLIENT COMMUNICATION

Careful client assessment and vigorous supportive care are required. To minimize weight gain, edema, and hypertension, a diet high in protein and potassium but low in calories, carbohydrates, and sodium is important. When replacement therapy is necessary, advise clients how the medications are to be taken. Carrying a medical ID card or wearing a medical alert bracelet is helpful for clients because any physiologically stressful situation likely will require increased medication.

Prognosis

The prognosis for Cushing syndrome depends on the etiology and on how far the disease has progressed before the institution of treatment. The prognosis is poor for an individual with Cushing syndrome caused by a carcinoma of the adrenal cortex. The prognosis is generally good if the condition is caused by a localized adenoma of the pituitary gland.

Prevention

Iatrogenic forms of Cushing syndrome are preventable. Individuals receiving glucocorticoid steroids or ACTH preparations to treat other diseases should be carefully monitored for symptoms of Cushing disease.

ADDISON DISEASE

ICD-10: E27.1, E27.2, or E27.40

Description

When the adrenal glands produce insufficient amounts of cortisol and androgen, adrenal insufficiency—or Addison disease—results. Addison disease is more common between ages 30 and 50 and can be life-threatening.

Etiology

The primary and most common cause of adrenal insufficiency is autoimmune. Other causes may be infections or bleeding of the adrenal glands, cancer that has metastasized to the adrenal glands, or tuberculosis. The secondary cause of Addison disease occurs if the pituitary gland is diseased and cannot produce

ACTH. Adrenal insufficiency may also result when individuals must cease to take corticosteroids for other diseases.

Signs and Symptoms

The signs and symptoms readily mimic many other ailments and include muscle weakness and pain, weight loss, **hypoglycemia,** craving for salt, hypotension, nausea, and vomiting. Acute renal failure or Addisonian crisis appears suddenly with severe vomiting and diarrhea leading to dehydration, pain in lower back and abdomen, hypotension, **hyperkalemia** (high blood levels of potassium), and unconsciousness.

Diagnostic Procedures

Blood tests are performed to determine the levels of potassium, sodium, cortisol, and ACTH. An ACTH stimulation test and an insulin-induced hypoglycemia test may also be ordered. A CT scan of the adrenal glands and/or the pituitary gland may detect any tumors or enlargements.

Treatment

Hormone replacement therapy is the treatment for early diagnosis of Addison disease. These medications are usually taken daily, but the primary care provider may indicate that dosages should be increased when facing surgery, stressful situations, or serious illness. The Addisonian crisis is a medical emergency requiring immediate IV hydrocortisone, saline, and dextrose.

Complementary Therapy

No significant complementary therapy is indicated.

⊙ CLIENT COMMUNICATION

Remind clients to keep adequate medications on hand in case they need to take additional amounts. Remind them, too, that missing a day of medications is dangerous. Advise clients to wear a medical alert bracelet or carry a medical alert card with them at all times. Clients may be advised to carry an emergency dose of intramuscular hydrocortisone.

Prognosis

With appropriate hormone replacement therapy, most individuals with Addison disease are able to lead a relatively normal life.

Prevention

There is no known prevention for Addison disease; however, persons who have the disease may be able to prevent the life-threatening Addisonian crisis by understanding the disease and recognizing the symptoms of a crisis. Rigid adherence to a hormone therapy regimen is necessary.

CHAPTER EPISODE—PART III

Susan's grandmother assures Susan and says, "Well, I had your mom, didn't I? Pregnancy is quite possible. Even though we had some difficulties, look how well it turned out." When Susan asked what kind of difficulties, her grandmother said, "Well, I miscarried before I got pregnant with your mom. Even though the only doctor in the rural area where we lived was just a general practitioner, he was understanding. He had seen the disease before and was smart enough to test my blood for glucose and hormone levels. Once my hormones were regulated and glucose levels returned to normal, he suggested your grandpa and I try again to get pregnant. And sure enough, it worked."

- Are there any other symptoms for Susan to address?

Pancreas and the Islets of Langerhans Diseases and Disorders

The pancreas lies behind the stomach, in front of the spine, and is surrounded by the intestines and liver. The pancreas serves both as an endocrine gland and an exocrine gland. It secretes the hormones insulin and glucagon through a specialized cluster of pancreatic cells known as the islets of Langerhans. Alpha cells release glucagon that breaks down **glycogen** in the liver, causing blood glucose levels to rise. Beta cells release insulin, making it possible for cells to use blood glucose for energy. Type 1 and type 2 diabetes, the most common endocrine diseases of the pancreas, are caused by lack of insulin or insulin deficiencies.

 ## DIABETES MELLITUS

ICD-10: E10.XX (Type 1), E11.XX (TYPE 2)

Description

Diabetes mellitus is a chronic disorder of carbohydrate metabolism resulting from insufficient production of insulin or from inadequate utilization of this hormone by the body's cells. Insulin is produced by the beta cells within structures called the *islets of Langerhans* scattered throughout the pancreas. Insulin acts to lower the levels of glucose in the blood by enabling glucose absorption by body cells. When the beta cells cannot produce sufficient levels of insulin, the glucose concentration in the blood rises to abnormally high levels, a condition called **hyperglycemia.**

Deprived of glucose, the principal fuel of the body's cells, they begin to metabolize fats and proteins, depositing unusually high levels of wastes called **ketones** in the blood and causing a condition called diabetic **ketoacidosis.** These two conditions, hyperglycemia and diabetic ketoacidosis, are responsible for the host of troubling and often life-threatening symptoms of diabetes mellitus. There are four types of diabetes mellitus:

- *Immune-mediated diabetes type 1.* This form of the disease has an abrupt onset, usually appearing before age 30. Type 1 diabetes mellitus is frequently marked by the complete absence of insulin secretion, making this form of the disease difficult to regulate.
- *Type 2 diabetes.* The more common form of the disease typically has a gradual onset, usually appearing in adults over age 40. In type 2 diabetes mellitus, the pancreas generally retains some insulin-secreting ability, but the body is resistant to it. The management of this disease is less problematic than that of type 1 diabetes mellitus.
- *Gestational diabetes mellitus (GDM).* This type of diabetes develops during pregnancy but most often resolves after delivery; however, GDM places women at increased risk for the development of type 2 diabetes later in life.
- *Other specific types of diabetes.* This group refers to diabetes in persons with genetic defects of beta-cell function and persons with pancreatic dysfunction caused by drugs, chemicals, and infections.

Etiology

The exact causes of type 1 and type 2 diabetes mellitus are still not known. However, type 1 (formerly known as *insulin-dependent diabetes*) seems to be autoimmune or related to genetics. Individuals who develop this form of diabetes mellitus inherit a defective gene that renders them susceptible to the disease. At some point early in life, a triggering event occurs—perhaps a viral infection; this leads to the production of antibodies that destroy the beta cells of the islets of Langerhans. Risk factors of type 1 diabetes include genetics, viral infections, and perhaps low levels of vitamin D. Being born with jaundice or respiratory problems may be potential risk factors as well.

For type 2 diabetes mellitus (formerly known as non-insulin-dependent diabetes), little is known about how this form of the disease arises; however, obesity and inactivity are primary factors. Other risk factors include a family member with diabetes, gestational diabetes, advancing age, and race. African Americans, Native Americans, Hispanics, and Asian Americans have a higher risk of developing type 2 diabetes.

The American Diabetes Association (ADA) reports that about 9% of pregnant women develop gestational diabetes (GDM). The cause is unknown, but it is believed that hormones from the placenta block the action of the mother's insulin at a time when more insulin is needed. When the body is not able to make or use all the insulin it needs, glucose builds up in the blood, creating hyperglycemia. This condition usually goes away after delivery.

Other specific types of diabetes mellitus occur secondary to other diseases or conditions, such as chronic pancreatitis, pancreatic neoplasms, or drug-induced suppression of insulin production. Other endocrine disorders, such as Cushing syndrome, also may induce diabetes mellitus. In addition, the disease may be caused by genetic abnormalities that render the body's cells insensitive to insulin.

Signs and Symptoms

The classic symptoms of most cases of diabetes mellitus are **polyuria** (excessive formation and discharge of urine), **glycosuria** (glucose in the urine), and **polydipsia** (excessive thirst). In addition to these symptoms, individuals usually experience weight loss and **polyphagia** (eating abnormally large amounts of food at mealtimes). Those with type 1 diabetes are susceptible to an unusually high level of ketone bodies in the blood (ketoacidosis). Those with type 1 and 2 diabetes can experience additional symptoms such as repeated or hard-to-heal infections of the skin, gums, vagina, or bladder due to poor blood circulation; blurred vision; and pruritus. Other generalized symptoms of both forms of the disease may include muscle weakness and fatigue. Because type 2 diabetes has such a gradual onset, individuals with this form of the disease often are still asymptomatic when the disease is discovered during routine screening.

Diagnostic Procedures

An international committee—comprised of experts from the ADA, the European Association for the Study of Diabetes, and the International Diabetes Federation—recommended that testing for type 1 and type 2 diabetes include the following:

- *Glycated hemoglobin (A1c) test.* This blood test shows the average level of blood glucose for the past 2 to 3 months. It measures the percentage of blood glucose attached to **hemoglobin,** the part of red blood cells that carries oxygen. The higher the blood glucose level, the more hemoglobin will have glucose attached to it. An A1c level of 6.5% or higher on two separate tests indicates diabetes.
- *Random blood glucose test.* A blood test randomly taken (sometimes used during a regular checkup) with a blood glucose level of 200 mg/dL or higher suggests diabetes.
- *Fasting blood glucose test.* A blood test taken after an overnight fast with a blood glucose level of 126 mg/dL on two separate tests indicates diabetes. It is most accurate when administered in the morning.

(Blood glucose of 100 to 125 mg/dL is considered prediabetes.)

- *Oral glucose tolerance test.* Two blood tests are used to measure blood glucose. The first is given after a person fasts for at least 8 hours. If the blood glucose level is between 140 and 199 mg/dL, the person is said to have prediabetes with impaired glucose tolerance. The person is then tested 2 hours after drinking a liquid containing 75 grams of glucose dissolved in water. If the 2-hour glucose level is 200 mg/dL or above, this means the person has diabetes (Table 11.2).

Treatment

A combination of diet and exercise is used to treat most forms of diabetes mellitus. Individuals with type 1 diabetes need insulin therapy to survive. These clients typically need to follow a consistent pattern of monitoring blood glucose levels after an injection of insulin. A consistent routine of exercise, healthy food choices, and healthy weight can lessen the need for insulin. Those with type 2 diabetes follow the same regimen and may require medications or insulin therapy at some point. Diet therapy alone may control the symptoms. If not, hypoglycemic drugs may be prescribed. These drugs act to stimulate insulin production or make body cells more sensitive to insulin. In some instances, those with type 2 diabetes also may require injected insulin.

The goal for both type 1 and type 2 diabetes is to keep the blood glucose level as close to normal as possible. If necessary, an insulin pump is used to provide continuous insulin delivery. The pump can be attached to a thin plastic infusion set that releases insulin at a programmed and constant rate into the body, usually the abdomen. Newer devices are placed directly on the skin and insulin is made through a personal digital assistant (PDA) device that must be within a 6-foot range of the insulin delivery service. Even newer glucose sensing technology is known as an *artificial pancreas* that gives insulin based on the actual glucose levels determined by a glucose sensor. See http://www.medtronicdiabetes.com/treatment-and-products/minimed-530g-diabetes-system-with-enlite for information on one of the most common insulin pump systems.

Self-management of the disease is the treatment goal for all forms of diabetes mellitus. Education and client compliance are essential for the control of diabetes. Diabetic individuals can test their blood glucose levels and urine glucose and acetone at home so that they can make decisions about simple modifications to their diet, exercise, and insulin regimen. Regular medical supervision is required.

Complementary Therapy

A proper diet and effective weight control are essential for the treatment of both type 1 and type 2 diabetes. A diet high in complex carbohydrates and fiber, whole grains, legumes, and vegetables is essential. Exercise is a must. Yoga, meditation, guided imagery, and biofeedback training are often suggested for persons with diabetes.

➔ CLIENT COMMUNICATION

Teach clients how to pay special attention to the health of their teeth and feet, have a yearly eye examination, and carefully monitor their weight. Give information on support systems. Local hospitals often have diabetes education classes. Provide diet and exercise information and remind clients of the importance of careful monitoring of blood glucose levels. Diabetes mellitus is a chronic disease, requiring lifelong treatment and lifestyle changes.

Prognosis

The prognosis for an individual with diabetes mellitus can be uncertain. Even a well-motivated individual following a carefully balanced treatment regimen may eventually fall victim to one or more of the life-threatening late complications of the disease. In general, though, if diabetes mellitus is detected early and the affected individual's glucose levels can be stabilized to near normal levels, persons with diabetes can reasonably expect to live for many years with few complications. Client motivation and knowledge of the disease process contribute significantly to effective management of the disease.

Complications affecting the prognosis may be classified as acute or late. Acute complications include metabolic crises resulting from swings in the levels of blood glucose and blood pH. One such complication is diabetic coma. This condition may be triggered by skipping or delaying an insulin injection or consuming too much food. It also may be occasioned by a period of

Table 11.2	**Blood Test Levels for Diagnosis of Diabetes or Prediabetes**			
	A1c (PERCENT)	FASTING GLUCOSE (mg/dL)	ORAL GLUCOSE TOLERANCE (mg/dL)	RANDOM GLUCOSE (mg/dL)
Diabetes ↑	6.5 or above	126 or above	200 or above	200 or above
Prediabetes	5.7 to 6.4	100 to 125	140-199	140-199
Normal	About 5	99 or below	139 or below	139 or below

Adapted from American Diabetes Association by Carol D. Tamparo.

emotional or physical stress. Severe hyperglycemia induces polyuria and subsequent dehydration, whereas ketosis raises blood acidity. The affected individual may experience intense thirst and abdominal pain with nausea or vomiting and may become lethargic and drowsy. From that point, the individual may lapse into a coma. A person in a diabetic coma typically exhibits deep, slow breathing; has a "fruity" breath odor (from ketones in the blood transpiring through the lungs); and exhibits red, dry skin and a dry tongue. Individuals in a diabetic coma require emergency medical treatment consisting of a large dose of insulin and IV administration of fluids and sodium.

Another acute complication is insulin shock. This may occur from injecting too much insulin, inadequate food intake, or excessive exercise. As a result, hypoglycemia develops. The affected person may begin feeling faint and shaky and begin to perspire. Speech disturbances, double vision, and clouded consciousness may follow. From this point, the individual may become comatose. Regrettably, coma produced by insulin shock is often difficult to distinguish from diabetic coma. A few distinguishing features of insulin-induced coma include short, shallow breathing with no characteristic breath odor and moist, clammy skin. Individuals experiencing insulin shock require emergency medical treatment consisting of IV administration of glucose.

The late complications of diabetes mellitus typically appear only after many years or even decades. Over time, the lipids that are released into the blood as a consequence of ketosis may cause arteriosclerotic disease. The subsequent impairment of blood flow in the extremities may produce intermittent claudication or even tissue necrosis and gangrene, especially in the feet and lower legs. Other arteriosclerotic complications may include coronary artery disease and cerebrovascular accident.

The vascular system is not the only system subject to damage, however. Diabetes mellitus is a leading cause of kidney disease and renal failure, whereas diabetes-induced **retinopathy** (disease of the retina) is a leading cause of blindness. The nervous system also may be affected over time. Central nervous system damage may produce numbness, paresthesia, and intermittent but severe bouts of pain. Autonomic nervous system damage may produce difficulties in swallowing, constipation or diarrhea, and neurogenic bladder problems. Diabetes mellitus also may hamper an individual's immune response, causing slow wound healing and leaving the person open to frequent infections.

Prevention

There are currently no specific measures to prevent any form of diabetes mellitus. Effective weight management and an exercise regimen are essential and can help in the prevention of complications.

REALITY EPISODE

Colin was diagnosed with type 2 diabetes when he was 40. The first steps for treatment were to change his diet and reduce his weight. It was not easy. Colin is a long-haul truck driver who eats in restaurants most of the time and loves fried food and beer. He always avoids fruits and vegetables, because he only likes cream corn and an occasional summer watermelon slice. He is 45 pounds overweight and gets no exercise.

When diet and weight reduction were unsuccessful, Colin began to inject insulin twice daily. It wasn't long until Colin began skipping his injections. His aversion to the needle was severe, and there was no one on the road to make certain he followed his regimen. Further, his schedule was erratic. Sometimes he would drive long hours to make a delivery, sleeping only an hour or two along the way. It was not long before complications set in.

Colin's vision changed, he developed diabetic neuropathy, his cholesterol was dangerously high, and he sometimes suffered uncontrollable diarrhea.

With the complications described, can Colin continue his work? Explain.

Rewrite these paragraphs describing the outcome if Colin is successful in managing his diabetes.

Gonadal Diseases and Disorders

The hormones produced by the ovaries in the female—estrogen, progesterone, and inhibin—are essential for secondary sex characteristics, menstruation, and preparation for pregnancy as well as the pregnancy and delivery. The hormones produced by the testes in the male—testosterone and inhibin—are important for secondary sex characteristics and maturation of sperm. While authorities may identify a number of disorders or diseases that result when one or more of these hormones malfunctions, there is little agreement about whether the cause of the malfunction is hormone difficulties, genetic tendencies, disease, or totally unknown. Only one gonadal disorder is identified here. Other reproductive diseases and disorders are discussed in Chapter 16.

POLYCYSTIC OVARY SYNDROME

ICD-10: E28.2

Description

Polycystic ovary syndrome (PCOS) affects about 1 in 40 women in the United States and is a leading cause of infertility. Numerous cysts in the ovaries disrupt the monthly reproductive cycle, often causing irregular menstrual periods, excess hair growth, and obesity.

Etiology

In PCOS, the body produces an excess of androgens (usually made in only small amounts by the ovaries), and the ratio of LH to FSH is abnormally high. Either ovulation occurs less frequently than the usual 28-day cycle or the ovaries do not ovulate at all (anovulation). This imbalance causes either a very irregular menstrual cycle or no menstrual cycle. There appears to be a connection between excess amounts of insulin produced in the islets of Langerhans and excess amounts of androgen production in the ovaries. The cause of PCOS is essentially unknown. It is possible that PCOS is genetic in origin.

Signs and Symptoms

Women with PCOS usually have one or more of the following symptoms:

- Amenorrhea or irregular menses—periods at intervals of longer than 35 days or fewer than eight times a year
- Enlarged polycystic ovaries
- Obesity
- Infertility
- Prediabetes or type 2 diabetes
- **Hirsutism,** acne, or **alopecia**
- Hypertension and elevated blood cholesterol
- Sleep apnea

Diagnostic Procedures

A complete physical examination, including a pelvic examination, is performed. Blood tests are ordered to measure hormone levels and to test for diabetes (hemoglobin A1c and fasting glucose). An ultrasound can check ovaries and the thickness of the uterine lining.

Treatment

Medications to regulate the menstrual cycle are most likely prescribed. Treatment is also dependent upon whether pregnancy is being sought. To regulate the menstrual cycle, there are low-dose oral contraceptives that combine synthetic estrogen and progesterone and that decrease androgen production. Progesterone can be given for 7 to 10 days each month as an alternative, or an oral medication for type 2 diabetes may be prescribed. The oral medication treats insulin resistance but also improves ovulation and reduces androgen levels. Long-term treatment considers methods to reduce the risk of diabetes, hypertension, and cardiovascular disease. Exercise and diet to promote weight reduction are important.

Complementary Therapy

No significant complementary therapy is indicated.

CLIENT COMMUNICATION

PCOS is quite frustrating, especially to women who want to become pregnant. It is also frightening to know the possible complications, but remind clients that with proper treatment and regular follow-up examinations, PCOS can be managed.

Prognosis

Women with PCOS should be monitored regularly for lipid profiles and glucose levels. This disorder likely progresses until menopause. It also can lead to cardiovascular disease and cerebrovascular accident, type 2 diabetes, and endometrial cancer.

Prevention

There is no known prevention for PCOS, but early diagnosis and treatment can help to prevent long-term complications.

CHAPTER EPISODE—PART IV

The conversation continues with Susan's grandmother's comments. "It seems that you and I are pretty fortunate, Susan. We don't have some of the other symptoms that women with PCOS often suffer. It can be very embarrassing to have hair grow on your chest and abdomen like a man because of such high levels of testosterone. Many women, especially if they are overweight, have great difficulties losing the excess weight, but a healthy weight and a diet filled with fruits and vegetables are essential. You don't have that problem. And look, at my age, I do not have any of the complications many women suffer."

- What complications might Susan's grandmother be referring to?
- How can Susan make certain that she stays healthy and strong?

COMMON SYMPTOMS OF ENDOCRINE SYSTEM DISEASES AND DISORDERS

Individuals may present with the following common symptoms that are often related to one or more diseases or disorders and deserve attention from health-care professionals:

- Mental abnormalities
- Unusual change in energy level
- Changes in skin, nails, or hair
- Muscle atrophy

- Growth abnormalities
- Polyuria or polydipsia
- Cold or heat intolerance
- Unusual weight gain or loss
- Nausea or vomiting
- Irregular menstruation
- Erectile dysfunction

Carefully listen to what clients say about their symptoms, and do not make assumptions without careful consideration and proper diagnostics.

SUMMARY

The endocrine system provides a second and very important control center for the body, with the only exception that its function works more slowly than the nervous system. Hyperfunctioning or hypofunctioning of even one gland's hormones can affect the entire endocrine system. The glands and their hormones are so interrelated that diagnosis may be difficult, thus requiring patience and persistence on the part of health-care professionals.

 For more resources and to sharpen your skills with interactive exercises, visit DavisPlus at http://davisplus.fadavis.com. Keyword *Tamparo*.

ONLINE RESOURCES

Diabetes mellitus
http://www.diabetes.org

Hormone Health Network
www.hormone.org

Hypopituitarism
http://www.pituitary.org/disorders/hypopituitarism.aspx

National Endocrine and Metabolic Diseases Information Service
http://endocrine.niddk.nih.gov/pubs/addison/addison.htm

Polycystic Ovarian Syndrome Association
http://www.pcosupport.org

CASE STUDIES

Case Study 1

Robyn O'Donald, a young woman who makes many of her own clothes, notices that she must increase the size of the neck in her dresses and blouses. A recent photograph suggests to her that her eyes are almost bulging. She complains that she "fidgets" a lot and constantly feels compelled to be doing something. During the general physical examination, she reports that she has recently gained weight.

Case Study Questions

1. What do these signs and symptoms suggest?
2. What diagnostic procedures might the primary care provider perform or order?
3. What additional information about Robyn would be helpful?

Case Study 2

A mother calls for an appointment for her 12-year-old son, Daniel. He eats enormous amounts of food and seems to be thirsty all the time. His mother notes that Daniel seems to be going to the bathroom more frequently, and his soccer coach has relayed to her his concern that the boy is tired all the time.

Case Study Questions

1. What endocrine dysfunction is suggested by these signs and symptoms?
2. If Daniel does have the indicated dysfunction, what are the likely treatments?
3. What might be the prognosis for Daniel?

REVIEW QUESTIONS

Matching

Match each of the following definitions with its correct term:

_____ 1. Gigantism

_____ 2. Acromegaly

_____ 3. Hypopituitarism

_____ 4. Diabetes insipidus

_____ 5. Thyroid cancer

_____ 6. Cushing syndrome

_____ 7. Myxedema

_____ 8. Hypoparathyroidism

_____ 9. Diabetes mellitus

_____ 10. Cretinism

a. Bilateral hyperplasia of adrenal glands

b. Often caused by pituitary or hypothalamus tumors

c. Comes in four types

d. Hypothyroidism in adults

e. Hypersecretion of hGH before puberty

f. Disorder caused by insulin lack or resistance

g. Results in hypocalcemia

h. Hypersecretion of hGH after puberty

i. Classic symptom is polyuria

j. Excessive glucocorticosteroid hormones

k. Congenital hypothyroidism

Short Answer

1. A round, moon-shaped face is a classic symptom of _____.

2. The thyroid gland secretes the hormones _____ and _____.

3. A potentially fatal complication of Graves disease is _____.

4. Insufficient secretion of _____ by the posterior pituitary gland causes central diabetes insipidus.

5. In diabetes mellitus, injecting too much insulin, not receiving adequate food intake, or exercising excessively can cause the complication _____.

Multiple Choice

Place a checkmark next to the correct answer.

1. Which of the following identifies polycystic ovary syndrome?

_____ a. Is a leading cause of infertility

_____ b. Causes serious weight loss

_____ c. Occurs when the body produces too much androgen

_____ d. Results in amenorrhea or irregular menses

2. How is thyrotoxicosis explained?

_____ a. It is a mild illness from untreated hyperthyroidism.

_____ b. It is serious but is never fatal.

_____ c. It is a known complication of Addison disease.

_____ d. It is marked by sweating, fever, tachycardia, and pulmonary edema.

3. What is very specific about gestational diabetes mellitus?

_____ a. It is always referred to as GMD.

_____ b. It is a form of type 1 diabetes.

_____ c. It develops during pregnancy.

_____ d. It is more common in women over age 40.

4. What does complementary therapy for type 1 and type 2 diabetes suggest?

_____ a. Effective weight control and a regular exercise regimen

_____ b. A regular exercise program especially designed around long-distance running

_____ c. A diet low in complex carbohydrates, fiber, whole grains, vegetables, and fruit

_____ d. Hyperglycemic drugs to stimulate insulin production

5. What is known about hypercalcemia?

_____ a. Affects men twice as frequently as women

_____ b. Occurs when phosphorus is increased and calcium is decreased

_____ c. May be either primary or secondary in etiology

_____ d. Is often the result of chronic obstructive pulmonary disease

Discussion Question/Personal Reflection

1. Discuss the interrelatedness of the endocrine diseases and why hyperfunction or hypofunction of one gland often affects the other endocrine glands.

_____

_____

_____

_____

_____

_____

_____

_____

_____

_____

_____

_____

> *Nobody has ever measured, not even poets, how much the heart can hold.*
> —ZELDA FITZGERALD

Cardiovascular and Lymphatic System Diseases and Disorders

Albumin (ăl•bū'mĭn)
Aneurysm (ăn'ū•rĭzm)
Blast (blăst)
Bradycardia (brăd"ē•kăr'dē•ă)
Bruit (brwē)
Cardiac tamponade
    (kăr'dē•ăk tăm"pŏn•ād')
Cardioversion
    (kăr'dē•ō•věr"zhŭn)
Cellulitis (sěl"ū•lī'tĭs)
Claudication
    (klaw"dĭ•kā'shŭn)
Cryoablation (krī"ō•a•blā'shŏn)
Diastole (dī•ăs'tō•lē)
Dilatation (dĭl"ă•tā'shŭn)
Dyspnea (dĭsp•nē'ă)
Effusion (ě•fū'zhŭn)

Embolus (ěm'bō•lŭs)
Fibrillation (fĭ"brĭl•ā'shŭn)
Fibrinogen (fĭ•brĭn'ō•jěn)
Globulin (glŏb'ū•lĭn)
Hematemesis (hěm"ă•těm'ě•sĭs)
Hematopoietic
    (hē"mă•tō•poy•ět'ĭk)
Hemoglobin (hē"mō•glō'bĭn)
Hemostasis (hē"mŏs'tă•sĭs)
Idiopathic (ĭ"dē•ō•pă'thik)
Induration (ĭn"dū•rā'shun)
Lacteal (lăk'tē•ăl)
Lymphangitis (lĭm"făn•jī'tĭs)
Lymphocytopenia
    (lĭm"fō•sīt"ō•pē'nē•ă)
Megakaryocyte
    (měg"ă•kăr'ē•ō•sīt")

Menorrhagia (měn"ō•rā'jē•ă)
Orthopnea (or•thŏp'nē•ă)
Pericardiocentesis
    (pěr"ĭ•kăr"dē•ō•sěn•tē'sĭs)
Petechiae (plural) (pē•tē'kē•ē)
Prothrombin (prō•thrŏm'bĭn)
Reticulocyte (rě•tĭk'ū•lō•sīt)
Systole (sis'tō•lē)
Tachycardia (tăk"ē•kăr'dē•ă)
Thrombus (thrŏm'bŭs)
Tinnitus (tĭn•ī'tŭs)
Uremia (yù-'rē-mē-ə)
Vasodilator (văs"ō•dī•lā'tŏr)
Videoplethysmography
    (vid'ē•ō•pleth"iz•mog'ră-fē)

● *learning outcomes*

Upon successful completion of this chapter, you will be able to:

- Define the key terms.
- Recall anatomy and physiology of the cardiovascular and lymphatic systems.
- Describe three infectious heart diseases and the tests used in diagnosis.
- Explain transesophageal echocardiogram.
- Identify and contrast the three types of aneurysms.
- Discuss precautions to be taken with pericarditis.
- Discuss the etiology of the valvular heart diseases and disorders.
- Explain heart murmurs.
- Identify the signs and symptoms of essential hypertension.
- Recall the pressure readings for stage 1 hypertension.
- Identify individuals at high risk for developing hypertension.
- Identify those at risk and the diagnostic procedures and possible treatment suggested for coronary artery disease.
- Describe angina pectoris and recall the safe time of duration.
- Describe atrial fibrillation.
- List the classic signs and symptoms of myocardial infarction.

- Describe congestive heart failure and its treatment.
- Compare and contrast cardiac arrest with myocardial infarction.
- Discuss the use of automated external defibrillators for cardiac arrest.
- Identify and contrast three types of aneurysms.
- Compare atherosclerosis with arteriosclerosis.
- Discuss possible prevention techniques for thrombophlebitis.
- Identify the primary location for and the treatment of varicose veins.
- Compare and contrast four anemias.
- Recall the descriptions of the four main types of leukemias.
- Discuss the various treatments of leukemias.
- Restate the prognosis for the four types of leukemias.
- Define *lymphedema*.
- Compare non-Hodgkin and Hodgkin lymphomas.
- Recall the three types of bone marrow transplants.
- List at least six common symptoms of cardiovascular and lymphatic diseases and disorders.

CHAPTER EPISODE—PART I

Barney, a 61-year-old dentist, has been experiencing fatigue that does not disappear after sleep. He has difficulty breathing, difficulty catching his breath, and profuse sweating. He retired early from his years as a dentist due to a viral infection that caused heart muscle damage, but he is truly alarmed when he is unable to walk across the backyard to his wonderful rose garden. He figures it is time for another check with his cardiologist.

- What might these symptoms tell the cardiologist?
- What tests might be ordered?

CARDIOVASCULAR AND LYMPHATIC SYSTEMS ANATOMY AND PHYSIOLOGY REVIEW

The cardiovascular system is composed of the heart and blood vessels. The heart pumps blood through blood vessels in a closed system. Arteries carry blood from the heart to capillaries in the body tissues, whereas veins carry blood back to the heart. The heart and blood vessels function to transport oxygen, nutrients, and hormones to cells and to remove waste products and carbon dioxide from cells. The heart and blood vessels work together to pump and circulate the equivalent of 7,200 quarts of blood through the heart every 24 hours.

Heart

The heart, about the size of a human fist, is made of muscle and valves (Fig. 12.1). There are four chambers—two atria and two ventricles. The walls of the heart chambers have a thick cardiac muscle tissue called the *myocardium* that contracts, providing the force behind the pumping action of the heart. The endocardium, a single layer of epithelium, lines the chambers of the heart and covers the heart valves. The epicardium is a thin membrane that attaches to the exterior surface of the myocardium. The atria walls are separated by the interatrial septum, and the ventricle walls are separated by the interventricular septum.

The four valves of the heart—the tricuspid or right atrioventricular, pulmonary, bicuspid or mitral, and aortic valves—allow the blood to flow in only one direction (see Fig. 12.1B). Contraction of the heart is called **systole,** and relaxation of the heart is called **diastole.** When the atria contract (atrial systole), the ventricles relax (ventricular diastole). Then the ventricles contract (ventricular systole), and the atria relax

(atrial diastole). There is a short interval when *both* atria and ventricles relax. This whole process constitutes the cardiac cycle.

Blood and Blood Vessels

The blood vessel network of the body is composed of arteries, arterioles (small arteries), veins, venules (small veins), and capillaries. Arteries carry blood from the heart; veins carry blood to the heart; capillaries link the arteries and the veins. Blood transports hormones, nutrients, and waste products; it defends the body against infection; and its ability to clot prevents blood loss. Blood circulation is either pulmonary or systemic. Pulmonary circulation pumps blood from the heart into the lungs (Fig. 12.2); systemic circulation pumps blood from the heart to the remainder of the body (Figs. 12.3 and 12.4).

Blood is made of plasma and blood cells. Although thicker than water, blood is about 92% water. Plasma is the transportation system for the hormones, nutrients, and waste products. It also consists of important proteins, including **prothrombin** and **fibrinogen,** important in blood clotting; **albumin,** which helps to keep blood from leaking out of the blood vessels; and three types of **globulins** that assist in the immune response. The blood cell types are the erythrocytes, leukocytes, and platelets. Erythrocytes, or red blood cells (RBCs), carry oxygen on the protein **hemoglobin.** The leukocytes, or white blood cells (WBCs), protect the body from infection and provide immunity against some diseases. The five types of WBCs are neutrophils, eosinophils, basophils, lymphocytes, and monocytes. The platelets or thrombocytes are pieces of cells that contribute to blood clotting and **hemostasis.**

Lymph and Lymph Vessels

The lymphatic system is composed of lymph capillaries, **lacteals** (capillaries in the villus of the small intestine), nodes, vessels, and ducts. The lymphatic system transports fluids, nutrients, and wastes exuded from tissues back to the bloodstream through connections with major veins. Figure 12.5 shows the relationship between lymphatic vessels and the cardiovascular system. Without the lymphatic system, fluid would accumulate in tissue spaces, and "foreign" particles, such as infection, microorganisms, and viruses, would cause disease. The lymphatic system also functions to attack toxins and cancer cells. The thymus and spleen are two important lymphatic organs whose function is similar to the lymphatic system.

Lymph nodes are masses of lymphatic tissue found singly or in groups along the route of lymph vessels. They serve as a filter by destroying microorganisms and abnormal cells harmful to the body through a process

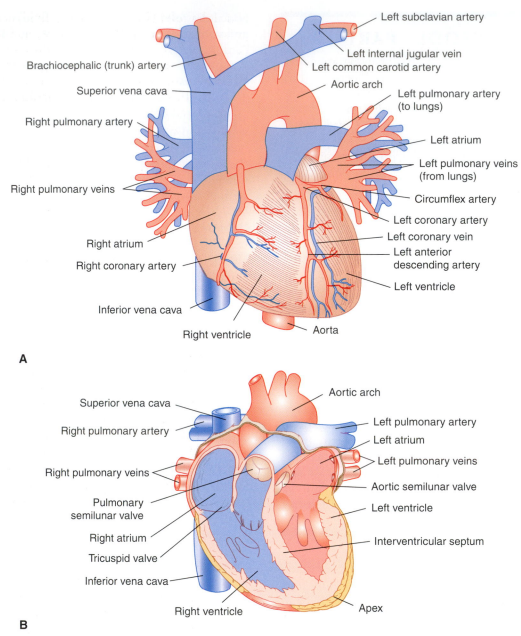

Figure 12.1 (A) Anterior view of the heart and major blood vessels. (B) Interior view of the heart.
(Adapted from Scanlon, VC, and Sanders, T: Essentials of Anatomy and Physiology, ed. 5. Philadelphia: F.A. Davis, 2007, p 276, with permission.)

called *phagocytosis*. An increase in the size of the nodes usually indicates a high level of phagocytosis. Three pairs of lymph nodes that are relatively easy to palpate are the cervical nodes (side of the neck), axillary nodes (in the armpit), and inguinal nodes (in the groin region).

The spleen, usually considered a part of the lymphatic system, helps to store platelets and destroys platelets and old RBCs when they are no longer necessary. It also destroys some foreign microorganisms and produces antibodies to foreign antigens. The thymus gland produces T lymphocytes in its stem cells. These cells move to the spleen, lymph nodes, and lymph tissue where they help control cell-mediated immunity.

Diseases of the Heart Muscle

While *heart disease* is the term often used to describe many diseases of the heart, in this section, it refers to diseases of the heart muscle itself. The majority of heart muscle diseases are related to inflammation or infection—thus the term *carditis*.

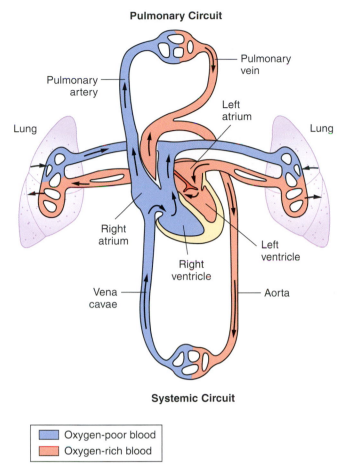

Pulmonary Circuit

Pulmonary vein

Pulmonary artery

Lung

Left atrium

Lung

Right atrium

Left ventricle

Right ventricle

Vena cavae

Aorta

Systemic Circuit

■ Oxygen-poor blood
■ Oxygen-rich blood

Figure 12.2 Pulmonary circulation circuit showing oxygen and carbon dioxide exchange to and from the lungs.

PERICARDITIS

ICD-10: I31.9

Description

Pericarditis is an inflammation of the pericardium, the saclike membrane that surrounds and protects the heart muscle. The disease can be acute or chronic.

Etiology

Pericarditis is usually **idiopathic,** meaning it is of unknown cause. It also may be caused by bacterial, fungal, or viral infection of the pericardium. The disease may be caused by metastasized neoplasms, rheumatic fever, **uremia,** or hypothyroidism. Trauma, heart surgery, myocardial infarction (MI), or any injury that causes blood to leak into the pericardial sac also may incite pericarditis.

Signs and Symptoms

The classic symptom of pericarditis is a sharp and often sudden pleuritic pain that increases with deep inspiration. The fluctuating nature of pericardial pain clearly differentiates it from the pain produced by an MI. If

pericardial **effusion** (an escape of fluid) occurs in acute pericarditis, **orthopnea, dyspnea,** and **tachycardia** (abnormally rapid heart rate) typically result. If the fluid accumulates rapidly, the pressure against the heart may result in clammy skin, pallor, and a decrease in blood pressure. This condition, called **cardiac tamponade,** is considered life-threatening.

Diagnostic Procedures

Auscultation may reveal a grating sound heard as the heart beats or pericardial friction rub, a classic symptom. Inflammation may be reflected in laboratory data showing elevated WBC count, erythrocyte sedimentation rate (ESR), and cardiac enzyme levels. An electrocardiogram (ECG) will show changes and may detect cardiac arrhythmias or irregularities in the force or rhythm of heart action. An ultrasound may be given to detect the presence of fluid in the pericardial sac. An echocardiogram also can detect the buildup of fluid.

Treatment

Underlying causes of the pericarditis must be treated and symptomatic relief provided. Bed rest, with the upper body elevated, may be prescribed, along with analgesics. If the cause of pericarditis is bacterial, antibiotic therapy may be started. The drug colchicine is the first-line treatment for and prevention of pericarditis by reducing inflammation in the body. NSAIDs and corticosteroids are also often prescribed. If heart function is seriously compromised by excess fluid around the heart, **pericardiocentesis**—surgical puncture or tapping to promote drainage—may be part of the treatment.

Complementary Therapy

Integrative medicine practitioners will work closely with the primary care providers (PCPs) to alleviate any infection. A nutritious, well-balanced diet that includes minimal amounts of saturated fats and is high in complex carbohydrates and whole grains, fruits, and vegetables is recommended to enhance the body's ability to fight the infection.

⊕ CLIENT COMMUNICATION

Having clients in a sitting position or leaning forward helps relieve the chest pain. Such pain causes fear in clients, so take measures to alleviate the fear. Listening and allowing clients to talk about their concerns might prove helpful.

Prognosis

The prognosis is determined by the etiology of the particular case, but generally it is good. Pericarditis typically lasts from 1 to 3 weeks but can recur, usually within a few months of the original episode. Recurrent pericarditis is difficult to treat and occurs in as many as 15% of cases.

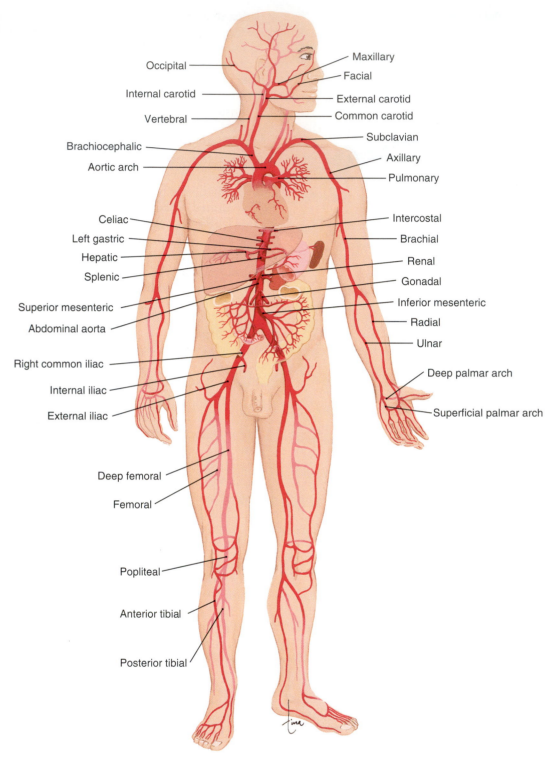

Figure 12.3 Systemic arteries. The aorta and its major branches are shown in anterior view. *(From Scanlon, VC, and Sanders, T: Essentials of Anatomy and Physiology, ed. 6. Philadelphia: F.A. Davis, 2011, p 321, with permission.)*

Prevention

Because pericarditis can result from a number of problems, there are no routine guidelines to prevent the condition. In general, however, help prevent heart-damaging infection by advising clients to practice good hygiene and get recommended immunizations. Wearing a seat belt helps reduce the risk of any trauma-related pericarditis. Measures to reduce the risk of coronary artery disease by not smoking, eating a healthy, weight-conscious diet, and exercising should be taken.

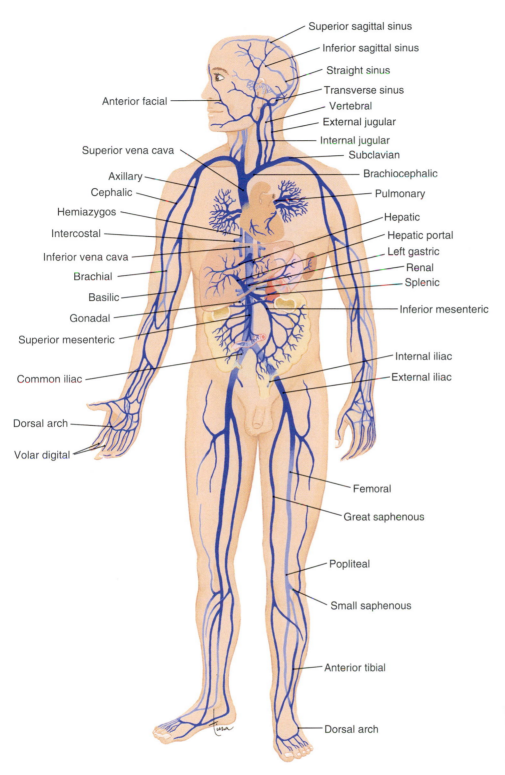

Figure 12.4 Systemic veins shown in anterior view. *(From Scanlon, VC, and Sanders, T: Essentials of Anatomy and Physiology, ed. 6. Philadelphia: F.A. Davis, 2011, p 322, with permission.)*

MYOCARDITIS

ICD-10: I51.4

Description

Myocarditis is inflammation of the cardiac muscle and conduction system without evidence of MI. The condition may be acute or chronic.

Etiology

Myocarditis may be caused by viral or bacterial infection, with viral infection being most common. Myocardial inflammation also may be caused by various toxins, or it may be a side effect of certain drugs or radiation therapy.

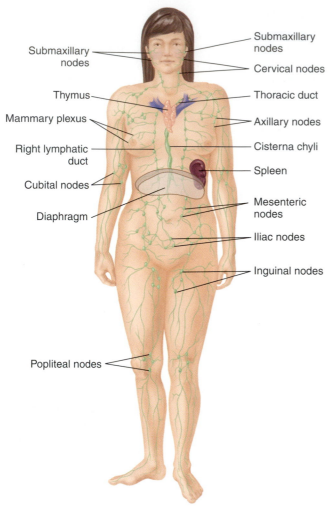

Submaxillary nodes

Submaxillary nodes

Cervical nodes

Thymus

Thoracic duct

Mammary plexus

Axillary nodes

Right lymphatic duct

Cisterna chyli

Cubital nodes

Spleen

Diaphragm

Mesenteric nodes

Iliac nodes

Inguinal nodes

Popliteal nodes

Figure 12.5 System of lymph vessels and major groups of lymph nodes, showing spleen and thymus glands.

Signs and Symptoms

The signs and symptoms of myocarditis are often non-specific, but they may include dyspnea, palpitations, fever, myalgia, and fatigue. Pleuritic pain and chest discomfort are often reported. Shortness of breath and tachycardia are common.

Diagnostic Procedures

A medical history may reveal a recent upper respiratory infection. Laboratory tests may show elevated cardiac enzyme, WBC, and ESR levels. An ECG typically shows diffuse ST-segment and T-wave abnormalities, conduction defects, and other supraventricular arrhythmias. If an ECG does not show a problem, then a Holter monitor may be worn for a few days to hopefully provide a clear picture of the problem. A chest x-ray, an echocardiogram, and magnetic resonance imaging (MRI) are helpful in further identifying myocarditis. An endomyocardial biopsy is a useful tool in diagnosis in some cases.

Treatment

Treatment is aimed at managing symptoms, treating any underlying conditions, and preventing myocardial damage. Bed rest is helpful in allowing the body to fight infection, and antibiotics may be needed in the case of a bacterial infection. Oxygen therapy and sodium restriction may be recommended to decrease the heart's workload. Agents such as diuretics that increase urine output and agents to increase the heartbeat, making it stronger, may be prescribed. Commonly prescribed today are angiotensin-converting enzyme (ACE) inhibitors, angiotensin II receptor blockers or inhibitors, and beta blockers. These medications work to relax heart blood vessels, helping blood to flow more easily or to regulate the heartbeat.

Complementary Therapy

See "Pericarditis."

⊖ CLIENT COMMUNICATION

Initially, it is important to help clients understand the necessity for bed rest and the need to lead a sedentary lifestyle for 6 to 12 months to allow the heart to heal. Dietary information to help clients reduce sodium intake is beneficial.

Prognosis

The prognosis for an individual with uncomplicated myocarditis is usually good. When complications include congestive heart failure, pulmonary edema, or left or right ventricular failure (cardiogenic shock), the prognosis is less promising.

Prevention

There is no specific prevention for myocarditis; see "Pericarditis."

ENDOCARDITIS

ICD-10: I38

Description

Endocarditis, also known as *infective endocarditis,* is inflammation of the membrane lining the valves and chambers of the heart. It can be acute, subacute, or chronic. The disease is characterized by the formation of abnormal growths called *vegetations* on the heart valves in the endocardial lining or in the endothelium of a blood vessel. A vegetation forms as the infected tissue is covered by a layer of platelets and fibrin. These vegetations may embolize to the spleen, kidneys, central nervous system, or lungs.

Etiology

Endocarditis is most frequently caused by infection from group A nonhemolytic streptococcal bacteria following septic thrombophlebitis; open-heart surgery for prosthetic valves; or bone, skin, and pulmonary infections. Bacteria can enter the bloodstream through catheters and IV drug injections. It also may arise as a consequence of sexually transmitted diseases or sores in the mouth caused by poor gums and teeth. Infecting organisms more readily establish themselves on the endocardium of a heart already damaged by congenital or acquired defects, although healthy endocardial tissue may be infected as well.

Signs and Symptoms

Symptoms vary according to the etiology and portion of the heart affected. There may be weakness and fatigue, night sweats, chills, and an intermittent fever that persists for weeks. A loud regurgitant heart murmur may be heard that was not previously detected. Additional symptoms may arise if the vegetations break off into the bloodstream to form embolisms that lodge in other organs. Paralysis can occur if a large embolus or mass of nondissolved matter lodges in the brain. If an **embolus** obstructs circulation in the kidney, there may be blood in the urine. If tiny vegetations lodge in the small vessels of the skin, subcutaneous ruptures called **petechiae** (pinpoint hemorrhagic spots on the skin) may appear.

Diagnostic Procedures

The medical history may reveal predisposing factors of endocarditis and a new heart murmur. Blood cultures will identify the bacteria in the bloodstream. A transesophageal echocardiogram (TEE) (see Client Communication) may reveal the presence of vegetative growths. Also commonly used in diagnosis are the chest x-ray and an ECG.

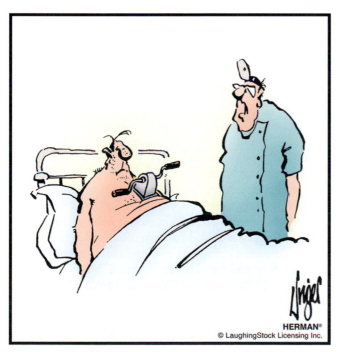

"It's just a back-up system for your pacemaker."

HERMAN®
© LaughingStock Licensing Inc.

HERMAN© is reprinted with permission from LaughingStock Licensing Inc., Ottawa, Canada. All rights reserved.

Treatment

It is important to eliminate the infecting organism. Treatment may require IV antibiotic therapy in a hospital followed by antibiotic therapy to continue over several weeks. Bed rest, analgesics, and increased fluid intake are helpful. Surgery may be necessary to repair severe valvular damage or to replace a valve with an artificial one.

Complementary Therapy

See "Pericarditis." Client should consider carrying a wallet card to identify risk of endocarditis. A sample can be downloaded from the American Heart Association's website at http://www.americanheart.org.

⊸ CLIENT COMMUNICATION

Explain the TEE to clients. The throat is numbed with an anesthetic spray. Then an IV sedative is given to help in relaxation. An ultrasound device is passed through the mouth into the esophagus. A tiny TEE transducer is placed at the end of the thin flexible tube that will transfer the images from the transducer to the monitor. This tube is swallowed with minimal discomfort as the transducer is positioned in the esophagus, directly behind the heart. By rotating and moving the transducer tip, the specialist can examine the heart from different angles.

Prognosis

If caused by bacteria, the disease is curable when treated early with antibiotics. Complications can be serious, however, and may cause death. These complications include congestive heart failure (CHF) and damage to vital organs as a result of embolism.

Prevention

Individuals at high risk should receive antibiotic therapy before undergoing surgery or certain procedures. High-risk individuals are those with an artificial heart valve, a previous endocarditis episode, congenital heart defects, and heart transplants. The procedures that may require this antibiotic therapy are:

- Dental procedures that will manipulate gum tissue and teeth
- Procedures for respiratory tract diseases
- Procedures for infected skin or musculoskeletal tissue

Valvular Heart Diseases and Disorders

Diseased heart valves may malfunction in two ways: The opening formed by a valve may be too large to close completely, so blood leaks back past the valve into the heart chamber from which it was pumped. Or the valve opening may be too narrow, a condition called *valvular stenosis,* so it impedes the flow of blood through the valve when it should be open and allows blood to leak back when it should be closed (regurgitation). Either condition can cause heart failure. The two most commonly affected valves are the mitral and the aortic valves, whereas the pulmonary and tricuspid valves rarely are affected. Diseased valves, the result of rheumatic heart disease, are far less common today because the incidence of rheumatic heart disease is now considered rare in the United States.

Heart murmurs—periodic sounds heard during auscultation with a stethoscope—are generated by blood flow through the heart when there is an anomaly. Murmurs can be caused by blood leaking back through an incompetent or deformed valve, by blood forcing its way through a narrowed valve, by **dilatation** (enlargement of the heart), or by a rapid diastolic flow. Exercise and tachycardia increase the intensity of any murmur.

Murmurs are graded on the basis of intensity, with grade 1 for the least intense and grade 6 for the most intense. Detecting and interpreting heart murmurs help to estimate their severity and diagnose valvular heart disease. Certain murmurs are consistently associated with severe heart dysfunction. Others may be insignificant.

MITRAL INSUFFICIENCY/STENOSIS

ICD-10: I34.0 or I34.8

Description

In mitral insufficiency, blood from the left ventricle flows back into the left atrium. In mitral stenosis, blood flow is obstructed from the left atrium to the left ventricle. In both cases, the result is an enlarged left atrium.

Etiology

Mitral insufficiency, or stenosis, is usually secondary to untreated streptococcal infection, MI, or infective endocarditis in which vegetations on the heart valves cause stenosis. In the past, rheumatic fever was a leading cause. Severe left-sided heart failure, or mitral valve prolapse, a falling or dropping down of the valve tissue, may occur (Fig. 12.6).

Signs and Symptoms

In both conditions, there may be orthopnea, dyspnea, fatigue, palpitations, peripheral edema, atrial **fibrillation,** pulmonary hypertension, and distention of the jugular veins. Abnormal heart sounds can be identified during auscultation.

Diagnostic Procedures

In both conditions, transthoracic echocardiography and electrocardiography may establish the diagnosis,

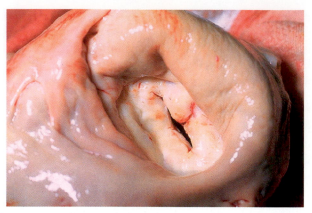

Figure 12.6   Gross pathology showing mitral stenosis. The left atrium has been opened to show thickened mitral valve leaflets from above. *(Centers for Disease Control and Prevention. Dr. Edwin P. Ewing, Jr. Creation date 1973.)*

as can a chest x-ray. Cardiac catheterization may be necessary to fully identify the severity of the problem. The results of auscultation will be specific to each condition.

Treatment

The treatment approach depends on the severity of the symptoms. Balloon valvuloplasty (also called *percutaneous balloon valvuloplasty*), a surgical procedure to open a narrowed heart valve, may be performed. In the most serious cases, the treatment of choice is surgical replacement with an artificial valve.

Complementary Therapy

It is important to remember to practice good oral health by brushing and flossing daily and seeing a dentist on a regular basis. Limit intake of caffeine, salt, alcohol, and maintain a healthy weight. Exercise regularly.

⟳ CLIENT COMMUNICATION

If surgery is necessary, prepare clients both preoperatively and postoperatively. You can tell them that with balloon valvuloplasty, a thin tube or balloon-tipped catheter is inserted through the skin in the groin area into a blood vessel. The tube is threaded up to the opening of the narrowed heart valve where the balloon is inflated to stretch the valve open. The procedure is performed in a cardiac catheterization laboratory and takes about 4 hours.

Prognosis

The prognosis is good. The disease usually is not progressive, and many clients live a long time without surgery. Both mitral insufficiency and stenosis can lead to right ventricular hypertrophy and right ventricular failure.

Prevention

There is no known prevention for mitral insufficiency/stenosis other than the prevention of rheumatic fever, infections, and MI.

AORTIC INSUFFICIENCY/STENOSIS

ICD-10: I35.X*

Description

Aortic insufficiency results in blood flowing back into the left ventricle, eventually causing left ventricular hypertrophy and failure. Aortic stenosis causes increased ventricular pressure as a result of a greater cardiac workload. Left ventricular failure may result.

Etiology

Aortic stenosis is a fairly common congenital heart defect in children. Stenosis of the aortic valve, illustrated in Figure 12.7, can occur in individuals in their 40s and 50s and is a fairly common ailment among elderly people when there is calcium buildup on the valve. Aortic insufficiency or stenosis can also be the result of rheumatic fever, but that is much less likely today.

Signs and Symptoms

Aortic insufficiency/stenosis may be asymptomatic until the problem progresses. Dyspnea, syncope, angina, fatigue (especially on exertion), and palpitations then become common symptoms. Congestion in the pulmonary vein, CHF, and pulmonary edema may occur on failure of the left ventricle.

Diagnostic Procedures

Auscultation may reveal a characteristic diastolic murmur in aortic insufficiency and a systolic murmur in aortic stenosis. As in most of the valvular heart diseases, common diagnostic procedures include chest x-ray, ECG, and cardiac catheterization.

Treatment

The person may need only to be assessed on a yearly basis with an ECG and an echocardiogram. Most cases require balloon valvuloplasty or surgical replacement of the aortic valve.

Complementary Therapy

See complementary therapy for mitral insufficiency.

⊙➔ CLIENT COMMUNICATION

Tell clients to limit strenuous exercise. If surgery is necessary, help clients understand the procedure. Prevention of further heart damage is important. It can be helpful for clients to monitor their blood pressure to keep hypertension under control.

Prognosis

The prognosis varies depending on the nature and severity of the disease. Complications include arrhythmias; cardiac failure; and ventricular fibrillation, an involuntary quivering of the heart muscle fibers.

Prevention

There is no known prevention for aortic insufficiency/stenosis other than avoiding endocarditis and hypertension.

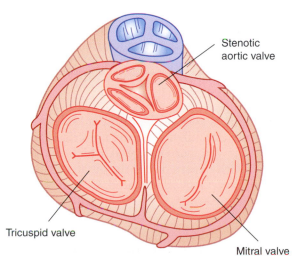

Figure 12.7 Stenosis of aortic valve. Prevents blood from flowing freely from the left ventricle to the aorta.

- Stenotic aortic valve
- Tricuspid valve
- Mitral valve

CHAPTER EPISODE—PART II

When Barney makes a call to his cardiologist, the receptionist makes certain to schedule his appointment for as soon as possible. The examination includes both an ECG and an echocardiogram performed in the facility, and Dr. Block also orders a chest x-ray and some blood work. Dr. Block has a frank discussion with Barney, revealing that he is certain his congestive heart failure has now reached the critical phase. Dr. Block further explains that if Barney really wants to continue to walk out into his garden, his only hope is a heart transplant. After discussion with his wife, Barney agreed to have his name placed on the list for a heart transplant.

- In the meantime, what must Barney do to stay healthy?
- What medications might be prescribed?

*The X represents the fourth digit that is often required and supplied once more detailed information about the disease or disorder is made known to the provider.

Hypertensive Heart Disease

 ESSENTIAL HYPERTENSION

ICD-10: I10

When the heart must work against increased resistance in the form of high blood pressure, hypertensive heart disease often results. About 75 million people in the United States suffer from hypertension. What constitutes hypertension—high blood pressure—may be different for each person and varies with a person's age, gender, race, and any concomitant disease; it quite often goes undetected. However, the medical community generally agrees that stage 1 hypertension exists if systolic pressure (contraction) persists over 140 mm Hg and diastolic pressure (relaxation) persists over 90 mm Hg. The most severe hypertension, stage 2 hypertension, is a systolic pressure of 160 mm Hg or higher or a diastolic pressure of 100 mm Hg or higher. Many persons with hypertension live long, vigorous lives. Others do not respond well to treatment and eventually die of heart failure, a cerebrovascular accident (CVA), or kidney dysfunction.

Description

Essential hypertension is persistently elevated blood pressure that develops without apparent cause and often progresses over a number of years. It affects nearly everyone eventually.

Etiology

Although essential hypertension is idiopathic, some persons are at a higher risk than others. They include African Americans, chronically stressed individuals, the obese, and those who consume a diet high in salt and saturated fats. Genetic factors are assumed to play an important role in hypertension. Insulin resistance and hyperinsulinemia may be possible causes of hypertension. Older persons, those with sedentary lifestyles, smokers, and women taking oral contraceptives also have a higher risk of hypertension.

Signs and Symptoms

Persons with hypertension may remain asymptomatic for months or years or until vascular changes in the heart, brain, or kidneys occur. There may be vague symptoms of light-headedness, **tinnitus** (ringing in the ears), nocturia, a tendency to tire easily, and palpitations.

Diagnostic Procedures

Diagnosis is relatively easy and usually occurs during a medical examination. Blood pressure readings taken on at least two separate occasions after the individual has rested will show pressure greater than 140/90 mm Hg.

It is important that a history of blood pressure readings be kept for comparison, because blood pressure can vary according to various situations. An abnormal sound called **bruits** may be heard on auscultation. ECG and chest x-ray will help detect cardiovascular damage.

Treatment

Although there is no cure for essential hypertension, a change in lifestyle (no smoking and limited alcohol consumption) and diet, along with antihypertensive drug therapy, can help to control the condition. A diet low in salt and fat and high in potassium that promotes a consumption of fruits, vegetables, and low-fat dairy products is recommended. Regular exercise, maintaining a healthy weight, and a reduction in stress are helpful. Diuretics or **vasodilators** (drugs to relax and expand blood vessels) also may be prescribed.

Complementary Therapy

Focusing on a nutritional diet low in fat and high in fruits, vegetables, and omega-3 fatty acids is essential. Some supplements have shown validity. They include ground flaxseed, calcium, and cod liver oil tablets. It is recommended that clients discuss any supplements with their PCP because some may interact with medications and cause harmful side effects. If obesity is an issue, a program of weight loss should begin. Biofeedback, relaxation, meditation, yoga, and hypnotherapy may help reduce stress. All practitioners should emphasize the importance of an exercise regimen.

⊙ CLIENT COMMUNICATION

Because the client's lifestyle likely needs modification, stress reduction and weight loss should begin. A nutritionist can assist with diet modification. Encourage regular physical activity. It may be helpful for clients to purchase a home blood pressure kit in order to regularly monitor their blood pressure.

Prognosis

The prognosis is good if the disorder is detected early and if clients carefully follow the prescribed treatment regimen. The younger the age at which the person is diagnosed with hypertension, the greater is the reduction in life expectancy if untreated. Complications may include atherosclerosis, CVA, heart failure, and kidney failure.

Prevention

Prevention includes minimizing controllable risk factors, such as diet, stress, obesity, and sedentary lifestyle. It is recommended that clients limit alcohol and salt intake and not smoke.

Coronary Diseases and Disorders

CORONARY ARTERY DISEASE

ICD-10: I25.9

Description

The American Heart Association indicates that coronary heart disease (CHD) is the single leading cause of death in America, affecting more than 13 million Americans. CHD causes heart attack and angina. More specifically, coronary artery disease (CAD) is the narrowing of the coronary arteries to such an extent that there is an inadequate blood supply to portions of the myocardium (Fig. 12.8). As the opening or lumen of the coronary artery narrows, the reduced blood flow deprives cells in the myocardium, causing them to weaken and die, a condition called *ischemia*. The myocardial cells are then replaced with scar tissue.

Etiology

The leading cause of CAD is atherosclerosis, a condition in which the lumen of the coronary arteries is narrowed by fatty, fibrous plaque that is formed by the abnormal accumulation of fat, cholesterol, calcium, and other cellular waste (see "Atherosclerosis"). Many factors seem to predispose individuals to this condition, including age, heredity, obesity, elevated serum cholesterol, decreased serum high-density cholesterol, diabetes mellitus, hypertension, smoking, and stress. The condition is more common in men, in postmenopausal women, and in middle-aged and elderly persons.

Signs and Symptoms

An immediate result of inadequate blood supply to the myocardium is angina, a burning, squeezing, tightness in the chest that may radiate to the neck, the shoulder blade, and the left arm. Women are apt to also experience abdominal and/or back discomfort. Nausea, vomiting, sweating, shortness of breath, and a feeling of panic may accompany these symptoms. A complete discussion of angina pectoris follows.

Diagnostic Procedures

The medical history may reveal one or more of the risk factors for CAD and a pattern of angina. An ECG is taken. Stress testing is likely to occur, with or without an echocardiogram. A computed tomography (CT) scan may be ordered. A magnetic resonance angiogram (MRA) or cardiac catheterization also may be necessary to determine the amount of heart damage.

Treatment

The goal of treatment is to lessen the angina by reducing myocardial oxygen demand or increasing oxygen supply. Treatment addresses lifestyle changes, beneficial medications, or surgery. Nitroglycerin preparations are helpful in increasing the oxygen supply to the heart by dilating the coronary arteries. Cholesterol-reducing medications can be beneficial. Primary care providers often advise clients to take one aspirin daily to reduce the hazard of blood clots occluding the coronary arteries. Beta

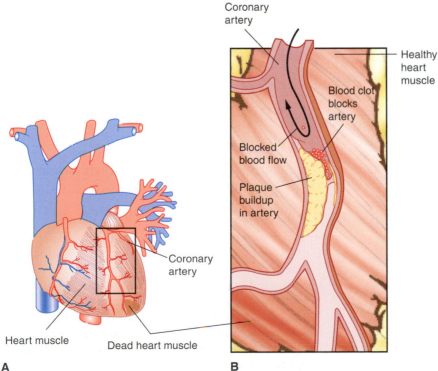

A

Coronary artery

Coronary artery

Healthy heart muscle

Blood clot blocks artery

Blocked blood flow

Plaque buildup in artery

Heart muscle

Dead heart muscle

B

Figure 12.8 Coronary artery vessels in anterior view revealing plaque buildup in the left coronary artery of coronary artery disease.

blockers can reduce high blood pressure, and calcium channel blockers help dilate vessels, increasing the blood flow to the heart. Coronary artery bypass surgery may be necessary to bridge obstructive lesions. There may be an attempt to compress the fatty plaque deposits in the coronary arteries by cardiac catheterization or by laser angioplasty, both of which correct occlusion by vaporizing fatty deposits. ACE inhibitors and angiotensin II receptor blockers (ARBs) decrease blood pressure and may help prevent progression of CAD. When a heart attack occurs, ACE inhibitors reduce the risk of future attacks. Dietary restrictions may be necessary, and persons are encouraged to refrain from smoking. A regular exercise regimen is encouraged.

Complementary Therapy

See "Essential Hypertension." The *American Journal of the Medical Sciences* has reported that at a recent symposium on nutrition and heart diseases, vitamin D deficiency was identified as an increased risk factor for cardiovascular disease. Primary care providers can easily check vitamin D levels, and if there is a deficiency, it should be corrected.

Clients who have any of the coronary diseases are likely to experience additional stress that comes from worry about quality of life and fear that comes from the threat of another episode. Accompanying depression is likely. Referral to support systems or counseling may be helpful, as well as any of the mind-body practices to help reduce stress.

⊕ CLIENT COMMUNICATION

It is paramount to teach clients the importance of addressing risk factors to include stress reduction, weight reduction, and engagement in a physical activity, such as walking, running, or swimming. If the person smokes, recommend cessation.

Prognosis

The prognosis varies greatly depending on the amount of arterial blockage, the extent of damage to the heart muscle, and the success of lifestyle changes. Possible complications include a serious heart attack or myocardial infarction.

Prevention

The best way to prevent CAD is to minimize controllable risk factors.

ANGINA PECTORIS

ICD-10: I20.8 or I20.9

Description

Angina pectoris is uncomfortable squeezing, pressure, fullness, or pain in the chest resulting from ischemia to a part of the myocardium. It is identified in three forms:

- *Stable angina* (the most common) is predictable and usually occurs during times of stress or exercise.
- *Unstable angina* is unexpected, may occur at rest, does not readily respond to nitroglycerin treatment, and often signals a blood clot creating blockage of one of the coronary arteries. Unstable angina is a medical emergency.
- *Variant or Prinzmetal's angina* (the least common) is spontaneous, usually occurs at rest, and often is the result of an artery spasm. It affects more women than men.

Etiology

Angina pectoris, a signal that the heart muscle is not getting sufficient blood and oxygen, is usually a clinical syndrome accompanying arteriosclerotic heart disease. Less frequently, it may be produced by a coronary spasm and severe aortic stenosis or aortic insufficiency. Angina attacks are frequently triggered in susceptible individuals by any condition that increases myocardial oxygen demand, such as stress, eating, exertion, or even extremes of temperature and humidity.

Signs and Symptoms

The classic signs of an angina attack are burning, squeezing, and tightness in the chest; these may radiate to the neck and the left arm and shoulder blade, generally after exertion. Women may have abdominal and back pain as well. Sometimes there is nausea and vomiting. Acute anxiety may accompany angina, especially in the person who is already aware of having a heart problem and is worried about whether this episode of angina is a precursor to an MI. An angina attack usually lasts less than 15 minutes and not more than 30 minutes; the average is 3 minutes.

Diagnostic Procedures

An ECG taken during the angina attack may indicate ischemia, and a medical history usually reveals a history of angina. Additional procedures include those detailed under "Coronary Artery Disease."

Treatment

The first step is to make lifestyle changes. It is important to stop smoking and avoid secondhand smoke, maintain a healthy weight, keep any diabetes under control, and avoid overexertion by taking rest breaks. Avoid large meals and learn how to reduce stress levels. Establish an exercise plan approved by your PCP. Medications may include nitrates, aspirin, clot-preventing drugs, beta blockers, statins, and calcium channel blockers. A coronary disease that causes disabling angina pectoris and does not respond to treatment may require a surgical procedure, such as percutaneous coronary intervention (PCI) with or without stent placement, minimally invasive heart surgery such as laser angioplasty or atherectomy, or coronary artery bypass graft surgery.

Complementary Therapy

See "Coronary Artery Disease."

⊕ CLIENT COMMUNICATION

Because angina pectoris pain can be excruciating, it is important to educate clients to have their nitroglycerin preparation with them at all times and to know when to take it. Reviewing all prescribed medications with clients is essential. Any surgery will require careful explanation of the procedure(s); allow clients the opportunity to address any questions they may have.

Prognosis

The prognosis depends on the severity of myocardial ischemia. Angina pectoris usually is considered a warning to the person to lessen exertion and stress that might bring on an MI and heart failure. If the pain persists longer than 30 minutes, immediate medical attention should be sought. These more severe symptoms are a manifestation of more serious and progressive narrowing of the coronary arteries.

Prevention

Prevention of angina pectoris includes avoidance of precipitating factors in the presence of ongoing CAD.

ATRIAL FIBRILLATION

ICD-10: I48.91

Description

Atrial fibrillation affects about 2.7 million Americans. In this condition, the two atria in the heart beat irregularly, often quite rapidly, and out of rhythm with the lower ventricles. The heart rate can be as high as 175 beats per minute. Because of the complications of atrial fibrillation, it is considered a medical emergency. During fibrillation, blood can stagnate in the atria and clot. If a clot travels to the brain, a CVA may occur.

Etiology

Injuries to the heart or abnormalities of the heart are likely the cause. These include hypertension, congenital birth defects, hyperthyroidism, previous episodes of heart problems, MI, abnormal or diseased heart valves, some viral infections, and sleep apnea. The incidence is greater when there is a family history of atrial fibrillation, when there has been binge drinking, and when a person ages.

Signs and Symptoms

Signs and symptoms can be sporadic or chronic. Because the heart is not beating efficiently, clients often feel a "racing" heart and palpitations. Confusion, chest pain, weakness, and shortness of breath occur. Chest pain with the atrial fibrillation is the signal to seek medical assistance immediately.

Diagnostic Procedures

Primary care providers will seek and treat the underlying cause of the atrial fibrillation. Common tests include ECG and a Holter monitor (worn only 1 or 2 days) or event recorder (worn for up to 1 month) to record the pattern of the heart's actions and any abnormality that occurs. Chest x-ray, blood tests, and an echocardiogram may be part of the diagnostic process, also. Very recently, the University of Rochester School of Medicine and Dentistry and Xerox introduced a new technology using a web camera and software algorithms to record subtle changes in the skin color of an individual, the result of uneven blood flow caused by atrial fibrillation. This new method, which researchers are calling **videoplethysmography,** can detect atrial fibrillation in a person in 15 seconds. A person sits in front of a camera while it scans the face. Algorithms built into the software can detect changes in skin color, which otherwise go undetected by the naked eye.

Treatment

On occasion, a client can reverse the fibrillation by coughing. Treatment of any underlying cause is important, and when successful, may end the episodes. Some PCPs attempt to slow the heartbeat with beta blockers or calcium channel blockers. Other treatment is aimed at resetting the heart's rhythm to normal sinus rhythm. This procedure, done electrically or with medication, is known as **cardioversion.** If medications are to be administered, a TEE is first performed to check for blood clots in the heart. If there are clots, blood-thinning medications are prescribed for a period of time. Also, many of the medications for cardioversion have serious side effects that need to be carefully considered. If these procedures are unsuccessful, surgery is the next step and may include **cryoablation.**

Complementary Therapy

At the time of the irregular heartbeat, there is no complementary therapy other than to advise clients to try coughing a number of times. Long-term therapy includes modifying diet, reducing weight, keeping alcohol consumption to moderate amounts, and stopping smoking. Moderate but regular exercise under the direction of a specialist is recommended.

CLIENT COMMUNICATION

Explain to clients the need for medical attention and what constitutes a medical emergency. Clients are often quite fearful. A calm, reassuring yet "direct and take control" attitude can be helpful in putting clients at ease.

Prognosis

Atrial fibrillation can increase the likelihood of a CVA or MI fivefold. Long-term monitoring is likely, especially if blood-thinning medications are prescribed on a long-term basis. Prognosis is better if the underlying cause can be treated.

Prevention

Elimination of any causative factors is recommended. Some over-the-counter medications act as stimulants to the heart and are to be avoided. They include cold and cough medicines containing pseudoephedrine and ephedrine. Taking prescribed medications as suggested and having regular checkups are important.

MYOCARDIAL INFARCTION (HEART ATTACK)

ICD-10-I21.X

Description

Myocardial infarction is a life-threatening condition and constitutes a medical emergency. The MI occurs when blood flow to a section of heart muscle becomes blocked, usually by a clot. If the flow of blood is not restored quickly, a section of heart muscle becomes damaged from lack of oxygen and begins to die. MI is a leading cause of death in both men and women in the United States.

Etiology

MI is caused by the occlusion of one or more coronary arteries and the subsequent necrosis of a section of the heart muscle tissue served by those arteries (Fig. 12.9). The predisposing factors of MI are the same as those for many other cardiovascular diseases and include heredity, obesity, aging, hypertension, elevated serum triglycerides, total cholesterol levels, low-density lipoprotein (LDL) levels, smoking, diabetes mellitus, a sedentary lifestyle, and chronic stress. Men and postmenopausal women are more susceptible than premenopausal women; however, the incidence of MI is rising, particularly among premenopausal women who smoke and use oral contraceptives.

Signs and Symptoms

The classic symptom of MI is crushing chest pain that may radiate to the left arm, neck, and jaw. The pain may be similar to angina pain but usually is severe and is not relieved by the same measures that relieve angina. Some individuals may exhibit few symptoms or confuse the pain with indigestion. There is growing incidence showing that symptoms for women are fatigue, nausea, vomiting, and shortness of breath. Individuals with CAD should be suspicious if angina occurs with increasing frequency and duration. For some, an MI is preceded by vague feelings of discomfort, fear, nausea, and vomiting.

Diagnostic Procedures

A medical history revealing CAD and episodes of chest pain will help in the diagnosis. Electrocardiography is

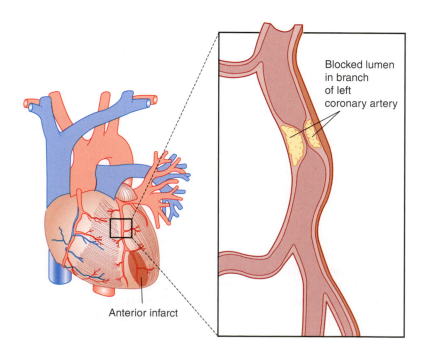

Figure 12.9 Myocardial infarction. The shaded area beneath the left coronary artery represents an area of infarct.

performed. Blood tests to detect elevated levels of cardiac enzymes—creatine phosphokinase (CPK) and creatine phosphokinase myocardial band (CPK-MB) levels—over a 72-hour period are useful in confirming MI. Cardiac imaging such as two-dimensional echocardiography may be useful.

Treatment

Prompt treatment can save lives and prevent disabilities. Treatment is most effective when started within 1 hour of the beginning of symptoms. If nitroglycerin has been prescribed, it should be taken while waiting for emergency personnel. Immediate hospitalization is important to relieve pain, stabilize heart rhythm, reduce cardiac workload, and preserve as much heart tissue as possible.

Complete bed rest with sedation and analgesia is usually instituted. In many cases, the affected individual is placed on a cardiac monitor to detect cardiac arrhythmias, a common problem during the first 48 hours after an attack. If cardiac arrest occurs, cardiopulmonary resuscitation (CPR) efforts are begun immediately. Cardiac surgical interventions may be necessary (see "Coronary Artery Disease").

A growing number of hospitals in the United States immediately place individuals suffering an MI in therapeutic hypothermia. Ice and coolants are applied to lower the body temperature while the individual is placed in a drug-induced coma for 24 hours before gradually being warmed to normal temperature. The cooling slows the body's metabolism and protects the brain from damage that occurs when the blood flow is restored.

Complementary Therapy

See "Coronary Artery Disease."

 CLIENT COMMUNICATION

Individuals experiencing an MI are generally restless and anxious; therefore, it is essential to help calm them and keep them quiet. A cardiac rehabilitation program may be ordered to include rest, exercise, and risk factor modification following an MI.

Prognosis

The prognosis for an individual experiencing an MI depends on the extent of damage to the myocardium but is usually guarded. Mortality is high if treatment is delayed; almost half of sudden deaths due to an MI occur before hospitalization, within 1 hour of symptoms. Complications of MI include arrhythmias; CHF; acute circulatory failure or cardiogenic shock; backward blood flow, or *mitral regurgitation*; breakage or tear in the septum between the left and right ventricles, a condition called *ventricular septal rupture*; pericarditis; and ventricular **aneurysm,** which is an abnormal saclike bulge in the heart.

 REALITY EPISODE

Wade is working out at the YMCA. He is about to wrap up his time on the treadmill. He feels a little funny, maybe a little dizzy. He steps off the treadmill and reaches for his water bottle. He has to hold on to the handle of the treadmill. He takes a drink of water and begins to wipe the sweat from his brow. He feels a hand on his shoulder and the words "Are you okay?" are fading as though they are coming from the end of a tunnel. He remembers nothing more until he hears emergency medical personnel tell him they are taking him to the hospital. Wade says, "I'm feeling fine. I'm not going to the hospital." The medics insist. He discovers at the hospital that immediate surgery is necessary to open a clogged coronary artery.

Identify the positive action and outcome of Wade's experience.

Prevention

Prevention includes avoidance of any predisposing factors, such as smoking, obesity, stress, and diets high in cholesterol.

CONGESTIVE HEART FAILURE

ICD-10: I50.9

Description

Congestive heart failure is a condition in which the pumping ability of the heart is progressively impaired to the point that it no longer meets bodily needs. When blood flow from the heart slows, blood returning to the heart backs up and causes congestion in the tissues. Circulatory congestion may occur in the systemic venous circulation, resulting in peripheral edema in the legs and ankles. Alternatively, the congestion may occur in the pulmonary circulation, causing pulmonary edema, an acute, life-threatening condition (Fig. 12.10). Heart failure also limits the kidneys' ability to dispose of sodium and water, which further increases edema.

Etiology

Either the left or right ventricle or both may be the source of the inadequate pumping action. Chronic CHF is the product of many cardiac and pulmonary disease processes, such as hypertension, CAD, and MI; degenerative conditions, such as cardiomyopathies, heart valve disease, and congenital birth defects; and any inflammation of the heart or its muscle.

Signs and Symptoms

Left ventricular failure may be manifested as dyspnea and fatigue and will result in primarily pulmonary

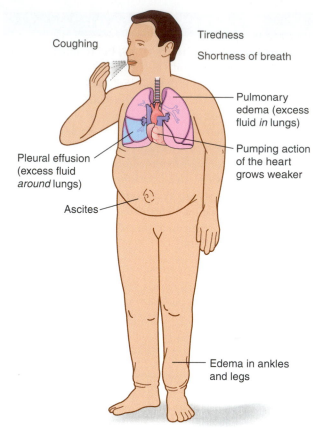

Coughing

Tiredness

Shortness of breath

Pulmonary edema (excess fluid *in* lungs)

Pleural effusion (excess fluid *around* lungs)

Pumping action of the heart grows weaker

Ascites

Edema in ankles and legs

Figure 12.10 Congestive heart failure indicating signs and symptoms.

symptoms. Right ventricular failure may cause distended neck veins and hepatomegaly and is more likely to result in systemic symptoms. Signs of advanced CHF may include tachypnea, palpitations, edema, weight gain, diaphoresis, and cyanosis. As the disease progresses, there may be hemoptysis, cyanosis, and pitting edema of the ankle (when an indentation in the skin remains a few minutes after the area is pressed with the finger).

Diagnostic Procedures

A complete history and physical examination will be conducted. An ECG, a chest x-ray, and an elevated central venous pressure will indicate the diagnosis. Blood tests ordered include complete blood count (CBC), electrolytes, glucose, blood urea nitrogen (BUN), and creatinine. Echocardiography with ejection fraction (a measurement showing how well the heart is pumping), cardiac CT and MRI, and cardiac catheterization may be ordered.

Treatment

The goal of treatment is to improve the heart's pumping function, relieve symptoms, and improve the client's quality of life. Treatment may involve the use of diuretics to reduce circulatory congestion by reducing total blood volume. Bed rest may be recommended. Drug therapy may include ACE inhibitors and ARBs.

Weight loss may be encouraged as well as no smoking. Salt intake may be restricted to combat edema.

Complementary Therapy

See "Coronary Artery Disease."

⊙➔ CLIENT COMMUNICATION

Counseling and continuous monitoring of lifestyle and limitations may be needed to help clients cope with their condition. Activities may be limited.

Prognosis

Acute CHF usually responds quickly to therapeutic measures. The prognosis is good, although it depends on the cause. If the congestion is severe and chronic, the prognosis is poor. The person usually must continue medication indefinitely and be carefully supervised by a PCP.

Prevention

Prevention consists of avoiding any predisposing factors. It is important to record weight daily and report any gain of 3 pounds or more to a PCP, limit sodium and alcohol, participate in an approved exercise program, reduce stress, consider sleeping with the head elevated 45 degrees, and not to smoke.

CHAPTER EPISODE—PART III

As time passed, Barney's congestive heart failure grew worse. Finally, Dr. Block had to tell Barney that he no longer was healthy enough for a heart transplant. Dr. Block, a University of Utah graduate, told him there might be one more possibility—an artificial heart. They discussed the procedure, which was just in its infancy, and the research around the procedure that was taking place at the University of Utah's medical school. Barney, the true scientist, was excited. Perhaps he could contribute something in the process. If he was going to die, why not contribute something to science in the process?

- What kind of discussion do you suppose Barney and his wife had about this idea of an artificial heart?
- If you were Barney, would you jump at this chance or be alarmed at the idea of your heart being removed and replaced by something artificial?

CARDIAC ARREST

ICD-10: I46.9

Description

Cardiac arrest is when a heart arrhythmia causes the heart to suddenly stop beating. **Cardiac arrest is a medical emergency.** Clients have no pulse, no respiratory effort, and are unresponsive. Cardiac arrest is different from an MI, in which the heart continues to beat.

Etiology

Cardiac arrest may result from CAD, MI, circulatory collapse due to various forms of shock, or ventricular fibrillation. Cardiac arrest also may result from massive hemorrhage, drug reactions or overdose, electrocution, drowning, or other forms of accidental physical trauma.

Signs and Symptoms

Before cardiac arrest, clients may have prolonged angina, acute dyspnea or orthopnea, light-headedness, or sustained tachycardia. The onset is precipitous and without warning. Symptoms of impending cardiac arrest may include sudden tachycardia or **bradycardia** (a slowed heartbeat), a drop in blood pressure, and respiratory failure. An individual experiencing cardiac arrest loses consciousness and ceases to breathe.

Diagnostic Procedures

The diagnosis of cardiac arrest is based on the absence of respiration and pulse and accompanying loss of consciousness. If medical support is immediately available, an ECG will show ventricular fibrillation or asystole.

Treatment

Summon emergency medical personnel immediately. CPR should be given while waiting for emergency personnel, who will use a defibrillation device to start the heart. Sudden cardiac arrest requires treatment with a defibrillator to send an electric shock to the heart. The electric shock may restore a normal rhythm to a heart that has stopped beating. As soon as possible, transport the client to a hospital where advanced life support can be received.

Complementary Therapy

There is no known complementary treatment.

⟳ CLIENT COMMUNICATION

If the client survives, the tips discussed under "Myocardial Infarction" should be followed. All medical personnel need to be able to perform CPR and manage a defibrillator. Automated external defibrillators (AEDs) are specially designed to allow even untrained bystanders to use them safely and effectively. AEDs are presently available in many public places, such as airports and shopping malls, and are programmed to give an electric shock *only* in the case of an arrhythmia such as ventricular fibrillation.

Prognosis

The prognosis is guarded at best. Persons may survive, especially if treatment begins within 3 minutes. Irreversible brain damage may occur after that time. Few attempts at resuscitation are successful after 10 minutes. Even with prompt treatment by emergency personnel, automated defibrillators, and improvements in CPR techniques, fewer than 10% of the 425,000 people who suffer cardiac arrest in the United States each year survive long enough to leave the hospital.

Prevention

The best prevention for cardiac arrest is receiving early treatment for cardiac symptoms, living a healthy lifestyle, and having the heart disease carefully monitored. Those with a known high risk of sudden cardiac arrest may consider an implantable cardioverter-defibrillator (ICD) as primary prevention. The ICD is placed under the skin in the chest. Its electrodes connect to the heart and monitor the heartbeat. If a dangerous heart rhythm occurs, the defibrillator gives an electric shock to restore the heart's normal rhythm.

Cardiac Advances

Cardiac surgeons are slowly moving toward angiogenesis through gene therapy. The gene coding for a protein called *vascular endothelial growth factor* is injected into the heart to encourage new blood vessels to grow from existing ones. Sometimes a virus is used as the delivery vehicle. The hope is that new vessels grow and restore the heart muscle within hours to a few days.

In another new form of cardiac therapy, a small incision is made in the chest through the left ventricle. A laser drills tiny holes through the muscle, and almost instantly, new vessels form around the injured area.

The most beautiful things in the world cannot be seen or even touched; they must be felt with the heart. —Helen Keller

Blood Vessel Diseases and Disorders

ANEURYSMS: ABDOMINAL, THORACIC, AND PERIPHERAL ARTERIES

ICD-10: I71.4 (ABDOMINAL)
ICD-10: I71.2 (THORACIC)
ICD-10: I72.8 (PERIPHERAL ARTERIES)

Description

An aneurysm (Fig. 12.11) is a local dilation of a blood vessel due to weakening of its walls. Aneurysms may be sacculated (shaped like a sac), fusiform (a spindle-shaped enlargement), or dissecting (the layers of the vessel wall are separated). Aneurysms may cause a blood clot or **thrombus** to form along the wall of a blood vessel, may hemorrhage from rupture, or may cause ischemia. (Cerebral aneurysm is discussed in Chapter 10.) Three additional types of aneurysms discussed here are abdominal aortic aneurysms (AAA), thoracic aortic aneurysms (TAA), and peripheral artery aneurysms (PAA). All three are more common in men over age 60. AAAs are a leading cause of death in the United States. Both AAAs and TAAs are life-threatening and constitute a medical emergency when the aneurysms are expanding or rupture. PAAs do not rupture as easily but can form clots that could block blood flow to a limb or the brain. All symptoms vary according to the size and location of the aneurysm and whether it has ruptured. See http://my.clevelandclinic.org/heart/disorders/aorta_marfan/aorticaneurysm.aspx for details related to aneurysms.

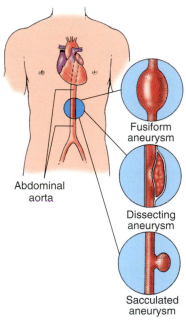

Figure 12.11 Aortic aneurysms. *(From Thomas, CL [ed]: Taber's Cyclopedic Medical Dictionary, ed. 21. Philadelphia: FA Davis, 2009, p 126, with permission.)*

Etiology

Aneurysms may be congenital or result from trauma, arteriosclerosis, inflammation, infection, and degeneration produced by atherosclerosis. Table 12.1 lists signs and symptoms and diagnostic procedures of aneurysms.

Signs and Symptoms

See Table 12.1 for a summary of common symptoms of each type of aneurysm.

Diagnostic Procedures

If an aneurysm is suspected, common tests ordered may include chest x-ray, CT scan, MRI, echocardiography, ultrasound, and angiography.

Treatment

If aneurysms are quite small, many PCPs recommend a wait-and-watch approach to treatment and prescribe antihypertensives or beta blockers and analgesics. Surgery is the treatment of choice when an aneurysm is likely to rupture or increases in size. Open chest or abdominal surgery can be performed for the AAA or the TAA, but endovascular (stent-graft) surgery is less invasive and easier for clients. The stent-graft surgery is recommended for treatment of PAAs also. There are risks to any surgery, but aneurysms do not go away on their own and pose a serious threat.

Complementary Therapy

Once an aneurysm has formed, there is no known complementary treatment.

⊕→ CLIENT COMMUNICATION

Teaching is minimal in most cases except to encourage clients to minimize their risk of aneurysms.

Prognosis

The prognosis is guarded for persons with AAA or TAA. If rupture occurs, many do not survive long enough to get to a hospital. Death results from rupture of the aneurysm, causing hemorrhage and shock. A possible complication, especially of PAAs, includes

Table 12.1	**Aneurysms**	
TYPE	**SIGNS AND SYMPTOMS**	**DIAGNOSTIC PROCEDURES**
AAA	Sudden, severe, constant back, flank, abdominal, and groin pain; if ruptured, cyanosis, tachycardia, hypotension, and altered mental status	X-ray, ultrasonography, CT scan, MRI, angiography; diagnosis often confused with other disorders
TAA	Chest, back, and abdominal pain; dysphagia, dyspnea, cough, and **hematemesis;** if ruptured, shock, hypotension, and tachycardia	CT scan, MRI, angiography, transesophageal echocardiography; chest x-ray
PAA	Commonly occurring in popliteal artery; also in femoral, carotid, or arm arteries; pulsing lump, claudication, painful sores of fingers and/or toes; limb numbness	CT scan, MRI, angiography, ultrasonography

formation of a thrombus along the wall of an aneurysm. A piece of the thrombus may break off, producing an embolus that may block the flow of blood to vital organs.

Prevention

The best prevention is to take steps to lower blood pressure and cholesterol, stop smoking, and manage weight.

ARTERIOSCLEROSIS/ ATHEROSCLEROSIS

ICD-10: I70.91 or I70.90

Description

Arteriosclerosis is widespread thickening of the walls of small arteries and arterioles with a resulting loss of elasticity. One type of arteriosclerosis is atherosclerosis, which is characterized by the accumulation of yellowish plaques of cholesterol, lipids, and cellular debris on the inner layers of the walls of large and medium-sized arteries. The vessel walls become thickened, fibrotic, and calcified, narrowing the arterial lumen (Fig. 12.12). It is fairly common even in the medical community to use the terms *arteriosclerosis* and *atherosclerosis* interchangeably. The most commonly affected vessels include the coronary and cerebral arteries. Circulatory impairment is the consequence of both conditions but is especially serious when the atherosclerosis is in major arteries that supply vital tissues. Atherosclerosis begins insidiously, with symptoms not appearing for 20 to 40 years.

Etiology

The etiology is unclear, complicated, and multifaceted. It may include trauma or the accumulation of lipids due to dietary excesses, faulty carbohydrate metabolism, a sedentary lifestyle, cigarette smoking, or a genetic defect. Both diseases are seen with aging and are often associated with diabetes mellitus, hypertension, obesity, scleroderma, and nephrosclerosis (a hardening of connective tissues within the kidney).

Signs and Symptoms

The signs and symptoms depend on the vessels involved and the extent of vessel obstruction. Often the person is asymptomatic until an artery is so narrowed it cannot supply adequate blood to the organs and tissues. If symptomatic, typical signs and symptoms include intermittent **claudication,** changes in skin temperature and color, bruits over the involved artery, headache, dizziness, and memory defects. Pain may be present, especially at night, due to sepsis or ischemia. Muscle cramping may occur. The effects of atherosclerosis are gradual lumen obstruction, thrombosis, and subsequent weakening of the vessel with dilation.

Diagnostic Procedures

A diagnosis is often made during a routine physical examination. Blood tests indicate elevated cholesterol, triglyceride, and lipid levels. A Doppler ultrasound that measures blood pressure in the arm or leg can help determine blockages and the speed of blood flow in the arteries. The ankle-brachial index, which compares blood pressure in the ankle with blood pressure in the arm, can show atherosclerosis in the limb arteries. ECG and angiogram are useful in determining where the blockage is occurring. A CT scan allows visualization of hardening or narrowing of the large arteries.

Treatment

Exercise and a diet low in saturated fats, cholesterol, and calories is important. Any infections, ulcers, or gangrene of the toes and feet need immediate attention.

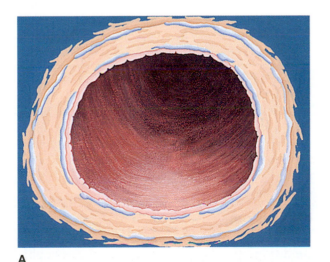
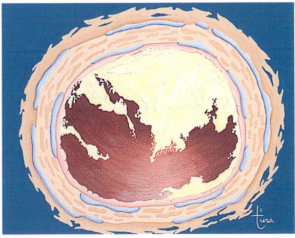

A

B

Figure 12.12   (A) Cross-section of normal coronary artery. (B) Coronary artery with atherosclerosis narrowing the lumen.
(From Scanlon, VC, and Sanders, T: Essentials of Anatomy and Physiology, ed. 6. Philadelphia: FA Davis, 2011, p 302, with permission.)

Medications can be effective in slowing atherosclerosis, especially those that decrease LDL cholesterol (the "lethal" cholesterol) and raise the level of high-density lipoprotein cholesterol. Aspirin, heparin, or warfarin may be prescribed to reduce the risk of blood clots in narrowed arteries. Blood pressure must be controlled. Surgery may be necessary. Angioplasty (using laser technology) with stent placement is common. An endarterectomy can remove fatty deposits within a narrowed artery. Thrombolytic therapy involves inserting a clot-dissolving drug into the artery at the point of the clot to break it up. Surgery to create a graft bypass allows blood to flow around the blockage.

Complementary Therapy

Integrative medical practitioners will suggest that clients lose weight, cease smoking, and exercise regularly. Increased fruit and vegetables in the diet and management of stress are helpful.

 CLIENT COMMUNICATION

It is imperative that clients understand the relationship of diet, exercise, and stress to the disease process. Lifestyle modifications are essential.

Prognosis

The prognosis varies and depends on the site and amount of arterial occlusion and the person's overall physical condition. Complications include infection, CAD, MI, CVA, aneurysms, and gangrene.

Prevention

Prevention includes moderate exercise, avoidance of stress, adequate rest, and a diet low in calories, cholesterol, and saturated fatty acids.

THROMBOPHLEBITIS

ICD-10: I80.9

Description

Thrombophlebitis is inflammation of a vein in which a clot is formed from the streaming blood constituents. An abnormal mass of platelets is formed and deposited on the vascular surface. The affected vein may be either partially or completely obstructed. The condition usually occurs in an extremity, most frequently in a leg, and can affect both superficial and deep veins.

Etiology

Thrombophlebitis is caused by a blood clot that may be related to trauma, reduced or turbulent blood flow, infection, chemical irritation, or prolonged immobility, or it may be idiopathic. Smoking, the use of oral contraceptives or hormone replacement therapy, and being overweight predisposes an individual to thrombophlebitis.

Signs and Symptoms

Clients may be asymptomatic. Signs and symptoms, however, depend on the site of the affected vein and may include a dull aching, warmth, and tight feeling at the site. There can be **induration** (hardness), redness, and tenderness along a superficial vein. If swelling becomes severe and there is shortness of breath, a deep vein thrombosis (DVT) may exist that requires immediate attention to prevent a dislodged clot from traveling to the lungs.

Diagnostic Procedures

Physical examination may reveal the inflammation. Blood tests may show an elevated clot-dissolving substance and a Doppler ultrasound may indicate a clot. Phlebography (which shows filling defects and diverted blood flow) and ascending venography may be used to diagnose thrombophlebitis. CT scan and MRI are likely ordered as well.

Treatment

In superficial thrombophlebitis, clients may be advised to rest in bed, elevate the affected limb, and apply heat over the site. In DVT, the affected limb may be elevated and possibly wrapped with elastic bandages. Lysin, a dissolving substance, may be injected for acute DVT in a process called *lysis*. Anticoagulant therapy may be prescribed. Surgical procedures, such as vein ligation and femoral vein thrombectomy, may be used in cases of DVT. Through-the-skin or percutaneous insertion of intracaval devices has mostly replaced surgical intervention.

Complementary Therapy

No significant complementary therapy is indicated.

 CLIENT COMMUNICATION

Postsurgery, it is important for clients to ambulate early and exercise the legs to improve venous flow. Support hose may be advised. Elevating the legs 15 to 20 degrees may be helpful.

Prognosis

If only superficial veins are involved, the condition may be self-limiting, and the prognosis is good. When deep veins are involved, the prognosis is less optimistic. A serious complication of thrombophlebitis is the formation of a pulmonary embolism, a life-threatening condition.

Prevention

Individuals with a history of varicose veins or other conditions predisposing them to thrombophlebitis should wear elastic support hose. It is advisable to allow for walking after long periods of sitting, such as when traveling or working.

VARICOSE VEINS

ICD-10: I83.XX

Description

Varicose veins are enlarged, twisted, superficial veins and may be referred to as *venous reflux disease*. They may occur in almost any part of the body, but most frequently they occur in the lower legs, involving the greater and lesser saphenous veins (Fig. 12.13). The condition is most common after age 50 and in obese persons, affecting more women than men. Varicose veins tend to be inherited.

Etiology

Defective or damaged valves in the veins prevent the blood from flowing freely toward the heart. This buildup of pressure in the superficial veins causes varicosities. Varicose veins may be due to an inherited defect or to venous diseases. They also may be produced by conditions such as multiple pregnancies or jobs requiring prolonged standing or heavy lifting. Many factors can aggravate the situation, including obesity.

Signs and Symptoms

Clients may be asymptomatic even though the varicose vein condition is severe. Quite frequently, however, the affected veins are visually evident. Characteristic symptoms of varicose veins in the legs include dull, aching heaviness or a feeling of fatigue after standing. Cramping may occur, followed by edema and stasis pigmentation, a tan discoloration of the skin.

Diagnostic Procedures

In most cases, visual observation may be all that is necessary. Phlebography may be performed for diagnosis. Doppler ultrasonography detects possible backflow in deep or superficial veins.

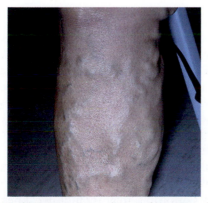

Figure 12.13 Varicose veins and stasis dermatitis of the ankle. *(From Thomas, CL [ed]: Taber's Cyclopedic Medical Dictionary, ed. 21. Philadelphia: F.A. Davis, 2009, p 2437, with permission.)*

Treatment

The use of elastic stockings, a moderate exercise program, and avoidance of prolonged periods of standing or lifting are recommended initially. Minimally invasive procedures, usually performed in an outpatient setting under local anesthesia, include radiofrequency ablation and endovenous laser therapy. Both use ultrasound to position a catheter or guide a laser into the diseased vein. The catheter, powered by radio-frequency energy or laser, delivers heat to the vein wall, shrinking the vein and sealing it closed. Blood is rerouted to other healthy veins. The procedure takes about 40 minutes. More severe varicose veins may require stripping and ligation, but clients must have patent deep venous channels.

Complementary Therapy

It is recommended that clients elevate the legs as much as possible, wear support stockings, lose weight, and avoid alcohol. They should not massage directly over the varicose veins.

CLIENT COMMUNICATION

Tell clients not to cross their legs when sitting; rather, they should cross their ankles. Wearing support hose and getting up frequently to walk is helpful. Remind clients to sit with their legs elevated if possible.

Prognosis

The prognosis is good; however, further varicose veins may develop, requiring additional treatment.

Prevention

Prevention of varicose veins includes avoiding prolonged standing or lifting, avoiding constrictive clothing, and elevating the legs when possible. If obesity is a problem, have the client begin a weight-loss plan.

Anemias

Anemias are a very common blood disorder affecting more than 3 million Americans. Anemia is the result when there is either insufficient red blood cells or red blood cells not working properly. The most common anemias appear here, except for sickle cell anemia that appears in Chapter 6.

IRON-DEFICIENCY ANEMIA

ICD-10: D50.9

Description

Iron-deficiency anemia is characterized by inadequate reserves of iron in the body and the formation of unusually small, hemoglobin-poor RBCs. These cells are smaller and lighter in color than normal cells because RBCs derive their color and oxygen from hemoglobin. Iron-deficiency anemia occurs more frequently in premenopausal women and in adolescents. It is a common chronic disease and the most common blood condition in the United States.

Etiology

The cause of iron-deficiency anemia is excessive blood loss. In healthy men and postmenopausal women, excessive blood loss most likely results from gastrointestinal (GI) bleeding. In premenopausal women, menstrual flow that is excessive in number of days or amount, a condition called **menorrhagia,** is a common cause. Pregnancy increases the risk of iron-deficiency anemia. Breastfeeding, chronic intestinal diseases associated with malabsorption of iron, or low dietary intake of iron-rich foods can cause the anemia. Overuse of NSAIDs, which can cause GI bleeding, may be a cause.

Signs and Symptoms

Common signs and symptoms include extreme fatigue, pallor, headache, cold hands and feet, and irritability. If the anemia progresses, symptoms become more severe and may include dyspnea, tachycardia, increased infections, and brittle nails.

Diagnostic Procedures

A detailed health history may reveal multiple pregnancies or GI bleeding. Blood testing typically indicates abnormally low hemoglobin and hematocrit values. Levels of serum iron and serum ferritin (the protein that helps to store iron in the blood) may be low as well. The RBC count typically reveals unusually high numbers of microcytic red cells. If it is necessary to rule out other difficulties, an endoscopy can look for GI bleeding, a colonoscopy can check for tumors or cancer of the colon, and ultrasound may be able to determine reasons for excessive menstrual flow. In extreme cases, bone marrow aspiration may be performed to differentiate iron-deficiency anemia from closely related blood disorders.

Treatment

Treatment depends on the severity and cause of the anemia. Iron-deficiency anemia may be treated with oral or parenteral (intramuscular or intravenous) iron supplements. Dietary modifications are often sufficient to restore lost bodily iron reserves.

Complementary Therapy

Stress to clients the importance of eating foods high in iron, such as red meat, pork, poultry, seafood, eggs, seeds and nuts, green leafy vegetables, barley, oats, beans, and peas. Some practitioners may prescribe vitamin C and calcium. It is recommended that clients limit sugar, alcohol, and caffeine.

 CLIENT COMMUNICATION

Because iron-deficiency anemia can be asymptomatic for a period of time, practitioners may regularly have occult stool specimens tested to determine if colorectal bleeding is occurring. Periodic colonoscopies are recommended for clients over age 50. Educate clients about foods high in iron and eating well-balanced meals.

Prognosis

The prognosis for iron-deficiency anemia is good if the underlying cause such as unusual bleeding is detected and treated. However, the condition may be chronic in some cases, making the treatment long-term. Untreated iron-deficiency anemia can cause heart irregularities, growth difficulty in children, and premature or low-weight births.

Prevention

Prevention for iron-deficiency anemia includes a diet with adequate iron for daily needs and identification of high-risk individuals. It is best to feed infants breast milk or iron-fortified formula for the first year.

FOLIC ACID DEFICIENCY ANEMIA

ICD-10: D52.X

Description

Folic acid deficiency anemia is characterized by the appearance of large abnormal red blood cells (megaloblasts), which form when there are inadequate stores of folic acid within the body. Folic acid is one of the B complex vitamins that help the body make new blood cells.

Etiology

The cause of this anemia is insufficient folic acid. The disease also may arise from increased utilization of folic acid, such as needed during pregnancy, in infancy, or as a result of other blood disorders. Impaired absorption of folic acid by the body and drug-related folic imbalances also may produce the disease. The disease may be due to poor diet or a consequence of alcoholism. The deficiency is more common in pregnant women, infants, children, and adolescents.

Signs and Symptoms

Signs and symptoms may include weakness, fatigue, anorexia, pallor, forgetfulness, irritability, and diarrhea.

Diagnostic Procedures

A physical examination and blood tests are ordered. A CBC often reveals the megaloblasts. Serum folate and vitamin B_{12} levels are typically decreased. Bone marrow studies may be done to determine if there is a secondary cause of the disease.

Treatment

Folic acid supplements may be given orally, or they may be administered parenterally if the client's condition indicates that more immediate intervention is needed. A diet high in folic acid is prescribed.

Complementary Therapy

Folic acid supplements are essential. Natural sources of folic acid are citrus fruits, any kind of beans, green leafy vegetables, beef, poultry, pork, eggs, seafood, and asparagus.

CLIENT COMMUNICATION

Refer clients to a dietitian to learn how to prepare a diet high in folic acid. Pregnant women are counseled to take folic acid supplements. If alcoholism is a problem, treatment should be recommended, and clients may need to remain on folic acid supplements indefinitely.

Prognosis

The prognosis depends on the underlying cause of the folic acid deficiency. For most, the prognosis is good. Medical professionals recommend a folic acid supplement both before and during pregnancy to prevent certain birth defects.

Prevention

Prevention of folic acid deficient anemia includes a diet with adequate sources of folic acid.

PERNICIOUS ANEMIA

ICD-10: D51.0

Description

Pernicious (megaloblastic) anemia is characterized by the appearance of large, abnormal RBCs, which form when there are inadequate levels of vitamin B_{12} in the body. The condition is called *pernicious anemia* because it was often fatal before the cause was discovered to be a lack of vitamin B_{12}. Other names for the disorder are *megaloblastic* or *vitamin B_{12}–deficiency anemia*.

Etiology

Pernicious anemia is caused by the failure of certain cells in the gastric mucosa to secrete adequate levels of a protein called *intrinsic factor* (IF). This protein is necessary for the absorption of dietary vitamin B_{12}, which is essential for RBC formation. Certain forms of the disease appear to be inherited; other forms appear to be autoimmune disorders. Persons with other autoimmune diseases such as Crohn disease are more likely to develop pernicious anemia. Insufficient vitamin B_{12} in the body may be due to alcoholism; it is also more common in individuals who are strict vegetarians.

Signs and Symptoms

The onset of signs and symptoms is usually insidious because the body stores vitamin B_{12} and compensates so well. By the time signs and symptoms appear—such as fatigue, dyspnea, palpitations, sore and bright red tongue, and numbness and tingling of the extremities—the damage can be severe. Weakness, nausea, vomiting, neuritis (inflammation of nerves), impaired coordination, altered vision, light-headedness, and tachycardia also may be present. The neurological signs and symptoms progress even though a client may experience remissions and exacerbations.

Diagnostic Procedures

A thorough medical history and physical examination are essential in the diagnosis of pernicious anemia. Usually, the first test used to diagnose anemia is a CBC. Laboratory studies may reveal decreased levels of hemoglobin, folic acid, and serum levels of vitamin B_{12}. Bone marrow aspiration and gastric analysis may be done.

Treatment

Pernicious anemia is initially treated with vitamin B_{12} injections daily or weekly at first, then one injection every month. Vitamin B_{12} given as pills or in a nasal gel or spray may be prescribed along with the injections. Vitamin B_{12} treatment may be necessary for life.

Complementary Therapy

Other than administering vitamin B_{12} as prescribed in traditional treatment, no significant complementary therapy is indicated. See "Folic Acid Deficiency Anemia" for dietary suggestions.

CLIENT COMMUNICATION

If neurological symptoms are severe, clients need instructions on coping. For example, if coordination and gait are affected, physical and occupational therapy will help maximize functioning. Remind clients to return regularly for treatment and monitoring of their vitamin B_{12} level.

Prognosis

The damaged IF-secreting cells in the gastric mucosa will not regenerate, but if treatment is prompt and properly maintained, clients with pernicious anemia typically are able to lead a normal life. Pernicious anemia can cause permanent damage to nerves and other organs if treatment is delayed. Clients have a higher incidence of gastric cancer than the general population.

Prevention

There is no known prevention for pernicious anemia.

APLASTIC ANEMIA

ICD-10: D61.9

Description

Aplastic anemia is characterized by insufficient or totally absent RBC production. The bone marrow stops producing RBCs, WBCs, and platelets. The result is that clients cannot fight infection and have a tendency to bleed.

Etiology

Aplastic anemia is the result of injury or destruction of the blood-forming tissue in the bone marrow. In over half of cases, aplastic anemia is idiopathic. Other causes include exposure to toxins, radiation and chemotherapy, and certain drugs. Medications used to threat rheumatoid arthritis, autoimmune disorders, and viral infections such as HIV and hepatitis may cause aplastic anemia. Infections and pregnancy can trigger the disease. Fortunately, aplastic anemia is uncommon.

Signs and Symptoms

The onset may be insidious or may occur slowly over a period of time. Signs and symptoms can include fatigue, pallor, shortness of breath upon exertion, irregular heart rate, purpura, nosebleeds and bleeding gums, infections, headache, and dizziness. Pancytopenia, a decrease in all cellular components of the blood, may occur if the bone marrow is damaged to the point that healthy blood-forming tissues are replaced by fatty abnormal tissue.

Diagnostic Procedures

Blood tests will show the RBC, WBC, and **reticulocyte** (immature form of RBCs) counts are low in the majority of cases. Bone marrow studies may show evidence of fatty tissue with **megakaryocytes,** large bone marrow cells with large or multiple nuclei. A medical history may provide evidence of recent exposure to any of the identified etiologies.

Treatment

Without treatment, aplastic anemia may progress and become fatal. Exposure to any known cause must be discontinued. Bone marrow or peripheral stem cell transplant is the treatment of choice in young persons with severe aplastic anemia. Immunosuppressive therapy may be tried. Transfusions of RBCs and platelets may be necessary.

Complementary Therapy

Exposure to known toxins must be avoided; otherwise, no significant complementary therapy is indicated.

➔ CLIENT COMMUNICATION

It is recommended that clients be taught to protect themselves from infection, to be aware of the signs and symptoms of bleeding, and to know when to seek immediate treatment.

Prognosis

The prognosis is poor for individuals with aplastic anemia. Death results in about 50% of cases. Those who live with the condition may go into partial or complete remission or need to be treated with transfusions for years. Complications include infections, hemorrhage, and transfusion-related problems.

Prevention

Prevention of aplastic anemia includes avoiding any chemical or physical agents, such as insecticides, herbicides, organic solvents, and paint removers that have the capacity to damage bone marrow.

CHAPTER EPISODE—PART IV

Barney and his wife made the decision. The medical professionals at the University of Utah accepted Barney as a prime candidate, knowing that he had only a short time to live without the transplant. Barney and his wife made the temporary move to Utah. The surgery was performed on December 2, 1982. Barney survived the surgery and the heart worked, but it was not an easy road. The plastic and aluminium heart functioned with two air-powered heart-shaped pumps that were implanted into Barney's chest. These pumps were connected to an external pneumatic compressor, about the size of a refrigerator, weighing over 400 pounds. The pump was noisy and the compressor made it impossible for Barney to move around much.

- You have probably guessed by now that this patient is Dr. Barney Clark, the first person to receive an artificial heart—the Jarvik 7. Do you think Dr. Clark was a pioneer for medical science or simply crazy to undergo such a surgery?
- What was the success/failure of this transplant?

Leukemias

ACUTE MYELOID LEUKEMIA, ACUTE LYMPHOBLASTIC LEUKEMIA, CHRONIC MYELOID LEUKEMIA, CHRONIC LYMPHOCYTIC LEUKEMIA

ICD-10: C92.0X (ACUTE MYELOID LEUKEMIA)
ICD-10: C91.0X (ACUTE LYMPHOBLASTIC LEUKEMIA)
ICD-10: C92.1X (CHRONIC MYELOID LEUKEMIA)
ICD-10: C91.1X (CHRONIC LYMPHOCYTIC LEUKEMIA)

Leukemias are progressive, malignant diseases of the blood-forming organs and are marked by the unrestrained growth of abnormal leukocytes and their precursors in the blood and bone marrow. The term *leukemia* refers to a neoplasm of **hematopoietic** tissue or tissue that is related to the blood cells in the bone marrow. At first, the leukemia cells function almost normally; however, over time they crowd out normal WBCs, RBCs, and platelets. The leukemia cells infiltrate the bone marrow and lymph tissue and then advance into the bloodstream and the various organs of the body. There may or may not be a rise in circulating WBCs, depending on whether the white cells are confined to the bone marrow.

Leukemia is classified according to the dominant abnormal cell type and the severity of the disease. Except for chronic lymphocytic leukemia (CLL), leukemia is not staged numerically (I, II, III, or IV) the way many other cancers are staged. Rather, it is classified as acute (usually fatal in less than 6 months if not treated) or chronic (develops more slowly), depending on the maturity of the cell. This classification gives some indication as to the seriousness of the disease. In addition, various prognostic factors, such as the blood counts, cytogenetic, and a person's general health, help to guide treatment decisions. Although other variants occur, the four more common leukemias are described here: acute myeloid (myelogenous) leukemia, acute lymphocytic (lymphoblastic) leukemia, chronic myeloid (myelogenous) leukemia, and chronic lymphocytic (lymphoblastic) leukemia.

Description

Acute myeloid (myelogenous) leukemia (AML) is a neoplasm characterized by the hyperproliferation of abnormal, immature white cell precursors called **blasts.** These abnormal cells accumulate in the bone marrow, blood, and body tissues. In AML, the white cells are immature, so there is rapid accumulation of myeloid precursors called *myeloblasts*. It accounts for about 18,860 new cases each year and is the most common type of nonlymphatic leukemia, occurring most frequently in men over age 50.

Acute lymphocytic (lymphoblastic) leukemia (ALL) is similar to AML except that there is abnormal growth of lymphocyte precursors called *lymphoblasts*. ALL accounts for about 6,020 new cases per year and is the most common type of leukemia in young children ages 2 to 5. Children account for about 80% of the ALL cases.

Chronic myeloid (myelogenous) leukemia (CML) is characterized by the proliferation of abnormal white cell precursors called *granulocytes* in the bone marrow. These granulocytes later enter the blood and invade other body tissues. CML accounts for about 5,980 cases of leukemia each year and usually affects older adults.

Chronic lymphocytic (lymphoblastic) leukemia (CLL) is characterized by the accumulation of immature, immunologically ineffective B lymphocytes. These cells accumulate to an enormous extent in the lymphoid tissue, blood, and bone marrow. CLL accounts for about 15,720 new cases of leukemia each year. It is the most common form of leukemia in the United States, usually affecting people over age 55. It almost never affects children.

Etiology

The exact cause of leukemia is unknown. Sometimes primary care providers are able to explain why a particular person gets leukemia; more often, the risk factors may include the following:

1. Exposure to high levels of certain chemicals, such as formaldehyde or benzene.
2. Chemotherapy, especially in those with cancer who are treated with alkylating agents.
3. Exposure to very high levels of radiation (the atomic bomb in World War II and nuclear power plant accidents such as that at Chernobyl, Ukraine). Radiation treatments may be another source of high-level exposure.
4. Certain genetic diseases caused by abnormal chromosomes such as Down syndrome. Chromosomal alterations are often evidenced in ALL.
5. Human T-cell leukemia virus-1 can cause a rare type of leukemia.
6. Myelodysplastic syndrome, which causes defects in blood cell formation, has been linked to an increased incidence of leukemia.

Some people who are diagnosed with leukemia may have no known risk factors.

Signs and Symptoms

In the acute forms of leukemia, the signs and symptoms appear and worsen quickly. Sometimes symptoms do not appear until the leukemia is in its chronic form, and when the symptoms do appear, they may be mild at first and then worsen gradually. Presenting signs and symptoms include fever or night sweats; frequent infections; feeling weak or tired; headache; bleeding, especially bleeding gums, and easy bruising; purplish patches in the skin; petechiae, or tiny red spots on the skin; pain in the bone or joints; swelling or discomfort in the abdomen from an enlarged spleen; swollen lymph nodes, especially in the neck or armpit; and weight loss. Other signs and symptoms may include prolonged menses, anorexia, vomiting, confusion, loss of muscle control, and seizures. As the disease progresses, tachycardia, palpitations, and increased incidence of infection are common.

Diagnostic Procedures

A complete physical examination may be the mechanism whereby leukemia is initially suspected. Laboratory tests are ordered to check the level of blood cells. These levels may reveal thrombocytopenia, leukocytosis, anemia, and neutropenia (the presence of abnormally small numbers of neutrophils in the circulating blood). A biopsy of the bone marrow from the hip bone or another large bone is necessary to diagnose leukemia. Further, laboratory personnel may look at the chromosome cells from samples of peripheral blood, bone marrow, or lymph nodes. In the case of CML, the Philadelphia chromosome can be detected. A spinal tap and chest x-rays may be ordered.

Treatment

Treatment depends on the type of leukemia, the extent of the leukemia, and the person's general health status and age. Chemotherapy, biological therapy, radiation therapy, or bone marrow transplant may be ordered either alone or in combination. Those with acute leukemia need immediate treatment with the hope of bringing about a remission and a possible cure. Those with the chronic forms may require no treatment, especially if they exhibit no symptoms and can be monitored closely. Chemotherapy is given in cycles with alternating treatment and recovery periods. Biological therapy is given via IV to encourage the immune system to kill leukemia cells in the blood and bone marrow. Biological therapy uses substances known as *biological response modifiers (BRMs)*. They include interferons, interleukins, colony-stimulating factors, monoclonal antibodies, vaccines, gene therapy, and nonspecific immunomodulating agents. Radiation therapy may be specifically focused or consist of total body radiation. Stem cell transplant allows clients to be treated with high doses of drugs, radiation, or both. The high doses of the treatment kill normal blood cells and the leukemia cells in the bone marrow. Later, clients receive more stem cells to stimulate formation of new blood cells.

Complementary Therapy

Because leukemias, especially the acute forms, are treated aggressively, the client's body is bombarded with treatment modalities that are quite harmful. Integrative medicine attempts to balance the aggressive treatment with as many complementary life-enhancing measures as possible. Conflict may occur when PCPs outline aggressive treatment without carefully identifying the risks and the physical, emotional, and personal difficulties that will result from treatment. In cooperation with primary care providers, complementary medicine can assist in the following:

- Identify steps to reduce nausea, vomiting, and diarrhea.
- Provide energy boosts when exhaustion is severe.
- Suggest recipes to boost nutrition when there is no desire to eat and food does not taste as it should.
- Recommend comfort and relaxation techniques to help clients cope.

CLIENT COMMUNICATION

The shock of the diagnosis may prevent clients from understanding the disease process and treatment. Clients need time to assess their options. It is essential to work closely with clients, teaching them what they can handle. As treatment progresses, side effects will increase, and encouragement is needed. Support systems, especially those with other clients with leukemia, may be helpful.

Prognosis

The prognosis of AML is highly variable. Clients with AML have a potentially curable disease; however, older clients and those individuals with other medical issues tend to have a poorer prognosis, generally surviving for only 1 year after diagnosis. One- to 2-month remissions may occur in half of childhood cases. In ALL, the treatment may induce remissions in the majority of cases; the remission lasts an average of 5 years. Children who undergo intensive treatment have the best survival rate. In CML, the disease is rapidly fatal after the onset of the acute phase. The average survival time is 3 years. In CLL, the progression is slow, but the prognosis is guarded and depends on the progression of disease and the person's age. If the person has anemia, death usually occurs within 2 years. Various immunologic disorders may accompany CLL, worsening the prognosis.

Prevention

Addressing the risk factors of leukemia is essential.

Bone Marrow Transplant

Bone marrow transplant (BMT) is a special treatment for clients with cancer or other diseases affecting the bone marrow and blood cell production (see Chapter 5). BMT involves taking stem cells from the bone marrow, filtering them, and giving them back to the donor or to another person. It transfuses healthy bone marrow cells into a person after his or her own unhealthy bone marrow has been eliminated. BMT has been used successfully to treat leukemias, lymphomas, aplastic anemia, immune deficiency disorders, and some solid tumor cancers.

In one form of BMT, stem cells are removed from you before you receive high-dose chemotherapy or radiation treatment. The stem cells are stored in a freezer (cryopreservation). After high-dose chemotherapy or radiation treatments, your stems cells are put back in your body to make (regenerate) normal blood cells. There are three types of BMT:

1. *Autologous BMT,* wherein the donor is the client. A person's blood cells are removed prior to receiving chemotherapy or radiation, stored in a freezer, and later returned to the body following treatment so normal blood cells can be regenerated. Often the term *bone marrow rescue* is used for this procedure because it replaces and restores bone marrow following high doses of chemotherapy or radiation.
2. *Allogeneic BMT,* wherein the donor and the recipient have the same genetic type—usually a sibling, parent, identical twin, or unrelated donor found through the national bone marrow registry.
3. *Umbilical cord blood transplant,* wherein stem cells come from an umbilical cord immediately after delivery. The stem cells are tested, typed, and frozen until they are transplanted.

Finding a matching donor is not easy. Voluntary marrow donors are registered in a number of national and international registries. A BMT is most successful when the donor's blood most closely resembles or matches that of the recipient.

Lymphatic Diseases and Disorders

LYMPHEDEMA

ICD-10: I89.0

Description

Lymphedema, or lymphatic insufficiency, is an abnormal accumulation of lymph, usually in the extremities. It is the most common lymphatic disease.

Lymphedema is identified as either primary (occurs alone) or secondary (occurs as a result of another disease or disorder). There is no cure, but it can be controlled.

Etiology

Lymphedema occurs when lymph vessels are unable to adequately drain lymph fluid from extremities (Fig. 12.14). Primary lymphedema is a rare, inherited condition occurring more frequently in women and usually affects the legs. Secondary lymphedema may arise directly as a result of surgery, trauma, burns, radiation, infections, neoplasms, allergic reactions, or thrombus formation.

Signs and Symptoms

The affected limb, in part or whole, is typically swollen and hypertrophied, with thickened and fibrotic skin. Lymphedema is usually painless, and it may be accompanied by episodes of **lymphangitis** (inflammation of the lymph vessels) and **cellulitis** (inflammation of the connective tissue). Some clients may experience a chronic dull, heavy sensation in the affected limb as well as some aching and discomfort. The edema may be either pitting or nonpitting.

Diagnostic Procedures

It is important to rule out other reasons for the swelling. A thorough client history and physical examination are

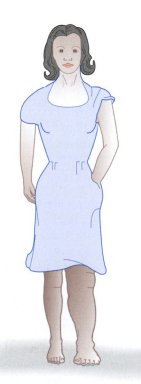

Figure 12.14 Lymphedema.

necessary. When the cause of lymphedema is not obvious, imaging tests are conducted. MRI, CT scan, and Doppler ultrasound may be ordered. Lymphoscintigraphy with radioactive dye moving through lymph vessels identifies blockage.

Treatment

Treatment attempts to lessen the swelling by moving the lymph out of the affected limb and reduce any aching and discomfort. These include the following:

- *Gentle exercise* of the affected limb following recommendations of a physical therapist.
- *Bandaging* the affected limb in such a way as to squeeze lymph toward the trunk.
- *Massage* for manual lymph drainage that is performed by a professional who understands the contraindications.
- *Pneumatic compression* that involves a sleeve connected to a pump placed over the affected limb. The sleeve intermittently inflates, placing pressure on the limb to move lymph fluid away from the fingers or toes to reduce swelling.
- *Compression garments* that include sleeves or stockings worn to compress the limb and reduce swelling.

Surgery to correct lymphatic obstruction and promote drainage may be necessary in some instances.

Complementary Therapy

The services of a physical therapist and a massage therapist can be beneficial, but the contraindications must be understood.

➔ CLIENT COMMUNICATION

Help clients understand why skin hygiene is important and that the application of emollients may prevent dry skin. Remind them to look for signs of trouble, such as cracks and cuts in the affected limb.

Prognosis

The prognosis for lymphedema depends on the cause. Infection worsens the prognosis.

Prevention

There is no known prevention for lymphedema.

Lymphomas

Lymphoma is the general term used to specify cancers of the lymphatic system. Lymphomas are cancers that begin with a malignant transformation of a lymphocyte. The two major categories are Hodgkin lymphoma and non-Hodgkin lymphoma.

HODGKIN LYMPHOMA

ICD-10: C81.9X

Description

Hodgkin lymphoma is a neoplastic malignancy of the lymphatic system characterized by painless enlargement of the lymph nodes, spleen, and other lymphatic tissues. It has two peaks of incidence: one in the early 20s and the other after age 50. It is slightly more common in men than in women. The National Cancer Institute reported 9,190 cases in 2014.

Etiology

The exact cause of Hodgkin lymphoma is not known. Infections such as the Epstein-Barr virus are suspected causes. Individuals with a compromised immune system are more likely to have the disease. Some individuals or families may have a genetic predisposition to the disease.

Signs and Symptoms

Abnormal B cells called Reed-Sternberg develop in Hodgkin lymphoma. Reed-Sternberg cells are giant connective-tissue cells that usually possess two large nuclei. They grow abnormally large and are a specific characteristic of Hodgkin lymphoma; these cells do not experience cell death. The usual presenting symptom is enlarged, firm, nontender, painless regional lymph nodes, generally in the neck, axilla, or groin. Fever, fatigue, weight loss, diaphoresis, and pruritus may follow.

Diagnostic Procedures

A thorough physical examination is conducted. Laboratory findings may reveal **lymphocytopenia** (abnormally small numbers of lymphocytes in the circulating blood) and anemia. Definitive diagnosis is established by identifying the presence of Reed-Sternberg cells in lymphatic tissue. A lymph node biopsy and bone marrow biopsy help to establish a diagnosis. X-rays, CT scan, and MRI may be conducted to identify the extent and involvement of the disease. It is important that the extent of the disease process be known and that it be staged before therapy is initiated.

Treatment

Treatment depends on the stage of the disease. The goal is to destroy as many malignant cells as possible, bringing the disease into remission. Treatment can range from some combination of short-term chemotherapy, followed by radiation mostly in the early stages, to combination chemotherapy in the later stages. If Hodgkin lymphoma recurs, usually chemotherapy is instituted, followed by autogenous bone marrow or stem cell transplant.

Complementary Therapy

See Complementary Therapy for leukemia.

CLIENT COMMUNICATION

It is important to educate clients that Hodgkin lymphoma is curable, but careful and frequent follow-up is essential. Prevention of recurrences is aimed at treating infections and keeping the immune system healthy.

Prognosis

The prognosis varies with the staging. When the Hodgkin lymphoma is at stages I and II, the prognosis is good if there are no manifestations for the first 5 years. It should be noted, however, that there are long-term effects of treatment. They include immune defects and lingering aftereffects of radiation and chemotherapy. These defects and aftereffects can include hypothyroidism, Graves disease, risk of solid tumor development, coronary artery changes, and infertility.

Prevention

There is no known prevention for Hodgkin lymphoma.

NON-HODGKIN LYMPHOMA (LYMPHOSARCOMA)

ICD-10: C85.8X

Description

Non-Hodgkin lymphomas, or lymphosarcomas, are a group of malignant diseases of the lymphatic system that can occur at any age. They are far more common in the United States than Hodgkin lymphoma. There were nearly 70,800 cases in 2014. They are categorized as follows:

1. Well-differentiated lymphatic
2. Poorly differentiated lymphocytic
3. Histiocytic (formerly called *reticulum cell sarcoma*)
4. Mixed lymphocytic and histiocytic
5. Undifferentiated or stem cell malignant lymphoma

Etiology

Abnormal lymphocytes grow and divide uncontrollably, gathering in the lymph nodes and causing swelling. What causes this phenomenon is essentially unknown, but researchers believe that activation of certain abnormal genes may be involved. About 85% of non-Hodgkin lymphomas occur in the B cells that help to fight infection in the body.

Signs and Symptoms

Usually a person is asymptomatic until the disease progresses. Swollen lymph nodes in the neck, axilla, and groin are common presenting symptoms. Coughing, dyspnea, fatigue, sweating, fever, and weight loss may follow.

Diagnostic Procedures

Non-Hodgkin lymphomas are to be distinguished from Hodgkin disease. Diagnosis includes a complete physical examination, CBC, lymph node biopsy, and/or bone marrow biopsy. CT scans, x-rays, MRI, and occasionally cerebrospinal fluid analysis are used to determine the extent of the disease.

Treatment

Staging is important before beginning any treatment. Refer to Chapter 5 for further information on staging, and check out "Stages of Adult Non-Hodgkin Lymphoma" on the National Cancer Institute website (www.cancer.gov/cancertopics/pdq/.../adult-non-hodgkins/.../page2_) for an excellent and detailed description of cancer staging. Treatment can include chemotherapy, radiation, combination chemotherapy and radiation, stem cell transplant, biotherapy and radioimmunotherapy used separately or in combination with chemotherapy, and interferon therapy.

Complementary Therapy

See Complementary Therapy for leukemia.

 CLIENT COMMUNICATION

Educate clients about the side effects of chemotherapy and radiation. The risk of infection is great, so prevention of infection is essential. Secondary malignancies can occur. Encourage routine checkups.

Prognosis

Prognosis depends largely on the stage of the cancer, its type, and the age and general health of the client. Liver function tests that check for lactate dehydrogenase (LDH) levels help to determine prognosis. Prognosis also depends on whether the lymphoma is newly diagnosed or has recurred. The prognosis is good if the person is in remission; however, if treatment cannot produce a remission, the prognosis is poor.

Prevention

There is no known prevention for non-Hodgkin lymphoma.

COMMON SYMPTOMS OF CARDIOVASCULAR AND LYMPHATIC SYSTEMS DISEASES AND DISORDERS

Individuals with cardiovascular diseases may present with the following common complaints, which deserve attention from health-care professionals:

- Fatigue
- Dyspnea, orthopnea

- Fever
- Weakness
- Tachycardia and palpitations
- Pallor
- Hypertension
- Chest pain
- Night sweats
- Edema
- Nausea, vomiting, or anorexia
- Anxiety
- Headache
- Claudication

SUMMARY

Cardiovascular and lymphatic diseases and disorders can affect the normal functioning of the heart with its vessels and valves, or the blood, blood vessels, and the lymphatic system. Many of the diseases and disorders can be prevented with proper diet, exercise, and reduction of stress; however, others are related to genetics, of which there is little control. Medical research has identified new and more efficient treatment modalities in the past few years. Cardiovascular and lymphatic diseases may alarm individuals, further complicating already complex disease processes. Health-care professionals can help calm clients and families by offering information when requested. Teaching is an important aspect of treatment for both the client and the family.

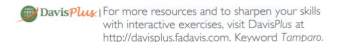

DavisPlus | For more resources and to sharpen your skills with interactive exercises, visit DavisPlus at http://davisplus.fadavis.com. Keyword *Tamparo*.

ONLINE RESOURCES

American Heart Association
http://www.americanheart.org

Aplastic anemia, folic acid deficiency anemia, pernicious anemia
http://www.nhlbi.nih.gov/health/dci/Diseases

Coronary artery disease
http://www.nhlbi.nih.gov/health/dci/Diseases/Cad/CAD_WhatIs.html

Endocarditis
http://www.endocarditis.org/index.html

Hodgkin lymphoma
http://www.cancer.gov/cancertopics/types/hodgkin

Lymphedema
http://www.lymphnet.org

Medical Daily
http://www.medicaldaily.com/facetime-your-heart-your-face-can-help-diagnose-atrial-fibrillation-300470

Myocarditis Foundation
http://www.myocarditisfoundation.org

National Cancer Institute (cancer staging)
http://www.cancer.gov

CASE STUDIES

Case Study 1

Mary Beth Plummer calls the medical clinic where you are employed to make an appointment for her 80-year-old husband, Jim. Jim has been complaining of shortness of breath and fatigue. Mary Beth has noticed prominent pulsations in the artery in his neck. She also reports that his ankles tend to swell.

Case Study Questions

1. How soon will you set the requested appointment? Identify the reason.
2. Is age a factor in Jim's condition? Explain.
3. What dietary restrictions, if any, might be recommended for Jim?

Case Study 2

Vicki Gabrielli, a single woman who is active both socially and professionally, complains of light-headedness and palpitations. She is about 70 pounds overweight, smokes two packs of cigarettes a day, and enjoys fine dining.

Case Study Questions

1. What circulatory condition might Vicki's circumstances and symptoms suggest? What are the contributing factors?
2. What diagnostic procedures might be called for in this situation? What treatment might be indicated?

Case Study 3

Fred and his wife, Marion, both in their mid to late 80s, lived in a motor home and traveled extensively, towing their car along for local driving when they stayed in a place for any length of time. Both had congestive heart failure, although Marion seemed to experience more medical complications than Fred. They had been grocery shopping and were putting away the groceries when Fred remembered their prescription medications were still in the car. He left to get them. When Marion noted it had been some time since Fred had gone, she looked out the window of the motor home. Fred was flat on his back on the ground just outside the car. She rushed to his side and noted that he was not breathing and seemed to be turning blue. She ran to the manager's office, and they called 911.

Case Study Questions

1. What action should take place immediately?
2. Describe the possible complications of congestive heart failure.
3. What is the prognosis if Fred had a myocardial infarction?

Case Study 4

Ron is 57 years old, and he is moderately obese. He is happily married and has two teenagers, one of whom is close to being expelled from school. He is the mediator between his daughter and her mother, who is very anxious about their daughter's future. Ron's job is even more stressful and affords little or no opportunity for change. Ron is diagnosed with hypertension and notes that his blood pressure drops within a "more normal" range on weekends away from work and when the kids spend the weekend with friends.

Case Study Questions

1. What steps might Ron take to reduce his hypertension?
2. Are there any steps the family might take to relieve this situation?

REVIEW QUESTIONS

Matching

Match each of the following definitions with its correct term.

_____ 1. Inflammation of cardiac muscle

_____ 2. Inflammation of the sac surrounding the heart

_____ 3. Inflammation of the heart valves and chambers

_____ 4. Heart suddenly ceases to pump

_____ 5. Local dilation of a blood vessel

_____ 6. Inflammation of vein with thrombus formation

_____ 7. Dilated, tortuous veins

a. Endocarditis

b. Pericarditis

c. Myocarditis

d. Thrombophlebitis

e. Cardiac arrest

f. Aneurysm

g. Varicose veins

h. Aplastic anemia

i. Lymphedema

Short Answer

1. Can you describe the four types of anemias?

   a. Iron deficiency anemia

   b. Folic acid deficiency anemia

   c. Pernicious anemia

   d. Aplastic anemia

2. What are the identifying characteristics of the four types of leukemia?

   a. Acute myeloid (myelogenous) leukemia

   b. Acute lymphocytic (lymphoblastic) leukemia

   c. Chronic myeloid (myelogenous) leukemia

   d. Chronic lymphocytic (lymphoblastic) leukemia

3. How would you compare/contrast the following?

   a. Atherosclerosis

   b. Arteriosclerosis

4. What are five risk factors for CAD?

   a. _____

   b. _____

   c. _____

   d. _____

   e. _____

   f. _____

5. Can you list the three forms of angina pectoris and label the form that is most serious?

   a. _____

   b. _____

   c. _____

6. How would you describe the two stages of essential hypertension?

   a. _____

   b. _____

Multiple Choice

Place a checkmark next to the correct answer.

1. According to the medical community, what constitutes stage 1 essential hypertension?

   _____ a. 120 systolic pressure and 80 diastolic pressure

   _____ b. Over 140 systolic pressure and over 90 diastolic pressure

   _____ c. Obesity, sedentary lifestyle, and being African American

   _____ d. Over 160 systolic pressure and over 100 diastolic pressure

2. What is the classic symptom of myocardial infarction, especially in men?

   _____ a. Hematemesis, dysphagia

   _____ b. Crushing chest pain that may radiate to the left arm, neck, and jaw

   _____ c. Tachypnea and heart palpitations

   _____ d. Claudication, limb numbness

3. What is the common medication taken sublingually or topically for angina pectoris?

   _____ a. Nitroglycerin preparations

   _____ b. Specific antibiotics

   _____ c. Antidiuretics

   _____ d. Antispasmodic medication

4. What is the other name for non-Hodgkin disease?

   _____ a. Lymphedema

   _____ b. Lymphocytopenia

   _____ c. Lymphosarcoma

   _____ d. Lymphadenitis

5. When someone is having atrial fibrillation, what might they try to reverse the fibrillation?

_____ a. Coughing

_____ b. Taking an aspirin and resting

_____ c. Establishing a cardioversion

_____ d. Drinking a strong cup of coffee

6. Lymphedema is most likely caused by which of the following?

_____ a. Hypertension

_____ b. Epstein-Barr virus

_____ c. Chemotherapy and exposure to toxic chemicals

_____ d. Surgery, trauma, burns, radiation, allergic reactions

7. What condition may now be diagnosed with a facial scan?

_____ a. Congestive heart failure

_____ b. Angina pectoris

_____ c. Atrial fibrillation

_____ d. Thoracic aortic aneurysm

8. What phrase best describes mitral insufficiency?

_____ a. Blood from the left ventricle flows back into the left atrium.

_____ b. Blood cannot flow from the left atrium to the left ventricle.

_____ c. Blood flows back into the left ventricle, causing hypertrophy.

_____ d. Blood from the right ventricle flows back into the right atrium.

9. What characterizes endocarditis?

_____ a. Serious pleuritic pain

_____ b. Severe left-sided heart failure

_____ c. Abnormal vegetations on the heart valves

_____ d. Blood flowing back into the left ventricle causing hypertrophy

10. What is the primary purpose of lymph nodes?

_____ a. They help to carry blood to and from the heart.

_____ b. They filter microorganisms and abnormal cells from the body.

_____ c. They destroy old RBCs when no longer necessary.

_____ d. They produce T lymphocytes to help control cell-mediated immunity.

Discussion Questions/Personal Reflection

1. Consider the discussion of complementary therapy for the leukemias. Why might the integration of traditional and complementary therapies be important? What does traditional therapy offer that complementary therapy does not? Vice versa?

_____

_____

_____

_____

_____

_____

_____

_____

_____

_____

2. Discuss the advantages and disadvantages of bone marrow transplant. Consider availability, side effects, and potential for success. Would you choose a bone marrow transplant? Justify your response.

_____

_____

_____

_____

_____

_____

_____

_____

_____

_____

Good timber does not grow with ease. The stronger the wind, the stronger the trees.

—J. Willard Marriott

13

Respiratory System Diseases and Disorders

● *chapter outline*

key words

Alveoli (pulmonary)
(ăl•vē'ō•lī)
Apnea (ăp•nē'ă)
Biotin (bī'ō•tĭn)
Blastomycosis
(blăs'tō•mī•kō'sĭs)
Bleb (blĕb)
Clubbing (klŭb'ĭng)
Coccidioidomycosis
(kŏk•sĭd'ē•oi'dō•mī•kō'sĭs)
Diaphoresis (dī'•ă•fō•rē'sĭs)
Empyema (ĕm'pī•ē'ma)
Endophthalmitis
(ĕn'dŏf-thəl-mī'tĭs)
Exudate (ĕks'ū•dāt)
Hemoptysis (hē•mŏp'tĭ'•sĭs)
Histoplasmosis
(hĭs'tō•plăz•mō'sĭs)

Hypersomnia (hī"pĕr•sŏm'•nē•ă)
Hypoxia (hī•pŏks'ē•ă)
Hypoxemia (hī•pŏks•ē'•mē•ă)
Kyphoscoliosis
(kī"fō•skō"lē•ō'sĭs)
Malaise (mă•lāz')
**Maxillomandibular
advancement**
(măk"sĭ•lō•măn•dĭb'ū•lăr
ăd•văns'mĕnt)
Nosocomial (nŏs"ō•kō'mē•ăl)
Orthopnea (ŏr•thŏp'nē•ă)
Percussion (pĕr•kŭsh'ŭn)
pH (pē•āitch')
Pleurectomy (ploo•rĕk'tō•mē)
Polycythemia vera
(pŏl"ē•sī•the'mē•a vē'ră)

Postural drainage
(pŏs'tū•răl drā'nĭj)
Pulmonary infarction
(pŭl'mō•nĕ•rē ĭn•fark'shŭn)
Rhonchi (rŏng'kī)
Septic (sĕp'tĭk)
Sputum (spū'tŭm)
Stridor (strī'dŏr)
Thoracentesis (thō"ră•sĕn•tē'sĭs)
Thoracotomy (thō"răk•ŏt'ō•mē)
Thrombocytosis
(thrŏm"bō•sī•tō'sĭs)
Transillumination
(trăns"ĭl•lū"mĭ•nā'shŭn)
Transudate (trăns'ū•dāt)
Uvulopalatopharyngoplasty
(ū"vū•lō•păl"ă•tō•fă•rĭn"gō•plăs'tē)

learning outcomes

Upon successful completion of this chapter, you will be able to:

- Define key terms.
- Recall anatomy and physiology of the respiratory system.
- Recall the signs and symptoms and the treatment of allergic rhinitis.
- List the causes of sinusitis and possible complementary therapy.
- Name the most common throat disorder and its etiology.
- Describe the treatment for laryngitis.
- Describe epiglottitis and restate its danger.
- Identify the cause and the confirming diagnosis of infectious mononucleosis.
- Contrast the three types of pneumonia.
- Recall the etiology of *Legionella* pneumonia.
- Describe the two diseases identified in chronic obstructive pulmonary disease (COPD).
- Recall the three stages of COPD.
- Discuss the treatment and prognosis for asthma.
- Describe the conditions under which a lung abscess may occur, where they likely occur, and how they might be prevented.
- Explain the growth of the tuberculosis bacteria in the lungs.
- Compare the four pneumoconioses, their treatments, and prognoses.
- Name the three respiratory mycoses.

- Explain treatment modalities for pneumothorax.
- Compare and contrast pneumothorax and atelectasis.
- Define pleurisy and describe its etiology and symptoms.
- Differentiate between transudate and exudate fluid and how it relates to pleural effusion.
- Identify the diagnostic tests for pulmonary hypertension.
- Discuss how pulmonary edema may be a medical emergency.
- Recall the description and the prognosis of cor pulmonale.
- Describe the etiology of pulmonary embolism and how it is a complication of hospitalized individuals.
- Compare and contrast respiratory acidosis and respiratory alkalosis.
- Identify the treatment therapies for sleep apnea.
- Recall the incident statistics for lung cancer.
- List the stages of non–small cell lung cancer.
- Review the etiology of sudden infant death syndrome.
- Report the treatment of choice for chronic tonsillitis and adenoid hyperplasia.
- Restate the symptoms of thrush and those at greatest risk.
- Describe the signs and symptoms of croup.
- Recall at least four common symptoms of respiratory diseases and disorders.

CHAPTER EPISODE—PART I

Amanda was on the venture of a lifetime. At 22, she found her dream job working for an environmental firm in the great state of Alaska. She was making the move and traveling by car to Anchorage, Alaska, from Olympia, Washington. Her brother, Paal, was accompanying her on this trek. Because money was short, they camped most of the way, unless the weather was really bad. Paal, aged 24, felt proud to be "the leader" in this venture, looking out for his little sister. The problem, though, was that Paal smoked like a chimney. Although Amanda kept her window down a bit, the smoke was really getting to her.

• What are the possible stresses that Amanda might be feeling?
• What dangers are there from Paal's smoking?

RESPIRATORY SYSTEM ANATOMY AND PHYSIOLOGY REVIEW

Respiration is essential for life. The body can survive a fair length of time without food, a few days without water, but only minutes without air. Figure 13.1 shows the structure of the respiratory system.

There are two stages involved in the respiratory process: external and internal respiration. External respiration is the exchange of two gases within the lungs. Oxygen that is present in inhaled air is exchanged for carbon dioxide that diffuses from the blood, across cell walls, into the air spaces of the lungs. The carbon dioxide is then exhaled from the lungs. Internal respiration is the exchange of oxygen and carbon dioxide at the cellular level within the organs of the body. Carbon dioxide is a waste product that results when oxygen and nutrients are metabolized within body cells.

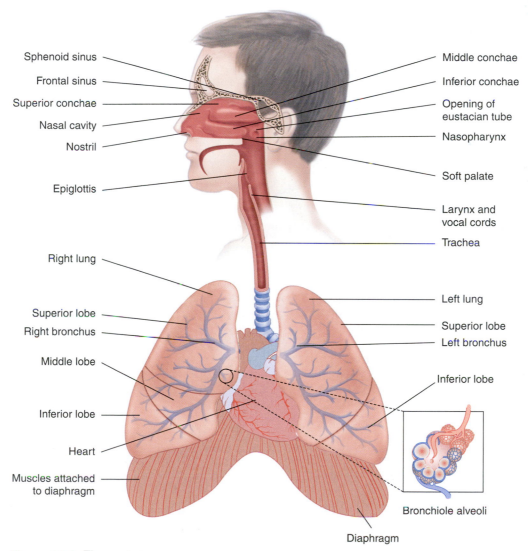

Sphenoid sinus
Frontal sinus
Superior conchae
Nasal cavity
Nostril
Epiglottis
Right lung
Superior lobe
Right bronchus
Middle lobe
Inferior lobe
Heart
Muscles attached to diaphragm

Middle conchae
Inferior conchae
Opening of eustacian tube
Nasopharynx
Soft palate
Larynx and vocal cords
Trachea
Left lung
Superior lobe
Left bronchus
Inferior lobe
Bronchiole alveoli
Diaphragm

Figure 13.1 The respiratory system.

The respiratory system is divided between the upper respiratory tract and the lower respiratory tract. The upper tract is composed of the organs located outside the chest cavity: the nose and nasal cavities, pharynx, larynx, and upper trachea (Fig. 13.2). The lower tract is composed of the organs located inside the chest cavity: the lower trachea, bronchi, bronchioles, alveoli (microscopic air sacs in the lung), and lungs. Additional parts of the lower tract are the pleural membranes and the respiratory muscles that form the chest cavity (see Fig. 13.1).

Air enters the nose, which is composed of bone and cartilage and contains ciliated epithelium and cells where the air is humidified and warmed. Tiny hairs just inside the nostrils help prevent particles of dust from entering the nasal cavities. The nasal septum separates the two sides of the nose. The nasal cavities are lined with a membrane that creates mucus designed to further trap bacteria and air pollutants. The upper nasal cavities contain the olfactory receptors that detect odors. Olfactory nerves pass through the ethmoid bone into the brain. The paranasal sinuses, the air cavities in the maxillae, frontal, sphenoid, and ethmoid bones, function to lighten the skull and provide resonance for the voice. These sinuses contain several drainage openings where mucus drains into the nasal cavity.

The pharynx, or throat, is divided into three parts: the nasopharynx, the oropharynx, and the laryngopharynx.

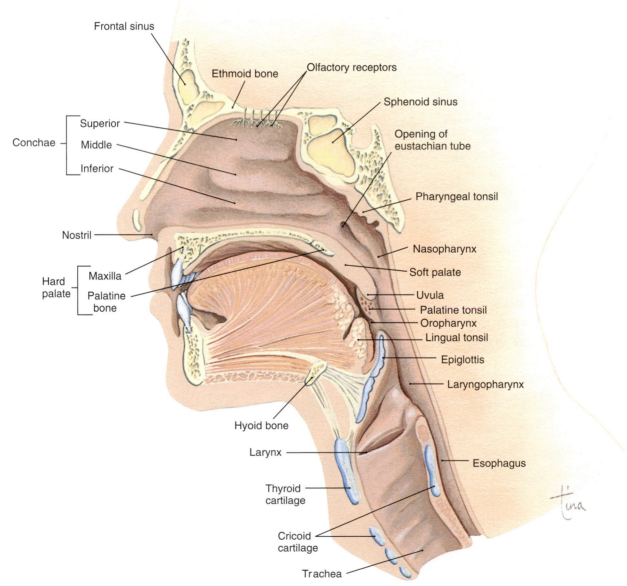

Figure 13.2 Midsagittal section of the head and neck showing the structures of the upper respiratory tract. *(From Scanlon, VC, and Sanders, T:* Understanding Human Structure and Function, *ed. 5. Philadelphia: F.A. Davis, 2007, p 345, with permission.)*

The nasopharynx is the passageway for air only. The adenoids are located in the nasopharynx. The soft palate within the nasopharynx prevents food from going up into the nasopharynx. The oropharynx contains the palatine tonsils at the base of the tongue, and the laryngopharynx opens into the larynx and into the esophagus.

The larynx, or voice box, serves as an air passageway and allows for speaking. Cartilage in the larynx prevents the collapse of the larynx, which must stay open for air passage. The epiglottis, located at the top of the larynx, closes over to prevent the entry of food into the larynx. The vocal cords are located on either side of the glottis.

The trachea contains C-shaped cartilage that keeps the windpipe open for air passage yet allows food to pass through to the esophagus, which is located behind the trachea. The trachea extends downward into the chest cavity where it splits into the right and left bronchus. These bronchi branch into secondary bronchi leading into the right and left lungs to form the bronchial tree. The branches become smaller, forming bronchioles that terminate in clusters of **alveoli,** the air sacs of the lungs (see Fig. 13.1). The millions of tiny alveoli (only one cell thick) in each lung are important for respiration. They house macrophages to phagocytize any foreign pathogens that might have made it all the way to the lungs. They also permit the diffusion of gases between air in the alveoli and blood in the pulmonary capillaries (also only one cell thick).

The lungs, located on either side of the heart, are protected by the rib cage and rest on the diaphragm. They are lined with pleural membranes. The parietal pleura lines the chest wall, while the visceral pleura is on the surface of the lung. Pleura serve to prevent friction and keep the two membranes together during breathing. The lungs are soft and cone-shaped and take up most of the thoracic cavity. The lobes of the lung (three on the right and two on the left) contain the bronchial tree.

Upper Respiratory Diseases and Disorders

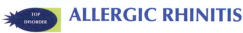

ALLERGIC RHINITIS

ICD-10: J30.9

Description

Rhinitis is inflammation of the nasal membranes. Allergic rhinitis is the most common type of rhinitis, affecting about 40 to 50 million people in the United States. It occurs when there is an allergic reaction to particles in the air. The immune system attacks the particles, causing sneezing and rhinorrhea. The eyes, ears, sinuses, and throat can become inflamed as well. It can be acute or chronic.

Etiology

The inflammation resulting from rhinitis is triggered by an immunoglobulin E (IgE)–mediated response to an allergen, such as pollen, dust, animal dander, smoke, or mold. When the reaction is caused by pollen, the name *hay fever* is often used. Pollens that cause a reaction vary among persons and regions. Hot, dry, windy weather with increased amounts of pollen in the air from trees, grasses, and ragweed produce the most symptoms. Allergic rhinitis can coexist with eczema, asthma, and nasal polyps. There is a strong genetic component to allergic rhinitis, especially if a parent has the same problem.

Signs and Symptoms

Commonly there is nasal congestion, sneezing, and rhinorrhea. Coughing, headache, and itching of the nose, mouth, eyes, throat, or skin may be seen. Some have a sore throat and their eyes tear. Others have what is called "allergic shiners," or dark circles under their eyes from vasodilation and nasal congestion.

Diagnostic Procedures

A physical examination should identify a history of the symptoms. Primary care providers (PCPs) will

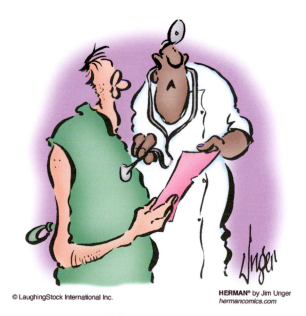

© LaughingStock International Inc.

HERMAN® by Jim Unger
hermancomics.com

"Breathe deeply and take a quick look at my bill."

HERMAN© is reprinted with permission from LaughingStock Licensing Inc., Ottawa, Canada. All rights reserved.

want to know whether the symptoms vary according to time of day or the season, exposure to pets or other allergens, and diet changes. Allergy testing may be performed to determine the cause. Skin testing is most likely and may include the prick or patch method. Blood testing may reveal elevated IgE levels and an elevated eosinophil count, which further supports the diagnosis.

Treatment

The management of allergic rhinitis consists of environmental control measures and allergen avoidance, medications, and immunotherapy or desensitization treatment. Controlling the environment and avoiding the allergen can be difficult but is worth the effort once the allergen has been identified. Medications are frequently prescribed and may include some over-the-counter drugs. Oral antihistamines, decongestants, or both may be necessary. Regular use of an intranasal steroid spray (even when symptoms are not present) may be appropriate for some clients with chronic allergic rhinitis. Immunotherapy treatment with allergy shots helps reduce symptoms and medication requirements. It can take as long as 6 to 12 months to notice a difference, however, and therapy may need to continue for a few years.

Complementary Therapy

Integrative medicine practitioners recommend the easiest route of treatment first, which includes removing or avoiding the allergen as much as possible. They also recommend following an anti-inflammatory diet, decreasing dairy protein and total protein intake, and increasing hydration. Cromolyn sodium nasal spray (NasalCrom), available over the counter, is recommended.

⊙ CLIENT COMMUNICATION

Clients with allergic rhinitis may be quite miserable by the time they seek medical attention. The disease can lead to otitis media or acute sinusitis. Explain to individuals how to protect their homes and environment from allergens as much as possible.

Prognosis

The prognosis for allergic rhinitis is usually good when clients respond to the steps identified in treatment. Prevention of recurrence and complications is important.

Prevention

Avoidance of known allergens and treatment management, even when symptoms are not present, is important.

Understanding Nosebleeds

Nosebleed, or epistaxis, is more likely a symptom rather than a disorder or disease. Bleeding from the nose is more common in winter months, which are likely cold and dry. It is more common in children and older adults. Nosebleeds are usually not considered serious, but some circumstances call for medical attention because of possible underlying causes:

• Repeated nosebleeds
• Syncope
• Hematemesis or hemoptysis

Nosebleeds commonly occur due to nose picking or nose trauma but may be secondary to rhinitis, hypertension, chemotherapy treatment, certain illnesses, and blood-thinning medications. Secondary nosebleeds should be reported to a medical professional.

To treat a nosebleed, have the client lean forward and press the soft portion of the nostrils against the septum for 10 minutes (pinch the nose). Apply cold, wet compresses. A vasoconstricting agent such as epinephrine on a cotton ball may be applied to the bleeding site. Cauterization or petrolatum gauze nasal packing may be needed. After the bleeding has stopped, instruct the client to try to prevent any further irritation to the nose for as long as possible. This includes avoiding sneezing, nose blowing, and coughing.

SINUSITIS

ICD-10: J32.9

Description

Sinusitis is inflammation of the paranasal sinus. The condition may be acute, subacute, chronic, allergic, or hyperplastic. Acute sinusitis generally is caused by the common cold and lingers in the subacute form in about 10% of cases. Chronic sinusitis follows a viral or bacterial infection. Allergic sinusitis often accompanies allergic rhinitis. Hyperplastic sinusitis is a combination of purulent acute sinusitis and allergic sinusitis.

Etiology

Sinusitis is usually caused by pneumococcal, streptococcal, or *Haemophilus influenzae* bacterial infections. The infection may spread to the sinuses when an individual has a cold, usually because of excessive nose blowing. Sinusitis also can result from swimming or diving, dental abscess or tooth extractions, or nasal allergies. Chronic sinusitis may be caused by the same etiologic factors as acute sinusitis but more frequently is caused by staphylococcal and gram-negative bacteria. These bacteria may be seen in hospital intensive care clients. Fungi are becoming an increasing cause of chronic sinusitis, especially in individuals with weakened immune systems.

Signs and Symptoms

Signs and symptoms depend on which sinuses are affected and whether the sinus infection is acute or chronic, but an individual with acute or chronic sinusitis may exhibit the following symptoms: nasal congestion; pain; tenderness, redness, and swelling over the involved sinus; purulent nasal discharge or postnasal drip; headache; generalized feeling of illness, or **malaise;** and a nonproductive cough. A low-grade fever also may be present. Allergic sinusitis may be accompanied by watering eyes and sneezing. Purulent nasal discharge lasting more than 3 weeks following an acute infection suggests subacute sinusitis.

Diagnostic Procedures

A nasal examination is commonly performed. A specimen of nasal secretions may be taken for culture to identify any infectious agent. X-rays and inspection of a cavity by passing a light through its walls, or **transillumination,** may show clouding of the involved sinus. A computed tomography (CT) scan, which is more sensitive than routine x-rays, aids in diagnosing suspected complications.

Treatment

Analgesics for pain relief, decongestants, and antibiotics for control of bacterial infection are typically the treatments of choice. Clients are encouraged to drink plenty of fluids to help liquefy secretions. The application of heat over the affected sinus may be helpful.

Complementary Therapy

Advise clients to drink plenty of water and hydrating beverages. Recommend hot herbal tea. Tell clients to inhale steam two to four times per day for about 10 minutes by leaning over a bowl of hot water or using a steam vaporizer. Also suggest that taking a hot, steamy shower may also help provide relief. Encourage clients to reduce stress and to eat a diet rich in antioxidants, especially fresh, dark-colored fruits and vegetables to help strengthen their immune system.

 CLIENT COMMUNICATION

Discuss any prescribed antibiotic therapy with clients. Encourage resting, drinking plenty of fluids, and reducing stress as much as possible.

Prognosis

The prognosis is good. Sinusitis is an uncomfortable condition, but with proper care, it usually does not last long.

Prevention

Prevention of a sinus infection depends on its cause. Remind clients to avoid contracting upper respiratory tract infections by maintaining strict hand-washing habits and avoiding those with a cold. Clients should have a yearly Hib (influenza) vaccination and should be prepared for seasonal allergy attacks.

PHARYNGITIS

ICD-10: J02.9

Description

Pharyngitis, inflammation of the pharynx, is the most common throat disorder and may be acute or chronic. On average, children experience sore throats about five times a year, adults twice a year.

Etiology

Acute pharyngitis can be caused by any number of bacterial or viral infections, with viral infections being the most common. *Streptococcus pyogenes* (which causes strep throat) is the most common of many possible bacterial pathogens; influenza virus and common cold viruses are the most common viral pathogens causing the condition. Less common is infection with bacteria from gonorrhea or chlamydia spread during oral sex. Acute pharyngitis also may arise secondary to systemic viral infections, such as measles or chickenpox. Noninfectious causes of the disease include trauma to the mucosa of the pharynx from heat, sharp objects, or chemical irritants. Chronic pharyngitis is more likely to have a noninfectious origin and is often associated with persistent cough, allergy, or acid reflux.

Signs and Symptoms

The hallmark of acute pharyngitis is a sore throat. The pain may be mild or of such severity that swallowing becomes difficult. Accompanying symptoms may include malaise, fever, headache, muscle and joint pain, coryza or cold, and rhinorrhea.

Diagnostic Procedures

Physical examination of the pharynx typically reveals red, swollen mucous membranes. In severe cases, pustular ulcerations of the pharyngeal wall may be evident. See Figure 13.3 for an example of strep throat. A throat culture is usually performed to identify the infecting organism. This culture generally takes up to 24 hours for results, but a 10- to 15-minute in-clinic rapid test (not quite as reliable) can also be obtained.

Treatment

Antibiotics are generally prescribed if the source of the infection is determined to be bacterial. Otherwise, treatment is symptomatic and typically includes the use of warm saline gargles, analgesics, and drugs to relieve fever (antipyretics). Bed rest and adequate fluid intake may be advised.

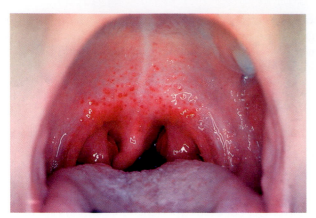

Figure 13.3 Inflammation of the oropharynx and petechiae, or small red spots on the soft palate caused by strep throat. *(Hardin MD. University of Iowa and the Centers for Disease Control and Prevention. http://www.lib.uiowa.edu/hardin/Md/cdc/3185.html.)*

Complementary Therapy

Gargling with warm water, one-quarter teaspoon of turmeric powder, and a pinch of salt may help. Aromatherapy that includes inhalation with lavender, thyme, eucalyptus, and sandalwood is often used. The client should drink herbal teas, diluted fruit juices, and broth.

⊛ CLIENT COMMUNICATION

A sore throat caused by a streptococcal infection must be identified and treated to prevent such complications as rheumatic fever, tonsil abscess, or acute glomerulonephritis.

Prognosis

The prognosis for most forms of pharyngitis is generally good. Uncomplicated pharyngitis usually subsides in 3 to 10 days. Serious complications, such as rheumatic fever and glomerulonephritis, may result from untreated acute streptococcal pharyngitis. Therefore, antibiotic therapy must be continued until the medication is gone.

Prevention

There are no specific preventive measures for pharyngitis. Some of the common ways to protect against strep throat are covering the mouth when sneezing or coughing, maintaining strict hand-washing habits to avoid contracting upper respiratory tract infections, and avoiding those with a cold. The use of both male and female condoms can prevent the spread of the bacteria during oral sex. Irritating substances, such as cigarette smoke and any known allergens, should be avoided.

LARYNGITIS

ICD-10: J04.0

Description

Laryngitis is inflammation of the laryngeal mucosa and the vocal cords, causing a hoarse voice; it may be acute or chronic. Most of the time, laryngitis comes on quickly and lasts no more than 2 weeks. Chronic cases last 2 weeks or longer.

Etiology

Acute laryngitis may result from bacterial or viral infections, with colds and influenza being the most common. It may occur as a complication of acute rhinitis or pharyngitis. Excessive use of the voice or the inhalation of dust and chemical irritants is also a cause. Acid reflux, or gastroesophageal reflux disease (GERD), causes the most common type of chronic laryngitis—*reflux laryngitis.* Chronic laryngitis also may be caused by more severe problems, such as nerve damage, sores, polyps, or hard and thick lumps (nodules) on the vocal cords.

Signs and Symptoms

Hoarseness or a complete lack of normal voice is a common sign. Also, there may be pain, dry cough, fever, and malaise.

Diagnostic Procedures

A physical examination includes information about when and how the laryngitis began. Laryngoscopy typically reveals red, inflamed, and possibly hemorrhagic vocal cords.

Treatment

Resting the voice is necessary for successful treatment. Any underlying disease or disorder must be diagnosed and treated. Antibiotic therapy may be necessary if a bacterial infection is causing the condition. Medications to reduce acid reflux may be prescribed. Analgesics and cough suppressants may provide symptomatic relief.

Complementary Therapy

See "Pharyngitis."

⊛ CLIENT COMMUNICATION

Maintaining adequate humidity in a room can be helpful. Speech training may be necessary if the laryngitis is caused by the way a person speaks or sings.

Prognosis

The prognosis for acute laryngitis is good with proper treatment. The prognosis for chronic laryngitis varies according to the underlying cause and its prevention.

Prevention

Preventive measures for acute or chronic laryngitis include avoiding misuse or overuse of the voice and avoiding irritants, such as cigarette smoke, alcohol, and extremes of air temperature.

EPIGLOTTITIS

ICD-10: J05.11

Description

Epiglottitis occurs when the epiglottis covering the windpipe swells and blocks the flow of air into the lungs. It is life-threatening.

Etiology

Infection with *Haemophilus influenzae* type b (Hib) is the most common cause, followed by burns from hot liquids and direct injury to the throat. Other bacteria and viruses that cause epiglottitis are pneumococcus; streptococcus A, B, and C; *Candida albicans;* and varicella zoster. Swallowing a foreign object and smoking crack cocaine and heroin may also cause epiglottitis.

Signs and Symptoms

Onset of symptoms is sudden. Likely symptoms include sore throat, painful swallowing, fever, drooling, hoarseness, dyspnea, and cyanosis.

Diagnostic Procedures

Once the airway is open and the condition is stable, the throat is examined with a flexible fiberoptic tube. A blood test and throat culture are likely taken to establish the cause of any infection.

Treatment

The first priority is to establish a clear passage for air; this may include a mask to deliver oxygen to the lungs or a breathing tube placed into the windpipe through the nose or mouth. In severe cases, a tracheotomy may be performed. If infection is the cause, antibiotics will be given.

Complementary Therapy

There is no known complementary therapy.

⊙ CLIENT COMMUNICATION

Explain procedures to clients; reassurance is helpful to calm the anxiety felt by clients when they have difficulty breathing.

Prognosis

Epiglottitis is a medical emergency. Fortunately, the availability of routine Hib immunization has greatly reduced the number of instances of epiglottitis. Those with weakened immune systems are more susceptible.

Prevention

Immunization with the Hib vaccine is an effective way to prevent epiglottitis. It is always best not to share personal items and to wash hands frequently in order to prevent infection of any kind.

INFECTIOUS MONONUCLEOSIS

ICD-10: B27.90

Description

Infectious mononucleosis is an acute infectious disease characterized by sore throat, fever, and swollen cervical lymph glands. The disease primarily affects adolescents and young adults. It is also called glandular fever.

Etiology

Infectious mononucleosis is caused by the Epstein-Barr virus (EBV). This virus is shed in the saliva of infected individuals and is usually spread through the oropharyngeal route (this is why it's called the "kissing disease"). Once in the body, EBV infects B lymphocytes, a type of white cell found in the lymph, blood, and connective tissue; these are important components of the body's immune system. Infectious mononucleosis is most likely contagious for a period before symptoms develop until the fever subsides and the oropharyngeal lesions disappear.

Signs and Symptoms

Initial symptoms are usually vague, mimic those of other diseases, and may include malaise, anorexia, and chills. After 3 to 5 days, sore throat, fever, and swollen lymph glands in the throat and neck occur. Early in the infection, a rash that resembles rubella sometimes develops.

Diagnostic Procedures

A thorough client history and physical examination are essential to rule out closely related disorders and will reveal the triad of symptoms: sore throat, fever, and swollen lymph glands. A blood test is necessary to confirm the diagnosis. It will show increased numbers of leukocytes, lymphocytes, monocytes, and antibodies to EBV.

Treatment

Treatment is supportive because mononucleosis resists prevention and antimicrobial treatment. Bed rest may be indicated during the acute phase, but clients may still need to lessen their activities in order to avoid potential injury to the softened and enlarged spleen until the disease completely subsides. Analgesics may be recommended for headache and sore throat. Warm saline gargles are also helpful.

Complementary Therapy

Bed rest is especially important in the acute phase of the infection. It is recommended that clients drink plenty of water, filtered to remove chlorine, heavy metals, benzene, lead, and mercury, and eat organic meats, eggs, milk, and poultry that contain no growth hormones or antibiotics. Vitamin supplements may be recommended.

 CLIENT COMMUNICATION

Stress adequate rest and reduction of activities. Clients may suffer from ongoing fatigue during much of the period of infection and tend to resume normal activity too quickly.

Prognosis

The prognosis is excellent, but recovery may take several weeks or months. Once infected with EBV, the virus remains—usually in a dormant state—for life. If the virus does reactivate, it does not cause illness. Mononucleosis sometimes leads to a serious condition called *chronic active EBV infection,* which causes illness more than 6 months after the initial diagnosis.

Prevention

The best prevention is to avoid oral-pharyngeal contact with a known EBV-infected person. The EBV virus is spread when saliva from an infected person gets into another person's mouth, so do not share dishes or eating utensils with someone who has mononucleosis.

SLEEP APNEA

ICD-10: G47.XX*

Description

Sleep apnea is potentially dangerous and occurs when an individual's breathing during sleep repeatedly stops and starts. The condition often is accompanied by snoring loud enough to disturb partners. There are three forms: *obstructive sleep apnea,* in which the throat muscles relax; *central sleep apnea,* in which the brain does not send the proper signals to the muscles that control breathing; and *complex apnea,* which is a combination of both. It is more common in males and in older adults.

Etiology

In obstructive sleep apnea, when the muscles in the back of the throat relax, the airway narrows and breathing temporarily stops. The brain senses the inability to breathe and causes the individual to awaken and take a breath. This occurrence may happen as many as 30 times per hour all night long. Repeated incidences cause the oxygen level in the blood to fall. Because sleep is so disturbed (even though most do not recall waking up to breathe), individuals may feel sleep deprived and have difficulty functioning throughout the day. Obstructive

sleep apnea is the most common form. In central sleep apnea, the most common cause is heart disease. Complex sleep apnea shares the cause in both obstructive and central sleep apneas.

Signs and Symptoms

The symptoms are loud snoring; **hypersomnia;** observed periods of breathing cessation during sleep; abrupt awakenings with shortness of breath; morning headache, dry mouth, sore throat; and insomnia.

Diagnostic Procedures

During a history and physical examination, the primary care provider likely will refer the client to a sleep specialist. The most common testing includes a nocturnal polysomnography or sleep study, oximetry to measure the level of oxygen in the blood, and portable cardiorespiratory monitoring. These steps are generally performed in a sleep center when individuals are carefully observed during their sleep.

Treatment

A continuous positive airway pressure (CPAP) machine is often prescribed. The machine delivers air pressure through a mask over the nose during sleep to keep airway passages open, thus preventing sleep apnea and snoring. Most CPAP units offer adjustable airway pressure and a humidifier. Sometimes the client is referred to a dental specialist who makes an oral appliance to be worn at night. The appliance opens the throat by bringing the jaw forward. If surgery is necessary in extreme causes, it will involve **uvulopalatopharyngoplasty** (UPPP), **maxillomandibular advancement,** or tracheostomy.

Complementary Therapy

While no complementary therapy is recognized, most health-care practitioners agree that losing weight is the first step to decreasing incidences of sleep apnea.

 CLIENT COMMUNICATION

Remind clients about losing weight, avoiding alcohol, sleeping on their sides, and properly using any medications that may also have been prescribed. Sleep apnea is frustrating, and many individuals do not do well with the CPAP machine. They report having difficulty getting comfortable, the noise of the machine disturbing their sleep, and taking it off before the night has ended.

Prognosis

The prognosis for sleep apnea is complicated. Because treatment is not always successful, clients often give up trying. Some sleep specialists report that 4 hours a night

---

The X represents the fourth digit that is often required and supplied once more detailed information about the disease or disorder is made known to the provider.

using the CPAP is a success. Dental specialists who design oral appliances report that their oral appliances are effective throughout the entire night in most cases. The surgeries suggested are extensive, have their own complications, and are not always successful in creating a cure for sleep apnea. Untreated sleep apnea can cause cardiovascular difficulties, daytime fatigue, and complications with medications and surgery. Anyone receiving any type of sedation for a surgical procedure must notify surgeons of their sleep apnea in order to prevent the risks from anesthesia.

Prevention

There is no prevention for sleep apnea other than to lose weight, avoid alcohol and tranquilizers, sleep on the side or abdomen, and keep nasal passages open at night. Sleep apnea worsens with age.

Lower Respiratory Diseases and Disorders

PNEUMONIA

ICD-10: J18.9

Description

Pneumonia is an acute inflammation of the respiratory bronchioles, alveolar ducts, alveolar sacs, and alveoli of the lung. The inflammation may be either unilateral or bilateral and involve all or a portion of the affected lung. Pneumonia once was the leading cause of death in the United States, but modern antibiotics greatly lessened the incidence of the disease. However, pneumonia still affects close to 4 million people each year and causes death for almost 60,000 individuals yearly in the United States. People over age 65 and those with depressed immunity are at greater risk. Pneumonia is often further identified as follows:

Lobar pneumonia: affects one or more lobes of the lung
Bronchopneumonia: also known as *lobular pneumonia;* bacterial form of the disease
Interstitial pneumonia: characterized by progressive scarring of both lungs

Etiology

Pneumonia may be caused by microorganisms, such as bacteria, viruses, fungi, protozoa, or rickettsiae. Viral and bacterial pneumonia are the two main types, with bacterial pneumonia being more serious. The most common cause of bacterial pneumonia is *Streptococcus pneumoniae* followed by *Haemophilus influenzae*. The disease also may arise secondary to other systemic diseases or may be induced by a variety of noninfectious agents, such as chemicals and dusts. Most of the microbial and noninfectious agents that cause pneumonia are either inhaled from the air or aspirated from the nasopharynx and oropharynx. The term *aspiration pneumonia*, however, is usually reserved for pneumonia caused by irritation from large quantities of foreign matter, especially gastric contents, drawn into the lungs. In children, viral pneumonias occur more frequently than bacterial pneumonias and often follow an upper respiratory viral infection.

Certain pneumonias are far more likely to be acquired during hospitalization and are called **nosocomial,** or hospital-acquired, infections. Other pneumonias occur more frequently in school environments or military settings.

Signs and Symptoms

Symptoms vary greatly; however, the cardinal symptoms are coughing, **sputum** production (substance produced by coughing), pleuritic chest pain, shaking chills, and fever. Accompanying symptoms may include an abnormal crackling sound heard on auscultation of the lungs. This sound is often referred to as *rales* but more accurately is called *coarse* or *fine crackles*. There will be dyspnea or labored and difficult breathing, cyanosis, and generalized weakness.

Diagnostic Procedures

A medical history and complete physical examination are performed. A chest x-ray, taken in most suspected cases of pneumonia, typically indicates the presence of infiltrates, the extent of lung involvement, and any complications present (Fig. 13.4). Sputum smears and blood cultures usually are done to isolate the suspected microorganism.

Treatment

The treatment varies with the etiology. Antibiotics are prescribed for bacterial pneumonia and antifungal medications if fungus is the cause. Supporting therapy for most types of pneumonia may include humidified oxygen therapy, mechanical ventilation, a high-calorie diet, increased fluid intake, bed rest, and analgesics. Bronchial hygiene or chest physiotherapy using a variety of noninvasive techniques to help improve the gas exchange in the lungs and remove secretions is instituted. Bronchial hygiene likely includes **postural drainage** with percussion and vibration. In postural drainage, the individual is required to assume a variety of positions to facilitate drainage of secretions in the lobes of the lungs or the bronchial passages. Percussion and vibration consists of tapping, clapping, or shaking the chest area over the lung segment to force secretions into larger airways.

Complementary Therapy

Supplements that strengthen the immune system can help shorten pneumonia infections, decrease their severity, and reduce lingering symptoms.

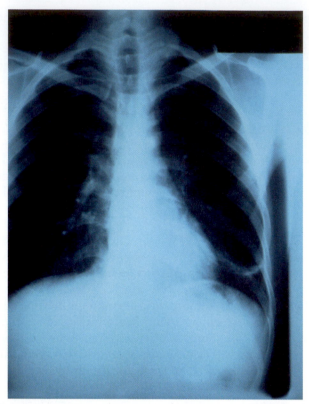

Figure 13.4 The anteroposterior chest x-ray reveals early left lower lobe pneumonia with unknown etiology. *(Centers for Disease Control and Prevention. Dr. Thomas Hooten, 1978.)*

⊘ CLIENT COMMUNICATION

Caution clients on the seriousness of the illness. Remind them to seek additional treatment if there are any complications. Show clients how to cough and to perform deep-breathing exercises. Teach them to properly dispose of tissues in which they have sneezed or coughed. Encourage frequent hand washing.

Prognosis

The prognosis varies with etiology. If the pneumonia is secondary to another disease or if clients are already debilitated, the prognosis may be poor. A similar prognosis exists for influenza-caused pneumonia, especially among elderly persons. A frequent complication of influenza-caused pneumonia is lung abscess. When the cause of pneumonia is bacterial, that same bacteria may enter the bloodstream, causing other infections.

Prevention

Those who are at higher-than-normal risk, such as elderly clients; those with a chronic illness; and those with a weakened immune system should receive the pneumococcal vaccine.

Understanding ARDS

Acute respiratory distress syndrome (ARDS) is sudden, life-threatening lung failure. ARDS occurs when the alveoli become inflamed and filled with liquid, causing their collapse. Gas exchange ceases, and the body is starved for oxygen. ARDS is a syndrome rather than a disease. It most often occurs within 24 to 48 hours of injury or illness, and the intensity and duration varies from person to person. The mortality rate ranges from 35% to 50%, in most cases as a result of underlying disease or mechanical ventilation complications.

LEGIONELLA PNEUMONIA (LEGIONNAIRES DISEASE)

ICD-10: A48.1

Description

A *Legionella* infection is an acute bronchopneumonia disease. There are two forms of the condition: Legionnaires disease and Pontiac fever. Legionnaires disease is named after an epidemic outbreak of the illness that killed 34 people and sickened more than 200 attending an American Legion convention in Philadelphia in July 1976. The disease may be mild and self-limiting, as in the case of Pontiac fever, or may produce a pneumonia severe enough to be fatal. According to the Centers for Disease Control and Prevention (CDC), between 8,000 and 18,000 people are hospitalized with Legionnaires disease each year in the United States.

Etiology

Legionella infection is caused by the gram-negative bacillus *Legionella pneumophila*. Other closely related bacteria within the genus *Legionella* also can produce outbreaks of the disease that are clinically indistinguishable from classic Legionnaires disease. The *Legionella* bacteria thrive primarily in warm aquatic environments such as in hot tubs, cooling towers, hot water tanks, large plumbing systems, or parts of the air-conditioning systems of large buildings. Individuals get the infection from inhaling a mist or vapor from aerosolized water droplets that house the bacteria. The bacteria does not spread from person to person. The bacteria for Legionnaires disease has an incubation period of about 1 week. Predisposing factors include smoking and prior physical debilitation, especially among those with chronic obstructive pulmonary disease, individuals with suppressed immune systems, and alcoholism.

Signs and Symptoms

The early symptoms of *Legionella* infection usually develop within 2 to 10 days after exposure and are nonspecific. Symptoms may include malaise, headache, nausea, aching muscles, and high fever. A nonproductive cough develops, which later produces grayish and nonpurulent sputum. Persons with Pontiac fever usually recover in 2 to 5 days without treatment.

Diagnostic Procedures

Fine crackles are heard on auscultation. A chest x-ray reveals pneumonia. The most commonly used laboratory test for diagnosis is the urinary antigen test, which detects *Legionella* bacteria from a urine specimen. Sputum direct fluorescent antibody (DFA) stains show *Legionella*. Laboratory studies may show elevated leukocytes, erythrocyte sedimentation rate (ESR), and liver enzyme activity. Bronchial washings and blood and pleural fluid cultures rule out other pulmonary infections.

Treatment

Antibiotic therapy is typically started even before the disease is definitely diagnosed. Antipyretics, fluid replacement, and oxygen therapy may be used.

Complementary Therapy

See "Pneumonia."

 CLIENT COMMUNICATION

Remind clients to take all the prescribed antibiotics, tell them the disease is not contagious, and have them return for follow-up to make certain the infection is gone.

Prognosis

The prognosis is usually good if treatment is initiated early in the course of the disease and if individuals are in good health otherwise. Even so, response to treatment is usually slow. Complications may include pneumonia, **hypoxia** (insufficient oxygenation of the blood), delirium, heart failure, and shock. Shock usually is fatal.

Prevention

Prevention includes detecting and eradicating *Legionella* bacteria from environments that may potentially infect people. Because smokers are much more likely to contract *Legionella* pneumonia, smoking cessation is recommended.

CHAPTER EPISODE—PART II

Amanda's car was making the trip fine. With help from their parents, she and her brother had planned well. They had food and water in the car, they had AAA plan their route with appropriate stops, and they were seeing wonderful things—a golden eagle by the road on an old tree stump, herds of elk, tons of trucks on the Alcan highway, and many hunters. But all was not good. Paal thought Amanda didn't drive fast enough; Amanda knew Paal drove way too fast around the curves with no centerlines when he was at the wheel, and the nonstop smoking continued. Amanda thought she was catching a cold; her nose was stuffy and she had a cough.

- Amanda's symptoms might signal what problem?
- What can Amanda do about any of those possibilities?

CHRONIC OBSTRUCTIVE PULMONARY DISEASE: PULMONARY EMPHYSEMA AND CHRONIC BRONCHITIS

ICD-10: J44.1 (COPD)
ICD-10: J43.9 (PULMONARY EMPHYSEMA)
ICD-10: J41.0 (CHRONIC BRONCHITIS)

Description

Chronic obstructive pulmonary disease (COPD) is a functional diagnosis given to any pathological process that decreases the ability of the lungs and bronchi to perform their function of ventilation. It is an umbrella term that includes pulmonary emphysema and chronic bronchitis. COPD affects 15 million Americans. The disease has declined some for men but has remained steady for women. It is a common cause of death and disability in the United States.

Pulmonary emphysema is the permanent enlargement of the air spaces beyond the terminal bronchioles resulting from destruction of alveolar walls (Fig. 13.5). As a consequence of this destruction, the lungs slowly lose their normal elasticity. Air reaches the alveoli in the lungs during inhalation but may not be able to escape during exhalation. Evidence suggests that some forms of emphysema may be hereditary. In rare instances, emphysema is associated with a deficiency of a_1-antitrypsin, a protein that plays a role in maintaining lung elasticity.

Chronic bronchitis is inflammation of the bronchial mucous membranes, causing the lining to thicken and generating a chronically productive cough. It is characterized by hypertrophy and hyperplasia of bronchial mucous glands, damage to the microscopic hairlike extensions of cells lining the interior of the bronchi (bronchial cilia), and narrowing of the bronchial airways. The passageways become clogged with mucus.

Etiology

Other diseases that may lead to COPD include chronic asthma, bronchiectasis, silicosis, and pulmonary tuberculosis. Smoking, prolonged exposure to polluted air,

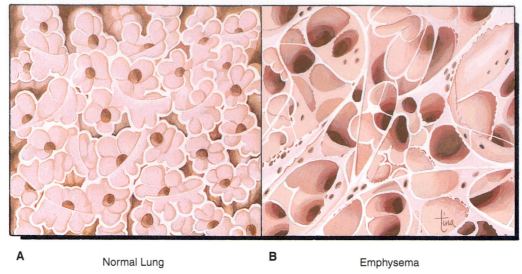

A   Normal Lung   **B**   Emphysema

Figure 13.5 (A) Lung tissue with normal alveoli. (B) Lung tissue with emphysema. *(From Scanlon, VC, and Sanders, T: Essentials of Anatomy and Physiology, ed. 6. Philadelphia: F.A. Davis, 2011, p 379, with permission.)*

respiratory infections, and allergies are predisposing factors in this disease. Occupational risk factors include exposure to textile dust fibers and certain petrochemicals.

Signs and Symptoms

COPD tends to develop insidiously, so no symptoms may be present initially until lung damage has already occurred. Later, a person may tire easily while exercising or doing strenuous work. The chest tightens and dyspnea on minimal exertion then develops. Chronic cough, chest tightness, and increased mucus production are exhibited.

A chronic cough with sputum production is the classic symptom of chronic bronchitis. A client with chronic bronchitis may have only a minimal increase in airway resistance. As the disease progresses, the airway resistance becomes greater. Weight gain due to edema and cyanosis, tachypnea, and wheezing may also be evident.

A characteristic "barrel chest" is often seen in pulmonary emphysema. The appearance of the barrel chest is the result of lungs chronically overinflated with air, causing the rib cage to stay partially expanded.

Two identifiers common in COPD are "blue bloater" and "pink puffer." A blue bloater describes a person with chronic bronchitis whose body responds to the increased obstruction by decreasing ventilation and increasing cardiac output. This leads to **hypoxemia** (oxygen deficiency in the blood) and polycythemia (excessive red blood cells). Together with retention of carbon dioxide, individuals show signs of cardiac failure.

A pink puffer describes a person with emphysema who has the decreased inability to oxygenate the blood. The body compensates with lower cardiac output and hyperventilation, causing a reddish complexion and a "puffing" appearance when breathing.

Diagnostic Procedures

A physical examination, chest x-ray, pulmonary function tests, arterial blood gases, sputum analysis, and CT scan are the procedures used to diagnose COPD, chronic pulmonary emphysema, and chronic bronchitis.

Treatment

Treatment is aimed at preventing further lung damage, relieving symptoms, and preventing complications. Persons diagnosed with COPD should be advised not to smoke. Bronchodilators may be used to open the air passages in the lungs, inhaled corticosteroid medications can reduce airway inflammation and help make breathing easier, and antibiotics may be prescribed in the event of respiratory infections. Administration of oxygen may eventually be necessary. Diuretics may be required. Surgery is an option for some. Lung volume reduction surgery removes small wedges of damaged lung tissue, creating extra space in the chest cavity. A single lung transplant may work for certain people with severe emphysema. Either surgery, however, may not prolong life and has a number of complicated risks.

Comprehensive pulmonary rehabilitation may be able to improve quality of life. The combination of education, exercise, nutrition, and counseling likely comes from physical therapists, respiratory therapists, physical fitness specialists, and dietitians who create a program for individual client needs.

Complementary Therapy

People with COPD need proper nutrition. So much energy is spent on breathing that ventilatory muscles can require up to 10 times the calories required of a healthy person's muscles. The client should eat foods from the basic food groups and limit salt and caffeine intake. If the client is using oxygen, the cannula should be worn while eating. Proper diet will help clients feel better and enable them to better fight infection.

 CLIENT COMMUNICATION

It is essential for clients to avoid cigarettes, cigarette smoke, dust, air pollution, and work-related fumes. Advise clients to avoid excessive heat, cold, and high altitudes.

Prognosis

The prognosis for COPD is difficult. The disease cannot be cured, and lost pulmonary function cannot be restored. However, COPD can be managed, controlled, and slowed. The degree of disability produced by COPD varies but tends to increase with time. The clinical development of COPD is described in four stages: (1) only mild airflow limitation; (2) progressing airflow limitation, shortness of breath, disease is now chronic; (3) severe airflow limitation and reduced exercise capacity; and (4) very severe airflow limitation—exacerbations can be life-threatening. Progressive diminution of pulmonary function leading to respiratory failure accounts for most deaths.

Prevention

Prevention includes not smoking, especially if other family members have a history of the disease. Early diagnosis is helpful. Periodic physical examinations to evaluate the development of COPD are recommended. Such a chronic disease often calls for evaluation from a pulmonary specialist.

ASTHMA

ICD-10: J45.XX

Description

Asthma is a respiratory condition marked by recurrent attacks of labored breathing accompanied by wheezing. Asthma is an inflammatory disorder of the airways that causes spasms of the bronchial tubes or swelling of their mucous membranes. Extrinsic asthma occurs when the bronchospasm is the result of an allergic response to environmental irritants. Intrinsic asthma is present when the client suffers attacks without evidence of allergic response. Extrinsic asthma is most common in childhood; intrinsic asthma more often begins in adulthood. Asthma affects 18.7 million Americans, 6.8 million of whom are children under age 12.

Etiology

The etiology of asthma is uncertain. There is often a family history of allergy and an individual history of hypersensitivity. Persons with asthma have very sensitive airways that react to "triggers" that cause asthma symptoms to start or worsen. Common triggers include upper respiratory infections; allergens, such as pollens, mold spores, pet dander, and dust mites; irritants, such as strong odors from perfume, cleaning solutions, or air pollution; tobacco smoke; exercise or exertion; change in temperature or humidity; and strong emotions, such as anxiety and stress.

Signs and Symptoms

Coughing caused by asthma is usually worse at night. During an acute episode, there is pronounced wheezing due to difficulty exhaling air from the lungs. Dyspnea, tachypnea, and chest tightness also may occur. The person experiencing an asthma attack may perspire profusely, exhibit pallor, and have difficulty speaking more than a few words. The person is usually anxious, feels exhausted, and complains of a "tight chest."

Diagnostic Procedures

A physical examination, chest x-ray, sputum analysis, pulmonary function tests, determination of arterial blood gases, and electrocardiography may suggest the diagnosis. Blood tests to measure eosinophils and IgE levels may be ordered. Allergy testing may identify suspected allergens. Symptoms vary widely among clients, so it is essential that clients and their primary care providers determine the severity of the disease and develop the best plan for treatment. New guidelines classify asthma into four categories: (1) mild intermittent, (2) mild persistent, (3) moderate persistent, and (4) severe persistent.

Treatment

Once clients are diagnosed with asthma, the goal of treatment is for them to avoid substances that trigger symptoms and to control airway inflammation. Treatment is directed toward achieving adequate oxygenation, providing bronchodilation, and decreasing airway inflammation. Reducing exposure to whatever is triggering the asthma is essential. There are two types of asthma medications: long-term preventive "controllers" and quick-relief "rescuers." Controller medications are taken daily to prevent attacks. Quick-relief rescuers are used when asthma symptoms occur. Acute asthma attacks may require high doses of bronchodilators and corticosteroids. If asthma attacks persist, bronchial thermoplasty is a technique often identified for adults with serious asthma that has provided much relief.

Complementary Therapy

Diet and nutrition, neurobiofeedback, and hydrotherapy have shown positive results in the treatment of asthma. Enhancing the immune system is the goal of alternative therapy as well as removing all known triggers to the disease. Air-conditioning can help reduce outside pollens; it is recommended to keep windows and doors closed

REALITY EPISODE

While standing in the shower, Diane's chest constricts. She begins to panic. She has difficulty getting her breath. She steps from the shower, grabs a towel, and goes to grab her inhaler. She does the best she can to inhale deeply, but relief takes a while. In fact, it takes too long this time. She breaks out in a sweat. Later she wonders what brought on the attack. She is never sure, but it exhausts her. Extensive testing has shown that she has no allergies. She didn't seem stressed by anything in particular, but she knows that it is now time for another assessment from her asthma specialist.

What questions might Diane have for her specialist?

during high-pollen days, reduce pet dander, and reduce dust that may aggravate nighttime symptoms. Pillows, mattresses, and box springs encased in dust/mite-proof covers are beneficial. Hardwood or tile flooring is better than carpet and should be cleaned with a damp mop.

➔ CLIENT COMMUNICATION

Assist clients in identifying asthma triggers, and encourage them to asthma-proof their homes. Have a specific place to keep all asthma-related medications for easy access. Stress the importance of taking medications as directed. A well-client examination with a pulmonologist helps in making a plan for long-term preventive measures.

Prognosis

Prognosis is good with proper attention and care. Asthma cannot be cured, but it can be controlled. Many asthmatic children become asymptomatic after reaching adulthood, but children with onset of symptoms after age 15 typically have persistent disease in adulthood.

Prevention

Among those with the condition, avoiding known allergens as much as possible may reduce the frequency of asthmatic attacks. Education about the use of medications and medication side effects is helpful in encouraging the person to lead an active, independent lifestyle. Encourage clients to develop an asthma plan, monitor their breathing, and take their medications consistently and regularly.

LUNG ABSCESS

ICD-10: J85.X

Description

A lung abscess is an area of necrotized lung tissue containing purulent material. Abscesses are more frequent in the lower dependent portions of the lungs and in the right lung, which has a more vertical bronchus.

Etiology

Lung abscesses caused by infectious organisms may be a complication of pneumonia. Aspiration of infectious material is the most frequent etiology; however, aspiration due to dysphagia or compromised consciousness (e.g., seizure, cerebrovascular accident, head trauma, alcoholism) appears to be a predisposing factor. Poor oral hygiene, dental infections, and gingivitis are also common indicators. Antibiotic therapy has greatly decreased the number of deaths caused by lung abscess. However, the increased use of corticosteroids, immunosuppressive drugs, and chemotherapeutic agents in the past couple of decades has changed the natural environment of the oropharyngeal cavity and contributed to increased frequency of opportunistic lung abscesses. The major determinant in developing a lung abscess, as opposed to developing pneumonia only, is the causative microorganism's ability to necrotize lung tissue. A lung abscess also may be produced by a **septic** (disease-causing organism or its toxins) embolism being carried to the lung in the pulmonary circulation.

Signs and Symptoms

Lung abscesses produce a cough accompanied by bloody, purulent, or foul-smelling sputum and breath. Chest pain, sweating, chills, headache, tachycardia, fever, dyspnea, and tachypnea often are present.

Diagnostic Procedures

Chest auscultation reveals crackles and decreased breath sounds. A chest x-ray is necessary to localize the affected portions of the lung. Percutaneous aspiration or fiberoptic bronchoscopy may be used to obtain cultures to identify the causative organism. Sputum culture also is used to detect possible infectious microorganisms. Blood culture may be used to assist in the diagnosis.

Treatment

Antibiotic therapy of fairly long duration (usually 4 to 6 weeks) is the treatment of choice until the abscess is gone. Surgical resection of the lesion is rarely required today.

Complementary Therapy

No significant complementary therapy is indicated.

➔ CLIENT COMMUNICATION

Teach clients coughing and deep-breathing techniques. Remind clients to increase fluid intake to help loosen secretions.

Prognosis

The prognosis is good with proper care and follow-up. About one-third of individuals develop **empyema,** or pus in the pleural space. Another complication may be the development of a brain abscess if infected materials are carried by the blood into the brain.

Prevention

Adequate dental care is important. Chronic illness and hospitalization make some people more susceptible. Prevent aspiration through proper care of anyone who is unconscious. Provide physical therapy to individuals to assist them in coughing up material in the bronchials and airways.

PULMONARY TUBERCULOSIS

ICD-10: A15.X

✔ **REPORTABLE DISEASE**

Description

Pulmonary tuberculosis (TB) is a slowly developing bacterial lung infection characterized by progressive necrosis of lung tissue. An inflammatory response begins with phagocytosis. Growths of inflamed, granular tissue (granulomas) form, and when they calcify, they leave lesions that may be visible on an x-ray. The lymph and blood generally are affected.

Pulmonary TB is a common cause of death in the world. Since its peak in 1992, the incidence of TB in the United States has steadily declined. In 2014, 66% of reported TB cases occurred among foreign-born persons; that is 13 times higher than among U.S.-born persons. The incidence of TB also is apparent in those who are homeless, those who abuse substances, and those with HIV infection—all related to individuals who are less likely to receive adequate medical attention. In general, TB is more common among elderly persons, the urban poor, and members of minority groups.

Etiology

Pulmonary TB is caused by *Mycobacterium tuberculosis.* The infected individual's immune system usually is able to wall the bacteria into a tubercle or tiny nodule. The bacteria can lie dormant for years and then reactivate and spread when conditions are favorable. The disease is transmitted in aerosol droplets exhaled by infected individuals. *Note:* Although the lungs are the organs most commonly infected, the bacteria can infect other parts of the body as well.

Signs and Symptoms

Pulmonary TB may be asymptomatic. The onset generally is insidious. When symptoms are present, they are often vague and may include cough, lassitude, malaise, fatigability, night sweats, anorexia, afternoon fever, weight loss, pleuritic chest pain, **hemoptysis,** and wheezing.

Diagnostic Procedures

A thorough physical examination, chest x-ray or CT scan, bronchoscopy, and positive tuberculin test often confirm the diagnosis (Fig. 13.6). The tuberculin test of choice is the Mantoux test, which consists of an intradermal injection of a purified protein derivative (PPD) of the tuberculin bacillus. The TB skin test cannot determine if the disease is active. This determination requires sputum analysis (smear and culture) in the laboratory. TB blood tests (also called *interferon-gamma release assays,* or IGRAs) measure how strong a person's immune system reacts to TB bacteria by testing the blood. The bacteria may be identified in the client's sputum, urine, body fluids, or tissues. Pulmonary and pleural biopsies may be ordered.

Treatment

Drug therapy is indicated in every case of pulmonary TB. There are many TB drugs, and these can be used in many different ways. To prevent the development of resistance, TB drugs are administered in combinations of two or more (usually four) in most instances. Prolonged use of about 6 to 9 months is essential. Bed rest and isolation are indicated until the person is strong enough to resume activities.

Complementary Therapy

A whole-foods and nutritious diet combined with vitamin supplements can be helpful. Enhancing the body's immune response with fresh air, rest, light exercise, and relaxation will prove beneficial.

⊕ **CLIENT COMMUNICATION**

Teach clients to cough and sneeze into tissues and to properly dispose of all secretions. Remind them of the importance of taking all their medications. Teach family members about the infectious nature of the disease and proper medication regimen. Individuals exposed to someone with pulmonary TB should contact their primary care provider or local health department about getting a TB skin test.

Prognosis

The prognosis for an individual with active pulmonary TB is good if the disease is detected early and if the client follows the prescribed drug therapy. However, if strains of bacteria are resistant to two or more of the major antituberculosis agents, mortality rates increase.

Prevention

Preventive measures include proper infection control, tuberculin testing of individuals known to have been in close contact with infected persons, and treatment of those reacting to the tuberculin testing. Generally, a person with a positive tuberculin reaction is put on

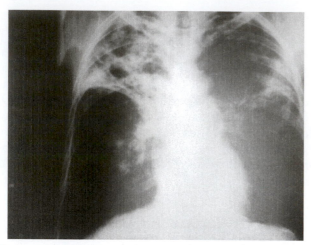

Figure 13.6 Anteroposterior x-ray of a patient diagnosed with advanced bilateral pulmonary tuberculosis. *(Centers for Disease Control and Prevention, 1972.)*

1 year of isoniazid prophylactically. Use of the bacille Calmette-Guérin (bCG) vaccination should be considered only for very select persons who meet specific criteria and in consultation with a TB expert.

CHAPTER EPISODE—PART III

Amanda and Paal had an argument about his smoking and how poorly Amanda was feeling. Finally Paal agreed to smoke only when they stopped for a rest. That helped a little, but when they camped that night, Amanda was in trouble. She woke in a panic. She could not catch her breath. She was scared, so she slipped out of the tent to go sit in the car for a bit. In time, the panic eased, and she was able to breathe more easily.

• What likely happened? Should she tell Paal?

PNEUMOCONIOSIS

ICD-10: J64

Pneumoconiosis is a disease of the respiratory tract caused by inhaling inorganic or organic dust particles or chemical irritants over a prolonged period. It is an occupational disorder associated with mining and stonecutting. Four of the most frequently seen varieties of pneumoconiosis are silicosis (most common), asbestosis, berylliosis, and anthracosis.

SILICOSIS

ICD-10: J62.8

Description

Silicosis, also known as *grinder's disease* and *potter's rot*, results from the inhalation of crystalline silica dust.

Silica is a common mineral found naturally in sand and rock. Silica scars lungs and creates small, discrete nodules in the upper lobes. As the disease advances, a dense fibrosis of the lungs develops, and emphysema with respiratory impairment may result. The disease is chronic and progressive.

Etiology

Silica exposure is common in mines and quarries and in a number of occupations, such as sandblasting, foundry work, ceramics, and glassmaking. The occupations most prone to silica exposure are mining, drilling, blasting, grinding, and abrasive manufacturing. Required exposure varies from 2 to 30 years; the average is 10 years.

Signs and Symptoms

The disease may be asymptomatic even though x-rays exhibit evidence of nodule formation. Dyspnea on exertion generally is the first symptom. A chronic dry cough that later turns productive, tachypnea, pulmonary hypertension, and malaise may result.

Diagnostic Procedures

A thorough medical history revealing exposure to silica dust is essential. Chest x-rays and CT scans show small, discrete, nodular lesions throughout the lung but concentrated in the upper areas of the lung. Arterial blood gas analyses and pulmonary function tests confirm the diagnosis.

Treatment

Silicosis is irreversible and cannot be cured. Therefore, treatment is symptomatic. Clients should remove themselves from further exposure to silica and other lung irritants, including tobacco smoking. Cough suppressants may help. Antibiotics are used to prevent TB, which is a common occurrence in silicosis. Chest physiotherapy or bronchial hygiene helps drain the bronchial tubes and bronchioles of mucus. Bronchodilators and oxygen administration can help breathing. Lung transplant may be an option for some.

Complementary Therapy

Steam inhalation, chest physiotherapy, and controlled coughing can help clients clear secretions. A whole-foods diet is recommended.

⊙ CLIENT COMMUNICATION

Prevention of infections is very important. Influenza and pneumococcal vaccines are essential.

Prognosis

The prognosis for an individual with silicosis varies unless the disease has progressed to the fibrotic form. The disease can be rapidly fatal, depending on the quantity and quality of the silica entering the lungs. Silicosis is always life-shortening.

Prevention

Prevention involves minimizing exposure to silica dust in the work environment. Water spray is often used where there is dust. Air filtering can also reduce dust particles.

ASBESTOSIS

ICD-10: J61

Description

Asbestosis is a form of pneumoconiosis resulting from exposure to asbestos fibers. The disease is characterized by a slow, progressive, diffuse fibrosis of the lung tissue. Despite recent health and safety regulations limiting workplace exposure to asbestos, asbestosis is still a frequently occurring form of pneumoconiosis. The Mesothelioma Cancer Alliance reports that as of 2013, there are still some 30 million pounds of asbestos used each year in the United States (http://www.mesothelioma.com/asbestos-cancer/asbestos-facts-statistics.htm#ixzz3DtlI8XJ1).

Etiology

Those at greatest risk for asbestosis include people who fabricate asbestos fibers, remove asbestos insulation from plumbing and buildings, or live within the area of an industry that discharges the fibers into the air. Family members of asbestos workers are also at risk of contracting the disease if they handle the worker's clothing. Twenty years or more of moderate exposure to asbestos dust usually is required before the characteristic lesions of the disease become evident.

Signs and Symptoms

The first symptom is dyspnea on exertion, which worsens until dyspnea occurs even while at rest. Pleuritic chest pain, dry cough, and recurrent respiratory infections are common as the fibrosis extends.

Diagnostic Procedures

A thorough medical history and physical examination revealing asbestos exposure are essential. Chest x-rays show a "honeycomb" or "ground-glass" appearance. Pulmonary function studies and arterial blood gas analyses will confirm the diagnosis. A CT scan may be ordered. It is more sensitive than the x-ray and may detect asbestosis before it appears on the x-ray.

Treatment

As with all pneumoconioses, treatment is to relieve symptoms. Refer to the treatment for silicosis.

Complementary Therapy

See "Silicosis."

 CLIENT COMMUNICATION

See "Silicosis."

Prognosis

There is increased incidence of bronchogenic carcinoma even after brief exposure. If the person with asbestosis smokes, the incidence of cancer is about 90%, making for a poor prognosis.

Malignant pleural mesothelioma, a cancer of the sac lining the pleural cavity, is a complication of asbestosis. Mesothelioma has been found in individuals who worked with asbestos for as little as 1 or 2 months, but its latency period can be as long as 30 years before diagnosis. Fortunately, the disease is rare, with about 3,000 cases per year in the United States.

Prevention

Prevention involves avoidance of asbestos dust. Federal law requires employers who work with asbestos products to monitor exposure, create regulated areas for asbestos work, and provide their employees with training, protective gear, and decontamination facilities. Individuals exposed to asbestos should be vigilant about regular checkups and inform their primary care provider of their exposure.

BERYLLIOSIS

ICD-10: J63.X

Description

Berylliosis is beryllium poisoning, usually of the lungs. The skin and other bodily organs also may be affected. The acute form of the disease is characterized by the onset of pneumonia-like symptoms and other respiratory tract disorders. The more common, chronic form is characterized by granuloma formation and diffuse interstitial pneumonitis.

Etiology

Those at risk of contracting berylliosis include workers in primary production, metal machining, and reclaiming scrap alloys. Other high-exposure occupations are in the nuclear power, aerospace, and electronics industries. The metal may be either inhaled or directly absorbed through the skin in the form of dusts, salts, or fumes. As with asbestosis, berylliosis can affect family members who are exposed to dust in the worker's clothing.

Signs and Symptoms

After exposure, dry cough and nasal mucosal swelling with ulceration occur. As the condition worsens, substernal pain, tachycardia, dyspnea, weight loss, and pulmonary insufficiency result.

Diagnostic Procedures

A thorough medical history and physical examination are essential and will reveal exposure to beryllium dust, mist, or fumes. Chest x-rays, pulmonary function studies, and arterial blood gas analyses are ordered. A positive beryllium patch test establishes hypersensitivity to beryllium, not the disease. An in vitro lymphocyte transformation test can diagnose berylliosis.

Treatment

Beryllium skin ulcers need to be excised. Chronic berylliosis is usually treated with corticosteroid therapy. Oxygen, bronchodilators, and chest physical therapy methods may be required.

Complementary Therapy

See "Silicosis."

 CLIENT COMMUNICATION

See "Silicosis."

Prognosis

The prognosis depends on the severity of the disease. Individuals must modify their lifestyle. The disease is progressive, and with each acute exacerbation, the prognosis worsens.

Prevention

The best prevention is avoidance of beryllium fumes or dusts.

ANTHRACOSIS

ICD-10: J60

Description

Anthracosis, also called *black lung disease* or *coal worker's pneumoconiosis,* is caused by the accumulation of carbon deposits in the lungs. Simple anthracosis shows small lung opacities. Complicated anthracosis exhibits massive fibrosis in the lungs.

Etiology

Anthracosis results from inhaling smoke or coal dust. Workers in the coal mining industry are most likely to develop the disease. Anthracosis frequently occurs with silicosis. Exposure of 15 years or longer is usually required before symptoms develop.

Signs and Symptoms

Exertional dyspnea, productive cough with inky-black sputum, and recurrent respiratory infections are common symptoms.

Diagnostic Procedures

A thorough medical history and physical examination revealing exposure to coal dust are essential and may reveal a barrel chest, rales or crackling sounds in the lungs, **rhonchi** (a rattling in the throat), and wheezing. Chest x-rays, pulmonary function studies, and arterial blood gas analyses will confirm the diagnosis.

Treatment

Treatment is strictly symptomatic and typically includes the use of bronchodilators and corticosteroid drugs. Chest physiotherapy will help remove secretions, and careful management of respiratory complications, such as TB or silicosis that usually occur in association with anthracosis, is important.

Complementary Therapy

See "Silicosis."

 CLIENT COMMUNICATION

See "Silicosis."

Prognosis

The prognosis varies. Simple anthracosis is self-limiting. The complicated form is chronic, progressive, and worsens the prognosis. Complications can be disabling.

Prevention

Prevention of anthracosis involves avoidance of coal dust.

RESPIRATORY MYCOSES

ICD-10: B49

Description

Mycoses (fungal infections) are classified as either superficial or deep. Superficial mycoses affect only the skin and are discussed in Chapter 8. Deep mycoses are systemic and may complicate other illnesses. The mycoses considered here are deep, systemic fungal infections that extensively affect the lungs: **histoplasmosis, coccidioidomycosis,** and **blastomycosis.**

Etiology

Histoplasmosis, also called *Darling disease,* is caused by *Histoplasma capsulatum.* The fungus is found in soil, especially soil contaminated by bird and chicken droppings. The spores become airborne when the contaminated soil is disturbed. The disease is transmitted when the fungal spores are inhaled or penetrate the skin following injury. The primary lesion is in the lungs.

Coccidioidomycosis, also called *San Joaquin Valley fever,* is caused by *Coccidioides immitis,* a fungus common in the dry desert soils of California, New Mexico, Nevada, and Arizona. The disease is transmitted by inhalation of fungal spores and commonly affects migrant farm laborers. **Coccidioidomycosis is a reportable disease in California, New Mexico, Nevada, and Arizona.**

Blastomycosis, specifically North American blastomycosis, is caused by *Blastomyces dermatitidis*. It can cause a cutaneous infection, but usually it affects the lungs. In rare instances, a serious progressive systemic infection may occur.

Signs and Symptoms

The signs and symptoms of all three diseases may be mild and similar to those of a common cold. More severe signs and symptoms include malaise, fever, myalgia, headache, cough, and chest pain. In coccidioidomycosis, however, the only symptom may be a persistent fever of several weeks' duration. In blastomycosis, nonpruritic and painless papules or macules may appear on exposed body surfaces.

Diagnostic Procedures

In histoplasmosis, chest x-ray, a positive *Histoplasma* skin test, sputum culture, or special stains of biopsied tissue confirm the diagnosis. In coccidioidomycosis, a positive coccidioidin skin test and special serological tests are necessary for confirmation. In blastomycosis, cultures to isolate the fungus from sputum or skin lesions are necessary. Tissue biopsy from the skin or lungs may be ordered.

Treatment

High-dose, long-term antifungal medications and supportive treatment for respiratory symptoms are used to treat histoplasmosis and blastomycosis. Coccidioidomycosis may heal spontaneously within a few weeks. Bed rest and symptomatic treatment may be all that are necessary. In some cases, surgery may be necessary to remove lung lesions.

Complementary Therapy

No significant complementary therapy is indicated.

CLIENT COMMUNICATION

Remind clients to watch for early signs of infection if they live in endemic regions and to consistently wear protective gear when exposure is possible. Encourage bed rest and adequate fluid intake.

Prognosis

The prognosis for an individual with histoplasmosis or coccidioidomycosis is usually excellent. Blastomycosis in its primary, acute form is self-limiting. If it progresses to a systemic infection, however, the prognosis is more difficult.

Prevention

Prevention includes following proper sanitary measures, wearing a face mask during exposure to potentially contaminated soil, and protecting exposed skin from invasion by the spores.

PNEUMOTHORAX (COLLAPSED LUNG)

ICD-10: J93.XX

Description

A pneumothorax is a collection of air or gas in the pleural cavity. It typically results in atelectasis, the complete or partial collapse of the lung (Fig. 13.7). One or both lungs may be affected. The condition is characterized as either spontaneous or traumatic.

Etiology

Spontaneous pneumothorax is caused by the rupturing of a small **bleb,** commonly called a *blister,* along the surface of the lung. What causes these blebs to form is not known, but they tend to form near the apex (bottom tip) of each lung. Changes in atmospheric pressure (flying, scuba diving, mountain climbing) can put individuals at risk. Smoking marijuana is a risk factor when individuals inhale deeply, then slowly breathe out against partially closed lips, forcing the marijuana smoke deeper into the lungs. Pneumothorax also may be secondary to other lung diseases, such as asthma, emphysema, lung abscess, or lung cancer. Traumatic pneumothorax may result from inserting a central venous line, from thoracic surgery, or from penetrating chest trauma, such as a knife wound or fractured rib. A perforated esophagus or use of mechanical ventilators also can cause pneumothorax. This disorder is further classified as open or closed. In open pneumothorax, air flows between the pleural space and the outside of the body. In closed pneumothorax, air reaches the pleural space directly from the lung.

Signs and Symptoms

Classic symptoms include sudden, sharp pleuritic pain that worsens with chest movement, coughing, or breathing. There may be shortness of breath and cyanosis. In moderate to severe pneumothorax, there may also be profound respiratory distress accompanied by pallor, weak and rapid pulse, and anxiety.

Diagnostic Procedures

Physical examination may reveal asymmetric expansion of the chest during inspiration. Auscultation typically reveals diminished breath sounds on the affected side. A chest x-ray usually provides confirmation, showing air in the pleural space. A CT scan may be ordered, and blood tests can reveal the amount of oxygen in the blood.

Treatment

In spontaneous pneumothorax with no signs of increased pleural pressure or dyspnea, or in which the lung collapse is less than 20%, the treatment of choice

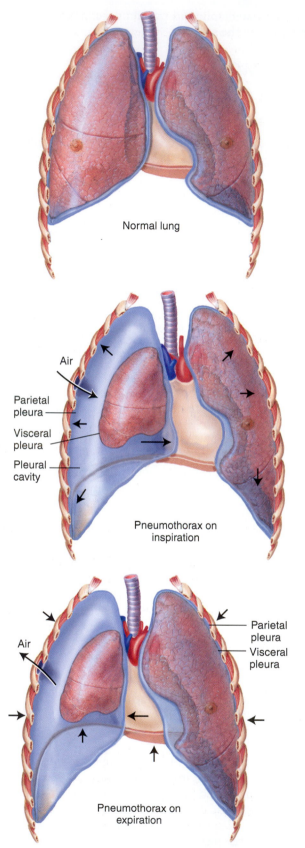

Normal lung

Pneumothorax on inspiration

- Air
- Parietal pleura
- Visceral pleura
- Pleural cavity

Parietal pleura
Visceral pleura
Air

Pneumothorax on expiration

Figure 13.7 **Pneumothorax.** *(From Thomas, CL [ed]: Taber's Cyclopedic Medical Dictionary, ed. 22. Philadelphia: F.A. Davis, 2009, p 1838, with permission.)*

is bed rest and careful monitoring of vital signs. In traumatic pneumothorax, a chest tube is inserted for drainage and to allow the collapsed lung to expand. A thoracoscopy procedure allows a surgeon to place a fiberscope into a tube between the ribs and surgical instruments into another tube to close the leak. Small incisions are made, and a tiny video camera is used to guide the surgery. In this procedure, two or three tubes are placed between the ribs under general anesthesia. Rarely, when this is not successful, a surgical procedure with an incision in the chest wall (**thoracotomy**) and surgical excision of a portion of the pleura (**pleurectomy**) may be necessary.

Complementary Therapy

No significant complementary therapy is indicated.

⊖ CLIENT COMMUNICATION

Reassure clients by explaining the disease process and identifying precautions to take to avoid recurrence.

Prognosis

The prognosis for pneumothorax is generally good with effective treatment. Spontaneous pneumothorax, however, tends to be a recurrent condition. A large pneumothorax can impair cardiac function and result in pulmonary and circulatory impairment without proper treatment.

Prevention

Individuals with a history of spontaneous pneumothorax should not subject themselves to extremes of atmospheric pressure such as would be encountered by flying in a nonpressurized aircraft or during scuba diving. It is best that clients do not smoke.

ATELECTASIS

ICD-10: J98.11

Description

Atelectasis is a collapsed lung or an airless condition of all or part of a lung that allows unoxygenated blood to pass unchanged through the area; this produces hypoxia. The condition may be acute or chronic.

Etiology

The condition may be caused by obstruction of the lung by foreign matter, mucus plugs, or excessive secretion. It is seen in many clients with COPD or cystic fibrosis and those who smoke heavily. Compression of the lung by tumors, aneurysms, enlarged lymph nodes, or pneumothorax also may cause lung collapse (see "Pneumothorax"). Atelectasis is sometimes a complication of abdominal surgery or a general consequence of postoperative immobilization.

Signs and Symptoms

Chronic atelectasis may be marked only by the gradual onset of dyspnea. Acute atelectasis typically includes marked dyspnea, cyanosis, fever, tachycardia, anxiety, and **diaphoresis** (profuse sweating). There may be a decrease in chest motion on the affected side. Chronic atelectasis may be marked only by the gradual onset of dyspnea.

Diagnostic Procedures

A thorough medical history, physical examination, and chest x-ray are essential for diagnosis. Sound on percussion may be dull, and auscultation will reveal decreased breath sounds. A bronchoscopy and arterial blood gas analysis may be ordered.

Treatment

The goal of treatment is to reexpand the collapsed lung tissue. Postural drainage, incentive spirometry, chest percussion, and frequent coughing and deep breathing are advised. Early postoperative ambulation is recommended. Bronchodilators may be prescribed.

Complementary Therapy

No significant complementary therapy is indicated, but measures to enhance the body's immune system will benefit a client's recovery during the treatment process.

⊕ CLIENT COMMUNICATION

Teach clients about respiratory care, including postural drainage, deep breathing, and coughing. As needed, it is recommended that clients stop smoking and lose weight.

Prognosis

The prognosis in postoperative atelectasis usually is good, especially if the area of collapse is not large. Death may result, however, if the condition is untreated or there is total collapse of the lung. In all other types of atelectasis, the prognosis is dependent on the cause.

Prevention

Prevention includes postoperative exercise and prompt treatment of any pulmonary problems. Movement and deep breathing are to be encouraged in anyone who is bedridden for long periods.

PLEURISY (PLEURITIS)

ICD-10: R09.1

Description

Pleurisy is inflammation of the visceral (inner) and parietal (outer) pleural membranes that envelop each lung.

The saclike membrane enveloping each lung and lining the adjacent portion of the thoracic cavity or the pleura of one or both lungs may be affected. The two layers are lubricated with pleural fluid. The condition may be either primary or secondary and is often associated with pleural effusion.

Etiology

Primary pleurisy is caused by infection of the pleura by bacteria, fungus, parasites, or viruses. It can be the result of inhaled toxins or chemical fumes. The condition is often secondary to pneumonia, heart failure, pulmonary infarction, neoplasm, systemic lupus erythematosus, pulmonary embolism, and chest trauma.

Signs and Symptoms

The lung's pain fibers are located in the pleura, so when the tissue becomes inflamed, the sharp stabbing pain can be so severe that it limits movement on the affected side when breathing. Clients often believe they are having a heart attack. Other symptoms may include coughing, fever and chills, and chest pain that is greater during inspiration. Dyspnea also may occur.

Diagnostic Procedures

Chest auscultation reveals a pleural friction rub ("squeaky leather" or grating sound) during respiration. Additional information can be obtained from a chest x-ray, ultrasound, and CT scan if necessary. Blood tests may show signs of any infection.

Treatment

Treatment is aimed at the underlying cause but is otherwise symptomatic. Such treatment may include the use of strong analgesics and anti-inflammatory agents. Bed rest is usually indicated. **Thoracentesis** (removing chest fluid) can relieve the pain and shortness of breath, but caution should be exercised because it can temporarily worsen the pleurisy if the two inflamed pleural surfaces rub directly on each other.

Complementary Therapy

Treatment of the underlying cause is essential, along with natural analgesics and anti-inflammatory agents. Getting plenty of rest is important.

⊕ CLIENT COMMUNICATION

Stress the importance of bed rest, and encourage clients to apply firm pressure at the site of pain during coughing to minimize discomfort.

Prognosis

Prognosis is dependent on etiology but is usually good. Pleural effusion, a collection of fluid in the pleural space, may develop.

Prevention

Early treatment of any respiratory disease is the best prevention.

PLEURAL EFFUSION

ICD-10: J91.8

Description

Pleural effusion is an excess of fluid between the parietal and visceral pleural membranes enveloping each lung. The accumulating fluid may be characterized as **transudate,** which has little or no protein, or **exudate,** which is rich in protein.

Etiology

Pleural effusion may occur regardless of whether there is a pathological process affecting the pleurae themselves. Transudative pleural effusions frequently result from congestive heart failure, hepatic disease with ascites, and peritoneal dialysis. Exudative pleural effusions more often are seen with inflammation of the pleura, TB, rheumatoid arthritis, pancreatitis, respiratory neoplasms, and bacterial pneumonia.

Signs and Symptoms

The person may be asymptomatic. When signs and symptoms are manifested, they may include cough, dyspnea, and chest or pleuritic pain. The symptoms of pleural effusion will typically accompany those of any underlying condition.

Diagnostic Procedures

Auscultation of the chest reveals decreased breath sounds. **Percussion,** or tapping body surfaces, elicits dull sounds over the effused area that indicate size, position, and general condition of the area. A chest x-ray may indicate pleural effusion. Thoracentesis and analysis of the extracted fluid are necessary to distinguish transudative from exudative effusions.

Treatment

Thoracentesis to alleviate fluid pressure may be necessary if the fluid is not reabsorbed. It is also important to treat the underlying cause of the pleural effusion.

Complementary Therapy

No significant complementary therapy is indicated.

⟳ CLIENT COMMUNICATION

Explain thoracentesis to clients. Encourage deep-breathing exercises and treatment of the underlying causes of pleural effusion.

Prognosis

The prognosis is dependent on the underlying disease. Excessive pleural effusion for a long time may cause lung collapse. Infected pleural fluid may create an abscess called an *empyema.* Pneumothorax can be a complication of the thoracentesis procedure.

Prevention

There is no specific prevention for pleural effusion other than prompt treatment and management of disorders that may lead to the condition.

PULMONARY HYPERTENSION

ICD-10: J80

Description

Pulmonary hypertension occurs when the pulmonary arteries and capillaries become narrowed or blocked, making the blood flow through the lungs difficult. As the pulmonary arteries' blood pressure rises, the right ventricle of the heart must work harder to pump the blood through the lungs. This causes the heart muscle to weaken.

Etiology

Pulmonary hypertension is either primary (idiopathic) or secondary. Primary pulmonary hypertension (PPH) has no underlying cause, although there may be a genetic predisposition. Secondary pulmonary hypertension is the result of an underlying problem, such as COPD, pulmonary embolus, sleep apnea, chronic liver disease, and AIDS. Older adults are more at risk, as are those who live above an altitude of 8,000 feet. Those who climb at high altitudes may develop a temporary form of pulmonary hypertension called *transient reversible pulmonary hypertension* unless they first acclimate to the altitude.

Signs and Symptoms

Signs and symptoms of the disease may go undetected for quite some time and may include dyspnea, fatigue, chest pain, edema in ankles and legs, cyanosis, tachypnea, and syncope.

Diagnostic Procedures

The symptoms are common to many diseases, making diagnosis difficult. Often, the disease is discovered during testing for some other problem. The results of a Doppler or transesophageal echocardiogram, pulmonary function test, perfusion lung scan, CT scan, or magnetic resonance imaging (MRI) may indicate pulmonary hypertension. Blood testing, chest x-ray, and right heart catheterization may be performed.

Treatment

Once a diagnosis has been made, the World Health Organization (WHO) suggests four classifications for identifying the disease: (1) diagnosis with no symptoms; (2) fatigue, shortness of breath, some chest pain with normal activity, and no symptoms at rest; (3) symptoms during activity are intensified and still comfortable at rest; and (4) all the symptoms are present even during rest.

Correcting any underlying cause is the first step in treatment. A number of medications may be successful: vasodilators, endothelin receptor antagonists (which help reverse the effect of endothelin, a substance in the blood vessel walls causing them to narrow), calcium channel blockers, anticoagulants, and diuretics. Oxygen therapy may be necessary. For young people with PPH, a heart-lung transplant may be an option.

Complementary Therapy

A diet that is low in sodium is recommended. Getting plenty of rest, reducing stress, and maintaining a healthy body weight are encouraged. It is important not to smoke; to avoid becoming pregnant, using birth control pills, or traveling to high altitudes; and to follow a nutritious diet.

 CLIENT COMMUNICATION

Because pulmonary hypertension cannot be cured, it is important to remind clients to continue medical care in order to lessen symptoms.

Prognosis

Pulmonary hypertension is a serious illness that is sometimes fatal. The disease becomes progressively worse over time. Right-sided heart failure (cor pulmonale) may occur as well as heart arrhythmias.

Prevention

There is no known prevention of pulmonary hypertension other than to treat any of the secondary causes of the disease.

PULMONARY EDEMA

ICD-10: J81.X

Description

Pulmonary edema is a diffuse extravascular accumulation of fluid in the pulmonary tissues and air spaces. Most commonly, it represents the projection of cardiac disease processes, such as atherosclerosis, hypertension, or valvular disease. The condition is usually a direct consequence of left ventricular failure. Pulmonary edema can occur as a chronic condition, or it can develop quickly. Pulmonary edema is considered a medical emergency.

Etiology

When the alveoli fill with fluid instead of air, preventing oxygen from being absorbed into the bloodstream, more blood is added to the pulmonary circulation than can be adequately removed. In addition to the cardiac problems already mentioned, pulmonary edema may also be the result of lung infections, living at high altitudes, smoking, certain toxin exposure, pneumonia, and acute respiratory diseases.

Signs and Symptoms

The onset of pulmonary edema frequently occurs at night, after the person has been lying down for a while. In the more acute form, clients exhibit dyspnea, coughing, and difficulty breathing unless sitting erect or standing (**orthopnea**). Tachycardia, tachypnea, diffuse rales, and frothy bloody sputum also may occur. A decrease in blood pressure, a fine, barely perceptible thready pulse, and cold, clammy skin occur as cardiac output fails. These symptoms of cardiac output failure constitute a medical emergency.

Diagnostic Procedures

Clinical features indicate the diagnosis. Arterial blood gas analyses and chest x-rays are useful in diagnosing this condition. Electrocardiogram, regular echocardiogram, and transesophageal echocardiogram are often performed. Pulmonary artery catheterization may be used to confirm left ventricular failure.

Treatment

Oxygen is typically administered along with bronchodilators and diuretics. Nitroglycerin is often prescribed as well as medication to relieve anxiety. Blood pressure medications may be given. Fluid intake may be limited, and mechanical ventilation may be necessary.

Complementary Therapy

No significant complementary therapy is indicated.

 CLIENT COMMUNICATION

Clients will be anxious, so reassure them as much as possible. Using a calm voice, explain all procedures. Provide emotional support to all family members. Remind clients to report any weight gain of even 2 to 3 pounds, to rest periodically during the day, and to avoid drinking alcohol.

Prognosis

Edema in the legs, abdomen, or pleural membranes is serious. Acute pulmonary edema can be fatal. The outcome depends on the condition of the heart and lungs before the edema develops. Drug-induced pulmonary edema can be a cause of death in individuals who abuse narcotics.

Prevention

There is no known prevention, but certain steps can reduce risk. They include lowering blood pressure and cholesterol, eating a healthy diet, exercising regularly, not smoking, managing stress, and making certain there is sufficient folic acid in the diet.

COR PULMONALE

ICD-10: I27.81

Description

Cor pulmonale, or right-sided heart failure, is hypertrophy and failure of the right ventricle of the heart. Lung disease may cause pulmonary hypertension. As a result, the workload of the heart is increased, and the right ventricle hypertrophies in an effort to force blood into the lungs. Eventually the right ventricle is weakened by this effort, and blood pools in the right ventricle.

Etiology

Cor pulmonale is caused by various disorders of the lungs, the pulmonary vessels, or the chest wall that impede pulmonary circulation. Disorders that may lead to cor pulmonale include COPD, bronchiectasis, pneumoconiosis, pulmonary hypertension, **kyphoscoliosis** (abnormal backward and lateral curvature of the spine), multiple pulmonary emboli, upper airway obstruction, and living at high altitudes. The condition may be acute but is more commonly chronic.

Signs and Symptoms

Signs and symptoms include shortness of breath; a productive, chronic cough; exertional dyspnea; fatigability; and wheezing respirations. Tachypnea, orthopnea, dependent edema, cyanosis, **clubbing** (bulbous swelling of the tips of the fingers and toes), and distended neck veins may occur as the condition worsens. The liver is enlarged and tender in advanced stages.

Diagnostic Procedures

A physical examination likely reveals wheezes and crackles on auscultation. There may be pitting edema. Chest x-rays and CT scan, echocardiography, and pulmonary function studies are useful diagnostic tools. Angiography and arterial blood gas analyses confirm the diagnosis.

Treatment

The goal of treatment is to reduce hypoxemia and to improve a client's exercise tolerance. Cor pulmonale is frequently treated with medications such as digitalis to stimulate heart action, antibiotics for secondary respiratory infections, pulmonary artery vasodilators, diuretics, anticoagulants, and bronchodilators. Oxygen may be necessary. Restriction of salt and fluids may be advised. The underlying cause needs to be treated.

Complementary Therapy

The primary goal is to help make clients more comfortable during treatment. Pulmonary rehabilitation provided by respiratory therapists is often useful.

> ⊙➤ **CLIENT COMMUNICATION**
>
> Help clients plan for small, frequent meals that restrict sodium intake. Instruct clients to take frequent rest breaks and to immediately report any signs of edema. Treatment of cor pulmonale is best monitored by primary care providers during regularly scheduled checkups.

Prognosis

The prognosis is typically poor for an individual with cor pulmonale, because it generally occurs late during the course of COPD and other irreversible diseases.

Prevention

There is no known prevention for cor pulmonale.

PULMONARY EMBOLISM

ICD-10: I27.82

Description

A pulmonary embolism is a mass of undissolved matter in the pulmonary artery or one of its branches. It is the most common pulmonary complication among hospitalized individuals, with about 250,000 incident cases occurring annually. It is not considered a disease itself but is a complication of venous thrombosis. It is potentially lethal.

Etiology

A pulmonary embolism generally originates in the pelvic veins or deep lower extremity veins and travels through the circulatory system until it blocks a pulmonary artery (Fig. 13.8). Those at high risk for pulmonary emboli include individuals immobilized with chronic diseases, those in body casts, persons with congestive heart failure or neoplasms, and postoperative clients. Also at risk are pregnant women, women taking oral contraceptives, and individuals with venous diseases, such as varicose veins; **polycythemia vera,** a chronic, life-shortening disorder of the bone marrow involving the tissue-producing blood cells; or **thrombocytosis,** a condition in which there is an abnormally small number of platelets in circulating blood.

Signs and Symptoms

Signs and symptoms depend on the size and location of the embolus. Total closure of the main pulmonary artery is quickly fatal. Acute symptoms may include dyspnea, tachypnea, pulmonary hypertension, and substernal

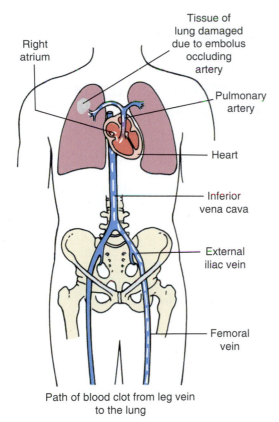

Figure 13.8 Embolism. *(From Thomas, CL [ed]:* Taber's Cyclopedic Medical Dictionary, *ed. 21. Philadelphia: F.A. Davis, 2005, p 744, with permission.)*

Labels on figure:
- Right atrium
- Tissue of lung damaged due to embolus occluding artery
- Pulmonary artery
- Heart
- Inferior vena cava
- External iliac vein
- Femoral vein

Path of blood clot from leg vein to the lung

pain. Other symptoms are productive cough, pleuritic pain, tachycardia, and low-grade fever. Apprehension is common.

Diagnostic Procedures

Client history is likely to indicate any predisposing conditions for pulmonary embolism and/or deep vein thrombosis. Pulmonary embolism is so common and so lethal that the diagnosis should be considered in every client with any chest symptoms that cannot be proven to have another cause. Diagnosing this condition is frequently difficult, but an electrocardiogram may reveal tachycardia, and a chest x-ray may indicate the location of the embolus. Blood tests, pulmonary angiography, or MRI may help in the diagnosis. Auscultation reveals crackling and a pleural rub near the area of the embolism. Ultrasound and CT scans may be used to identify the location of any clots within the legs.

Treatment

The goal is to maintain adequate cardiovascular and pulmonary function while clearing the obstruction. Treatment typically involves the use of anticoagulants, such as heparin and warfarin, to prevent clot formation and fibrinolytic therapy to dissolve the embolus. Surgical management may be indicated in exceptional cases. This involves removing the embolus completely. A filter may be placed into the inferior vena cava to block clots that might be carried to the lungs.

Complementary Therapy

Graduated compression stockings can reduce the chronic swelling that a blood clot in the leg may cause. The stockings are worn on the legs from the arch of the foot to just above or below the knee. They are tight at the ankle and become looser as they go up the leg. This causes a gentle compression up the leg to keep blood from pooling and clotting.

⊕ CLIENT COMMUNICATION

Remind clients to maintain adequate nutrition and fluid balance. They should never vigorously massage their legs and should not cross their legs; both actions encourage thrombus formation. Clients should report all medications before any surgery, because there are a number of herbal medications that complicate the blood flow and its coagulability.

Prognosis

The prognosis is guarded if the embolism is massive enough to trigger a **pulmonary infarction,** a condition in which lung tissues die and which occurs in about 10% of cases.

Prevention

Prevention includes early postoperative ambulation or initiating prophylactic anticoagulant therapy for clients deemed to be at risk. Other steps to lower the risk of pulmonary embolism include the following:

- Perform postsurgical leg exercises, early ambulation, and pneumatic leg compressions.
- Exercise lower leg muscles during long road or airplane trips.
- Take medicines to prevent clots as prescribed.
- Follow up with the primary care provider.

RESPIRATORY ACIDOSIS (HYPERCAPNIA)

ICD-10: E87.4

Description

Respiratory acidosis is excessive acidity of body fluids attributable to inadequate removal of carbon dioxide (CO_2) by the lungs. Whenever CO_2 cannot be adequately ventilated, the CO_2 dissolved in the blood rapidly increases. As the level of CO_2—called the *partial pressure of carbon dioxide* ($PaCO_2$)—rises, so does the amount of CO_2 that combines with water to form carbonic acid. Consequently, the **pH** (acidity or alkalinity) of the blood decreases. The condition may be acute or chronic.

Etiology

Acute respiratory acidosis occurs whenever there is a sudden impairment of ventilation resulting from airway obstruction. This may be due to such causes as a foreign object blocking the airway or to the effects of certain drugs, neuromuscular diseases, or cardiac arrest. Chronic respiratory acidosis is caused by pulmonary diseases that change the characteristics of lung tissue, impairing the ability to release CO_2, such as emphysema, bronchitis, and COPD. Chronic respiratory acidosis also may be a consequence of extreme obesity or obstructive sleep apnea.

Signs and Symptoms

Signs and symptoms vary with the etiology, but typically they include weakness, shallow respirations, confusion and/or anxiety, muscle tremors, and tachycardia. Clients may complain of headaches and exhibit dyspnea.

Diagnostic Procedures

Diagnosis of respiratory acidosis is usually evident from the clinical situation. Arterial blood gas testing to confirm elevated $PaCO_2$ levels is required to confirm the diagnosis. Chest x-ray, CT scan, MRI, and pulmonary function tests are also likely. In persons with no obvious source of respiratory acidosis, a drug screen should be performed.

Treatment

The only useful treatment for respiratory acidosis involves measures to correct the underlying cause. Bronchodilators, increased ventilation, and oxygen therapy often are prescribed.

Complementary Therapy

No significant complementary therapy is indicated.

⊕ CLIENT COMMUNICATION

Helping clients and family members understand the etiology is beneficial. In the case of hospitalization, staff will maintain airway, provide humidification, and alleviate the client's anxiety as much as possible.

Prognosis

The prognosis for an individual with respiratory acidosis varies with the cause. Respiratory acidosis can cause shock or cardiac arrest.

Prevention

There is no specific prevention other than treatment of the cause. Smoking cessation is an important aspect in the long-term treatment, especially when COPD is an issue. Weight loss is very helpful when clients are obese.

RESPIRATORY ALKALOSIS (HYPOCAPNIA)

ICD-10: E87.3

Description

Respiratory alkalosis is excessive alkalinity of body fluids attributable to the excessive removal of carbon dioxide (CO_2) by the lungs. When excessive amounts of CO_2 are ventilated by the lungs, the $PaCO_2$ in the blood decreases, initiating a series of chemical and metabolic changes that act to reduce the level of serum bicarbonate. Consequently, the pH of the blood increases. The condition may be acute or chronic.

Etiology

Respiratory alkalosis is caused by acute or chronic hyperventilation. Acute respiratory alkalosis may result from hyperventilation induced by anxiety or psychological trauma, fever, pain, salicylate poisoning, excessive exercise, or excessive use of mechanical ventilators. It is also associated with hypoxia due to pneumonia, asthma, or pulmonary edema. Chronic respiratory alkalosis from hyperventilation is typically associated with hypoxia due to chronic cardiopulmonary diseases or high altitudes.

Signs and Symptoms

The classic sign of respiratory alkalosis is deep, rapid breathing of as much as 40 breaths per minute. Symptoms vary with etiology, but they may also include tachycardia, numbness or tingling of the extremities, light-headedness, muscle spasms, and periods of **apnea**, the temporary cessation of breathing.

Diagnostic Procedures

Diagnosis of respiratory alkalosis usually is based on the clinical evidence presented, but it must be confirmed through arterial blood gas analysis revealing decreased levels of serum bicarbonate or decreased $PaCO_2$ levels. Complete blood count analysis, chest x-ray, and CT scan may also be ordered.

Treatment

Treatment is aimed at correcting the underlying cause. Short-term measures may involve having the client breathe into a bag or administering a sedative to relieve hyperventilation in very anxious clients.

Complementary Therapy

No significant complementary therapy is indicated.

CLIENT COMMUNICATION

Teaching clients about the cause of respiratory alkalosis is helpful. Help them learn to alleviate stress and anxiety as much as possible.

Prognosis

The prognosis of an individual with respiratory alkalosis varies with etiology but is generally good.

Prevention

There are no specific preventive measures for respiratory alkalosis.

CHAPTER EPISODE—PART IV

Amanda did tell Paal the next morning. They talked about what happened. Because Paal was studying to be a radiologist, he knew something about Amanda's symptoms. He thought she might be allergic to something or maybe was having an asthma attack. Amanda wasn't sure, though, because she had never had any signs of asthma, and there was none in the family. She agreed, however, to see someone as soon as they arrived in Anchorage. Paal did not smoke close to Amanda again, and their trip ended with no more episodes.

- What tests might a primary care provider order to check Amanda?
- What is the likely outcome and what treatment is ordered?

LUNG CANCER

ICD-10: C34.XX

Description

Lung cancer comprises various malignant neoplasms that may appear in the trachea, bronchi, or air sacs of the lungs. It is the leading cancer killer in both men and women. According to the U.S. National Cancer Institute (NCI), approximately 1 out of every 14 men and women in the United States will be diagnosed with cancer of the lung or airways at some point in their lifetime. There are two major types of lung cancer: non–small cell lung cancer (NSCLC) and small cell lung cancer (SCLC). NSCLC is more common, and it generally grows and spreads slower than SCLC. The three main types are squamous cell or epidermoid carcinoma, adenocarcinoma, and large-cell carcinoma. SCLC, or oat cell cancer, is less common, but it grows more quickly and is likely to spread to other body organs.

Etiology

Although the precise triggering mechanisms are not known, most lung cancers are caused either directly or indirectly by smoking, accounting for 87% of cases. Tobacco smoke contains a number of chemicals known to be carcinogenic. Radon is the second leading cause of lung cancer in the United States. Radon gas can come up through the soil under a building and enter through gaps or cracks in the foundation as well as through pipes and drains. It is a radioactive gas that cannot be seen and has no odor or taste. Long-term exposure to asbestos, uranium, arsenic, and some petroleum products is also associated with an increased incidence of lung cancer. Both lung cancer and mesothelioma (cancer of the pleura of the lung and the peritoneum) are associated with exposure to asbestos. Cigarette smoking greatly increases the chance of developing an asbestos-related lung cancer to those exposed.

Signs and Symptoms

Early-stage lung cancer usually produces no symptoms and is difficult to detect. When symptoms appear, they may include smoker's cough, hoarseness, weight loss, wheezing, chest pain, dyspnea, and hemoptysis.

Diagnostic Procedures

Chest x-ray, a sputum cytology test, and fiberoptic bronchoscopy are useful in diagnosing lung cancer. Tissue biopsy is required for definitive diagnosis. A helical low-dose CT scan is much more sensitive than a regular x-ray and can detect tumors when they are small. Several tests are used to accurately stage a lung cancer, including laboratory (blood chemistry) tests, x-rays, CT scans, bone scans, and MRI. Abnormal blood chemistry tests may signal the presence of metastases in bone or liver, and radiological procedures can document the size of a cancer as well as possible spread to other organs. NSCLC stages are as follows:

Stage I: Cancer is confined to the lung.
Stages II and III: Cancer is confined to the chest. Larger and more invasive tumors are stage III.
Stage IV: Cancer has spread from the chest to other parts of the body.

SCLCs are staged using a two-tiered system:

Limited SCLC: Cancer is confined to its area of origin in the chest.
Extensive SCLC: Cancer has spread beyond the chest to other parts of the body.

Treatment

Treatment most often involves a combination of surgery, radiation therapy, and chemotherapy, because lung cancer often metastasizes to other tissues by the time it is diagnosed. Metastasis to the brain, liver, and bone is common. Photodynamic therapy (PDT) is a type of laser therapy that injects a special chemical into the bloodstream and kills the cancer cells when a laser light is aimed at the cancer. PDT can be used to relieve breathing problems when the cancer cannot be removed by surgery. It is most likely used in treating very small tumors.

Complementary Therapy

Clients will find a fair amount of confusion in treating lung cancer with alternative therapies. Clients who seek information from their primary care provider and integrative practitioners and perform independent research are likely to be the most satisfied with their treatment choices. Clients should consider how far the cancer has advanced and what will be the likely response to traditional and complementary treatments. The American College of Chest Physicians reports that some therapies are helpful for people with lung cancer, including the following:

- *Acupuncture.* Acupuncture may relieve pain and ease cancer treatment side effects, such as nausea, vomiting, and dry mouth. However, acupuncture is not safe when blood counts are low or individuals are taking blood thinners.
- *Hypnosis.* Hypnosis may reduce anxiety, nausea, and pain in people with cancer, and it may improve appetite.
- *Massage.* Massage can help relieve anxiety, distress, fatigue, and pain in people with cancer. Some massage therapists are specially trained to work with people who have cancer. The massage should not be painful, and there should be no massage anywhere near the tumor or any surgical sites. Massage is not recommended when blood counts are low or when taking blood thinners.
- *Meditation and guided imagery.* Both may reduce stress and improve quality of life in people with cancer. Meditation and guided imagery can be done alone or with instructors.
- *Yoga.* Yoga may help people with cancer sleep better, and it is generally safe when taught by a trained instructor. Clients should not make any moves that hurt or do not feel right. Many fitness centers offer yoga classes.

➔ CLIENT COMMUNICATION

Follow-up care is very important. Regular checkups ensure that any health changes are noted and that if any cancer returns, it can be treated quickly. Cancer support systems can be particularly helpful to individuals with cancer in providing emotional support and practical information on the disease.

Prognosis

Despite advances in diagnosis, the overall survival rate for those with lung cancer has changed little during the past 30 years and is still only about 16% at 5 years after diagnosis.

Prevention

Lung cancer is largely preventable if individuals stop smoking. If smokers stop at the time of early precancerous cellular changes, the damaged bronchial tissues often return to near normal.

Childhood Respiratory Diseases and Disorders

SUDDEN INFANT DEATH SYNDROME

ICD-10: R99

Description

Sudden infant death syndrome (SIDS) is the completely unexpected and unexplained death of an apparently normal and healthy infant, usually at age 10 to 12 weeks. Most often, the death occurs when the infant is sleeping. SIDS occurs more frequently in male than in female infants, in premature infants, and during the winter months. The number of deaths has been greatly reduced in the last 2 decades, but it is a leading cause of death in infants aged 1 to 12 months. Approximately 2,000 infants die each year.

Etiology

The cause is unknown, but several possibilities have been suggested, including mechanical suffocation; prolonged apnea; lack of **biotin,** a component of the vitamin B complex essential for the metabolism of fat and carbohydrates in the diet; an unknown virus; immunoglobulin abnormalities; a defect in the respiratory mucosal defense; or an anatomically abnormal larynx.

Signs and Symptoms

There are no premonitory signs and symptoms. The infant generally does not cry out or show evidence of distress or struggle. When found, the infant is dead and may have mottled skin, indicating cyanosis. There may be blood-tinged sputum. The infant's diaper is likely to be wet or filled with stool.

Diagnostic Procedures

A diagnosis of SIDS is exclusionary—that is, it is made only after all other causes of death have been eliminated as possibilities. An autopsy is required to rule out other causes of death.

Treatment

There is no treatment. There are SIDS support systems for parents. Emotional support should be provided.

Complementary Therapy

No significant complementary therapy is indicated.

CLIENT COMMUNICATION

Families may need grief counseling and referral to SIDS support systems. All new parents should know that the American Academy of Pediatrics recommends that all infants be positioned on their backs for sleeping.

Prognosis

It is currently believed that children are no longer at risk of SIDS by age 1.

Prevention

Some home monitoring devices have been tried on infants who have experienced apneic periods, but their use remains controversial. Prevention of SIDS is largely aimed at trying to identify infants at risk and placing infants on their backs to sleep on a firm mattress.

ACUTE TONSILLITIS

ICD-10: J03.90

Description

Acute tonsillitis is inflammation of a tonsil, especially one or both of the palatine tonsils that lie on either side of the opening of the throat. It can be acute or chronic.

Etiology

Tonsillitis is most frequently caused by infection by the bacteria *Streptococcus pyogenes* or *Staphylococcus aureus*, although a variety of infectious agents may be involved. The condition is a common complication of pharyngitis.

Signs and Symptoms

Acute tonsillitis is typically manifested by the sudden onset of chills and a high-grade fever with a mild to severe sore throat. Additional symptoms may include malaise, headache, and dysphagia. Chronic tonsillitis causes a recurrent sore throat, tonsillar hypertrophy, and abscess.

Diagnostic Procedures

On physical examination, the tonsils appear red and swollen. In severe cases, abscesses may be visible on the affected tonsil's surface. Blood tests may reveal leukocytosis. A throat culture to detect bacteria typically is performed.

Treatment

Antibiotic therapy, especially penicillin, is prescribed for bacterial tonsillitis in its early stages. Symptomatic relief includes saline gargles, analgesics, and antipyretics. Bed rest is usually indicated. Recurrent bouts of tonsillitis may require tonsillectomy.

Complementary Therapy

Complementary therapy includes a diet with plenty of fluids—diluted fruit juices, warm broth, and light soups.

CLIENT COMMUNICATION

Remind clients or parents that the entire antibiotic course must be taken in order to be effective. Popsicles can help a child ingest sufficient fluids.

Prognosis

The prognosis for acute tonsillitis is usually good. In severe cases, however, the tonsils may swell sufficiently to interfere with breathing. Localized complications may include otitis media, mastoiditis, and sinusitis.

Prevention

There is no specific prevention for acute tonsillitis except for prompt treatment of any pharyngeal infection.

ADENOID HYPERPLASIA

ICD-10: J35.2

Description

Adenoid hyperplasia is the enlargement of the lymphoid tissue of the nasopharynx, causing partial breathing blockage.

Etiology

The cause is essentially unknown. Circumstances that may cause the adenoids to continue to grow when they normally would atrophy (approximately ages 5 to 8) may include repeated infection and nasal congestion, chronic allergies, and heredity.

Signs and Symptoms

The most common symptoms are chronic mouth-breathing, snoring, and frequent head colds. The child's speech has a nasal quality.

Diagnostic Procedures

Diagnosis is usually made by visualizing the hyperplastic adenoidal tissue or by the use of lateral pharyngeal x-rays.

Treatment

The treatment of choice is adenoidectomy, often performed in conjunction with a tonsillectomy.

Complementary Therapy

No significant complementary therapy is indicated.

CLIENT COMMUNICATION

Explain in simple terms the surgical procedure to a child. Be sympathetic to both parents and the child in preparation for surgery.

Prognosis

The prognosis is excellent with proper care and attention. If untreated, however, adenoid hyperplasia can lead to changes in facial features and complications such as otitis media, which carries an accompanying risk of hearing loss.

Prevention

There is no specific prevention for adenoid hyperplasia.

THRUSH

ICD-10: B37.X

Description

Thrush is a yeast infection of the mucous membrane lining the mouth and tongue. It is commonly seen in infants but occurs in individuals with diabetes, those taking antibiotics for a long period of time, individuals with poorly fitting dentures, and those receiving chemotherapy treatments. Persons with HIV or AIDS are also susceptible.

Etiology

When the immune system is weakened, the small amount of *Candida* fungus normally living in the mouth grows unchecked and becomes a problem. The "sweet" saliva in the mouth of diabetics feeds the *Candida*, and long-term use of antibiotics destroys healthy bacteria that prevents its growth.

Signs and Symptoms

Thrush appears as whitish, velvety lesions in the mouth and on the tongue. The tissue underneath the lesions easily bleeds. The lesions gradually increase in number and size. It is painful to eat or swallow.

Diagnostic Procedures

Diagnosis is easily determined by a primary care provider or dentist looking at the mouth and tongue. Microscopic examination of mouth scrapings or culture of mouth lesions may be performed to confirm the *Candida* organisms.

Treatment

Infants with thrush are seldom treated, because thrush disappears in less than 2 weeks. For others, eating yogurt or taking over-the-counter acidophilus capsules can help. Controlling blood sugar levels for diabetics is

often sufficient to clear up the problem. An antifungal mouthwash (nystatin) or lozenges (clotrimazole) to suck on may be prescribed for those with weakened immune systems. In severe cases, when the infection spreads throughout the body, medications such as fluconazole (Diflucan) or ketoconazole (Nizoral) may be ordered.

Complementary Therapy

Rinsing the mouth and using a soft toothbrush with diluted 3% hydrogen peroxide solution several times a day is beneficial.

 CLIENT COMMUNICATION

Thrush is uncomfortable. Remind clients with weakened immune systems to report any outbreak; they may want to take antifungal medication on a regular basis to avoid recurrent infections.

Prognosis

When left unchecked, candida can spread throughout the body, causing such complications as esophagitis, meningitis, endocarditis, and **endophthalmitis.**

Prevention

Sterilize or discard any pacifiers or bottle nipples to prevent reinfection. Replace toothbrushes often, and take antifungal medications when the immune system is weakened by other disease.

CROUP

ICD-10: J05.0

Description

Croup, a common childhood ailment, is acute and severe inflammation and obstruction of the upper respiratory tract, occurring most frequently from 3 months to 3 years of age. It is more common in male infants and children and usually occurs in the winter.

Etiology

The condition may be caused by parainfluenza virus, adenoviruses, respiratory syncytial viruses, and influenza and measles viruses. Croup generally follows an upper respiratory tract infection.

Signs and Symptoms

Common symptoms include hoarseness; fever; a distinctive harsh, brassy, barklike cough; respiratory distress; and persistent **stridor** during inspiration. Stridor is a harsh, high-pitched sound during respiration due to obstruction of the air passages. The infant or child may be anxious and frightened by the respiratory distress. The symptoms may last a few hours or persist for a day or two.

Diagnostic Procedures

The clinical picture is very characteristic, so a diagnosis is made fairly quickly. Cultures of the causative organism are performed. Neck x-ray and laryngoscopy may also be performed.

Treatment

Children are treated symptomatically at home in most cases with bed rest, liquids, and antipyretics. Cool humidification of the air is tried. Often children are more comfortable when in a sitting position; holding them or placing them in an infant seat may ease their breathing. If dehydration is suspected, hospitalization may be necessary and antibiotic therapy and oxygen therapy may be started.

Complementary Therapy

No significant complementary therapy is indicated.

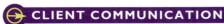

CLIENT COMMUNICATION

Keep the child as quiet as possible. Control fever with sponge baths and antipyretics. Water-based fruit juices and Popsicles can help soothe the throat. Use of a cool humidifier or vaporizer can be helpful.

Prognosis

The prognosis for croup is good with treatment.

Prevention

Prevention includes prompt treatment of any respiratory tract infections.

COMMON SYMPTOMS OF RESPIRATORY DISEASES AND DISORDERS

Individuals may present with the following common symptoms, which deserve attention from health-care professionals:

- Pain anywhere in the respiratory tract, especially sore throat
- Cough, productive or nonproductive, chronic or acute
- Breathing irregularities, such as dyspnea, wheezing, tachypnea, shortness of breath, or rales
- Hemoptysis or hematemesis
- Fever
- Malaise
- Headache
- Cyanosis

SUMMARY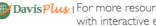

Many times, respiratory diseases and disorders are frightening to clients and their families because they affect their breathing. Some diseases become progressively worse with or without treatment. However, as with other body system diseases and disorders, many respiratory diseases are preventable with changes in lifestyle and/or early diagnosis and treatment intervention. The burden of respiratory diseases affects individuals and their families, schools, workplaces, neighborhoods, cities, and states and results in higher health insurance rates and lost productivity.

DavisPlus | For more resources and to sharpen your skills with interactive exercises, visit *DavisPlus* at http://davisplus.fadavis.com. Keyword *Tamparo*.

ONLINE RESOURCES

American Academy of Allergy, Asthma, & Immunology
http://www.aaaai.org

American Sleep Apnea Association
http://www.sleepapnea.org

COPD International
http://www.copd-international.com

Lung cancer
http://www.cancer.gov/cancertopics/types/lung

Pneumothorax (collapsed lung)
http://www.pneumothorax.org

Pulmonary hypertension
http://www.americanheart.org

CASE STUDIES

Case Study 1

Sam D'Onofrio, a 55-year-old naval shipyard worker, begins to experience a slightly irritating cough. His wife, Ginger, tells him that it is probably the result of smoking three packs of cigarettes a day. Ginger begs him to quit, as she did many years ago. He begins to experience trouble breathing even when at rest. Soon, however, Ginger also begins to experience symptoms of respiratory disease. Sam visits his primary care provider, who, based on the work and family history, suspects asbestosis. Because Ginger has washed his work clothes for 26 years, she is also advised to seek medical attention.

Case Study Questions

1. What causes or predisposing factors are apparent?
2. What is the pertinent symptom of this case?
3. What could have prevented the wife's involvement?
4. Comment on the role of smoking.

Case Study 2

A single mother of two young adults was always healthy and active. She was a nonsmoker. At age 56, she developed a dry lingering cough in late October. She was treated for asthma-like symptoms. She was well enough to prepare Thanksgiving dinner for 10 guests. Three weeks later, she was diagnosed with stage IV lung cancer. She lived only 2 months.

Case Study Questions

1. Do the history and symptoms indicate a neoplasm? Explain.
2. Why is it often so difficult to diagnose lung cancer?
3. What diagnostic tests might have picked up the neoplasm at an earlier date?
4. What implications does the person's age have in this case?

Case Study 3

Don Paladio had been a pharmacist in New York City. He retired to Florida and spent the better part of every day swimming in the Gulf. He was healthy and strong. Gradually, however, his years of smoking began to compromise his lung's capacity. Soon he could not swim at all. He enjoyed the beach from under his umbrella. Eventually, the trips to the beach were not possible. The diagnosis was pulmonary emphysema and COPD. Oxygen was needed, and his activities were diminished to cooking dinner for his wife and himself. Don was embarrassed about the oxygen tank and would no longer go out in public. He died when he was 85.

Case Study Questions

1. Discuss the impact of both diseases on Don's life.
2. What, if anything, could have been done to make his suffering less difficult?
3. Identify characteristics of such long-term chronic illnesses that are particularly difficult.

REVIEW QUESTIONS

Matching

Match each of the following definitions with its correct term.

_____ 1. Air in pleural cavity

_____ 2. Chronic obstructive pulmonary disease

_____ 3. Sore throat

_____ 4. Caused by Epstein-Barr virus

_____ 5. Excess fluid in pleural space

_____ 6. Black lung disease

_____ 7. Nosebleed

_____ 8. Lungs lose normal elasticity

_____ 9. Inflammation of the pleura

_____ 10. Hoarseness or loss of voice

_____ 11. Unexplained sudden death of an infant

_____ 12. Enlarged lymph tissue in nasopharynx

a. Epistaxis

b. Pharyngitis

c. Adenoid hyperplasia

d. Infectious mononucleosis

e. Pneumothorax

f. SIDS

g. Pleural effusion

h. COPD

i. Emphysema

j. Pulmonary anthracosis

k. Asthma

l. Cor pulmonale

m. Pleurisy

n. Laryngitis

Short Answer

1. What are the three major causes of sinusitis?

   a. _____

   b. _____

   c. _____

2. Treatment of acute tonsillitis and adenoid hyperplasia is apt to be _____.

3. What are the three major causes of pneumonia?

   a. _____

   b. _____

   c. _____

4. What is a complication that may result from a lung abscess? _____.

5. Can you name the classic symptom of sleep apnea?

   _____

6. What are the classic symptoms of asthma?

   a. _____

   b. _____

   c. _____

   d. _____

7. The diagnostic test of choice to confirm pulmonary tuberculosis is _____.

8. What is the best prevention for any of the pneumoconioses? _____.

9. Mycoses are what kind of infections?

   _____.

10. The most common pulmonary complication among hospital patients is _____.

Multiple Choice

Select the best answer.

1. What is known about allergic rhinitis?

   _____ a. It is controlled by avoiding known allergens.

   _____ b. It causes death usually during sleep.

   _____ c. It afflicts more females than males.

   _____ d. It is treated with medications and immunotherapy.

2. What are the symptoms of croup?

   _____ a. Profuse sweating and fever

   _____ b. Snoring and a barking cough

   _____ c. Barking cough, persistent stridor, hoarseness

   _____ d. Respiratory distress and cyanosis

3. What might complementary therapy for lung cancer treatment include?

   _____ a. Restriction of salts and fluids

   _____ b. The use of heparin and warfarin to reduce pain

   _____ c. Photodynamic therapy

   _____ d. Meditation, guided imagery, acupuncture, hypnosis

4. What is known about pulmonary edema?

   _____ a. It is diffuse extravascular accumulation of fluid in the left ventricle of the heart.

   _____ b. It commonly occurs during the daytime.

   _____ c. It is usually the direct consequence of right ventricular failure.

   _____ d. It causes the collapse of pulmonary arteries.

5. How is asthma, a condition marked by recurrent attacks, characterized?

_____ a. It affects 5 to 10 million Americans.

_____ b. Sufferers have sensitive airways that react to known "triggers."

_____ c. The intrinsic form is seen mostly in childhood.

_____ d. Produces a thick sputum during an acute episode.

Discussion Questions/Personal Reflection

1. Discuss with another individual how lifestyle choices that you have made might affect your respiratory health. Identify preventive measures that might be put in place. Is there anything that you could or would change?

_____

_____

_____

_____

_____

_____

_____

_____

_____

_____

2. Because secondhand smoke is dangerous to everyone, many cities in the United States have voted to make all public places smoke free. Some agencies have even created personnel policies that say any new hires must be smoke free 24 hours a day, 7 days a week. Discuss the health implications of these rulings. Discuss any potential discrimination problems that you see.

_____

_____

_____

_____

_____

_____

_____

_____

_____

_____

_____

14

Digestive System Diseases and Disorders

● *chapter outline*

key words

Anticholinergic
  (ăn"tĭ•kō"lĭn•ĕr'jĭk)
Ascites (ă•sī'tĕz)
Bilirubin (bĭl•ĭ•roo'bĭn)
Bilirubinuria
  (bĭl"ĭ•roo•bĭn•ū'rē•ă)
Cachexia (kă•kĕks'ē•ă)
Colectomy (kō•lĕk'tō•mē)
Coryza (kŏ•rī'ză)
Dysphagia (dĭs•fā'jē•ă)
Enteropathy (ĕn"tĕr•ŏp'ă•thē)
Epigastric (ĕp"ĭ•găs'trĭk)
Exudate (ĕks'ū•dāt)
Fecalith (fē'kă•lĭth)
Fissure (fĭ'shĕr)

Fistula (fĭs'tū•lă)
Gliadin (glī'ă•dĕn)
Hematemesis
  (hĕm"ă•tĕm'ĕ•sis)
Hematochezia
  (hĕm"ă•tō•kē'zē•ă)
Hemolysis (hē•mŏl'ĭ•sĭs)
Hepatomegaly
  (hĕp"ă•tō•mĕg'ă•lē)
Hyperchlorhydria
  (hī"pĕr•klor•hī'drē•ă)
Hyperglycemia
  (hī"pĕr•glī•sē'mē•ă)
Ileostomy (ĭl"ē•ŏs'tō•mē)
Jaundice (jawn'dĭs)

McBurney point
  (mĭk•bŭr'nē poynt)
Microbiome (mi"kro•bi'ōm)
Occult blood (ŭ•kŭlt')
Peristalsis (pĕr•ĭ•stăl'sĭs)
Polyposis (pŏl"ē•pō'sĭs)
Prebiotics (prē"bī•ŏt'ĭks)
Probiotics (prō"bī•ŏ'tĭks)
Reflux (rē'flŭks)
Sclerotherapy
  (sklĕr"ō•thĕr'ă•pē)
Tetany (tĕt'ă•nē)
Varices (văr'ĭ•sēz)
Villi (vĭl'ī)

learning outcomes

Upon successful completion of this chapter, you will be able to:

- Define key terms.
- Recall the anatomy and physiology of the digestive system and accessory organs.
- Compare and contrast the two types of stomatitis.
- Describe gastroesophageal reflux and its prognosis.
- Identify at least four causes of gastritis.
- Outline the etiology of peptic ulcers and their treatment.
- Discuss the signs and symptoms of gastroenteritis.
- Describe celiac disease, its diagnosis, and treatment.
- Review causes of irritable bowel syndrome.
- Discuss the inflammatory pattern of Crohn disease and why surgery may be necessary.
- List at least three predisposing factors of ulcerative colitis and compare to Crohn disease.
- Recall the cause and predisposing factors of diverticulitis disease.
- Describe the symptoms for acute appendicitis and how it is diagnosed.
- Compare and contrast the two types of hemorrhoids and their treatment.
- Explain what constitutes constipation.

- Recall treatment for diarrhea.
- Identify when to see a primary care provider for nausea and vomiting.
- Recall the description and treatment possibilities for infantile colic.
- Restate the cause of and treatment for hiatal and abdominal hernias.
- Explain the implications of pancreatitis for complications.
- Discuss the relationship between cholelithiasis and cholecystitis.
- Describe treatment protocol for cholecystitis.
- Identify the etiology of and the complications of cirrhosis.
- Discuss the different types of hepatitis.
- Recall the treatment protocol and prognosis for pancreatic cancer.
- Identify populations at risk for colorectal cancer and its survival rate.
- List at least five common symptoms of digestive system diseases and disorders.

CHAPTER EPISODE—PART I

Katy is a senior in high school. She has a passion for volleyball and is on the varsity volleyball team. She is happy, seemingly healthy, and has plans for going to the community college in the fall. Her life is about to change, however. She woke in the middle of the night with severe stomach cramps and rushed to the bathroom. The diarrhea was explosive, and to her horror, there was bright red blood in the toilet bowl as well. Her mom heard the distress and knocked on the door to see what was happening. When Katy told her what was happening, she, too, was alarmed.

- What might be the cause of these symptoms?
- What should Katy and her mother do?

DIGESTIVE SYSTEM ANATOMY AND PHYSIOLOGY REVIEW

The digestive system consists of the set of organs and glands associated with the ingestion and digestion of food and the absorption of nutrients (Fig. 14.1). It may be the system that is most taken for granted. Whether a person is eating foods of little value or a well-balanced diet, the task of the digestive system is the same—to nourish the cells of the body. The basic functions of the digestive system are to ingest, digest, and absorb the nutrients taken in, creating simple organic and inorganic molecules that can be transported to the body's cells through blood and lymph. This system also eliminates solid, mostly indigestible, wastes from the body through the large intestine.

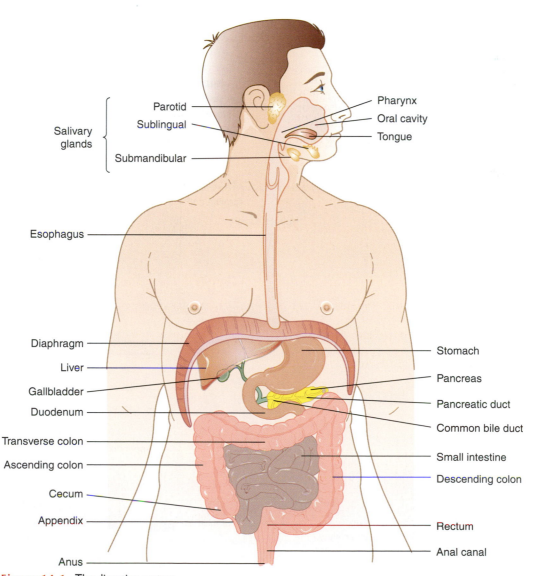

Figure 14.1 The digestive system.

Often the digestive system is divided into the upper gastrointestinal (GI) tract and the lower GI tract. The system is composed of the alimentary canal and the accessory organs of digestion. The canal is a tube that passes from the mouth to the anus. The parts of the alimentary canal are noted in Figure 14.1 and include the mouth, pharynx, esophagus, stomach, small intestine, and large intestine. The colon extends from the small intestine to the anus.

The following list briefly covers each digestive system organ in the alimentary canal:

Mouth or oral cavity: In the mouth, the first part of the canal, the teeth mechanically break down food that is mixed with saliva. The food is pushed about by the tongue; the tongue's taste buds provide the pleasurable sensation of taste.

Salivary glands: Three sets of salivary glands in the mouth secrete saliva (mostly water and amylase) in the mouth to moisten food for swallowing and begin digesting carbohydrates.

Pharynx: The pharynx, or throat, is the portion of the alimentary canal that carries the swallowed food product to the esophagus.

Esophagus: The food product is carried farther through the canal by **peristalsis** into the stomach. No digestion takes place in either the pharynx or the esophagus. The lower esophageal sphincter (LES), or cardiac sphincter, relaxes to allow food into the stomach; it then contracts, preventing the backup of stomach contents.

Stomach: The stomach sac holds the food for the digestion process to continue. A number of secretions occur in the stomach to form gastric juice. The secretions include mucus that coats and protects the stomach lining, hydrochloric acid and pepsin to digest proteins, intrinsic factor for the absorption vitamin B_{12}, and the hormone gastrin to stimulate further production of gastric juice. When the food becomes a thick liquid called *chyme*, the pyloric sphincter relaxes to allow small amounts of chyme to pass into the first portion of the small intestine.

Small intestine: Digestion is completed in the small intestine, a tube about 20 feet long. The first portion of the small intestine is called the *duodenum*. Bile secreted by the liver enters the duodenum to emulsify fats. The second portion, the *jejunum*, continues the digestion process, and absorption begins—glucose and amino acids go into blood capillaries and fats go into lymph capillaries (lacteals). The third portion, the *ileum*, is the final and longest segment of the small intestine. It is specifically responsible for the absorption of vitamin B_{12} and the reabsorption of bile salts.

Large intestine (colon): Any undigested food and water pass into the first part of the large intestine, called the *cecum* (Fig. 14.2). Peristalsis

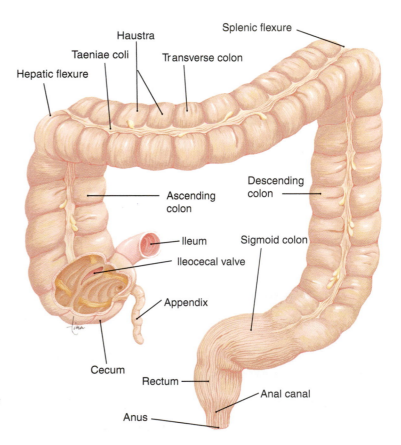

Figure 14.2 The large intestine shown in anterior view. The term *flexure* means a turn or bend. *(From Scanlon, VC, and Sanders, T: Essentials of Anatomy and Physiology, ed. 6. Philadelphia: F.A. Davis, 2011, p 399, with permission.)*

carries the waste to the ascending, transverse, and descending colon, the sigmoid colon, the rectum, and finally the anal canal. No digestion takes place in the colon. The colon absorbs water, minerals, and vitamins and eliminates the remaining waste products.

The accessory glands include the pancreas, liver, and gallbladder (Figs. 14.3 and 14.4). The pancreas is both an exocrine (produces digestive enzymes) and an endocrine (produces insulin and glucagon) gland. The liver, the largest organ in the abdominal cavity, produces bile and regulates the level of most chemicals in the blood. It plays a central role in cellular metabolism of the body. The gallbladder concentrates and stores bile that is received from the liver.

The two functions of the digestive system are digestion and absorption. In digestion, food is broken down into simpler molecules such as amino acids, fatty acids, and simple sugars through both mechanical and chemical processes. The mechanical process involves physically breaking down food as it is chewed and swallowed and moved to the stomach, where further chemical action takes place, creating chyme. The chemical process occurs when the enzymes act on the digested food to create simpler chemical molecules. This prepares the food for absorption, where simpler molecules, minerals, vitamins, and water move from the digestive tract across the digestive wall and into the blood to be carried into body tissue.

The various accessory organs secrete fluids into the digestive tube to help in the digestion and absorption of nutrients. The process of ingesting, digesting, and absorbing nutrients supplies the energy and chemical building blocks for growth and maintenance of the body.

Upper Gastrointestinal Tract

STOMATITIS (HERPETIC AND APHTHOUS)

ICD-10: K12.30 or K12.2

Description

Stomatitis, or inflammation of the oral mucosa, is a common inflammation that most often occurs in two forms: acute herpetic stomatitis (cold sore) and aphthous stomatitis (canker sores). Painful blisters or ulcers characterize both. Redness, swelling, and sometimes bleeding occur.

Etiology

Acute herpetic stomatitis is a highly contagious viral illness caused by herpes simplex virus type 1 (HSV-1). It often occurs in and lies dormant in nervous tissue with recurring lesions appearing throughout life. There may be a systemic illness with fever, blisters, and inflammation of the gums. The cause of aphthous stomatitis is essentially unknown, but lack of vitamin B_{12}, folic acid, and iron is suspect. Aphthous stomatitis is activated periodically as well. Stress, fatigue, anxiety, eating foods high in acid, and immunosuppression exacerbate both acute herpetic stomatitis and aphthous stomatitis.

Signs and Symptoms

Acute herpetic stomatitis begins suddenly. There is mouth pain, difficulty eating and swallowing, and fever. Gums are swollen, and the mucous membrane has

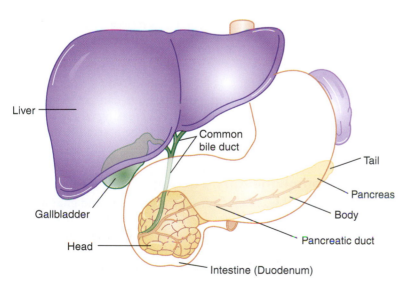

Figure 14.3 The liver and gallbladder with blood vessels and bile ducts.

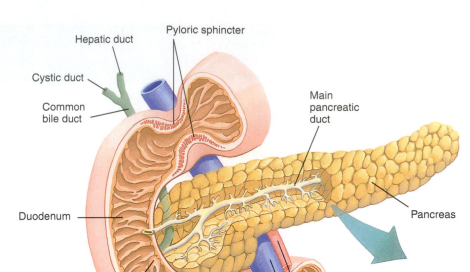

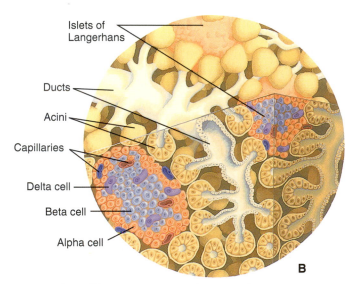

Figure 14.4 (A) The pancreas, sectioned to show the pancreatic ducts. The main pancreatic duct joins the bile duct. (B) Microscopic section showing acini with their ducts and several islets of Langerhans. *(From Scanlon, VC, and Sanders, T: Essentials of Anatomy and Physiology, ed. 6. Philadelphia: F.A. Davis, 2011, p 410, with permission.)*

blisters and ulcerating inflammatory lesions that heal in less than 2 weeks. In aphthous stomatitis, there is burning, tingling, and some swelling of mucous membrane. One or more shallow ulcers with white centers and red borders are present. The ulcers are discrete and shallow and gradually heal in 10 to 14 days.

Diagnostic Procedures

Diagnosis is based on physical examination.

Treatment

Supportive measures to relieve the pain are recommended, such as warm-water mouth rinses and topical anesthetics. Antiviral medications can treat herpetic stomatitis quite successfully. Increasing levels of iron, folic acid, and vitamin B_{12} may be started in treating aphthous stomatitis.

Complementary Therapy

A mouthwash made from steeped sage and chamomile may be helpful as a gargle. Clients are advised to avoid high-acid fruits, caffeine, alcohol, commercial mouthwashes, and smoking. Naturopaths believe that an allergy to wheat is a major cause of aphthous stomatitis.

⊕ CLIENT COMMUNICATION

Instruct individuals on the importance of meticulous oral hygiene and of avoiding any irritating foods. Remind clients that approximately 90% of the population carries herpes simplex virus and that nearly all children pick up the virus at some time during their childhood.

Prognosis

Both forms are self-limiting and usually clear within 10 days. When a high fever accompanies acute herpetic stomatitis, a primary care provider (PCP) should be contacted.

Prevention

Alleviation of precipitating factors can be helpful. Avoid spicy and acidic foods. Recurrence is likely for both forms. It is best to avoid close contact with people who have the herpetic form of stomatitis. Do not share utensils, drinking glasses, razors, and toothbrushes with actively infected individuals. If infected, remember to wash your hands after touching the cold sore and never touch your eyes after touching the cold sore to prevent its spread to the eyes.

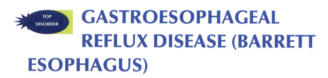

GASTROESOPHAGEAL REFLUX DISEASE (BARRETT ESOPHAGUS)

ICD-10: K21.9 (GERD)
ICD-10: K22.70 (BARRETT ESOPHAGUS)

Description

Gastroesophageal reflux disease (GERD) is the backup of gastric or duodenal contents into the esophagus and past the lower esophageal sphincter (LES) without belching or vomiting. The liquid contents can inflame and damage the lining of the esophagus. About one-third of Americans have GERD.

Etiology

The major cause is an abnormally weak contraction of the LES, reducing its ability to prevent **reflux.** The second cause is abnormal relaxations of the LES, or transient LES relaxations. The LES should create sufficient pressure to close the lower end of the esophagus yet relax after each swallow to allow food to pass into the stomach. Reflux, a flowing back or return flow of fluid, occurs when the LES pressure is deficient or when the pressure within the stomach exceeds the LES pressure. A person with reflux is unable to swallow fast enough or often enough to create sufficient peristaltic amplitude to clear the gastric acid from the lower esophagus. The result is prolonged acidity in the esophagus when reflux occurs. Some predisposing factors include pyloric surgery, long-term nasogastric intubation, certain foods, alcohol, smoking, obesity, and some drugs. Hiatal hernia and any position that increases intra-abdominal pressure may also cause GERD.

Signs and Symptoms

GERD symptoms may not always be present (especially in older clients), and it is not always possible to confirm physiological reflux. The most common symptoms, however, are heartburn, regurgitation, and nausea. For some, the first sign of GERD is a dry cough and laryngitis, or what is now called *reflux laryngitis.* Symptoms may be relieved by taking antacids or by sitting upright and are worsened by vigorous exercise, bending, or lying down.

Diagnostic Procedures

After a careful history and physical examination, medications to suppress the production of stomach acid are given. If the heartburn diminishes, the diagnosis of GERD is confirmed. Further tests to determine GERD include upper GI endoscopy, esophageal acid testing, esophageal probe, and esophageal manometry. Recurrent GERD after 6 weeks is abnormal. An acid perfusion test (Bernstein) can show reflux, but endoscopy and biopsy allow visualization and confirmation of any pathological changes in the mucosa.

Treatment

Decreasing esophageal irritation is helpful. This can be partially accomplished by eating low-fat, high-fiber foods and avoiding caffeine, tobacco, alcohol, chocolate, peppermint, and carbonated beverages. Elevating the head portion of the bed may decrease night symptoms. It is best to eat several small meals instead of two or three large meals. Antacids can neutralize gastric acid and relieve heartburn. Proton pump inhibitors (PPIs), a group of medications that decrease the amount of acid in the stomach and intestines, may be prescribed. Metoclopramide is a GI stimulant that improves gastric emptying and increases LES pressure. Surgery that creates an artificial closure of the gastroesophageal junction may be necessary in severe cases that do not respond to other treatment.

Complementary Therapy

Most practitioners suggest that avoiding trigger foods, especially chocolate, caffeine, spicy foods, and foods that have a lot of acid (like tomatoes and oranges), is the first step toward eliminating GERD. One recommendation includes chewing gum after meals. Another recommendation is to drink warm water with a meal to reduce reflux. Integrative practitioners agree that PPI medications may be the first choice of treatment.

CLIENT COMMUNICATION

It is best for clients to eat nothing within 3 hours of going to bed, avoid tight clothing, maintain a normal body weight, and avoid trigger foods. Clients are advised to avoid circumstances that increase intra-abdominal pressure.

Prognosis

The prognosis for GERD varies with the underlying cause; however, it is a chronic condition and a risk factor for developing Barrett esophagus, the predominant precursor to esophageal adenocarcinoma. In Barrett esophagus, there is a change in the epithelium of the distal esophagus that is often seen in cancerous tissue. A gastroenterologist will perform an esophagogastro-duodenoscopy (EGD) to look for abnormalities when symptoms of weight loss, **dysphagia,** blood in the stool, or anemia are present. If a diagnosis of Barrett esophagus is made, then periodic checks will be done as a precautionary measure against esophageal adeno-carcinoma, considered the fastest growing cancer in the Western world.

Prevention

Clients should avoid any offending foods; reducing fat and increasing fiber in the diet are also recommended. Clients are advised to not eat before going to bed and to elevate the head of the bed for increased comfort. Taking nonprescription medicines to reduce or block acid are helpful. These include antacids such as Tums, H2 blockers such as Pepcid, and PPIs such as Prilosec.

GERD in the News

Studies through the National Institutes of Health's Human Microbiome Project continue to indicate that GERD and other gastrointestinal diseases are associated with global alteration of the **microbiome** in the esophagus and along the GI tract. Human microbiome consists of all the microorganisms that reside in the human body—microbes, their genetic elements, and how they react in a particular environment. In the case of GERD, the esophagus is the environment. The lead author of the study, Shiheng Pei, MD, PhD, assistant professor of pathology and medicine at New York University's Langone Medical Center, said, "At this time, we don't yet know whether the changes in bacterial populations are triggering GERD or are simply a response to it. If changes in the bacterial population do cause reflux, it may be possible to design new therapies with antibiotics, **probiotic** bacteria or **prebiotics.**"

GASTRITIS

ICD-10: K29.XX*

Description

Gastritis, the most common stomach ailment, describes a group of conditions with one thing in common: inflammation and erosion of the gastric mucosa. Erosive gastritis destroys the stomach lining. Gastritis can be acute or chronic and can occur at any age.

Etiology

The etiology of gastritis is varied and complex. It usually develops when the stomach's protective mucus-lined layer is weakened or damaged, allowing digestive juices to damage and inflame the stomach lining. Irritating foods, alcoholic beverages, caffeine, overuse of NSAIDs, and ingested poisons can cause gastritis. Smoking worsens the irritation. It can be secondary to stress, bile reflux, and an autoimmune response. When *Helicobacter pylori* bacteria is present, stomach ulcers may also occur.

Signs and Symptoms

After exposure to the offending substances, the acute form of gastritis may feature **dyspepsia,** indigestion, cramping, belching, vomiting, and **epigastric** pain in the region of the abdomen over the pit of the stomach. There may be **hematemesis,** or vomiting of blood in erosive gastritis. A client with the chronic form of gastritis may exhibit similar symptoms, mild discomfort, or no symptoms. When symptoms do develop, they may be hard to pinpoint. A person may experience a loss of appetite or a "full" feeling in the stomach or have vague epigastric pain.

Diagnostic Procedures

A medical history that reveals exposure to a GI irritant may suggest this disorder. A blood test to check for the presence of *H. pylori* antibodies is likely ordered. A breath test and stool analysis can also check for *H. pylori* bacteria. Upper GI endoscopy with biopsy will help confirm the diagnosis when done before lesions heal, usually within 24 hours. GI x-ray with barium swallow is another commonly used tool.

Treatment

Treatment for gastritis and *H. pylori* infection depends on the cause. Symptoms are relieved by eliminating any known irritant, such as NSAIDs or alcohol. Chronic gastritis caused by *H. pylori* infection is treated by eradicating the bacteria. Medications to treat stomach acid and promote healing may be ordered. These include PPIs, antacids, and acid blockers.

*The X represents the fourth digit that is often required and supplied once more detailed information about the disease or disorder is made known to the provider.

In the event of ingestion of toxic substances, an antidote or antiemetic may be prescribed. Any hematemesis should be reported to the PCP.

Complementary Therapy

Practitioners are likely to encourage avoidance of irritants, especially alcohol and NSAIDs. Nutritional supplements and herbal remedies may be suggested to encourage repair of the stomach lining. None should be taken without first discussing with the PCP.

 CLIENT COMMUNICATION

Educating persons who have gastritis includes discussions of prevention; eating smaller, more frequent meals; and maintaining appropriate fluid levels in the body.

Prognosis

The prognosis of gastritis is good with proper treatment. Untreated, gastritis may be a precursor to gastric polyps and benign or malignant tumor.

Prevention

Prevention of gastritis includes avoiding gastric irritants. Advise clients to take prescribed medications with milk or food and avoid aspirin-containing substances. Also tell clients to avoid spicy foods, alcohol, caffeine, and tobacco.

PEPTIC ULCERS

ICD-10: K27.X

Description

Peptic ulcers can be found in the lower esophagus, the stomach, the pylorus, the duodenum, and the jejunum. However, these ulcers, or circumscribed lesions in the mucous membrane, are most likely found in the stomach and duodenum. Nearly 6 million individuals suffer from peptic ulcers in the United States. Gastric peptic ulcers affecting the stomach mucosa are found mostly in women over age 60. Duodenal peptic ulcers are most commonly found in men between ages 20 and 50. A gastric ulcer is a lesion in the mucosal lining of the stomach. In this disease, a patch of mucosal tissue becomes necrotic and is subsequently eroded by the acids and pepsins released within the stomach. Put simply, the stomach begins digesting itself (Fig. 14.5). A duodenal ulcer is a circumscribed, craterlike lesion in the mucous membrane of the short, wide segment of the small intestine called the *duodenum*.

Etiology

The three major causes of peptic ulcers are infection with *H. pylori,* use of NSAIDs, and pathological hypersecretion disorders. Just how ulcers develop is not entirely clear, but their development is believed to be related to increased gastric acid production and/or to factors that impair mucosal barrier protection. Such irritants as alcohol, aspirin, caffeine, and tobacco likely

CHAPTER EPISODE—PART II

Katy lives in a small apartment with her disabled mom. Funds are scarce, and their only source of health insurance is through Medicaid. Their PCP is a nurse practitioner, and when they call for an appointment, none is available until the end of the next day. Katy and her mom hoped the problem would go away before then, but it did not. Katy was unable to attend school prior to the appointment because she continued to have cramping and diarrhea accompanied by bright red blood. Her mom now believes there is internal bleeding somewhere and is truly frightened. Katy is in near panic. She missed one volleyball game and fears she will miss another game depending upon the PCP's diagnosis—enough to put her on probation with the team.

- Does the apparent stress in the household complicate Katy's condition? Explain your response.
- Could anything be done for Katy to see a professional sooner? If so, describe.

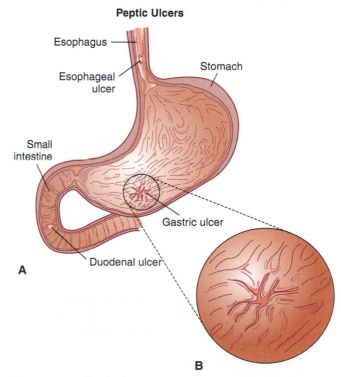

Figure 14.5 Peptic ulcers.

accelerate gastric acid production and the erosion of the mucosal barrier. Predisposing factors include blood type. Gastric ulcers appear most often in individuals with type A blood; duodenal ulcers tend to afflict persons with type O blood.

Signs and Symptoms

Persistent "heartburn" and indigestion are the classic symptoms; there may be nagging stomach pain as well. GI bleeding, **hematochezia** (bright red bloody stools), nausea, vomiting, and weight loss can occur. The chronic, periodic heartburn pain may radiate into the back region. Often, a peculiar sensation of hot water bubbling in the back of the throat occurs. The symptoms of both gastric and duodenal ulcers appear about 2 hours after eating or after consuming orange juice, caffeine, alcohol, or aspirin. Although most peptic ulcers are small, they can cause a considerable amount of discomfort.

Diagnostic Procedures

Diagnosis is made by EGD or upper GI barium swallow. Laboratory analysis to detect minute quantities of blood or **occult** blood in stools, serological testing to determine clinical signs of infection, studies of gastric secretions that show **hyperchlorhydria,** and a carbon 13 (^{13}C) urea breath test result will reflect activity of *H. pylori*.

Treatment

It is recommended that every person with an ulcer be treated at least once to eradicate *H. pylori* infection. Antibiotics prescribed to treat *H. pylori* include amoxicillin (Amoxil), clarithromycin (Biaxin), and metronidazole (Flagyl). Individuals who require NSAIDs may be given a prostaglandin analog to suppress ulceration, or a change of medication is ordered. Medications may be given to reduce acid secretion. Antacids and PPIs are likely prescribed. If GI bleeding occurs, EGD will reveal the site of bleeding, and coagulation by laser or cautery will control the bleeding. Surgery is indicated for perforation, suspected malignancy, or when conservative treatment is unsuccessful.

Complementary Therapy

Having clients eliminate food and drink irritants is helpful. Dietary changes, herbal medicines, and stress reduction are recommended. Therapy to treat infection is also recognized. Herbal medications should be taken only with the approval of the PCP.

⊕ CLIENT COMMUNICATION

Prompt treatment is important to prevent complications, as is avoiding offending foods and drugs. Remind clients that the combination of alcohol and NSAIDs is especially harmful.

Prognosis

Peptic ulcers tend to be chronic with remissions and exacerbations. From 5% to 10% of individuals develop complications that necessitate surgery. Complications of peptic ulcers include hemorrhage and perforation, both potentially life-threatening situations. Gastric ulcers are carefully monitored for signs of malignancy.

Prevention

No prevention is known, but the following suggestions can be made to clients to help lower the risk of developing peptic ulcers: Do not smoke, do not take NSAIDs longer than a few days, and limit alcohol intake. Careful adherence to treatment protocols may prevent recurrence.

GASTROENTERITIS

ICD-10: K52.89 or K52.9

Description

Gastroenteritis is the inflammation of the stomach and small intestine; it may also be known as intestinal flu, traveler's diarrhea, or food poisoning. It occurs in persons of all ages and is a major cause of death in developing countries.

Etiology

Causes of gastroenteritis include infection from bacteria, amoebae, parasites, and viruses. The ingestion of toxins, allergic reactions to certain foods, and drug reactions also may produce this disease. The bowel reacts to any of these agents with hypermotility, producing severe diarrhea and resultant depletion of intracellular fluids.

Signs and Symptoms

The etiology of the particular case determines, in part, the signs and symptoms, which may include diarrhea, cramping, nausea, vomiting, malaise, fever, and rumbling stomach sounds. More serious symptoms include hemoptysis, hematemesis, and dehydration. Hemoptysis and hematemesis occur when small blood vessels tear in the throat or esophagus from continuous and forceful vomiting.

Diagnostic Procedures

The medical history and physical examination may suggest gastroenteritis. A stool and/or blood culture will identify any bacteria or parasite. An endoscopy may be performed.

Treatment

Treatment is symptomatic and supportive. Fluid and nutritional support are important to minimize electrolyte and fluid imbalances. Antidiarrheals and antiemetics may be prescribed. Children and elderly persons are especially intolerant to fluid and electrolyte imbalance.

Complementary Therapy

Avoidance of the irritant is important. Diarrhea is the body's way of eliminating the irritant, but this symptom should be carefully monitored to prevent loss of electrolytes and fluids. Sucking on ice chips, sipping Sprite or 7UP, and drinking small amounts of clear broths are recommended.

 CLIENT COMMUNICATION

Discuss all methods of prevention, and encourage uninterrupted rest. Sitz baths for 10 minutes two or three times daily are helpful for perianal discomfort. Some primary care providers prefer that no over-the-counter medications be taken because they may mask a more serious problem. Any antibiotics or anti-infective agents prescribed should be taken until they are completely gone.

Prognosis

The prognosis varies with the etiology but is generally good once the cause has been isolated and treatment has begun. Gastroenteritis is a self-limiting disorder.

Prevention

To help prevent gastroenteritis, remind clients to properly refrigerate all perishable food and wash hands thoroughly before handling food. Instruct clients to cook all foods thoroughly. Flies and roaches need to be eliminated in the home. People traveling in developing countries should be especially cautious of contaminated water or food.

INFANTILE COLIC

ICD-10: R10.83

Description

Infantile colic is defined in infants who are healthy and well fed but have paroxysms of irritability, fussing, or crying lasting for 3 hours a day and occurring on more than 3 days in 1 week for a period of 3 weeks. The condition usually occurs during the first 3 months of life.

Etiology

Excessive fermentation and gas production in the intestines are thought to be the cause of colic. Other factors include too rapid feeding, overeating, swallowing air, or poor burping techniques. Many times the cause cannot be determined.

Signs and Symptoms

Loud crying and drawing of the legs up to the abdomen are typical behaviors of an infant experiencing colic. The crying usually begins suddenly, and often after a feeding.

The cry is loud and continuous and lasts from 1 to 4 hours. The infant's face often gets flushed or red.

Diagnostic Procedures

There is no specific diagnostic test for this disorder. The "rule of 3" is often used: crying occurs during the first 3 months, lasts longer than 3 hours a day, occurs more than 3 days a week, and continues for at least 3 weeks.

Treatment

The best treatment may be the availability of a calm setting for feeding time for both parent and child and gentle burping midway through the feeding and again at the end. Mothers who breastfeed should avoid eating foods that may cause gas. Swaddling the infant to decrease jerky movements and using a front carrier may be helpful. Taking the infant for a car ride or using an infant swing is often successful in soothing him or her. Walking or rocking works for some. Applying gentle pressure to the infant's abdomen or gentle massage to the infant's back while the infant is lying down may be tried.

Complementary Therapy

In addition to suggestions given, a steeped chamomile tea might be given to the infant with a little water.

 CLIENT COMMUNICATION

Infantile colic is stressful for parents. Reassure them and suggest ways they can get a break during this time.

Prognosis

The prognosis for infantile colic is good. The infant will continue to thrive and develop even with colic. Colic usually disappears spontaneously after 3 months of age.

Prevention

The best prevention of infantile colic includes frequent and smaller feedings and avoidance of gassy foods for nursing mothers.

Lower Gastrointestinal Tract

CELIAC DISEASE (GLUTEN-INDUCED ENTEROPATHY)

ICD-10: K90.0

Description

Celiac disease, or gluten-induced **enteropathy,** is a disease of the small intestine marked by malabsorption, gluten intolerance (gluten is a protein found in wheat, barley, and rye), and damage to and characteristic changes in the mucosal lining of the intestine. Because of the gluten intolerance characterizing celiac disease, it is sometimes referred to as *gluten-induced* enteropathy, a disease of the intestine. The incidence of celiac disease is high among siblings. More than 3 million individuals in the United States are afflicted.

Etiology

Celiac disease is an autoimmune disorder in response to the **gliadin** fraction of gluten. Gliadin is a water-insoluble protein present in the gluten of wheat, barley, and rye. Celiac disease most often surfaces in individuals with a genetic predisposition to the disease and an unusually permeable intestinal wall. The gluten-induced damage to the intestine mucosal lining may result from either a toxic or an immunologic reaction to this protein.

Signs and Symptoms

Symptoms of celiac disease may include weight loss, anorexia, abdominal distention, flatulence, intestinal bleeding, peripheral neuritis, dermatitis, and muscle wasting. The condition is also marked by the passage of abnormally large diarrheal stools that are characteristically light yellow to gray, greasy, and foul smelling. The resultant chronic malnutrition may cause mineral depletion that may be revealed in the musculoskeletal system as bone pain; tenderness; compression deformities; and sharp, painful, periodic muscle contractions called **tetany.** Anemia from the poor absorption of folate, iron, and vitamin B_{12} can also be a symptom. Neurological effects may include neuropathy and seizures. Dry skin, eczema, and psoriasis can be the result of celiac disease. Amenorrhea and hypometabolism are endocrine symptoms.

Diagnostic Procedures

The disease often is difficult to diagnose and to differentiate from other intestinal disorders. An initial serological test followed by biopsy is recommended. The serology includes testing for antigliadin antibodies (IgA), antiendomysium antibodies (EMA), and tissue transglutaminase (tTG) antibody to screen persons suspected of having celiac disease. If these antibody tests are positive, there is a 99.6% chance that the individual has celiac disease, and a biopsy is ordered to confirm the diagnosis. For a definitive diagnosis of celiac disease, the following are necessary: biopsy of the small intestine indicating destruction of the **villi,** tiny fingerlike projections lining the interior of the small intestine that absorb fluid and nutrients, and remission of symptoms and improvement in the condition of the villi after the institution of a gluten-free diet.

Treatment

Treatment consists of lifelong strict adherence to a gluten-free diet. A few persons who do not experience improved small bowel function after instituting a gluten-free diet may be treated with corticosteroid drugs. Supportive treatment may include supplemental iron, vitamin B_{12}, and folic acid. Research is currently under way to develop medications that prevent an immune response to gluten and block the action that makes the intestine permeable. Microbiome also plays a role in celiac disease. It is believed that the variance of microbiome from person to person enables many to go undetected for years. The microbiome seem able to influence which genes are active at any given time, thus allowing some to tolerate gluten for many years and then suddenly lose that ability, causing celiac disease to develop.

Complementary Therapy

It is essential that clients avoid all wheat, barley, and rye. A daily multivitamin and mineral supplement that includes 1,000 milligrams of calcium along with 400 milligrams of magnesium (note that too much magnesium can cause diarrhea) can be helpful to individuals with celiac disease.

⊕ CLIENT COMMUNICATION

Educate clients on careful reading of all food labels to detect offending ingredients. Encourage them to join a celiac disease support system to learn more about the disease, special recipes, and stores that sell gluten-free foods. A nutritionist can encourage diet alternatives. If persons go on and off the diet, tissue regeneration may no longer be possible.

Prognosis

With proper treatment and a lifelong gluten-free diet, the prognosis is good. Symptomatic relief often occurs within a few weeks, but improvement in tests of absorption function and small bowel tissue characteristics may not occur for months, sometimes years. Persons with celiac disease have an increased incidence of abdominal lymphoma and carcinomas later in life. Individuals who develop GI symptoms while in remission and on a gluten-free diet should be carefully evaluated for malignancy.

Prevention

There is no known prevention of the disease; however, if there is a strong family history of celiac disease, screening with the EMA and tTG is recommended for early diagnosis.

Trouble With Gluten in the Diet

For many years a person with celiac disease had great difficulty finding foods that were totally free of gluten. Today, the stores are full of products that are gluten-free. This is due mostly to a surge in popularity of the individuals who believe they are allergic to gluten. Thus, a new diagnosis "gluten sensitivity" has arisen. Symptoms may be similar, but more likely include disabling headaches and fatigue. Recent studies, however, reveal that the sensitivity may not be to gluten but rather to a group of distinct molecules in wheat and other grains, proteins, or even some carbohydrates. Evidence indicates that as many as 60% of individuals who underwent extensive testing to diagnose celiac disease discovered they were negative for the illness. Because of this research, some medical professionals believe the term *nonceliac wheat sensitivity* is more accurate than *gluten sensitivity*. Khamsi, Roxanne: "The Trouble with Gluten," *Scientific American*, February 2014, pp. 30–31.

IRRITABLE BOWEL SYNDROME

ICD-10: K58.9

Description

Irritable bowel syndrome (IBS) is a complex group of symptoms marked by abdominal pain and altered bowel function—typically constipation, diarrhea, or alternating constipation and diarrhea—for which no organic cause can be determined. The disorder is chronic, with the onset of symptoms usually occurring in early adulthood and lasting intermittently for years. IBS is a frequently occurring GI disorder in the United States. Its management often proves frustrating to clients and providers alike.

Etiology

The cause of IBS is unknown, but it is suspected that the disease may arise from a number of underlying disorders. What is known is that IBS is associated with an increase or decrease in colonic motility. The disease also tends to have a psychological component. Nervousness or poor diet is *not* the cause, but stress and intolerance of some foods can precipitate attacks.

Signs and Symptoms

The hallmark of IBS is abdominal pain with constipation or with constipation alternating with diarrhea. The totally diarrheal form of IBS is often painless. Heartburn, abdominal distention, back pain, weakness, and faintness also may accompany the primary symptoms. Stool may be reported as mucus covered. Symptoms usually are experienced as acute attacks that subside within 1 day, but recurrent exacerbations are likely. Women are more likely to have IBS during menstruation.

 REALITY EPISODE

For Francine, the feeling comes when she least expects it. Heat sears the intestines, and she has to go to the bathroom *now!* As she gets up from her office chair to move down the hall to the bathroom, the rush is more urgent. She pauses, hoping that if she stops walking, she can squeeze down and hold the urge a moment or two. But she cannot. Stool begins to gush from her body.

Now she hurries to the bathroom, swings the door open to the toilet. (Thank goodness there is no one waiting!) Francine pulls her clothes away, lowers herself to the stool, and the flow continues. There is release and relief. Her clothes are a mess. She wipes, washes, flushes two or three times, and prays that no one comes into the restroom to see her. She is so glad to see that none of her outer clothing is spoiled. She wraps her now-rinsed underwear in paper towels, goes back to her office, and puts the paper towels in a plastic bag and seals it. She is embarrassed but so glad that she has a change of underwear with her. This is not the first time, and she has learned to be prepared. She is learning not to feel shame. She has a disease—irritable bowel syndrome. Many others share this disease with her and have the same problem. She is grateful the restroom is nearby.

How might the outcome be different if it occurs while working on a construction site? Could this affliction preclude some occupations? Explain.

Diagnostic Procedures

The chronic, intermittent nature of the symptoms without obvious cause suggests the diagnosis; however, IBS must be differentiated from other GI diseases. A careful client history, especially of psychological factors, is essential. A complete blood cell count and stool examination for **occult blood,** ova, parasites, and pathogenic bacteria will help rule out closely related conditions. Colonoscopy, sigmoidoscopy, barium enema, and rectal biopsy may provide similarly useful information.

Treatment

There is no one successful treatment for controlling IBS. Dietary modification may be attempted, such as avoiding irritating foods or adding fiber if constipation is a symptom. Diet guidelines include avoiding caffeine and alcohol; limiting intake of fatty foods, dairy products, and artificial sweeteners; increasing fiber in the diet; and avoiding beans, cabbage, and uncooked cauliflower and broccoli. Clients are advised to get adequate sleep and exercise and alleviate as much stress as possible. A sedative or an antispasmodic drug may be ordered.

Complementary Therapy

Complementary therapy for clients aims to reduce irritation to the bowel, relying on dietary changes and stress reduction. Herbal medications should be taken only under the care of a primary care provider or an appropriate practitioner. On the other hand, there is some evidence that taking probiotics may help IBS sufferers. Probiotics are bacteria that naturally live in the intestine. The bacteria *Lactobacillus acidophilus* and *Bifidobacteria infantis* lessened the symptoms for some people after taking the probiotics for 4 weeks. Eating meals at regular intervals, chewing food slowly, and drinking eight glasses of water daily are helpful for clients. Biofeedback, acupuncture, and hypnosis have shown promise in reducing stress and relaxing intestinal spasms.

➔ CLIENT COMMUNICATION

An individual with chronic IBS should have regular checkups to monitor any major change in symptoms. Educate clients about the chronic nature of the disease and possible complications of the treatment process. Persons with IBS may experience an extra urgency in evacuating the bowel that requires immediate availability of a toilet. Advise clients that in a public setting where there are no restrooms, they can calmly and politely say to a proprietor, "I believe I am going to be sick." This statement may make an otherwise unavailable bathroom available. Suggest that clients carry extra undergarments in case of an accident.

Prognosis

Because IBS cannot be cured, the prognosis varies according to how successfully the symptoms can be controlled. IBS may disrupt an individual's lifestyle. It also can exacerbate hemorrhoids.

Prevention

There is no known prevention for IBS.

CHAPTER EPISODE—PART III

When Katy finally sees the PCP, she is referred to a GI specialist. The PCP orders blood work, and a prescription is given to help put a stop to the diarrhea. A bland diet is recommended. Even though, at her mom's insistence, the PCP personally made a phone call to the clinic of the only specialist who sees Medicaid clients, Katy had to wait more than 2 weeks to be seen.

- Identify what is positive about this exchange.
- Identify what is negative about this exchange.

Inflammatory Bowel Disease

Crohn disease and ulcerative colitis are both inflammatory bowel diseases, and while they may share similar symptoms with lower intestinal tract diseases, they are quite different as distinguished by their inflammatory pattern.

CROHN DISEASE (REGIONAL ENTERITIS, GRANULOMATOUS COLITIS)

ICD-10: K50.90

Description

Crohn disease, sometimes called *regional enteritis* or *granulomatous colitis*, is a serious, chronic inflammation, usually of the ileum, although it may affect any portion of the GI tract. Crohn disease is distinguished from closely related bowel disorders by its inflammatory pattern. The inflammation extending through all layers of the intestinal wall results in a characteristic thickening or toughening of the wall and narrowing of the intestinal lumen. The inflammation tends to be patchy or segmented. In Crohn disease, all layers of the intestine may be involved, with normal healthy bowel found between diseased sections of bowel. Crohn disease affects men and women equally and seems familial in nature. It is most often diagnosed in people between ages 20 and 30.

Etiology

The cause of Crohn disease is unknown. Researchers now believe that emotional stress and psychological changes are the *result* of chronic and severe symptoms of Crohn disease rather than the *cause*. Research is under way in the fields of immunology and microbiology. Many scientists believe that the interaction of a virus or bacterium with the body's immune system may trigger the disease or that such an agent may cause damage to the intestinal wall, initiating or accelerating the disease process. This triad of events—genetic susceptibility, environmental trigger, and a weakened or damaged intestinal wall—has the same effect as the microbiome action identified in other digestive system diseases and disorders.

Signs and Symptoms

Signs and symptoms include intermittent or steady abdominal pain in the right lower quadrant, diarrhea, lack of appetite, and weight loss. A variety of sores, **fissures** (grooves or deep furrows), or **fistulas** (abnormal tubelike passages) may appear in the anal area of some individuals.

Diagnostic Procedures

Crohn disease is diagnosed by differentiating its characteristic pattern of inflammation from those of other bowel disorders. A thorough medical history is essential. Barium enema, colonoscopy, and stool sample may be necessary. Only a biopsy provides a definitive diagnosis.

Treatment

Treatment of Crohn disease is symptomatic and supportive. Currently, there are five basic categories of medications used in the treatment of Crohn disease. Oral forms of mesalamine (the generic name for 5-aminosalicylic acid [5-ASA]) and sulfasalazine have been found beneficial in treating Crohn disease and in preventing relapses. Corticosteroids (given orally, rectally, or by injection) are given when symptoms are more severe. Immunomodulators help reduce the inflammatory response. Antibiotics can help control symptoms, reducing intestinal bacteria and suppressing the intestine's immune system. Biological therapies are targeted to particular enzymes and proteins that are abnormal in people with Crohn disease.

Surgical treatment of the disease is usually reserved for managing complications, but **colectomy** (surgical removal of all or a portion of the colon) or **ileostomy** (surgically creating an opening in the ileum, bringing it to the abdominal surface for the purpose of evacuating feces) may be necessary in persons with extensive disease. About 70% of individuals with Crohn disease eventually require surgery.

Complementary Therapy

Complementary therapy for Crohn disease is very similar to the recommendations in the treatment of IBS. Some herbal medications have proved beneficial, but the recommendation is that an individual with IBS or Crohn disease work cooperatively with two practitioners, a gastroenterologist and a naturally oriented practitioner, before taking any herbal remedies. It is important to make certain the body gets all the nutrients it needs. For example, sulfasalazine reduces the body's ability to absorb folate, and corticosteroids can reduce calcium levels.

⊙ CLIENT COMMUNICATION

Focus on supporting clients through acute attacks and teaching measures to prevent future complications. Adequate nutritional intake and fluid balance are essential. See Client Communication in IBS.

Prognosis

The prognosis depends on the severity of the initial onset of the disease and its clinical history but worsens over time. Complications may include intestinal obstruction and fistula formation, resulting in peritonitis and sepsis.

Prevention

There is no known prevention or cure for Crohn disease.

ULCERATIVE COLITIS

ICD-10: K51.90

Description

Ulcerative colitis is a chronic inflammation and ulceration of the colon, often beginning in the rectum or sigmoid colon and extending upward into the entire colon. Ulcerative colitis and Crohn disease are often referred to as inflammatory bowel disease (IBD). Ulcerative colitis is distinguished from closely related bowel disorders by its characteristic inflammatory pattern. The inflammation involves only the mucosal lining of the colon, which exhibits erythema and numerous hemorrhagic ulcerations. In addition, the affected portion of the colon is uniformly involved, with no patches of healthy mucosal tissue evident (compare with Crohn disease). Together, ulcerative colitis and Crohn disease affect approximately 500,000 to 2 million people in the United States. Men and women are affected equally.

Etiology

The etiology for ulcerative colitis is the same as for Crohn disease. Researchers believe that the body's defenses may be operating against some substance in the body, perhaps even the digestive tract, which is recognized as foreign. These foreign substances or antigens may stimulate the body's defenses to produce an inflammation. Researchers believe that microbiome actions are apparent in ulcerative colitis as well. Recent research shows that a high intake of linoleic acid, a polyunsaturated omega-6 fatty acid found in red meat and in many oils and some types of margarine, may be associated with nearly 33% of cases of ulcerative colitis.

Signs and Symptoms

The classic symptom is recurrent bloody diarrhea, often containing pus and mucus, accompanied by abdominal pain and severe urgency to move the bowels. Other symptoms may include fever, weight loss, and signs of dehydration. There is a tendency toward periodic exacerbation and remission of symptoms.

Diagnostic Procedures

The disease is diagnosed by the characteristics of the inflammatory process. Sigmoidoscopy may reveal the mucosal lining to be friable (easily broken or pulverized) with thick, inflammatory **exudate.** Colonoscopy may be necessary to determine the extent of the disease. A biopsy may be done at the same time to rule out carcinoma.

Treatment

The treatment program generally includes measures to suppress the inflammatory response, permit healing, and relieve the symptoms. Treatment of ulcerative colitis with medications is similar, though not always identical, to treatment of Crohn disease. Medications used to treat ulcerative colitis include (1) anti-inflammatory agents, such as 5-ASA compounds, systemic corticosteroids, topical corticosteroids in the form of suppositories, liquid or foam enemas, and (2) immunomodulators. Sulfasalazine (a compound derived from sulfapyridine and 5-ASA) is an effective anti-inflammatory agent used for mild to moderate episodes of ulcerative colitis. Oral forms of 5-ASA compounds appear to be effective in treating active ulcerative colitis and in preventing relapses. Corticosteroid treatment is also effective against ulcerative colitis. Surgical excision or resection of the entire colon is reserved for management of serious complications. This procedure necessitates an ileostomy. Removing or reducing all products with linoleic acid in the diet may prove beneficial for some clients.

Complementary Therapy

Early research suggests that prebiotics—natural compounds found in plants such as artichokes—can help fuel beneficial intestinal bacteria. Probiotics might help combat the disease as well. Fish oil, an anti-inflammatory, may be beneficial for some. Several studies have found acupuncture to be helpful to people with ulcerative colitis.

⊕ CLIENT COMMUNICATION

Provide coping skills and emotional comfort. Explain symptoms of complications, such as hemorrhage, bowel stricture, or infection. Encourage follow-up because of the high incidence of colon and rectal cancers in persons with ulcerative colitis. Refer to Client Communication in IBS.

Prognosis

Complications may be life-threatening and include anemia and perforated colon with resulting septicemia. The prognosis for a toxemic individual with ulcerative colitis depends on the severity of the acute episodes of the disease. Persons who have ulcerative colitis that involves the whole colon for 8 to 10 years are at an above-average risk for developing colorectal cancer.

Prevention

There is no known prevention and no known cure for ulcerative colitis. Regular checkups with periodic colonoscopy as advised by a primary care provider are important. Clients may have to take prescribed medications for life.

DIVERTICULAR DISEASE (DIVERTICULOSIS AND DIVERTICULITIS)

ICD-10: K57.XX

Description

Bulging pouches (diverticula) in the GI tract wall push the mucosal lining through surrounding muscle (Fig. 14.6). The sigmoid colon is the most common site for diverticula, but they may form anywhere along the intestinal tract. Diverticulitis is the acute inflammation of the small, pouchlike herniations in the intestinal wall. The presence of diverticula (diverticulosis) usually produces no symptoms; rather, it is the rupture and infection of the diverticula that produces the clinically significant condition.

Etiology

The cause of diverticular disease is not clearly understood. The colon walls thicken with age and increased pressure to eliminate feces. Sometimes the accumulation of intestinal matter within a diverticulum forms a small, hard, solid, intestinal mass around a core of fecal material called a **fecalith.** Bacteria multiply around the fecalith, attacking the inner surface of the diverticulum; the resulting inflammation may lead to perforation. The formation of diverticula and, hence, the incidence of diverticulitis may be due in part to a diet of highly refined, low-residue foods.

Signs and Symptoms

Diverticulosis usually exhibits no symptoms. The symptoms of diverticulitis vary from case to case in both intensity and duration. If a diverticulum ruptures, the

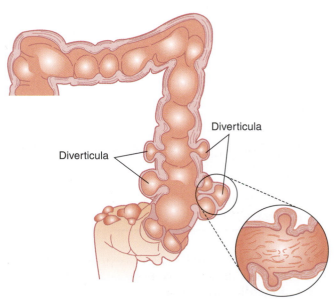

Figure 14.6 Multiple diverticula of the colon.

bacteria within the colon spread into the tissues surrounding the colon, causing diverticulitis. Such an attack is characterized by fever, and there is pain in the left lower abdomen that is relieved following a bowel movement and/or flatulence. Abdominal muscle spasms, guarding, and tenderness may occur. The person usually experiences alternating constipation and diarrhea.

Diagnostic Procedures

Abdominal x-rays, computed tomography (CT) scan, and stool specimen examination may be sufficient for diagnosis. A barium enema or a colonoscopy may be attempted but not if the disease is in the active phase because of the possibility of perforation and hemorrhage.

Treatment

Treatment of uncomplicated diverticular disease consists of a high-residue diet that includes bran, bulk additives, and stool softeners. Antibiotics or **anticholinergic** drugs may be ordered for diverticulitis. Anticholinergic drugs inhibit the action of the neurotransmitter acetylcholine, blocking parasympathetic nerve impulses, with consequent reduction in smooth muscle contractions and various body secretions. If diverticular disease is not relieved by conservative treatment and if perforation or hemorrhage occurs, hospitalization, surgery, and blood transfusions may be necessary. Surgery usually involves a colon resection with a temporary colostomy while the colon heals.

Complementary Therapy

A whole-foods, high-fiber diet as well as soluble fibers, such as ground flax, psyllium, and oat bran, are suggested. Integrative medical practitioners have long recommended 25 to 35 milligrams of daily fiber for bowel regularity and to prevent diverticulosis.

CLIENT COMMUNICATION

Help clients manage acute inflammatory episodes. Explain the connection between dietary habits and the disease. Refer clients to a dietitian who can help in adding more fiber to their diet.

Prognosis

The prognosis becomes less favorable with advancing age. Proper dietary measures can generally help forestall acute episodes of the disease. Chronic diverticulitis may cause fibrosis and adhesions that lead to bowel obstruction. Perforation of the intestinal wall in diverticulitis can lead to acute peritonitis, sepsis, and shock.

Prevention

There is no known prevention. Diets high in fiber increase stool bulk and reduce constipation, thereby assisting in the prevention of further diverticular formation or worsening of the condition.

ACUTE APPENDICITIS

ICD-10: K35.80 or K35.89

Description

Acute appendicitis is an inflammation of the vermiform appendix due to an obstruction. Between 7% and 8% of individuals in the United States have appendicitis each year.

Etiology

Appendicitis may be initiated by obstruction of the interior of the appendix by a fecalith, stricture, foreign body, or viral infection. In many cases, though, ulceration of the mucosal lining of the appendix appears to be the causative factor. Regardless of the etiology, the course of the disease is the same. Bacteria multiply and invade the appendix wall, compromising circulation to the organ. Necrosis of appendical tissue, gangrene, and eventually perforation occur. Perforation of the appendix is life-threatening because the infection then spreads into the peritoneal cavity, causing peritonitis, the most common and serious complication of appendicitis.

Signs and Symptoms

Pain usually starts near the belly button and moves slowly down to the lower right quadrant. The classic symptoms are generalized abdominal pain followed by pain localized in the upper right quadrant. Nausea, vomiting, and anorexia will likely occur. The pain eventually settles over the appendix in the right lower abdomen (**McBurney point**) with "boardlike" rigidity, increased tenderness, and abdominal spasms (Fig. 14.7). Fever, malaise, diarrhea or constipation, and tachycardia are among the later symptoms.

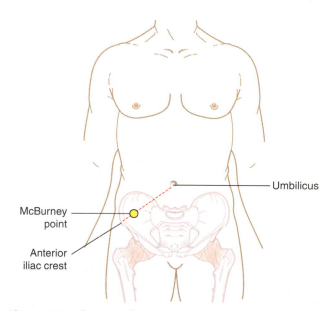

Figure 14.7 Pain at McBurney point is a symptom of appendicitis.

Focusing on Acute Appendicitis

It is common to confuse acute appendicitis with other diseases and disorders because the symptoms are so similar. Early diagnosis can be crucial in some cases because a delay may allow the appendix to burst its contents into the peritoneum. Surgeons also describe performing appendectomies after a confirmed diagnosis only to find a perfectly healthy appendix. Medicine is not always an exact science; it is often embraced by experience, trial and error, and a sixth sense. Diseases that share similar symptoms with acute appendicitis include the following:

- Pelvic inflammatory disease (PID)
- Endometriosis
- Ovarian cyst, ureterolithiasis, and renal colic
- Uterine leiomyoma
- Diverticulitis
- Crohn disease
- Colon cancer
- Cholecystitis
- Bacterial enteritis

Diagnostic Procedures

Physical examination and the characteristic symptomatology generally indicate appendicitis. Tenderness on pressure at the McBurney point and the client's ability to pinpoint the area of maximum tenderness are the strongest diagnostic indicators of appendicitis. Laboratory findings may reveal leukocytosis and pyuria. CT scan of the abdomen and pelvis can evaluate abdominal pain suspected of being caused by appendicitis. Ultrasound can identify enlarged appendix abscesses and is commonly used in small children to test for appendicitis. Children with appendicitis have a biomarker in their urine, leucine-rich alpha-2 glycoprotein (LRG) that may indicate acute appendicitis. A simple urine test, rather easy to obtain, would make diagnosis for children much easier. Studies need to be conducted to determine if the same biomarker is found in adults.

Treatment

Appendectomy is the only recommended treatment for acute appendicitis.

Complementary Therapy

No significant complementary therapies are indicated.

⊙ CLIENT COMMUNICATION

Advise clients of postoperative care, including instructions on lifting and any heavy labor.

Prognosis

With early diagnosis and treatment, the prognosis is good. If the appendix ruptures, however, peritonitis may ensue, greatly increasing the risk of further serious complications.

Prevention

No prevention for acute appendicitis is known.

CHAPTER EPISODE—PART IV

The medication and diet change help Katy some. For a time, the diarrhea ceases and there is little or no blood in her stool. Katy is able to play in one volleyball match, but she is now beginning to lose weight and her stamina is limited. Unfortunately, by the time Katy sees the specialist, she is worse and has missed several days of school.

- What diagnostic tests is the specialist likely to perform?
- What will the treatment be?

HEMORRHOIDS

ICD-10: K64.9

Description

Hemorrhoids are dilated, tortuous veins in the mucous membrane of the anus or rectum. They are common and usually insignificant unless they bleed or cause pain and itching. There are two kinds: external hemorrhoids, those involving veins below the anorectal line, and internal hemorrhoids, those involving veins above or along the anorectal line. About 50% of adults over age 50 have hemorrhoids, and they are common among pregnant women (Fig. 14.8).

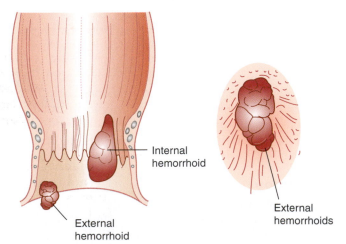

Internal hemorrhoid

External hemorrhoids

External hemorrhoid

Figure 14.8 Hemorrhoids.

Etiology

Straining to eliminate stool, chronic constipation or diarrhea, prolonged sitting, pregnancy, anal intercourse, and anorectal infections are factors that contribute to the development of hemorrhoids. Another factor may be loss of muscle tone due to advanced age.

Signs and Symptoms

There may be rectal bleeding, pruritus, and vague discomfort. In some cases, the hemorrhoids may protrude from the anus. There may be a discharge of mucus from the rectum, too.

Diagnostic Procedures

Physical examination will reveal external hemorrhoids. Proctoscopy will reveal internal hemorrhoids and rule out rectal polyps. If there is significant bleeding, red blood cell and hemoglobin levels may be low.

Treatment

Treatment generally includes measures to ease pain and discomfort such as taking warm sitz baths. A high-roughage diet and using stool softeners also may be recommended. Over-the-counter suppositories and creams can calm inflammation. Protruding hemorrhoids may be reduced manually with a lubricated gloved finger, by ligation, by **sclerotherapy,** or by cryosurgery. In the event of severe complications or chronic discomfort, complete internal or external hemorrhoidectomy may be advised.

Complementary Therapy

Sitz baths can relieve discomfort. Clients may apply aloe vera gel to the anal area frequently, and instead of using dry toilet paper, they may use a compress of witch hazel. A high-fiber diet is the most important component in preventing hemorrhoids.

⟳ CLIENT COMMUNICATION

Include information about over-the-counter local applications for comfort and a nutritional high-fiber diet when teaching clients about hemorrhoids.

Prognosis

With proper treatment, the prognosis is good. Complications may include fecal incontinence, anorectal infections, prolapse and strangulation of the hemorrhoidal vein, and secondary anemia due to chronic blood loss.

Prevention

Prevention of hemorrhoids includes avoiding straining to eliminate stool and adherence to a proper diet and exercise regimen.

Problematic Digestive System Symptoms

Two very common symptoms, constipation and diarrhea, are seen with many of the digestive system diseases. Often they are symptoms of a particular disease. However, both constipation and diarrhea can be problematic. Therefore, they are presented here.

Constipation

ICD-10: K59.00

Description

Constipation is considered a symptom, not a disease. Constipation is different for every individual but is generally described by professionals when any two of the following symptoms exist for at least 12 weeks:

- Straining at the toilet
- Lumpy or hard stool
- Bloating or feeling of a full bowel
- Fewer than three bowel movements per week

Etiology

When too much water is absorbed by the colon or an individual's muscle contractions are sluggish, the stool hardens, becomes dry, and constipation likely results. Lack of exercise, some medications, insufficient fiber in the diet, laxative abuse, food allergies, cerebrovascular accident or stroke, IBS, pregnancy, and aging all are potential causes of constipation.

Signs and Symptoms

Clients often complain of bloating, abdominal discomfort, and fewer than three bowel movements per week.

Diagnostic Procedures

A history and physical examination provide pertinent information for health professionals. A rectal examination to detect tenderness or obstruction is often sufficient for a diagnosis. Severe cases may require a colorectal transit study or anorectal function test. Internal obstruction can be viewed by barium enema x-ray, sigmoidoscopy, and colonoscopy.

Treatment

Dietary and lifestyle changes usually relieve symptoms. A diet high in fiber is recommended, as is consumption of plenty of water and fruit juice or vegetable juice. For more serious or long-term cases, temporary use of laxatives, stool softeners, lubricants, and stimulants may be necessary.

Complementary Therapy

Practitioners will advise clients to drink more water and fruit juice (not caffeine or alcohol, which tends to dry out the colon), eat a handful of prunes a day, eat an apple a day, and increase fiber in the diet. The dietary supplement acidophilus may help rebuild intestinal flora and aid in digestion.

Client Communication

Clients, especially older adults, can be embarrassed and sensitive about discussing their bowel habits. Help clients understand the importance of reporting any over-the-counter or home remedies to their primary care provider. Refer clients to a dietitian if diet modification is recommended.

Prognosis

Prognosis is generally good, but constipation can cause hemorrhoids.

Prevention

The best prevention for constipation is to follow the dietary suggestions indicated. Advise clients to allow specific time after meals for undisturbed toilet visits and not to ignore the urge to have a bowel movement.

DIARRHEA

ICD-10: R19.7

Description

Diarrhea is the frequent passage of feces, with an accompanying increase in fluidity and volume. Diarrhea is not a disease; it is a symptom of another underlying condition. "Normal" bowel habits vary widely; consequently, what is considered diarrhea in some individuals may be normal in others. This disorder is stressful and embarrassing, especially if the individual is unable to get to a bathroom quickly enough.

Etiology

Diarrhea is the result of an abrupt increase in intestinal motility. The highly liquid content of the small intestine is rushed through the colon without sufficient time for fluid reabsorption, resulting in the watery stools characteristic of diarrhea. Numerous diseases and conditions can cause such an increase in intestinal motility. Childhood diarrhea may be an inflammatory process of infectious origin or a toxic reaction to dietary indiscretions. Adult diarrhea may result from malabsorption syndrome, gastritis, lactose intolerance, IBS, Crohn disease, ulcerative colitis, GI tumors, diverticular disease, viral and bacterial infections of the intestine, parasitic infections, psychogenic disorders, food allergies, and a variety of medications.

Signs and Symptoms

The diarrhea may vary in fluidity and volume. It may be accompanied by flatulence, abdominal distention, fever, headache, anorexia, vomiting, malaise, and cramping.

Diagnostic Procedures

The clinical history of the diarrhea involves determining whether its onset was abrupt or gradual and whether it is acute or chronic. To help determine underlying causes, bacterial cultures and microscopic examination of the stool may be performed. Additional tests include proctoscopy, radiological studies, and tests for occult blood.

Treatment

Treatment goals in clients with diarrhea include relief of symptoms and correction of underlying disorders. Clear liquids may be prescribed for children.

Complementary Therapy

Identify any food allergies and replace fluids, mineral, and vitamin losses in clients with diarrhea.

Client Communication

Caution clients that while the disorder may be self-limiting, medical attention should be sought if diarrhea does not resolve in a few days.

Prognosis

The prognosis of diarrhea depends on the cause. Possible complications include dehydration and electrolyte imbalance. Severe childhood diarrhea may require hospitalization.

Prevention

Cases of diarrhea due to infectious agents can often be prevented by following proper hygiene and sanitation

Nausea and Vomiting

Another set of symptoms not considered a disease but is nevertheless quite troubling is nausea and vomiting. Both are common symptoms in gastrointestinal diseases. These conditions may be caused by certain medications, viral gastroenteritis, or morning sickness. Medical attention should be sought if nausea and vomiting are accompanied by chest pain, blurred vision, fainting, confusion, severe abdominal pain or cramping, cold and clammy skin, high fever, or if the vomit has a fecal odor. Any signs of dehydration such as dry mouth, excessive thirst, and dark-colored urine indicate immediate attention is necessary.

Except in an emergency, while waiting to see a primary care provider for the nausea and vomiting, it can be helpful to sip cold ginger ale, lemonade, or water. Try drinking herbal teas and eating soda crackers or toast. Spicy and fatty foods should be avoided.

procedures. Cases due to allergic reactions can be prevented by avoiding known allergens.

Hernias

There are several types of hernias. They occur when an organ or tissue squeezes through a weak spot in a muscle or connective tissue called *fascia*. The most common types covered here are hiatal, abdominal, and inguinal hernias. Other types include incisional hernias that result from an incision and the umbilical hernia near the belly button.

HIATAL HERNIA

ICD-10: K44.X

Description

A hiatal hernia is the protrusion of some portion of the stomach into the thoracic cavity through the opening in the diaphragm through which the esophagus passes (the esophageal hiatus). The two major varieties of hiatal hernia are (1) sliding hernias (most common), in which the gastroesophageal junction and the upper portion of the stomach slide upward through the esophageal hiatus, and (2) paraesophageal, or "rolling," hernias, in which the gastroesophageal junction remains fixed, but some portion of the stomach passes through the esophageal hiatus. Occasionally, a hiatal hernia exhibits characteristics of both the sliding and rolling hernia (Fig. 14.9).

Etiology

The cause of hiatal hernias is unclear. They may be due to intra-abdominal pressure or weakening of the gastroesophageal junction caused by loss of muscle tone or trauma. Risk factors include severe coughing or vomiting, lifting heavy objects, pregnancy, and straining at stool. The incidence of hiatal hernia increases with age. Prevalence is higher in women than in men, and obesity is a contributing factor.

Signs and Symptoms

Over half of hiatal hernias may remain asymptomatic. If symptoms are present, they commonly include heartburn—aggravated by reclining, belching, esophageal reflux or GERD, dysphagia, or severe pain if a large portion of the stomach is caught above the diaphragm.

Diagnostic Procedures

Diagnosis of hiatal hernias is made by chest x-ray, barium x-ray, endoscopy and biopsy, and pH studies of any reflux (to eliminate the possibility of gastric ulcer).

Treatment

The goal in treatment is to alleviate symptoms. Surgery is not the first choice of treatment unless strangulation of the hernia is evident or symptoms cannot be controlled. An attempt is made to reduce heartburn and reflux or GERD through dietary modification or by strengthening the LES with medication. Antacids, H2 blockers, and PPIs likely are prescribed. Activity restrictions may be indicated to reduce intra-abdominal pressure, and persons may be advised to avoid tight or restrictive clothing. Stool softeners and laxatives to prevent straining may be prescribed. Avoidance of food intake before sleep and elevation of the head of the bed may be suggested.

Complementary Therapy

Diet modifications include avoidance of spicy or fried foods, caffeine, carbonated drinks, citrus juices, alcohol, peppermint, and green and red peppers and strictly avoiding overeating. Deep breathing exercises to strengthen the diaphragm and expand the lungs may be helpful.

Sliding Hiatal Hernia

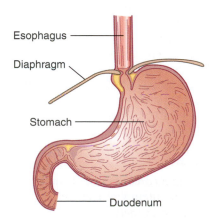

Paraesophageal or Rolling Hernia

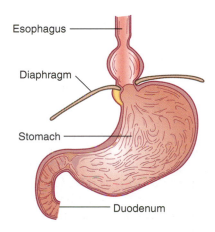

Figure 14.9 Types of hiatal hernias.

⊕ **CLIENT COMMUNICATION**

Explain diagnostic tests, treatment, and significant symptoms to clients. Describe dietary restrictions and warn against activities that increase intra-abdominal pressure.

Prognosis

The prognosis for a hiatal hernia is good with proper treatment. Complications include stricture, significant bleeding, pulmonary aspiration, or strangulation and require surgical repair. Strangulation is a medical emergency. It occurs when the hernia contents become swollen and compromise blood supply to the bowel. This causes significant abdominal pain and vomiting.

Prevention

There is no known prevention of hiatal hernias other than avoiding any of the risk factors.

ABDOMINAL AND INGUINAL HERNIAS

ICD-10: K41.X or K42.X

Description

An abdominal hernia is the protrusion of an internal organ, typically a portion of the intestine, through an abnormal opening in the musculature of the abdominal wall. Abdominal hernias are categorized according to the location of the herniation and include umbilical, inguinal, and femoral hernias (Fig. 14.10). Inguinal hernias are the most common type and occur in men more often than in women.

Hernias

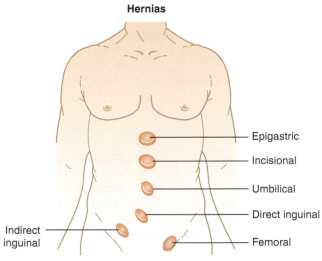

Indirect inguinal — Epigastric — Incisional — Umbilical — Direct inguinal — Femoral

Figure 14.10 Hernias and their locations.

Etiology

Hernias may result from a congenital weakness in the abdominal wall or muscle or increased pressure within the abdomen. Heavy lifting, pregnancy, obesity, and straining at stool are predisposing factors.

Signs and Symptoms

Inguinal and umbilical hernias are evidenced by the appearance of a lump over the herniated area that tends to disappear when the person is supine. Sharp, steady, accompanying pain may be present in the groin. Strangulation of a herniated portion of the intestine will cause severe pain and can cause bowel obstruction. Strangulation of the intestine is considered a medical emergency.

Diagnostic Procedures

Physical examination reveals the herniated area. A medical history of sharp abdominal pain when lifting or straining also may help confirm the diagnosis. An x-ray or CT scan is ordered if bowel obstruction is suspected.

Treatment

Umbilical hernias may require only taping or binding the affected area until the hernia closes. Femoral and inguinal hernias require reduction of the hernia and trussing the weakened portion of the abdominal wall. Herniorrhaphy and/or hernioplasty (possibly laparoscopically) are the corrective surgical procedures used.

Complementary Therapy

No significant complementary therapies are indicated.

⊕ **CLIENT COMMUNICATION**

Advise clients to be aware of their work and home environments and of how much lifting is required. Help clients learn proper lifting techniques, to wear supportive devices as indicated, and to maintain proper body weight.

Prognosis

The prognosis is excellent with proper treatment and care. Complete recovery time from surgery depends on the type of repair made. Clients should consult with the primary care provider before returning to normal activities.

Prevention

Preventive measures include following recommended guidelines for lifting objects, maintaining soft stool consistency, and practicing moderate exercise.

PANCREATITIS

ICD-10: K85.9

Description

Pancreatitis, or inflammation of the pancreas, may occur in acute or chronic forms. In this disease, pancreatic enzymes that normally remain inactive until reaching the duodenum begin digesting pancreatic tissue, causing varying degrees of edema, swelling, tissue necrosis, and hemorrhage. The pancreas is both an exocrine and endocrine organ; thus, if the islet cells are damaged, diabetes mellitus results (see Chapter 11). The disease can be mild and self-limiting or chronic and fatal. It is more common in men than in women.

Etiology

The causes of this autodigestive process in pancreatitis are not well understood, although a number of conditions are known to lead to the disease. Commonly, acute pancreatitis is caused by the presence of gallstones—small, pebblelike substances made of hardened bile—that cause inflammation in the pancreas as they pass through the common bile duct. The second most likely cause is alcoholism (mostly in men) and biliary tract disease (more common in women). Other conditions include trauma to the abdomen, viral infections, drug reactions, systemic immunologic disorders, pancreatic cancer, or complications from a duodenal ulcer.

Signs and Symptoms

The only symptom of mild pancreatitis is steady epigastric pain. The most important symptom of acute pancreatitis is the sudden onset of severe, persistent abdominal pain that is centered over the epigastric region and that may radiate toward the back. The abdomen is tender. Severe attacks of acute pancreatitis also may cause abdominal distention, persistent vomiting, fever, and tachycardia. Vital signs show rapid, shallow respirations, a fall in blood pressure, and an elevated temperature. Someone with acute pancreatitis usually looks and feels very ill and needs immediate medical attention.

Diagnostic Procedures

A clinical history of acute onset of the characteristic abdominal pain may suggest the diagnosis. A blood test revealing an elevated level of the enzyme amylase in the serum generally confirms the diagnosis and rules out many other disorders. Abdominal or endoscopic ultrasonography and abdominal CT scans may reveal pancreatic enlargement and bile duct involvement. Magnetic resonance cholangiopancreatography (MRCP) may be ordered. MRCP allows the provider to visualize the pancreas, gallbladder, and pancreatic and bile ducts.

Treatment

Treatment is largely symptomatic but may require hospitalization. The aim is to maintain circulation and fluid volume, decrease pain and pancreatic secretions, and control any complications. Treatment for acute pancreatitis requires IV fluids, antibiotics, and medication to relieve pain. The person should refrain from eating or drinking as much as possible for a few days to allow the pancreas to rest and recover. Unless complications arise, acute pancreatitis usually resolves in a few days. In severe cases, the person may require nasogastric feeding—a special liquid given in a long, thin tube inserted through the nose and throat and into the stomach—for several weeks while the pancreas heals.

Complementary Therapy

Complementary therapy should be conducted only in conjunction with traditional therapy and may include nutritional guidance and supplements. While complementary therapy cannot cure pancreatitis, it can help in the recovery process. Some evidence suggests that increasing intake of antioxidants (found in fruits and green vegetables) may help protect against pancreatitis or reduce symptoms. Studies have explored the role of free radicals, the by-products of metabolism harmful to the body's cells, in pancreatitis. Antioxidants can help rid the body of free radicals and increase levels of antioxidants in the blood. Alcohol-induced pancreatitis is linked to low levels of antioxidants as well.

CLIENT COMMUNICATION

Alcohol abuse counseling is indicated if that is the primary cause. Explain to clients the seriousness of complications and emphasize follow-up care. An individual with loss of pancreatic endocrine function requires extensive ongoing diabetic teaching.

Prognosis

Acute pancreatitis is a life-threatening medical emergency. Pancreatic function can eventually be restored, but a host of possible complications may worsen the prognosis. The prognosis is poor and the mortality rate is high for chronic pancreatitis that follows alcoholism. Possible complications include type 2 diabetes and shock due to toxins in the blood. In mild cases, where only the pancreas is inflamed, the prognosis is excellent. In chronic pancreatitis, recurring attacks tend to become more severe.

Prevention

There is no known prevention. If alcoholism is the cause, refraining from alcohol is necessary but often proves difficult.

CHOLELITHIASIS AND CHOLECYSTITIS

ICD-10: K80.20 (CHOLELITHIASIS)
ICD-10: K81.9 (CHOLECYSTITIS)

Description

Cholelithiasis is the formation or presence of stonelike masses called *gallstones* within the gallbladder or bile ducts. These stones may be formed of either cholesterol or calcium-based compounds and range from a few millimeters to a few centimeters in size. Cholelithiasis is a common condition in the United States, with women affected more than twice as frequently as men, until after age 50, when men and women are equally affected. Most individuals with gallstones remain asymptomatic. Clinically significant symptoms result when a gallstone obstructs a biliary duct. Acute cholecystitis is a severe inflammation of the interior wall of the gallbladder.

Etiology

The cause of cholelithiasis is not well understood. Any factors that cause the bile to become overladen with cholesterol may increase the likelihood that cholesterol-based gallstones will form. Such factors include obesity, high-calorie diets, certain drugs, oral contraceptives, multiple pregnancies, and increasing age. The production of calcium-based (pigmented) gallstones is even less well understood, but it may be related to genetic factors, hemolytic disease, alcoholic cirrhosis, or persistent biliary tract infections.

Most cases of acute cholecystitis are a consequence of gallstones obstructing bile ducts. The resulting inflammation may occur from the increased pressure of accumulating bile within the gallbladder, chemical changes in the bile that erode the gallbladder tissue, or secondary infection from multiplying bacteria. Some forms of the disease are not caused by obstructing gallstones. These cases may be due to obstruction of bile ducts by neoplasms or to vascular disease, diabetes mellitus, parasitic infections, and various systemic diseases.

Signs and Symptoms

As mentioned previously, many individuals with gallstones remain asymptomatic. If bile ducts are obstructed, a classic "gallbladder attack," more properly referred to as *biliary colic,* results. The telltale symptom is the acute onset of upper right quadrant abdominal pain radiating to the shoulder and back. Nausea and vomiting may accompany the attack. Flatulence, belching, and heartburn also may occur at intervals. Gallbladder attacks typically tend to follow ingestion of large meals or fatty foods. The pain and other symptoms of an attack gradually subside on their own over a period of several hours.

A characteristic symptom of acute cholecystitis is the gradual onset of upper right quadrant pain that usually remains localized over the area of the gallbladder. Unlike the pain of biliary colic, which ceases once the gallstones are passed, the pain of acute cholecystitis does not tend to subside after a few hours. Anorexia, nausea, vomiting, and a low-grade fever and chills also may accompany the pain. The pain may be severe enough to cause an individual to seek emergency treatment.

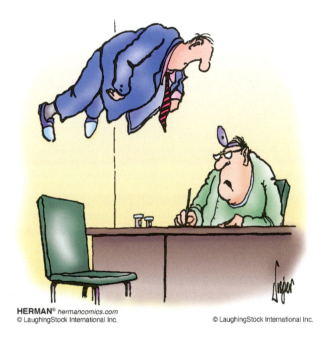

HERMAN® hermancomics.com
© LaughingStock International Inc.

© LaughingStock International Inc.

"I'll give you something for gas."

HERMAN© is reprinted with permission from LaughingStock Licensing Inc., Ottawa, Canada. All rights reserved.

Diagnostic Procedures

A clinical history of the characteristic pain of biliary colic suggests a diagnosis of gallstones. Various methods of visualizing the stones are used to provide a definitive diagnosis, typically including a gallbladder ultrasound, oral cholecystogram, IV cholangiogram, or a plain abdominal x-ray. A hepatobiliary iminodiacetic acid (HIDA) scan tracks production and flow of bile through the small intestine and will show any blockage. If the common bile duct is obstructed, the serum **bilirubin** is elevated. Oral cholecystography shows stones in the gallbladder and biliary duct obstruction.

Treatment

Hospitalization is often required. If the condition is asymptomatic, treatment is nonsurgical unless the symptoms appear or there is a history of previous gallstones with complications. Bowel rest, analgesia, and IV antibiotics and hydration may be necessary. In elective surgery, a laparoscopic cholecystectomy is performed. Cholecystectomy is the treatment of choice for symptomatic cholelithiasis. A nonsurgical treatment involves insertion of a flexible catheter, guided by fluoroscopy, directly to the stone. A Dormia (stone) basket is threaded through the catheter, opened, and twirled to entrap the stone. It is then closed and withdrawn. Another nonsurgical option is extracorporeal shock wave lithotripsy with litholytic therapy that fragments the stones.

Still another nonsurgical approach involves dissolving cholesterol-based stones through bile acid therapy. This therapy inhibits the synthesis and secretion of cholesterol within the liver, altering the composition of the bile. Existing stones may be decreased in size or dissolved entirely.

Complementary Therapy

Clients are advised to identify any food allergies that can be eliminated, reduce fat intake, and avoid refined carbohydrates. It is best for clients to eat frequent, smaller meals and avoid overeating. Increasing dietary fiber is beneficial. Clients should not avoid seeing a specialist if the pain is severe because surgery may be the first and best choice of treatment.

➔ CLIENT COMMUNICATION

Provide supportive care and advice on any postoperative instructions. Identify any food restrictions and instruct clients to notify their primary care provider if there is pain for longer than 24 hours, nausea, or vomiting.

Prognosis

The prognosis is generally good with prompt treatment. Complications can result when proper treatment is not sought, infection occurs, or peritonitis results from the gallbladder rupturing.

Prevention

No prevention for cholelithiasis and cholecystitis is known, but about 15% of the Caucasian population is affected. High-fat diets are to be avoided.

CIRRHOSIS

ICD-K74.60

Description

Cirrhosis is a chronic, irreversible, degenerative disease of the liver characterized by the replacement of normal liver cells with fibrous scar tissue and other alterations in liver structure. The hepatic cells become necrotic, causing a change in liver structure that impairs the flow of blood and lymph. Scarring impairs the liver's ability to control infections; remove toxins from the blood; process nutrients, hormones, and medications; make proteins to regulate blood clotting; and produce bile to help emulsify fats. Hepatic insufficiency results.

Etiology

Cirrhosis has a diverse set of etiologies. The most common cirrhoses are portal, nutritional, or alcoholic (Laennec). Cirrhosis is also caused by chronic hepatitis B, C, and D; nonalcoholic fatty liver disease; biliary cirrhosis (manifested by a halt in bile production and secretion by the liver); certain inherited diseases; some toxins; and congestive heart failure. Cirrhosis also may be idiopathic in origin. It is more common in men than in women.

Signs and Symptoms

The person may be asymptomatic for a prolonged period, or symptoms may be vague or unspecific. Symptoms may include nausea, vomiting, anorexia, dull abdominal ache, weakness, fatigability, weight loss, pruritus, peripheral neuritis, bleeding tendencies, edema of the legs, **ascites** (accumulation of fluid in the peritoneal cavity), and jaundice. **Jaundice** is a condition characterized by a yellowish discoloration of the skin, whites of the eyes, and bodily fluids that results from the accumulation of bilirubin in the blood.

Warning About Acetaminophen Use

Acetaminophen can cause liver damage and liver failure. Acetaminophen is an important medication that is effective in reducing pain and fever and is safe when taken as directed. However, the drug is often abused when clients believe misinformation such as the following:

- If one tablet only reduces the headache, then two must be better.
- When did I take the last capsule? Whenever it was, the pain is still intense; two more will help.
- When feeling "dull" or "a little off," a Tylenol will perk me up.
- Adding an over-the-counter acetaminophen product to flu or cold medicine will hasten getting well.
- It can help me sleep.

Very few individuals are able to adequately recall the safe dosage of acetaminophen in a 24-hour period. The result can lead to an overdose. The risk of liver damage increases with each dose taken too soon or taken with another medication containing acetaminophen. The risk is even higher when consuming alcohol at the same time.

To be safe, help clients understand the recommended dose and how much can be taken within a 24-hour period. Remind clients never to take more than one medication containing acetaminophen at a time. Instruct clients to write down the time and dosage of medications taken to help prevent accidental overdoses.

Diagnostic Procedures

Palpation reveals the liver to be enlarged and firm—if not hard—with a blunt edge. Laboratory findings may reveal anemia, folate deficiency, blood loss, and a rupturing of red blood cells with the resulting release of hemoglobin into the plasma, a process called **hemolysis.** Liver enzymes (alanine aminotransferase [ALT] and aspartate aminotransferase [AST]) are assayed to check for elevated enzyme levels. The bilirubin level will also be increased. CT scan, ultrasound, or magnetic resonance imaging (MRI) may be ordered.

Treatment

Treatment is aimed at what is causing the cirrhosis in an attempt to prevent further liver damage. Adequate rest and diet are essential, as is restriction of alcohol. Vitamin and mineral supplements may be prescribed. In the event of gastric upset or internal bleeding, antacids may be given. If there is ascites, the fluid is removed with the use of diuretics or through paracentesis. Liver transplantation may be an option for persons with end-stage liver disease. There is a 1- and 5-year survival rate of 70% and 60%, respectively. However, more than 17,000 people in the United States have been approved and are waiting for a liver transplant, and fewer than 6,500 liver transplants will be performed.

Complementary Therapy

A whole-foods, low-protein (although this remains controversial) diet that avoids processed fats is recommended. Alcohol is strictly forbidden. Overeating is discouraged, and drugs and herbs of any kind must be taken only under careful supervision of a primary care provider. Several herbal supplements have been found to cause liver damage, including black cohosh, comfrey, kava, mistletoe, pennyroyal, skullcap, some Chinese herbs such as ma-huang, and valerian.

 CLIENT COMMUNICATION

Refer client for alcohol treatment if indicated. Encourage regular follow-up care with a primary care provider.

Prognosis

The prognosis is poor in advanced cirrhosis, especially for alcoholic cirrhosis should the person continue drinking. With end-stage cirrhosis, the liver can no longer effectively replace damaged cells. Hematemesis, jaundice, and ascites are unfavorable signs. Elevated blood pressure in the portal vein, called *portal hypertension,* is a common complication of cirrhosis. Consequently, blood pressure increases within the spleen, causing enlargement of the spleen or splenomegaly, and blood bypasses the liver, producing ascites or esophageal **varices,** which are abnormally dilated and twisted veins or arteries. Hemorrhage of esophageal varices often requires emergency treatment. If cirrhosis is not treated, hepatic failure and death result.

Prevention

There is no known prevention unless alcohol is a contributing factor; then treatment for alcoholism may be necessary. Recommend that clients eat a healthy diet and maintain healthy weight. Advise clients to take precautions when using household chemicals and insect sprays. Stress the importance of following careful adherence to guidelines for acetaminophen.

VIRAL HEPATITIS (A, B, C, D, E)

✔ **REPORTABLE DISEASE**

ICD-10: B15.XX-B19.XX

Description

Viral hepatitis is the infection and subsequent inflammation of the liver caused by any one of several viruses. Most cases of hepatitis are caused by one of five viral agents: hepatitis A virus (HAV), hepatitis B virus (HBV), hepatitis C virus (HCV), hepatitis D virus (HDV), and hepatitis E virus (HEV). A sixth virus, hepatitis G virus (HGV), has been discovered, but little is known about it. The most common hepatitis viruses are types A, B, and C. Viral hepatitis destroys hepatic cells, causing them to become necrotic. When clients are generally healthy, hepatic cells can regenerate; however, this is less likely in elderly people. Viral hepatitis can be either acute or chronic. The disease is reported to the public health department for proper follow-up because of the possibility of contagion.

Etiology

There are six types of viral hepatitis:

1. HAV was formerly known as *infectious hepatitis.* It has an incubation period of 2 to 6 weeks. It is highly contagious through the fecal-oral route when food or water is contaminated with human waste in unsanitary conditions. It can be spread among household members, restaurants, and day-care centers because of poor sanitary conditions and inadequate hand washing. Once infected with HAV, clients are protected from further infections of the virus. HAV is an acute infection that is rarely fatal and does not become chronic. The rates of HAV have fallen to the lowest they have been in 40 years due to the HAV vaccine introduced in 1995.
2. Hepatitis B is caused by HBV, which causes over 780,000 deaths each year in the United States. It has a long incubation period of 5 weeks to 6 months and is transmitted by blood or serum.

Commonly, hepatitis B is spread through shared needles in those who abuse drugs, tattooing, body piercing, accidental needle sticks contaminated with infected blood in the health-care setting, and by infected mothers to their newborns. Health-care professionals are frequently exposed to HBV, which is more serious than HAV. Hepatitis B may become chronic. The HBV vaccine has been quite successful in vaccinating children and adolescents through childhood immunization schedules, but adults who are not vaccinated remain at risk.

3. HCV affects 3.2 million Americans and is the most common chronic blood-borne infection in the United States. It is transmitted through transfusions from asymptomatic individuals or through contaminated needles. It is spread similarly to hepatitis B, and its incubation period is 2 to 12 weeks. This disease often insidiously damages the liver for up to 20 years before symptoms emerge. Those with the chronic form of the disease can infect others. They are at high risk for cirrhosis, liver failure, and liver cancer.

4. HDV is also called *delta hepatitis*. It is a defective virus that needs HBV to exist. Its incubation period is 4 to 12 weeks. It occurs in persons frequently exposed to blood, such as hemophiliacs or IV drug users. If types B and D occur together, pulmonary complications are likely, and HBV infections may be increased in severity.

5. HEV is rarely seen in the United States. Outbreaks have been reported in India, Pakistan, Borneo, Sudan, Ivory Coast, Algeria, and Mexico. It is commonly seen in young to middle-aged adults and has a high mortality rate in pregnant women. Feces-contaminated water is the mode of transmission. Consumption of contaminated drinking water and the ingestion of raw or uncooked shellfish has been the source of sporadic cases in endemic areas. Its incubation period is 15 to 16 days.

6. HGV has been discovered, but little is known about it. It is a blood-borne virus; has frequent coinfections with HBV, HCV, and HIV; and is seen more commonly with injection drug users. There is little proof that HGV causes any liver damage; therefore, it may not be a true "hepatitis virus."

Signs and Symptoms

In many people, there may be no symptoms. When symptoms develop, they may be flulike and include malaise, fatigue, anorexia, myalgia, fever, dark-colored urine, clay-colored stools, rashes, hives, abdominal pain or tenderness, pruritus, and jaundice. Nausea, vomiting, headache, photophobia, cough, and **coryza** (cold) may precede jaundice. An aversion to smoking and certain foods is common.

Diagnostic Procedures

The specific type of hepatitis has to be established. Specific blood tests will show liver enzymes, the antibody-antigen type, and viral proteins or genetic material. A clinical history of exposure to infected persons, recent blood transfusions, or IV drug use may suggest a diagnosis of hepatitis. The liver may be enlarged and tender, and splenomegaly may occur. Liver biopsy helps to confirm the diagnosis. Laboratory findings in most forms of hepatitis include proteinuria and **bilirubinuria** (the presence of bilirubin in the urine). Increased levels of liver enzymes, alkaline phosphatase, and gamma globulin may also be evident. Gamma globulin is a class of proteins formed in the blood that function as antibodies.

Treatment

For the acute form of hepatitis, clients are treated with general supportive measures. Bed rest, adequate diet, and fluid intake are advised. Antiemetics may be ordered. In the recovery phase, the symptoms subside but the liver enlargement and abnormalities are evident. Recovery may take 1 to 4 months, depending on the individual and the type of hepatitis. Short-term protection from HAV is available from immune globulin (IgG) that can be given within 2 weeks of exposure. When the hepatitis is chronic, both HBV and HCV infections may respond to α-interferon. Adefovir dipivoxil and lamivudine are also licensed to treat HBV infection. Ribavirin may be effective with HCV infection and is usually given in combination with α-interferon.

Complementary Therapy

Recommend to clients a whole-foods diet consisting of small meals that are eaten throughout the day. Suggest they avoid refined sugars, alcohol, and caffeine and drink plenty of filtered water. Drinking fresh lemon juice in water every morning and evening, followed by a vegetable juice, is therapeutic for the liver. Vitamin supplements are suggested.

⊕ CLIENT COMMUNICATION

Remind clients to practice proper hygiene, especially when using needles for injections and when handling human secretions. Health-care practitioners are continually being reminded to always practice universal precautions.

Prognosis

The particular type of hepatitis and extent of liver damage determine the prognosis. Serious consequences include cirrhosis, liver cancer, and acute fulminant hepatitis. Acute fulminant hepatitis is a rare but severe inflammation that causes confusion or coma because the liver is unable to detoxify chemicals.

Prevention

When individuals are exposed to HAV, IgG may be administered as a preventive measure. Persons who abuse drugs and share contaminated needles are advised to seek treatment and rehabilitation. Vaccinations for HAV and HBV are highly recommended for everyone. There currently is no vaccine for HCV, HDV, or HEV.

In the News

Late in 2014, the FDA approved a drug to treat nearly 70% of the individuals infected with the genotype 1 of HCV. The problem, however, is that the 8- to 12-week regime required to cure this form of hepatitis will cost $1,000 a dose or $84,000 for the full 12 weeks. Members of the Senate have asked the pharmaceutical company, Gilead, to turn over its documents detailing the rationale for the price. Most insurers, outraged by the cost, likely will not pay such rates and will certainly require prior approval to do so.

CHAPTER EPISODE—PART V

Katy's diagnosis was ulcerative colitis. She was devastated. When she asked the PCP about treatment and how long she would have to be on medication, he drew a lifeline on a sheet of paper to indicate that in all probability she would take medications all her life if she wanted to get well and stay well. On a positive note, the PCP told Katy and her mom about the Crohn and Colitis Foundation of America and its work. He said he would check to see if the very expensive medications needed to get Katy healthy again might be subsidized. Katy was told to return to the specialist in 4 weeks.

- What likely is the prognosis for Katy?
- What advantages are there that the specialist is familiar with the Crohn and Colitis foundation?

Cancers of the Digestive System and Accessory Organs

A number of cancers are related to the digestive system, but by far the most common are colorectal cancer and pancreatic cancer. The prognosis of colon cancer is far better than for pancreatic cancer, especially when diagnosed early.

COLORECTAL CANCER

ICD-10: C19

Description

Colorectal cancer, almost always adenocarcinoma, is the collective designation for a variety of malignant neoplasms that may arise in either the colon or rectum (Fig. 14.11). Colorectal cancer afflicts men and women equally.

Etiology

The cause of colorectal cancer is unknown, but there is a higher incidence in societies that have a diet high in red meat and low in fiber. Other predisposing factors include diseases of the digestive tract, a history of IBS, and familial **polyposis.** Polyposis is the formation of numerous small growths or masses on a mucous membrane of the digestive tract. The incidence of colorectal cancer increases after age 40.

Signs and Symptoms

Symptoms are vague in the early stages. Rectal bleeding and blood in the stool may occur. The disease may metastasize to adjacent organs, such as the bladder, prostate, ureters, vagina, and sacrum. Later symptoms may include pallor, ascites, **cachexia** (a marked weakness of the body), lymphadenopathy, and **hepatomegaly** (enlargement of the liver). Any significant change in bowel habits should be regarded as suspicious; this may include alternating states of diarrhea and constipation and the presence of blood in the stool.

Diagnostic Procedures

Only tumor biopsy can verify colorectal cancer, but other tests can help in detection. Digital examination of the rectum may be sufficient to detect rectal tumors. Testing the blood for liver enzymes and the tumor markers CEA

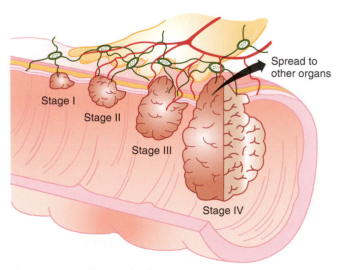

Figure 14.11 Stages of colon cancer.

and CA-19 is often done. Testing for occult blood in the stool, sigmoidoscopy, and colonoscopy to obtain a biopsy are helpful in detection. Ultrasound, MRI, and CT scanning help to show metastasis. Barium x-rays can locate lesions that are manually or otherwise visually undetectable.

Treatment

Surgery to remove the tumor, adjacent tissues, and any affected lymph nodes is the treatment of choice. Chemotherapy and radiation therapy also may be used if the cancer has deeply perforated the bowel wall or metastasized. Carcinoembryonic antigen testing (see Chapter 5) is helpful in monitoring clients before and after treatments to detect metastasis or recurrence.

Complementary Therapy

Complementary therapy should be partnered with a primary care provider. A number of complementary therapies may be most helpful in easing the side effects of chemotherapy and radiation. They include acupuncture, relaxation, and meditation. See Chapter 5.

 CLIENT COMMUNICATION

Provide information on postoperative procedures and expected adverse effects of chemotherapy and radiation.

Prognosis

The prognosis for colorectal cancer varies. This cancer tends to progress slowly and remains localized for a fair length of time. If diagnosed early and is localized, colorectal cancer is potentially curable in about 90% of cases.

Prevention

A high-fiber, low-fat diet may reduce the risk of colorectal cancer for some individuals. Early diagnosis and treatment provide a greater chance of cure.

PANCREATIC CANCER

ICD-10: C25.X

Description

Pancreatic cancer is usually an adenocarcinoma that occurs most frequently in the head of the pancreas. Pancreatic cancer is a leading cause of cancer deaths in the United States. The highest incidence is among people ages 60 to 70.

Etiology

The etiology is not known but is linked to inhalation or absorption of carcinogens. Cigarette smoking, exposure to occupational chemicals, and a diet high in

fats and protein are associated with an increased incidence of pancreatic cancer. Chronic pancreatitis and a family history of pancreatic cancer also have been suggested.

Signs and Symptoms

The classic symptoms are abdominal pain that may radiate to the back, anorexia, jaundice, and weight loss. Other symptoms include weakness, fatigue, diarrhea, nausea and vomiting, and low-back pain. If the disease affects the islets of Langerhans, symptoms of insulin deficiency appear. These symptoms include glucosuria; **hyperglycemia,** or abnormally high levels of sugar in the blood; and glucose intolerance.

Diagnostic Procedures

Percutaneous needle aspiration biopsy of the affected portion of the pancreas is used to confirm the diagnosis. Ultrasonography, CT scanning, MRI, and endoscopic retrograde cholangiopancreatography (ERCP) are useful in establishing a diagnosis. X-ray series and blood tests may be ordered to help in staging the cancer.

Treatment

Treatment for pancreatic cancer depends on the stage, the location of the cancer, the person's age, and overall health. Treatment quite often is palliative because most pancreatic cancers are diagnosed after they have metastasized to the lungs, liver, and bones. If surgical resection is possible, localized tumors are removed. Radiation therapy and multidrug chemotherapy may be administered, but pancreatic carcinomas usually respond poorly. It is important to manage the pain and to correct any nutritional defects.

Complementary Therapy

See Pancreatitis.

 CLIENT COMMUNICATION

Reinforce to clients the need for small, frequent meals and to avoid overeating at any one meal. Instruct clients to notify their primary care provider when signs of jaundice occur, when they experience significant weight loss, or when signs of bowel obstruction occur.

Prognosis

The prognosis is poor, because 80% to 85% of individuals have advanced disease at first diagnosis.

Prevention

There is no known prevention other than avoiding known carcinogens, reducing the amount of fat in the diet, and participating in a regular exercise program.

COMMON SYMPTOMS OF DIGESTIVE SYSTEM DISEASES AND DISORDERS

Individuals may present with the following common symptoms, which deserve attention from health-care professionals:

- Loss of appetite, weight loss, anorexia
- Nausea and vomiting
- Dehydration
- Any change in bowel habits, such as diarrhea, constipation, and flatulence
- Hemoptysis or hematemesis
- Blood or mucus in the stool
- Fever
- Pain in any area of the GI tract
- Heartburn, indigestion, dysphagia, and reflux
- Malaise, loss of strength, and fatigability
- Jaundice

CHAPTER EPISODE—PART VI

Unfortunately, Katy's difficulties are not over. The medication brought her back to decent health, but she found it necessary to drop the volleyball team. She was able to enroll in the community college the next fall and stayed at home with her mom. At the beginning of her second semester, however, the disease spiralled out of control again. She had to drop several classes and lost 20 pounds. She couldn't eat without running to the bathroom and she soon became depressed as well. Her social life dwindled to nothing and she felt chained to the bathroom. Katy and her doctor tried everything. Katy made diet changes, lifestyle changes, and they tried new medicines, but nothing worked. She was also receiving IV infusions every 6 weeks.

Finally she made a very difficult decision with her specialist—they decided to remove her colon. She was referred to the Cleveland Clinic where she woke symptom-free for the first time in a long time following the surgery. Without her colon, there was nothing for her immune system to attack. When she was finally able to eat her first full meal, she braced herself for the usual cramping, pain, and bathroom run, but nothing happened. She cried with happiness. Nine months later, Katy was back at the clinic for surgery that would create a new colon from her small intestine.

Today at age 22 she is symptom-free and finishing her associate in arts degree. She hopes to get into a nursing program.

- Is Katy's story unusual? Explain.
- What might the future hold for Katy? Would you attempt such a serious surgery if it were you?

SUMMARY

Proper nutrition is important to a healthy, functioning digestive system, which has the task of nourishing every cell in the body. Unbalanced food and fluid intake forces the digestive system to respond with the goal of bringing about homeostasis. When homeostasis fails, disease is the result. On the positive side of the coin, progress has been made in making foods safer and healthier. In 2013, when the U.S. Food and Drug Administration stated that partially hydrogenated oils—the primary source of trans fats—were no longer considered safe, there was a more than a 75% reduction of trans fats from the U.S. food supply. Diseases and disorders of the digestive system have a profound effect on the body and the individual in that they almost always interfere with the daily meal intake and nourishment for the body's cells.

DavisPlus | For more resources and to sharpen your skills with interactive exercises, visit *DavisPlus* at http://davisplus.fadavis.com. Keyword *Tamparo*.

ONLINE RESOURCES

Celiac disease
http://www.CeliacCentral.org

Crohn disease, IBS, and ulcerative colitis
http://www.ccfa.org

Viral hepatitis
http://www.medicinenet.com

CASE STUDIES

Case Study 1

George Payton, a 52-year-old man previously diagnosed with IBS, reports that he is having three to five bowel movements per day. The movements are runny and loose and filled with red blood. George has not experienced any constipation. His family practitioner refers him to a gastroenterologist.

Case Study Questions
1. Describe IBS.
2. Are the reported symptoms compatible with IBS?
3. Of these symptoms, which is most significant? Is any other disease suspected?
4. What tests is the gastroenterologist likely to order?

Case Study 2

A 35-year-old woman, Elaine Morrison, experiences flatus, weight loss, abdominal distention, and loss of appetite. Elaine has complained of these symptoms on several previous occasions. In response to her PCP's question, Elaine reports that her stool floats in the toilet bowl and is foul smelling.

Case Study Questions
1. What steps do you think the primary care provider might take?
2. How would a complete physical examination help in the diagnosis of this case?
3. What specific diagnostic tests might be ordered?

REVIEW QUESTIONS

Matching
Match each of the following definitions with its correct term.

_____ 1. Backup of gastric contents into the esophagus

_____ 2. Examination of colon using fiberoptic endoscope

_____ 3. Symptoms include pain that settles in the lower right quadrant of the abdomen

_____ 4. Irreversible chronic degenerative hepatic disease

_____ 5. Inflammation of the gallbladder

_____ 6. Acute infection and inflammation of the liver

_____ 7. Inflammation of the stomach and bowel

_____ 8. Associated with *Helicobacter pylori*

a. Gastroenteritis

b. GERD

c. Appendicitis

d. Irritable bowel syndrome

e. Colonoscopy

f. Cholecystitis

g. Cirrhosis

h. Viral hepatitis

i. Peptic ulcer

j. Hemorrhoids

Short Answer

1. Can you name the three functions of the GI tract?

   a. _____

   b. _____

   c. _____

2. What is the common name for aphthous stomatitis?

   _____

3. How do you describe the "rule of 3" in infantile colic?

   a. _____

   b. _____

   c. _____

   d. _____

4. What is the major distinction between IBS and IBD?

   a. _____

   b. _____

5. What is the likely surgical treatment for Crohn disease?

   a. _____

   b. _____

6. How do you compare and contrast the following?

   a. Diverticulosis

   b. Diverticulitis

Multiple Choice
Place a checkmark next to the correct answer.

1. What statement best describes hemorrhoids?

   _____ a. They are dilated, tortuous veins in the jejunum.

   _____ b. They are the result of gluten intolerance.

   _____ c. They can be internal or external.

   _____ d. They have a poor prognosis even with diet restrictions.

2. What is a "rolling" hiatal hernia?

   _____ a. It is the most common form of hiatal hernia.

   _____ b. It presents vomiting as its most common symptom.

   _____ c. It occurs when the gastroesophageal junction is fixed but some portion of the stomach passes through the esophageal hiatus.

   _____ d. It occurs when the gastroesophageal junction and the upper portion of the stomach slide upward through the esophageal hiatus.

3. How is acute appendicitis described?

   _____ a. It is a viral infection caused by stricture.

   _____ b. It exhibits classic symptoms of lower left quadrant pain.

   _____ c. It responds well to appendectomy, the only recommended treatment.

   _____ d. It is a circumscribed, craterlike lesion of the vermiform appendix.

4. What are the major causes of pancreatitis?

   _____ a. It is a severe, chronic inflammation of the ileum.

   _____ b. It is caused by cholelithiasis and/or alcoholism.

   _____ c. Multiple pregnancies are a common cause.

   _____ d. It is because of a congenital weakness in the abdominal wall.

5. What do you know about colorectal cancer?

_____ a. It afflicts more men than women.

_____ b. It is caused by a lymphoma.

_____ c. It rarely metastasizes.

_____ d. It is usually treated with surgery.

Discussion Questions/Personal Reflection

1. Compare and contrast the five main types of viral hepatitis.

_____

_____

_____

_____

_____

_____

_____

_____

_____

2. Crohn disease is a recognizable disability covered under the Americans with Disabilities Act (ADA). Explain why. What kinds of accommodations might be made in a place of employment? Can you think of other digestive diseases that could be included under the ADA regulations? If so, name them.

_____

_____

_____

_____

_____

_____

_____

_____

_____

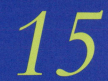

> *Everything is funny as long as it happens to somebody else.*
> —WILL ROGERS

15

Urinary System Diseases and Disorders

● *chapter outline*

URINARY SYSTEM ANATOMY AND PHYSIOLOGY REVIEW

INFECTIONS OF THE URINARY SYSTEM

Cystitis and Urethritis
Pyelonephritis (Acute)
Glomerulonephritis (Acute)

KIDNEY DISEASES AND DISORDERS

Renal Calculi (Uroliths or Kidney Stones)
Hydronephrosis
Acute Tubular Necrosis
Nephrotic Syndrome
Polycystic Kidney Disease
End-Stage Renal Disease

OTHER URINARY DISEASES AND DISORDERS

Neurogenic or Overactive Bladder

CANCERS OF THE URINARY SYSTEM

Bladder Cancer
Renal Cell Carcinoma or Kidney Cancer

COMMON SYMPTOMS OF URINARY SYSTEM DISEASES AND DISORDERS

SUMMARY

ONLINE RESOURCES

CASE STUDIES

REVIEW QUESTIONS

● *key words*

Antipyretic (ăn″tĭ•pī•rĕt′ĭk)
Ascites (ă•sī′tēz)
Azotemia (āz″ō•tē′mē•ă)
Bacteriuria (bak•tēr″ē•ū′rē•ă)
Calyx (kā′lĭks)
Creatinine (krē•ăt′ĭn•ĭn)
Cystectomy (sĭs•tĕk′tō•mē)
Dysuria (dĭs•ū′rē•ă)
Electrolyte (ē•lĕk′trō•līt)
Hematuria (hē″mă•tū′rē•ă)

Hyperkalemia (hī″pĕr•kă•lē′mē•ă)
Hyperlipemia (hī″pĕr•lĭp•ē′mē•ă)
Hyperparathyroidism (hī″pĕr•păr″ă•thī′roy•dĭzm)
Hypoalbuminemia (hī″pō•ăl•bū″mĭn•ē′mē•ă)
Incontinence (in-ˈkänt-ən-ən(t)s)
Ischemia (ĭs•kē′mē•ă)
Lipiduria (lĭp″ĭ•dū′rē•ă)
Micturition (mĭk•tū•rĭ′shŭn)

Nocturia (nŏk•tū′rē•ă)
Oliguria (ŏl•ĭg•ū′rē•ă)
Pallor (păl′ŏr)
Proteinuria (prō″tē•ĭn•ū′rē•ă)
Pyuria (pī•ūr′ē•ă)
Transurethral resection (trăns″ū•re′thrăl rē•sĕk′shŭn)
Urea (ū•rē′ă)
Uremia (ū•rē′mē•ă)
Urolith (ū′rō•lĭth)

- Define key terms.
- Recall anatomy and physiology of the urinary system.
- Explain urinalysis and what it indicates.
- Identify the major diseases of the kidney.
- Name the most common diagnostic procedures used to detect kidney and kidney-related diseases.
- Describe the prognosis of lower urinary tract infections.
- Explain why women are more prone than men to urinary tract infections.
- Compare and contrast pyelonephritis and glomerulonephritis.
- Recall infectious precursors to kidney-related diseases.
- Discuss the complications of renal calculi.

- Identify possible treatments for hydronephrosis.
- Describe how acute tubular necrosis occurs.
- List the characteristics unique to nephrotic syndrome.
- List at least three characteristics common to polycystic kidney disease.
- Name at least three causes of end-stage renal disease.
- Discuss kidney transplantation.
- Distinguish between the three types of kidney dialysis.
- Define neurogenic or overactive bladder.
- Recall the major cause of tumors of the bladder.
- Discuss treatment of renal cell or kidney cancer.
- List at least four common complaints of the urinary system.

CHAPTER EPISODE—PART I

Peter's diagnosis was devastating but not unexpected. He had been told long ago that his type 2 diabetes and serious hypertension might one day cause kidney failure. When the first kidney failed, he was still able to function for nearly a year. But now the second kidney was not doing its job. At only 60, Peter felt his life might be over.

- Identify the possible feelings that Peter is having right now.
- What might be his options?

URINARY SYSTEM ANATOMY AND PHYSIOLOGY REVIEW

The urinary system is responsible for the production and elimination of urine when a type of waste called *urea* is removed from the blood. **Urea** is produced when protein-containing foods are broken down in the body. It is then carried in the bloodstream to the two kidneys, where urine is formed. The two ureters, the urinary bladder, and the urethra are responsible for the elimination of urine. Figure 15.1 illustrates the urinary system in relationship to the body, and the insert illustrates the cross section of the kidney.

The kidneys, each about the size of a fist, help to regulate the water, **electrolyte** (ionized salt), and acid-base content of the blood, and they selectively filter the waste products of metabolism. They also play an important role in regulating blood pressure. Internal structures and blood vessels are illustrated in Figure 15.2 A and B. Each kidney contains more than 1 million nephrons (Fig. 15.3), which are the principal filtering units of the kidney. Each nephron houses a ball of tiny blood capillaries called the *glomerulus* and a renal tubule. It is here that the three-part process of selective filtration of wastes, reabsorption of vital minerals and fluid, and secretion of waste products and other substances takes place. As urine is formed, it passes through the nephrons into the renal tubules of the kidneys.

From the kidneys, urine travels into the ureters (thin tubes about 8 to 10 inches in length) on its way to the

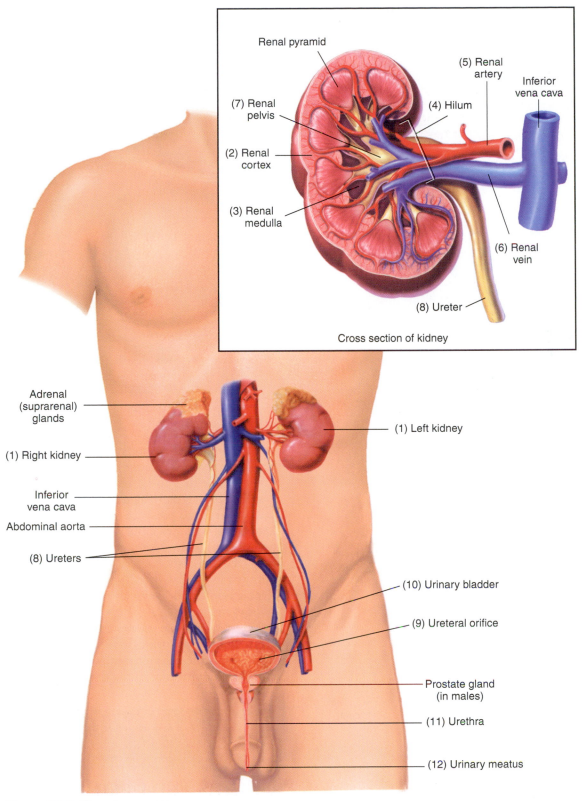

Figure 15.1 The urinary system.

urinary bladder. Small amounts of urine drip into the urinary bladder about every 12 seconds. The urinary bladder is a balloon-shaped muscular organ that stores urine until it is emptied. It can hold about 16 ounces of urine for 2 to 5 hours. Nerves in the urinary bladder indicate when it should be emptied. Sphincter muscles keep urine from leaking into the urethra too soon and relax when it is time to urinate.

It is worth emphasizing the reabsorption process of the kidneys' nephrons. Were it not for this process, the body

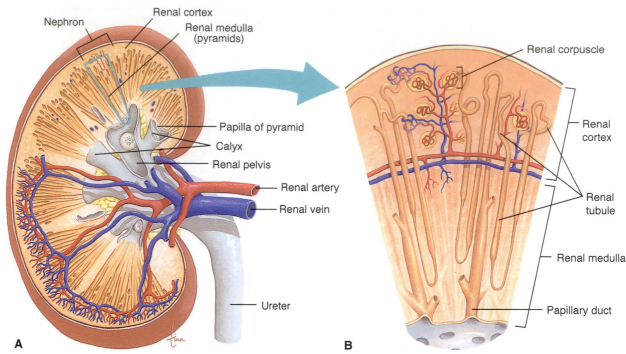

Figure 15.2 (A) Frontal section of the right kidney showing internal structures and blood vessels. (B) Magnified section of the kidney shows several nephrons. *(From Scanlon, VC, and Sanders, T: Essentials of Anatomy and Physiology, ed. 6. Philadelphia: F.A. Davis, 2011, p 450, with permission.)*

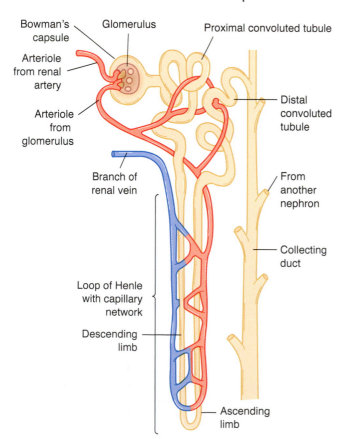

Figure 15.3 Nephron with associated blood vessels.

would rapidly be depleted of its fluid. Typically, only 1% of the fluid passing through a nephron is excreted as urine.

A routine diagnostic test for suspected urinary disease is a urinalysis, which includes testing the specific gravity; pH; and presence of protein, blood, sugar, and ketones. It includes a microscopic examination for the presence of white blood cells (WBCs) and red blood cells (RBCs), casts, bacteria, and crystals. Normal urine is amber in color with a slightly acid reaction, has a particular odor, and frequently deposits a precipitate of phosphates when fresh. The specific gravity varies from 1.005 to 1.030. The greater the rate of urine excretion, the lower is the specific gravity. Refer to Table 15.1 throughout the chapter, noting possible abnormalities and their significance to the disease in question.

Infections of the Urinary System

CYSTITIS AND URETHRITIS

ICD-10: N30.90, N30.91 (CYSTITIS)
ICD-10: N34.1, N34.2 (URETHRITIS)

Description

Cystitis (inflammation of the bladder) and urethritis (inflammation of the urethra) are common urinary tract

Table 15.1	Significance of Changes in Urine		
	NORMAL	ABNORMAL	SIGNIFICANCE
Quantity	1,000 to 1,500 mL (approx. 95% H_2O)		Depends on water and fluid, foods consumed, exercise, temperature, kidney function
		High (polyuria)	Diabetes mellitus, diabetes insipidus, nervous diseases, certain types of chronic nephritis (kidney disorder), diuretics (e.g., caffeine, digitalis) causing increased urinary excretion
		Low (oliguria)	Acute nephritis, heart disease, fever, eclampsia, diarrhea, vomiting, inadequate fluid intake
		None (anuria)	Uremia (nitrogenous wastes in blood), acute nephritis, metal poisoning (e.g., due to bichloride of mercury), complete obstruction of urinary tract
Color	Yellow to amber		Depends on concentration of pigment (urochrome)
		Pale	Diabetes insipidus; due to a very dilute urine
		Milky	Fat globules, pus in genitourinary infections
		Reddish	Blood pigments, drugs, or food pigments
		Greenish	Bile pigment, associated with jaundice
		Brown-black	Poisoning (mercury, lead, phenol), hemorrhage
Transparency	Clear		Normal
	Cloudy on standing		Precipitation of mucin from urinary tract; not pathological
	Turbid		Precipitation of calcium phosphate; not pathological
		Milky	Presence of fat globules; pathological
		Turbid	Presence of pus due to inflammation of urinary tract; pathological
Odor	Faintly aromatic		Normal
		Pleasant (sweet)	Acetone, associated with diabetes mellitus
		Unpleasant	Decomposition or ingestion of certain drugs or foods
	Peppermint		Menthol ingestion
	Acrid		Asparagus in diet
	Spicy		Ingestion of sandalwood oil or saffron
Proteinuria	Albumin and globulin		Excretion of 10 to 100 mg every 24 hours is normal, but this amount is not detected by usual tests
		Albumin	Evidence of altered renal function; may be due to renal pathology or a systemic disease such as diabetes mellitus
		Globulin	Bence-Jones proteins associated with multiple myeloma and diseases of globulin metabolism; other types of globulins may be present in acute and chronic pyelonephritis
Specific Gravity	1.010 to 1.025; can vary in absence of pathology		Ordinary; specific gravity inversely proportional to volume
		Low (chronic)	Dilution if volume is large; otherwise nephritis
		High (chronic)	Acute nephritis; concentrated if volume is small; otherwise, if light colored and volume is large, diabetes mellitus
Acidity	Acid (slight)		Diet of acid-forming foods (meats, eggs, prunes, wheat) overbalances the base-forming foods (vegetables and fruits)
		High acidity	Acidosis, diabetes mellitus, many pathological disorders (fevers, starvation)
		Alkaline	Vegetarian diet changes urea into ammonium carbonate; infection or ingestion of alkaline compounds

Source: Venes, D (ed): Taber's Cyclopedic Medical Dictionary, *ed. 19. Philadelphia: F.A. Davis, 2001, pp 2188–2189, with permission.*

infections (UTIs). Together these diseases account for the majority of health-care provider visits by individuals experiencing urinary tract problems. In fact, after upper respiratory tract infections, UTIs are the most common type of bacterial infection seen by health-care providers.

Etiology

The growth of bacteria in normally sterile urine causes infection. This infection usually starts at the urethral opening and is commonly the result of the bacteria *Escherichia coli*, which accounts for most cases of cystitis and urethritis. Other causative organisms include *Proteus, Klebsiella, Enterobacter,* and *Serratia* bacteria. These organisms typically ascend the urinary tract from the urethral opening, but they also may be introduced as a result of urinary tract catheterization. Urethritis also

may be caused by sexually transmitted organisms, such as *Chlamydia trachomatis* and *Neisseria gonorrhoeae*.

Women are 10 times more susceptible to ascending UTIs than are men, in part because of the shorter urethra in women and the comparative ease with which fecal contaminants can be spread from the anus to the urethral opening and up into the bladder. Women who are sexually active are more predisposed to cystitis, because sexual intercourse enhances the bacterial transfer from the urethra into the bladder. Finally, both women and men are more at risk of contracting a UTI as a complication of any disorder that obstructs normal urinary flow. Also at risk are individuals whose medical conditions cause incomplete emptying of the bladder, such as those with spinal cord injuries or bladder decompensation, individuals who take immunosuppressant medications, men with prostatitis, and those who are catheterized for long periods of time.

Signs and Symptoms

Signs and symptoms cannot be relied on for the diagnosis or localization of a UTI. Some individuals may present with few symptoms yet have significant **bacteriuria.** The person presenting with cystitis may complain of dysuria, urinary frequency and urgency, and pain above the pubic region. Cloudy, bloody, or foul-smelling urine also may be noted. The individual with urethritis typically presents with similar symptoms, except the quality of the urine is often not affected. Any other symptoms, such as fever, nausea, vomiting, and low back pain, may indicate problems such as pyelonephritis.

Diagnostic Procedures

The medical history may reveal past UTIs, recent catheterization, or a change in sexual partners. A clean-catch urine specimen is obtained to diagnose a UTI. This test involves cleansing the area around the urethral opening to prevent bacteria from contaminating the sample and collecting a midstream urine sample. A urine culture is necessary to identify the organism responsible for the infection. The presence of RBCs and WBCs in the urine sample is also an indicator. X-ray, ultrasonography, computed tomography (CT), and renal scans may be necessary to identify any abnormality in the urinary tract such as an obstruction.

Treatment

Antibiotics or sulfonamide (sulfa) drugs appropriate to combat the particular causative organisms may be prescribed; however, the type of antibiotic and the duration of treatment depend on circumstances. A primary care provider (PCP) determines whether a 1-day, 3-day, or 7-day course of antibiotic therapy is best. Fluid intake may be increased to promote urinary outflow. Analgesics may be prescribed for short-term pain relief. For persons (especially women) who are susceptible to repeated infections (at least two UTIs in 6 months or three UTIs in 1 year), the PCP may prescribe preventive antibiotic therapy or recommend one or more of the over-the-counter (OTC) products to treat mild symptoms at the first sign of infection.

Complementary Therapy

Naturopathic providers may prescribe an herbal preparation to be used three to four times per day during a UTI. They include the following:

- Goldenseal root, an herb with a long and well-documented history as an antimicrobial agent. It can be made as a tea using 1 teaspoon of dried herb per cup of hot water, in capsule form (1,000 mg), or as a tincture (1 to 2 teaspoons in warm water).
- Uva ursi, clinically shown to be useful as an antiseptic with soothing and strengthening properties. It can be made as a tea using 2 teaspoons of herb per cup of hot water or as a tincture (1 to 2 teaspoons in warm water).

In addition to these measures, advise clients that pure blueberry or cranberry juice (not sweetened) may be useful. Drinks that may irritate the bladder are to be avoided. These may include alcohol, caffeine, and citrus juices. Also tell clients that urinating after intercourse can help flush out any bacteria introduced.

⊸ CLIENT COMMUNICATION

Explain the purpose and course of the medication. Advise clients to drink plenty of fluids. Caution them that untreated UTIs can lead to more serious infections in the kidney and renal pelvis. A warm heating pad applied to the abdomen may help ease discomfort.

Prognosis

If no complications arise, the prognosis for complete recovery from cystitis and urethritis is quite good. Reinfection in susceptible individuals is likely.

Prevention

Preventive measures include complete emptying of the bladder and avoiding "holding urine." Proper feminine hygiene, including wiping the perineum from front to back and cleansing well after a bowel movement, will lessen the chance of introducing disease-causing microorganisms into the urethra. Women with a history of UTI also may be placed on a long-term course of antibiotics.

PYELONEPHRITIS (ACUTE)

ICD-10: N10

Description

Pyelonephritis, also called *infective tubulointerstitial nephritis* or *kidney infection,* is inflammation of the kidney and renal pelvis due to infection. One or both kidneys may be affected. The infection can destroy or scar renal tissue, impairing kidney function. It is the most common type of kidney disease and is more common in women than in men due in part to the anatomic difference between men and women.

Etiology

Pyelonephritis is most commonly due to infection by the *E. coli* bacteria. *E. coli* is a normal intestinal bacteria that grows rapidly and is found in fecal matter. *Proteus, Pseudomonas, Staphylococcus,* and *Enterococcus* bacteria are less frequent agents of the infection. The bacteria typically ascend to the kidneys from the lower urinary tract, but they also may enter the kidneys through the blood or lymph.

Women, particularly those who are pregnant or who practice poor genital hygiene, are at risk. In men, pyelonephritis may arise as a complication of prostate enlargement. Any catheterization of the urinary tract also increases the likelihood of infection.

Signs and Symptoms

The individual experiencing acute pyelonephritis may complain of a fever and lumbar, side, or groin pain. These symptoms may be accompanied by **pyuria** (pus in the urine), **dysuria** (difficult or painful urination), and **nocturia** (excessive urination at night). Clients often look quite ill and report that symptoms appeared rapidly.

Diagnostic Procedures

The physical examination may reveal tenderness during palpation of abdominal or lumbar areas. Culture and sensitivity tests are performed on a clean-catch urine specimen, which may appear cloudy and have a "fishy" odor. Urinalysis also may reveal casts, WBCs, bacteria, and hematuria. Men may have a digital rectal examination (DRE) to determine if a swollen prostate gland is blocking the neck of the bladder. An ultrasound or CT scan is frequently used to detect any obstruction in the urinary tract.

Treatment

Antibiotic therapy that is appropriate to the infecting organism is the treatment of choice. **Antipyretics** may be ordered to decrease the fever. An increase in liquids is helpful. It is important that clients are kept hydrated and that they take all the ordered medication. Generally, a follow-up culture is done 2 weeks after the person has finished the antibiotic therapy to ensure that the infection is gone.

Complementary Therapy

Refer to UTIs. Suggest to clients that applying heat to the abdomen can provide comfort. Pain medications may be ordered to relieve discomfort. Instruct clients to stay hydrated.

⊕ CLIENT COMMUNICATION

Remind individuals to practice proper genital hygiene to avoid introducing bacteria into the urinary tract. If the disease recurs, it may be necessary to determine any factor that might predispose a person to recurrent infection.

Prognosis

The prognosis is usually good with proper treatment and follow-up care. Acute pyelonephritis frequently subsides in a few days, even without treatment with antibiotics. Reinfection is likely, however, for persons of high risk such as those with prolonged use of an indwelling catheter. Repeated infection may lead to a chronic form of the disease, causing elevated blood pressure and sufficient destruction of kidney tissue to produce renal failure.

Prevention

The best prevention is avoidance of any infection and the use of proper genital hygiene. Remind clients to drink plenty of fluids, especially water, and empty their bladder after intercourse.

GLOMERULONEPHRITIS (ACUTE)

ICD-10: N00.9

Description

Glomerulonephritis, which is inflammation of the glomeruli in the kidney's nephrons, reduces the rate of blood filtration. Retention of water and salts follows, resulting in injury to the glomeruli, which allow RBCs and serum protein to pass into the urine. Both kidneys are affected.

Etiology

The cause is often unknown. However, it is also known as *acute poststreptococcal glomerulonephritis* (APSGN), following a streptococcal infection of the respiratory tract. This inflammation is a consequence of an infection elsewhere in the body, most frequently in the upper respiratory tract or the middle ear and caused by streptococcal bacteria. APSGN is more likely to occur in children but is less common today owing to the antibiotic therapy used for streptococcal infections. However, other bacteria and certain viruses and parasites, such as impetigo, mumps, Epstein-Barr virus, hepatitis B and C, and HIV/AIDS, may induce glomerulonephritis as well. The disease also may arise as a consequence of various multisystem diseases such as lupus erythematosus (see Chapter 9) or bacterial endocarditis (see Chapter 12).

Signs and Symptoms

The primary presenting sign is hematuria, and the urine may be the color of cola because of the RBCs and casts. If the urine is "foamy," it is likely an indication of **proteinuria** (excessive levels of serum protein in the urine). Usually the disease has an abrupt onset. There may be headaches from secondary hypertension; puffy eyes due to edema from leaky, inflamed capillaries; pain in the lumbar region from swollen kidneys; and **oliguria** (reduced urine secretion) due to the nephron damage. There also may be malaise, anorexia, and a low-grade fever.

Diagnostic Procedures

A detailed medical history is important and may reveal a recent streptococcal infection of the upper respiratory tract. Urine may also be described as "bloody," "coffee-colored," or "smoky." Urinalysis will show hematuria and proteinuria. Blood urea nitrogen (BUN), **creatinine,** and erythrocyte sedimentation rate (ESR) are measured and may show elevated levels. The nitrogen and creatinine are present in the blood because these final products of decomposition cannot be excreted in normal amounts. X-ray, ultrasound, CT scan, or a renal biopsy may be necessary to confirm the diagnosis.

Treatment

Treatment goals are generally dependent on the cause. The PCP may prescribe diuretics and/or angiotensin-converting enzyme (ACE) inhibitors or angiotensin II receptor agonists to control edema and hypertension. Bed rest is usually indicated. Dietary restrictions on salt, protein, and potassium may be advised. If an underlying infection can be confirmed, antibiotics are prescribed.

Complementary Therapy

No significant complementary therapy is indicated other than to maintain a healthy weight, quit smoking, and control blood sugar levels if diabetic.

⊙ CLIENT COMMUNICATION

Refer the client to a dietitian to develop a diet high in calories and low in protein and sodium. Referral to support systems may prove beneficial. The National Kidney Foundation (http://www.kidney.org) may provide a list of possible resources. Remind clients that follow-up examinations are necessary to prevent chronic glomerulonephritis.

Prognosis

The prognosis is generally good. Most clients with acute glomerulonephritis experience a resolution of symptoms within a few weeks of onset. Children generally recover more rapidly than adults. A few cases, though, may progress into a chronic form of the disease when repeated acute attacks occur.

Prevention

Most forms of glomerulonephritis cannot be prevented. Prompt treatment of any streptococcal upper respiratory tract infection is important. Take steps to reduce clients' hypertension. Instruct clients to practice safer sex to

prevent such infections as HIV and hepatitis. Advise clients to avoid IV drug use.

Kidney Diseases and Disorders

RENAL CALCULI (UROLITHS OR KIDNEY STONES)

ICD-10: N20.0

Description

Renal calculi are the most common cause of urinary obstruction. A renal calculus is a concentration of various mineral salts in the renal pelvis or the cuplike extension of the renal pelvis called the **calyx** (Fig. 15.4). They can be small like a grain of sand or very large. Most stones develop in the kidney and are formed from calcium salts, uric acid, cystine, and struvite, in descending order of frequency.

Etiology

Renal calculi form because of a disturbance in the kidney's delicate balancing act of preventing water loss while at the same time eliminating water-soluble mineral wastes. Many factors, such as prolonged dehydration or immobilization, can upset this balance. The balance also may be upset by underlying diseases, such as gout, **hyperparathyroidism** (disease caused by oversecretion of the parathyroid glands), Cushing syndrome, or urinary tract infections and neoplasms. A person may develop renal calculi because of an excessive

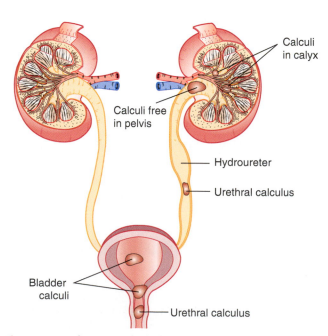

Figure 15.4 Location of calculi in the urinary tract.

intake of vitamin D or dietary calcium. The condition appears to be genetic for certain types of stones, with men much more commonly affected than women. In many instances, no specific cause can be pinpointed.

Signs and Symptoms

A person having renal calculi may remain asymptomatic for long periods. If a stone or calculus fragment lodges in a ureter, however, the individual may complain of intense flank pain and urinary urgency. Classic ureteral colicky pain is manifested by acute, intermittent, and excruciating pain in the flank and upper outer quadrant of the abdomen on the affected side. If calculi are in the renal pelvis and calyces, the pain is duller and more constant. Back pain and severe abdominal pain may occur. Other presenting symptoms include nausea, vomiting, chills and fever, hematuria, and abdominal distention.

Diagnostic Procedures

The history may reveal a familial tendency toward the formation of kidney stones. A urinalysis may be ordered to detect elevated levels of RBCs or WBCs in the urine or to check for the presence of protein, pus, and bacteria. CT scan and abdominal x-ray (or kidneys, ureter, bladder [KUB]) may be ordered to determine the locations of calculus formation. A noncontrast spiral CT scan of the ureters and kidneys is the preferred test for kidney stones. In this test, the scanner moves in a circle as the client moves through the machine. This test takes less time than a standard CT scan and provides better images of the kidneys and ureters. Blood testing may be helpful in confirming imbalances of minerals or the existence of other metabolic disorders.

Treatment

Treatment is directed at clearing obstructive stones and preventing the formation of new ones. Increased fluid intake (greater than 3 L/day) may enhance elimination of stones in some cases, but large stones may require surgical intervention, especially if renal function is threatened. Ureteroscopic removal with fluoroscopic guidance may be used to dilate the ureter to grasp and remove the stone. Techniques such as ultrasonic percutaneous lithotripsy and extracorporeal shock wave lithotripsy pulverize stones in place, allowing them to be passed in the urine or removed by suction. Lithotripsy via ureteroscope can also be used to remove urethral stones. Antibiotics may be prescribed if it is determined that the calculus buildup is due to bacterial infection. Analgesics may be necessary for the relief of intense pain.

Complementary Therapy

Complementary practitioners recommend drinking 8 or more glasses of water per day and eating a diet high in fiber and low in fat, with reduction of red meat consumption. Vitamins and minerals may be helpful, especially when coordinated with the PCP. Relaxation techniques may be beneficial to deal with the pain.

 CLIENT COMMUNICATION

Stress the importance of proper diet and completing any medicinal therapy. Explain any diagnostic or surgical procedures to clients. Encourage increased fluid intake.

Prognosis

The prognosis is good if urinary tract obstruction is prevented and underlying disorders are promptly treated. However, about 60% of people who have a calcium stone have further stone formation later.

Prevention

An adequate daily fluid intake is the best way to minimize the chance of stone formation, especially among individuals at risk. Fruit juices, especially unsweetened cranberry and blueberry juice, help acidify urine and may help prevent the formation of renal calculi.

CHAPTER EPISODE—PART II

Peter and his wife had partially prepared for when he might lose function of his kidneys. They had packed as much life into the time since his first kidney failed as was possible. They rode motorcycles together, did some hiking, and enjoyed the great scenery in their beloved Hawaii. However, they also spent time researching their options. Kidney dialysis (and what kind), kidney transplant, no treatment at all—they considered it all. Their research indicated that at age 60, he was still a viable candidate for dialysis and maybe even a transplant, but Peter also realized that the long wait for a kidney transplant could easily jeopardize his chances of a donor kidney.

- What is likely the first step for Peter at this point with the second kidney failing?
- Why does age play any part in either dialysis or kidney transplant?

HYDRONEPHROSIS

ICD-10: N133.0

Description

Hydronephrosis is the distention of the renal pelvis and calyces of a kidney due to pressure from accumulating urine. The pressure impairs, and may eventually interrupt, kidney function. One or both kidneys may be affected.

Etiology

Hydronephrosis is caused by a urinary tract obstruction. The ureters and renal pelvis dilate proximal to, or behind, the obstruction. This swelling causes the hydronephrosis with resultant destruction of functional tissue. In children, the obstruction is usually the result of some congenital defect in urinary tract structure. In adults, the obstruction is more often acquired, resulting from blockage by neoplasms or **uroliths,** commonly called *kidney stones* or *renal calculi.* Urinary tract obstruction in men may be produced by benign or malignant enlargement of the prostate. Women may experience urinary tract obstruction as a complication of pregnancy. Underlying disorders such as neurogenic bladder also may allow urine to accumulate to the extent that it produces hydronephrosis.

Signs and Symptoms

The signs and symptoms depend on the site of obstruction, the cause, and the rapidity with which the condition developed. If the obstruction is above the opening of the bladder, only one kidney may be affected and the person may be asymptomatic for a prolonged period ("silent" hydronephrosis). Symptoms may be severe, however, especially if both kidneys are affected. The person often complains of intense flank pain, nausea, vomiting, dysuria, oliguria or anuria, and hematuria. Clients may also complain of unexplained pruritus.

Diagnostic Procedures

Palpation and percussion of the abdomen may reveal distention of the kidney or urinary bladder. A history of changes in urinary volume, difficulty in voiding, and pain may be found. BUN can help assess kidney function. Ultrasound may be ordered to visualize obstructions. A noncontrast spiral CT scan or MRI may be ordered to further define the site of obstruction. Urinalysis may reveal hematuria, pus, and bacteria and may be helpful in determining the extent of any impairment of renal function.

Treatment

Treatment goals include draining excess urine from the kidney, removing any obstruction, preventing complications, and treating underlying disorders. Catheterization may be necessary for the immediate relief of urinary pressure. Analgesics may be prescribed. Antibiotics are required to treat infection. Surgery is sometimes required to dilate a ureteral stricture.

Complementary Therapy

No significant complementary therapy is indicated.

⊙ CLIENT COMMUNICATION

Encourage regular medical checkups, and explain symptoms of hydronephrosis so that the client can report them to the primary care provider as necessary.

Prognosis

The prognosis is variable, depending on whether one or both kidneys are affected, whether the obstruction can be removed, and whether permanent renal damage has occurred.

Prevention

There are no specific preventative measures. Prompt treatment of conditions that can cause hydronephrosis is important.

ACUTE TUBULAR NECROSIS

ICD-10: N17.0

Description

Acute tubular necrosis is the rapid destruction or degeneration of the tubular segments of nephrons in the kidneys. The disease is characterized by a sudden deterioration in renal function, with resulting accumulation of nitrogenous wastes in the body. Impaired or interrupted renal function from acute tubular necrosis is considered reversible.

Etiology

The majority of cases of acute tubular necrosis are due to renal **ischemia,** or the interruption or impairment of blood flow in and out of the kidneys. This disease is the most common cause of acute renal failure in critically ill persons. Although there can be numerous causes for such impairment, renal ischemia leading to acute tubular necrosis is most frequently produced by severe bodily trauma or as a complication following surgery. The renal tubules also can be damaged in other ways. Acute tubular necrosis may be toxin induced (as a result of exposure to solvents, heavy metals, or certain medications), may be caused by transfusion reactions, or may arise as a complication of pregnancy.

Signs and Symptoms

The individual with acute tubular necrosis may have a host of widely distributed symptoms. Principal symptoms include oliguria and an excessive amount of potassium in the blood, or **hyperkalemia.** Other generalized symptoms include weakness, mental confusion, and edema. The disease has four phases: (1) onset or initiating phase, (2) oliguria or anuric phase, (3) diuretic phase, and (4) recovery or convalescent phase. The onset phase lasts from the precipitating event until tubular injury results. The oliguria phase, with decreased urine output and increased fluid retention, lasts generally 10 to 14 days. The diuretic phase is when the nephrons recover to the point where urine excretion is possible. Then, during the recovery phase, renal function slowly recovers. Some kidney damage may persist.

Diagnostic Procedures

A history of chronic and debilitating illness, trauma, surgery, transfusion, or pregnancy complications may indicate a risk of acute tubular necrosis. Diagnostic tests ordered may include urinalysis, which reveals dilute urine with RBCs and casts. BUN and creatinine tests often indicate increased nitrogen and creatinine or reveal disturbances in the electrolyte balance of the blood. Most of the time, diagnosis occurs when the disease is more advanced.

Treatment

The main goal of treatment is to identify and correct the underlying cause. The primary care provider generally attempts to promote proper renal circulation if the acute tubular necrosis is due to ischemia. If the disease is toxin induced, dialysis may be attempted to cleanse the blood. Dialysis may also be indicated to allow the kidneys to rest and to improve conditions for regeneration. Otherwise, treatment is largely supportive until kidney function increases. Supportive treatment may include dietary modifications and careful control of fluid intake.

Complementary Therapy

No significant complementary therapy is indicated.

 CLIENT COMMUNICATION

Maintaining proper fluid and electrolyte balance is important. Providing emotional support for the client and family is helpful.

Prognosis

The prognosis is guarded. Before adequate renal function resumes (highly variable period), individuals with acute tubular necrosis may die from cardiovascular complications, gastrointestinal (GI) disorders, blood abnormalities, and infections.

Prevention

Prompt treatment of conditions that can lead to decreased blood flow and/or decreased oxygen to the kidneys can reduce the risk of acute tubular necrosis. Prevention includes avoiding exposure to toxins and careful monitoring of individuals known to be at risk, especially those with diabetes, liver disorders, and cardiac disorders.

NEPHROTIC SYNDROME

ICD-10: N04.9

Description

Nephrotic syndrome is a condition or a complex of signs and symptoms (syndrome) of the basement membrane of the glomerulus. (The basement membrane surrounds each of the many tiny capillaries comprising a glomerulus.) The disease is characterized by severe proteinuria, often to the extent that the body cannot keep up with the protein loss, which is known as **hypoalbuminemia.** The disease is further characterized by **hyperlipemia** (excessive levels of lipids in the blood), **lipiduria** (lipids in the urine), and generalized edema.

Etiology

Nephrotic syndrome may result from a variety of disease processes that can damage the basement membrane of the glomerulus. Between 70% and 75% of nephrotic syndrome cases result from some form of glomerulonephritis. The syndrome also may arise as a consequence of diabetes mellitus, systemic lupus erythematosus, neoplasms, or reactions to drugs or toxins. The disease is occasionally idiopathic in origin.

Signs and Symptoms

Edema around the eyes and in the feet and ankles is the most common symptom, and it may be either slow in onset or sudden. As body fluid accumulates, clients may experience shortness of breath and anorexia. **Ascites** (abnormal accumulation of fluid in the peritoneal cavity), hypertension, **pallor,** and fatigue may result.

Diagnostic Procedures

Nephrotic syndrome may be difficult to diagnose. Urinalysis may reveal proteinuria and increased waxy, fatty, granular casts. Blood serum tests may show decreased albumin levels and increased cholesterol. Renal biopsy may be important to reach a definitive diagnosis.

Treatment

Treatment is symptomatic and supportive and preserves renal function. An attempt is made to manage edema and hyperlipemia. A moderate-protein diet, vitamin supplementation, and salt restriction may be prescribed. Any underlying disease or condition determined to be responsible for the nephrotic syndrome must be treated as well. Corticosteroids, immunosuppressive, antihypertensive, and diuretic medications may be prescribed. Some people recover spontaneously; others require treatment for life.

Complementary Therapy

No significant complementary therapy is indicated.

 CLIENT COMMUNICATION

It is important to encourage clients to routinely check their urine protein level. A dietitian referral can assist with a diet. High activity and exercise are important, as is careful skin care, especially during the edema phase.

Prognosis

The prognosis varies according to the underlying cause and the client's age. The prognosis is good for children. With adults, nephrotic syndrome is frequently a manifestation of a serious, progressive kidney disorder or of a disorder elsewhere in the body leading to renal failure. Renal vein thrombosis is a complication that significantly worsens the prognosis.

Prevention

Nephrotic syndrome is sometimes avoided through prompt diagnosis and treatment of underlying disorders that can produce this syndrome.

POLYCYSTIC KIDNEY DISEASE

ICD-10: Q61.3

Description

Polycystic kidney disease is a developmental defect of the collecting tubules in the cortex of the kidneys. Groups of tubules that fail to empty properly into the renal pelvis slowly swell into multiple grapelike, fluid-filled sacs or cysts. The pressure from the expanding cysts slowly destroys adjacent normal tissue, progressively impairing kidney function. Both kidneys are usually affected and are grossly enlarged. Polycystic kidney disease is one of the most common hereditary diseases in the United States, affecting more than 500,000 people. It is the cause of nearly 10% of end-stage renal disease and affects men, women, and all races equally.

Etiology

There are two forms of the disease, each due to a genetic defect. The more common adult form, usually manifested during midlife, is an autosomal-dominant defect. The much less common infant and childhood forms, manifested at birth or during childhood, are autosomal-recessive defects. The following discussion pertains to the more frequently occurring adult form.

Signs and Symptoms

The disease is usually asymptomatic until midlife. Then clients may complain of colic and lumbar pain or mention seeing blood in the urine. The pain is generally from the enlarging cysts. Clients may complain of headaches, have UTIs, or pass renal calculi. The onset is insidious, or occurs slowly with few or unnoticeable symptoms.

Diagnostic Procedures

The history may reveal a family tendency toward renal disease. The physical examination may reveal palpably enlarged kidneys and **hypertension,** or persistently high arterial blood pressure. The primary care provider likely orders ultrasound examination or CT scan to detect enlarged kidneys and the presence of cysts. Ultrasonography and CT scans or MRI are able to detect small cysts. Urinalysis may be ordered to evaluate renal function and to detect **hematuria,** or blood in the urine.

Treatment

No treatment will stop the course of the disease; however, treatment attempts to minimize the symptoms. Treatment goals include preventing or managing UTIs and controlling secondary hypertension. Urine cultures should be performed at regular intervals to detect infection and allow for antibiotic therapy. In the event of renal failure, renal dialysis or kidney transplantation may be attempted to prolong life.

Complementary Therapy

No significant complementary therapy is indicated, but drinking lots of fluids may help prevent obstructive clots in the urinary tract.

 CLIENT COMMUNICATION

Ensure that clients understand the disease, and assist them to maintain a supportive environment. Inform clients and their families how to avoid UTIs; provide information on kidney dialysis and transplantation if requested.

Prognosis

The prognosis is variable yet poor because there is no cure. Kidney function is progressively impaired, leading to renal failure, a toxic condition, or **uremia** (creatinine and urea in the blood), and eventual death, usually within 10 years.

Prevention

No prevention is known. Genetic counseling is indicated for first-degree relatives of infected persons or for families at risk. Taking steps to avoid chronic UTIs can be helpful in delaying the disease progression. Managing hypertension is essential.

END-STAGE RENAL DISEASE

ICD-10: N18.6

Description

End-stage renal disease (ESRD), usually the result of chronic renal failure, is the gradual, progressive deterioration of kidney function to the point that the kidneys cannot sustain their necessary day-to-day life activity. As the kidney tissue is progressively destroyed, the kidney loses its ability to excrete the nitrogenous end products of metabolism, such as urea and creatinine, which accumulate in the blood and eventually reach toxic levels.

As kidney function diminishes, every organ in the body is affected, and dialysis or kidney transplantation is eventually needed for survival.

Etiology

Causes of ESRD include diabetes mellitus (leading cause), hypertension, chronic glomerulonephritis, pyelonephritis, obstruction of the urinary tract, congenital anomalies such as polycystic kidneys, vascular disorders, infections, medications, and toxic agents.

Signs and Symptoms

The early signs and symptoms are oliguria and **azotemia**, or the presence of nitrogenous compounds in increased amounts in the blood; electrolyte imbalance and metabolic acidosis follow. Eventually, clients may complain of drowsiness and lethargy, weight loss, easy bruising or bleeding, decreased sensation in the hands and feet, hiccups, pruritus, and decreased urine output. The individual with ESRD also may have decreased alertness and appear mentally confused. The skin may be pallid and scaly. The severity of signs and symptoms varies depending on the extent of the renal damage and remaining function, any underlying conditions, and the person's age.

Diagnostic Procedures

The client may have a long history of chronic renal disease or other predisposing disorder. The physical examination may reveal one or more of the presenting signs and symptoms, along with hypertension. Blood testing of creatinine and BUN typically reveals elevated serum creatinine and potassium levels, along with decreased hemoglobin and hematocrit. Urine output decreases or stops completely.

Treatment

Dialysis or kidney transplantation are the only treatments for ESRD. The client's physical condition and other factors determine which one is used. Other treatment is generally used to assist the body in compensating for the existing impairment and guarding against complications; however, this treatment is unlikely to work without dialysis or a transplant. Hypertension must be controlled, usually with an ACE inhibitor or angiotensin receptor blocker. Dietary restrictions of protein, sodium, and potassium intake may be necessary. Blood transfusions may be needed to control anemia.

Dialysis

The blood of an individual experiencing acute or chronic renal failure typically contains high concentrations of metabolic waste products. Dialysis may be attempted to remove these wastes. In its broadest sense, dialysis is a process in which water-soluble substances diffuse across a semipermeable membrane. Most clients undergo 9 to 12 hours of dialysis per week, equally divided among several sessions. Factors determining the amount of dialysis include the client's size, dietary intake, illnesses, and remaining renal function. Three methods are currently used to dialyze the blood: peritoneal dialysis, hemodialysis, and continuous renal replacement therapy (CRRT):

Peritoneal dialysis. This uses a person's own peritoneum as the dialyzing membrane. A plastic tube is inserted through the client's abdomen into the peritoneal cavity and sutured in place. A dialyzing fluid is passed through the tube into the person's peritoneal cavity and left there for a prescribed period. During this time, wastes diffuse across the peritoneal membrane into the fluid. The contaminated fluid is then drained and replaced with fresh solution. This process can be performed manually or automatically by machine; generally, it is repeated three times a week or as often as required. This type of dialysis may be continuous or intermittent and is easier for individuals to perform themselves than hemodialysis.

Hemodialysis (extracorporeal hemodialysis). In this process, blood is drawn outside the person's body for dialysis in an artificial kidney, or dialyzer, and then returned to the individual via tubes connected to the person's circulatory system. This form of dialysis treatment takes from 3 to 5 hours, about half the time of peritoneal dialysis. It is the most common form and the preferred dialysis method in cases of acute renal failure.

Continuous renal replacement therapy. There are several types of CRRT, which are generally used in critical care units. It is used in persons who are clinically unstable and can be started quickly in hospitals with dialysis machines. An extremely porous blood filter containing a semipermeable membrane is used in all methods.

Kidney Transplantation

Kidney transplantation has become the treatment of choice for ESRD. The donor of a kidney can be either a close relative of the person receiving the kidney or a recently deceased person (cadaver donor). If the donor and recipient are related, the graft has a better chance of survival.

Every transplanted kidney contains antigens foreign to the recipient unless it is donated by an identical twin. Once the donor antigens are in the recipient, a rejection process begins in which the recipient's immune system produces antibodies that lead to the destruction of the tissue of the transplanted kidney. Immunosuppressive drugs may be administered to combat this process. Still, some recipients may reject the kidney. Once rejection occurs, the donated kidney is removed, and the client must resume dialysis.

For those persons who do not reject the donor kidney, life can seem relatively normal. Immunosuppressive drugs must be continued indefinitely, however, making the person more susceptible to infections and other diseases. Sometimes, too, the underlying disease process that destroyed the original kidney will destroy the donor kidney.

There are not enough organs available for everyone who suffers from ESRD. In October 2014, the United Network for Organ Sharing, a national nonprofit organization (http://www.unos.org), reported that nearly 124,000 people are waiting for kidney transplants in the United States, but only 16,884 transplants had been performed by that same date.

Complementary Therapy

No significant complementary therapy is indicated.

> ### ⊙➔ CLIENT COMMUNICATION
>
> A dietitian will provide useful information on a "kidney-friendly" diet according to the progression of ESRD. There is often the need for low-sodium, low-protein, and low-potassium diet with vitamin supplements. Giving emotional support to the client and family is paramount. Make certain that clients are up-to-date on important vaccinations.

Prognosis

The prognosis is guarded even with transplantation because of the alteration in function of virtually every organ system in the body. A variety of complications often cause death before complete kidney failure occurs. Chief among these are infections; others include a spectrum of cardiovascular, blood, and GI abnormalities.

Prevention

No prevention is known other than prompt treatment of underlying disorders and chronic kidney disease that may eventually lead to ESRD.

CHAPTER EPISODE—PART III

Peter began to feel much better once dialysis began. He and his wife discussed their options with Peter's nephrologist and considered what they believed to be the best course of treatment at the time. They learned that some dialysis centers have a reputation of being unprofessional, even rough on their clients. They know others are filled with compassionate and well-trained individuals whose only thought is the very best care of their clients. Home dialysis might be an option down the road, but Peter's wife is still working and hopes to do so for 3 more years. Someone needs to be present while Peter is on home dialysis. Fortunately, Peter is a writer and he has made a pretty good living from it. He will still be able to continue his writing, perhaps not reducing any of it at all.

- What might Peter and his wife choose?
- What would you want to do if you found yourself in need of dialysis? Justify your response.

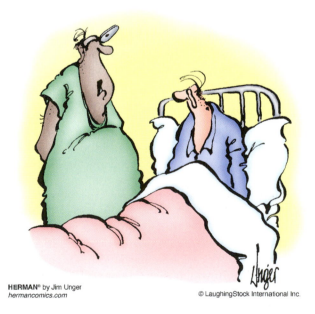

HERMAN® by Jim Unger
hermancomics.com   © LaughingStock International Inc.

"There's a guy in the next ward who wants to buy one of your kidneys."

HERMAN© is reprinted with permission from LaughingStock Licensing Inc., Ottawa, Canada. All rights reserved.

Other Urinary Diseases and Disorders

NEUROGENIC OR OVERACTIVE BLADDER

ICD-10: N31.9

Description

Neurogenic bladder refers to any loss or impairment of bladder function caused by central nervous system injury or by damage to nerves supplying the bladder. Overactive bladder function may be manifested as either **incontinence** (loss of voluntary control of **micturition**) or loss of the autonomic reflex, producing the sensation that the bladder is full. This is also referred to as *urinary incontinence*.

Etiology

Neurogenic bladder may present in one of the following two ways: (1) specific bladder dysfunction in which the neurological lesions are above sacral nerves S2 through S4 or (2) flaccid bladder dysfunction in which the lesions are below sacral nerves S2 through S4. Physical trauma to the spinal cord is a frequent cause of neurogenic bladder. This condition may also arise as a consequence of multiple sclerosis, dementia, and Parkinson disease or from chronic alcoholism or heavy-metal poisoning. Metabolic disorders (e.g., diabetes mellitus or hypothyroidism) and collagen diseases (e.g., systemic lupus erythematosus) may cause overactive bladder. UTIs, cancer, kidney stones, and an enlarged prostate can cause overactive bladder as well.

Signs and Symptoms

An individual may complain of mild to severe urinary incontinence or the inability to control the passage of urine, inability to empty the bladder completely, difficulty in starting or stopping voiding, and bladder spasms.

Diagnostic Procedures

A detailed history and a physical examination that includes a neurological evaluation are essential. Special tests that may be ordered include cystourethrography to evaluate bladder function, a urine flow study to assess urine flow, and sphincter electromyography to evaluate how well the bladder and urinary sphincter muscles work together. The skull, spine, and urinary tract may be imaged by x-ray, MRI, or CT scan to aid in diagnosis.

Treatment

Treatment goals include preventing complications from UTIs and controlling incontinence through learning special bladder evacuation techniques. The PCP may recommend one of two common methods of evacuation to clients who are unable to empty the bladder completely. In Credé method, the client presses on the lower abdomen while voiding. The second method, intermittent self-catheterization, requires the client to insert a catheter into his or her bladder through the urethra. Medications to relax the bladder may be prescribed to relieve episodes of incontinence. These drugs include tolterodine (Detrol), oxybutynin (Ditropan), trospium (Sanctura), solifenacin (Vesicare), and darifenacin (Enablex). Surgeries to aid in the control of urine may be necessary. Any underlying diseases that are detected will be treated.

Complementary Therapy

Biofeedback may be useful for teaching some aspects of bladder control.

REALITY EPISODE

Sadie has urinary incontinence. It is very embarrassing for her. She leaks urine every time she sneezes—a frequent occurrence during allergy season. Sometimes she must launder her bedding two to three times a week. She plans to visit her sister, who is recovering from surgery, and hopes to lessen the incontinence. She visits with the nurse-practitioner at her clinic about the issue.

What are some of the steps Sadie might take to lessen her incontinence?

CLIENT COMMUNICATION

Teach clients bladder evacuation techniques. Provide emotional support for both the client and family.

Prognosis

The prognosis depends on whether the damage to the nerves supplying the bladder is reversible. Such complications as UTIs and the formation of renal calculi worsen the prognosis. If the disorder is of the form in which sensation of a full bladder is lost, urine may back up, causing hydronephrosis and possible renal failure.

Prevention

There is no specific prevention other than prompt treatment of diseases that may produce the nerve damage that leads to neurogenic bladder.

Cancers of the Urinary System

BLADDER CANCER

 ICD-10: C67.X*

Description

Tumors of the bladder arise from the epithelial cell membrane lining the bladder interior. These neoplasms are almost always malignant, and they metastasize readily. Bladder tumors are staged according to their depth of penetration. Transitional cell carcinoma is the most common type of bladder cancer in the United States.

Etiology

The cause of bladder tumors is unknown; however, cigarette smoking is thought to be the predominant cause.

The X represents the fourth digit that is often required and supplied once more detailed information about the disease or disorder is made known to the provider.

Predisposing factors may include exposure to certain types of industrial chemicals and/or radiation. Individuals with chronic cystitis also seem prone to developing bladder tumors. The disease affects men three times more frequently than women and generally occurs between ages 50 and 70. Bladder cancer is the fourth most common cancer in men.

Signs and Symptoms

Many persons are asymptomatic until advanced stages of the disease. For those presenting with symptoms, however, painless, gross hematuria is the most common indicator. Less frequently, the individual may complain of dysuria, urinary frequency and urgency, or nocturia. UTIs are a common complication.

Diagnostic Procedures

The history may reveal occupational exposure to certain industrial chemicals and/or radiation. A complete physical examination and a urinalysis to detect hematuria are performed. Microscopic urinalysis may reveal cancer cells. Cystoscopy and biopsy of the suspected lesions are usually required to reach a definite diagnosis. A bone scan, CT scan, and MRI will help determine possible metastases and staging of the cancer.

Treatment

The choice of treatment is based on the extent of the disease. If the disease is superficial, an endoscopic resection may be all that is necessary. If it is invasive, further surgery is required. The tumor may be surgically removed through fulguration (electrical destruction) or **transurethral resection,** a surgical procedure in which cancerous tissue is removed from the bladder using an instrument passed through the urethra. For advanced cases, removal of the urinary bladder, or radical **cystectomy,** may be required, followed by radiation, immunotherapy, or chemotherapy treatment.

Complementary Therapy

Some therapies to help clients live more comfortably with both symptoms of the disease and side effects of treatment include meditation, whole-foods nutrition, yoga, tai chi, acupuncture, and guided imagery.

⊙ CLIENT COMMUNICATION

Inform clients of all options for treatment, possible surgical techniques, follow-up care, and the possibility of recurrence. Because of the risk of recurrence, bladder cancer survivors often undergo follow-up screening tests for years after treatment.

Prognosis

The prognosis varies depending on the depth of penetration of the tumor. Although the immediate prognosis for an individual with a superficial bladder tumor may be good, there is still a great likelihood of recurrence within 3 years. When the tumor penetrates the bladder more deeply or has metastasized, the prognosis is poor, with a low 5-year survival rate.

Prevention

The best prevention is to minimize risk factors by suggesting clients protect themselves from exposure to industrial chemicals, that they not smoke, and that they seek treatment for all UTIs.

RENAL CELL CARCINOMA OR KIDNEY CANCER

ICD-10: C64.X

Description

Renal cell carcinoma (RCC), also known as *renal cell adenocarcinoma,* is by far the most common type of kidney cancer, accounting for 90% of kidney cancers. RCC usually grows as a single mass within the kidney but can be found in more than one part of the kidney or in both kidneys. It occurs most often in individuals over age 40.

Etiology

The cause is essentially unknown; however, risk factors include smoking, obesity, hypertension, long-term dialysis, and exposure to chemicals and irritants, such as asbestos or cadmium in the workplace.

Signs and Symptoms

Symptoms may include hematuria, flank or side pain that does not go away, a lump or mass palpated in the side or abdomen, weight loss, and fever. Some clients report feeling listless and not well.

Diagnostic Procedures

A complete physical examination may reveal an enlarged mass. BUN and creatinine levels are checked. A CT scan or MRI using contrast media is often used in diagnosis, as is the intravenous pyelogram (IVP). A solid tumor can also be detected by ultrasound. In some cases, a biopsy to remove tissue cells is necessary.

Treatment

Treatment protocol most likely is determined by the stage and the spread of the cancer. Surgery is the most commonly chosen form of treatment, removing either part or all of the diseased kidney. Arterial embolization may be used. This treatment involves passing a catheter into the renal artery that supplies blood to the kidney. A substance is injected to block the flow of blood, preventing the cancer from receiving the oxygen it needs to grow. Radiation therapy, immunotherapy, and chemotherapy may also be considered.

Complementary Therapy

There is no known complementary treatment that will cure the cancer. However, a number of therapies may make traditional treatment easier to withstand. See Complementary Therapy under Bladder Cancer; also see Chapter 5.

 CLIENT COMMUNICATION

Help clients understand how important it is to maintain a nutritious and high-calorie diet even though food does not taste good to them. Provide recipe material or referral to the National Cancer Institute for their booklet "Eating Hints for Cancer Patients."

Prognosis

Prognosis for RCC or kidney cancer depends on how far the cancer has spread. In the early stage, the 5-year survival rate is 70% to 80%. If the cancer has spread to the lymph nodes, the 5-year survival rate drops to 5% to 15%. If it has spread to other organs, the 5-year survival rate is as low as 8%.

Prevention

The only possible prevention is for clients to avoid the risk factors. It is best if clients maintain a healthy weight and do not smoke.

COMMON SYMPTOMS OF URINARY SYSTEM DISEASES AND DISORDERS

Individuals may present with the following common complaints, which deserve attention from health-care professionals:

- Any change in normal urinary patterns, such as nocturia, hematuria, pyuria, proteinuria, dysuria, or urgency and frequency

- Pain in the lumbar region or flank pain, varying from slight tenderness to intense pain
- Fever
- Nausea and vomiting or anorexia
- Malaise, fatigue, and lethargy

Serious urinary system diseases also may produce circulatory system and respiratory system symptoms. These symptoms might include hypertension, edema, ascites, and shortness of breath.

SUMMARY

Diseases and disorders of the urinary system can be troubling and uncomfortable or very serious and debilitating in nature. Millions of individuals are affected by urinary diseases in the United States. Urologists (specialists in the field of urology) and nephrologists (kidney specialists) are often called into attendance for those affected by urinary diseases and disorders.

 DavisPlus | For more resources and to sharpen your skills with interactive exercises, visit DavisPlus at http://davisplus.fadavis.com. Keyword *Tamparo*.

ONLINE RESOURCES

Bladder cancer
http://www.cancer.gov/cancertopics/pdq/treatment/bladder/Patient

Cystitis and urethritis
http://www.onlinemedicare.org/diseases/cystitis-and-urethritis.html

Eating hints for cancer patients
http://www.cancer.gov/cancertopics/eatinghints

National Kidney Foundation
http://www.kidney.org

CASE STUDIES

Case Study 1

A 27-year-old man named Carlos Santiago comes into an ambulatory care facility complaining of extreme flank pain and frequent urination. The PCP asks if Carlos has noted any difference in the color or appearance of his urine, and Carlos reports that he has noted some bits that look like sand in his urine. Carlos also says he recently was treated for a urinary tract infection.

Case Study Questions
1. What diagnostic tests might be ordered?
2. What are some effective preventative measures for urinary disease?

Case Study 2

Trang Ngoc, a 35-year-old woman, reports pain on urination, pain in the pubic area, and the need for frequent urination. Trang also says that the need to urinate is urgent and that her urine is foul smelling.

Case Study Questions
1. When Trang comes to the ambulatory care setting, what questions will you ask?
2. What tests might be ordered for diagnosis?
3. What preventative measure might Trang take in the future?

REVIEW QUESTIONS

Matching

Match the following by placing the correct letter in the column.

_____ 1. Nocturia

_____ 2. APSGN

_____ 3. Ascites

_____ 4. Uremia

_____ 5. Micturition

_____ 6. Pruritus

_____ 7. Pyuria

_____ 8. Oliguria

_____ 9. Hematuria

a. Acute poststreptococcal glomerulonephritis

b. Accumulation of serous fluid in abdominal cavity

c. Blood in urine

d. Urination

e. Excessive urination at night

f. Scanty urine

g. Urine in the blood

h. Pus in urine

i. Itching

Short Answer

1. What is the name of a disease that exhibits multiple, grapelike, fluid-filled sacs or cysts in the kidney cortex?

   _____

2. When the body cannot keep up with the loss of protein in the urine, what is the result called?

   _____

3. What is another name for chronic renal failure?

   _____

4. Intense pain with urinary frequency, nausea, vomiting, fever, hematuria, and flank pain may indicate what disease? _____

5. A disorder, often difficult to diagnose, that is related to some kind of nerve dysfunction of the bladder is referred to by what name? _____

6. Can you name the most common type of kidney disease? _____

7. What might headaches from secondary hypertension and puffy eyes due to edema from leaky capillaries indicate? _____

8. What is the meaning of the abbreviation UTI?

   _____

Multiple Choice

Place a checkmark next to the correct answer.

1. What is the main function of the kidneys?

   _____ a. They regulate body fluids, blood pressure, and filter wastes.

   _____ b. They filter wastes from the urine.

   _____ c. They store urine until it is time to be emptied.

   _____ d. They house the renal tubules and the ureters for passage of waste products.

2. What percentage of the fluid that passes through the nephron becomes urine?

   _____ a. 50%

   _____ b. 5%

   _____ c. 10%

   _____ d. 1%

3. What is commonly known about urinary tract infections?

   _____ a. They are commonly caused by a virus.

   _____ b. They are often characterized by dysuria, urgency, and frequency.

   _____ c. They are more common in men due to the length of the urethra.

   _____ d. They only respond to long-term antibiotic therapy.

4. Can you name the three forms of dialysis?

   _____ a. Peritoneal, hemodialysis, and CRRT

   _____ b. Perineal, hemodialysis, and ESRD

   _____ c. Peritoneal, extracorporeal, and CRRT

   _____ d. Perineal, extracorporeal, and ATN

5. What is the term used to describe the inability to control urine excretion?

   _____ a. Ischemia

   _____ b. Micturition

   _____ c. Incontinence

   _____ d. Anuria

Discussion Questions/Personal Reflection

1. Research the cost of kidney transplantation and the involvement of Medicare. List and comment on at least three facts you learned.

_____

_____

_____

_____

_____

_____

_____

_____

2. Discuss the differences and similarities of the three types of dialysis and when a particular type might be chosen. Explain the rationale. Although not discussed in the text, what will the client need to do when traveling?

_____

_____

_____

_____

_____

_____

_____

_____

_____

_____

Nobody will ever win the battle of the sexes. There's too much fraternizing with the enemy.
—HENRY A. KISSINGER

16

Reproductive System Diseases and Disorders

● *chapter outline*

(chapter outline continued)

● key words

Anovulation (an"ov"yū•lā'shŏn)
Anuria (ăn•ū'rē•ă)
Cervicitis (sĕr•vĭ•sī'tĭs)
Chancre (shăng'kĕr)
Conization (kŏn•ĭ•zā'shŭn)
Cryoablation (krī"o•ab•la'shŭn)
**Dilation and curettage
(D&C)** (dī•lā'•shŭn ănd
kū'rĕ•tăzh)
Effacement (ē•făs'mĕnt)
**Epididymis (pl.
epididymides)**
(ĕp"ĭ•dĭd'ĭ•mĭs, ĕp"ĭ•dĭd'ĭ
•mĭ•dēz)

Hysterosalpingography
(hĭs"tĕr•ō•săl"pĭn•gŏg'ră•fē)
Leiomyoma (lī"ō•mī•ō'mă)
Lochia (lō'kē•ă)
Meiosis (mī•ō'sĭs)
Menarche (mĕn•ăr'kē)
Metrorrhea (me"trō•rē'ă)
Nystagmus (nĭs•tăg'mŭs)
Oogenesis (ō"ō•jĕn'ĕ•sĭs)
Orchiectomy (ŏr-kē-'ek-tə-mē)
**Panhysterosalpingo-
oophorectomy**
(păn•hĭs"tĕr•ō•săl"pĭng•gō-ō"
ŏf•ō•rēk'tō•mē)

Parturition (păr•tū•rĭsh'ŭn)
Primigravida (prī"mĭ•grăv'ĭ•dă)
Prostaglandin (prŏs"tă•glăn'dĭn)
Purulent (pūr'ū•lĕnt)
Rhonchus (pl. rhonchi)
(rŏng'kŭs)
Spermatogenesis
(spĕr"măt•ō•jĕn'ĕ•sĭs)
Teratoma (tĕr•ă•tō'mă)
Varicocele (văr'ĭ•kō•sēl)

● learning outcomes

Upon successful completion of this chapter, you will be able to:

• Identify key terms.
• Describe the anatomy and physiology of the reproductive system.
• Discuss sexual health.
• Recall the factors that contribute to infertility.
• Identify six sexually transmitted diseases (STDs).
• Compare and contrast the causes of STDs.
• Recall prevention strategies for STDs.
• Identify the diseases related to the prostate gland.
• Discuss the complications of prostate-related disorders.
• Restate the common causes of epididymitis.
• Describe the treatment for prostatic and testicular cancers.
• Differentiate premenstrual syndrome (PMS) from premenstrual dysphoric disorder (PMDD).
• Identify possible causes of amenorrhea.
• Discuss treatment for dysmenorrhea.
• Name the characteristic signs and symptoms of ovarian cysts or tumors.
• Identify a primary complication of endometriosis.

• Recall signs and symptoms of uterine leiomyomas.
• Name the causes of pelvic inflammatory disease.
• Discuss complementary therapy for menopause symptoms.
• Identify the advantages and disadvantages of hormone replacement therapy (HRT).
• Describe ovarian cancer and its signs and symptoms.
• Restate the description of fibrocystic breasts.
• Identify and describe benign fibroadenoma.
• Recall treatment protocols for breast cancer.
• Discuss breast reconstruction.
• Recall the possible causes of spontaneous abortion.
• Define *ectopic pregnancy.*
• Compare and contrast preeclampsia with eclampsia.
• Compare and contrast placenta previa with abruptio placentae.
• Describe premature rupture of membranes (PROM).
• Recall common symptoms of the reproductive system diseases and disorders.

CHAPTER EPISODE—PART I

Allison started having menses at the age of 12. The early years of her menses were extremely painful, and it was getting persistently worse. Now in her 20s, her periods are irregular and still extremely painful.

- What other symptoms might she be having?
- Should she seek medical attention?

REPRODUCTIVE SYSTEM ANATOMY AND PHYSIOLOGY REVIEW

The reproductive system functions to continue the human species; hence, the organs of the system are usually classified into two groups: gonads (testes and ovaries), which produce germ cells, and hormones within their duct system that are used for the transportation of the germ cells. Cell division, called **meiosis,** produces gametes, or the sperm and the ovum. The gametes each contain half the number of chromosomes (23) necessary to produce an offspring. If fertilization occurs, the nuclei of the sperm and ovum fuse and produce a zygote with the full chromosome complement (46). The ductal system of the female transports, nourishes, and grows the fertilized ovum.

Spermatogenesis is regulated by hormones and occurs in the seminiferous tubules in the testes. The follicle-stimulating hormone (FSH) from the anterior pituitary gland initiates sperm production. In addition, the anterior pituitary's luteinizing hormone (LH) stimulates the production of testosterone, which is secreted by the testes to promote the maturation of the sperm.

Beginning at puberty (ages 10 to 14 in males), millions of sperm are produced daily and are only gradually diminished in advancing age.

Oogenesis, also regulated by hormones, begins in the ovaries. FSH initiates the growth of the ovarian follicles and stimulates the follicles to secrete estrogen to mature the ovum. Ova production begins at puberty (ages 10 to 14 in females) and continues until menopause (ages 45 to 55) when the ovaries atrophy. A mature ovum is produced about every 28 days during this time period.

MALE REPRODUCTIVE SYSTEM

The male reproductive system consists of the testes and a series of ducts and glands (Fig. 16.1). During ejaculation, the sperm is transported through the epididymis, ductus deferens, ejaculatory duct, and urethra. The male reproductive glands—the seminal vesicles, prostate gland, and bulbourethral glands—produce fluid secretions that become part of the semen. The urethra is the final duct through which the semen passes, and its longest portion is enclosed within the penis, an external genital organ.

The testes are located in the scrotum where the temperature is about 96°F, the temperature necessary for viable sperm production. Each testis, about 1.5 inches long and 1 inch wide, is divided into lobes housing the seminiferous tubules. Spermatogenesis takes place in these tubules. The **epididymides** are tubes about 20 feet in length that are coiled on the posterior surface of the testes. In the epididymis, sperm maturation is completed and sperm is propelled into the vas deferens. The vas deferens ducts carry the sperm to the ejaculatory ducts where the secretions to create semen are received from the seminal vesicles (fructose for energy), the

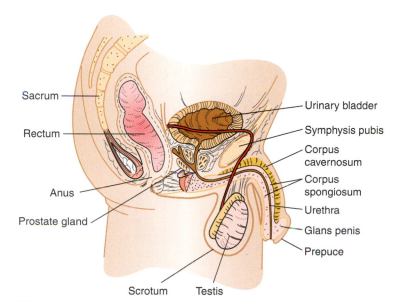

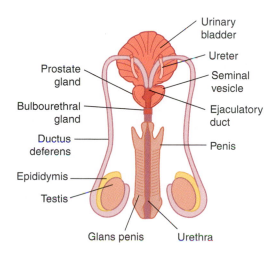

Figure 16.1 Male reproductive system.

prostate gland (alkaline fluid for motility), and the bul-bourethral glands (to coat the urethra and neutralize any acidic urine present). The urethra, enclosed in the penis, is the last duct through which semen travels. The urethra releases urine during micturition and expels semen upon ejaculation. The penis is the external genital organ that becomes engorged with blood during sexual stimulation, causing it to become erect and firm. The erect penis is able to enter the vagina during sexual intercourse to deposit semen. Approximately 2 to 4 milliliters of semen are expelled during ejaculation; each milliliter contains about 100 million sperm cells.

FEMALE REPRODUCTIVE SYSTEM

The female reproductive system consists of the paired ovaries and fallopian tubes, the uterus, the vagina, and the external genital structures (Fig. 16.2). The egg cells, or ova, are produced in the ovaries and travel through the fallopian tubes to the uterus, where a fertilized ovum can implant and grow. The ovaries produce hormones necessary for the secondary sex characteristics and for maintenance of pregnancy. The breasts or mammary glands are accessory organs of the reproductive system that are able to provide milk for the infant.

The ovaries are oval structures about 1 inch long, each housing several hundred thousand primary follicles present at birth. Close to 400 of these follicles will produce mature ova. The mature follicle responds to LH from the anterior pituitary, causing ovulation. During this time, the ruptured follicle, at this stage called the *corpus luteum,* secretes progesterone and estrogen. The corpus luteum, now called the *ovum,* is pulled into one of the two fallopian tubes where it is propelled toward the uterus. Each fallopian tube is about 4 inches in length and is composed of ciliated epithelial tissue capable of

moving the ovum toward the uterus. Fertilization usually occurs in the fallopian tubes; if it does not, the ovum dies within 24 to 48 hours. The fertilized ovum becomes a zygote and is swept into the uterus in about 4 to 5 days.

The uterus is pear shaped and is about 3 inches long and 2 inches wide. During pregnancy, the uterus expands significantly to allow the developing fetus to grow. The upper portion of the uterus is called the *fundus;* the *body* is the central part, and the *cervix* is the lower end of the uterus. The two-layer lining of the uterus is the endometrium. One layer is permanent, but the other layer, known as the *functional layer,* is regenerated and lost during each menstrual cycle. Under the hormonal action of estrogen and progesterone, blood vessel growth thickens the functional layer in preparation for a possible pregnancy. If fertilization does not occur, this layer sloughs off in menstruation. During pregnancy, the endometrium also forms the maternal portion of the placenta.

The vagina is a muscular tube about 4 inches in length that extends from the cervix to the vaginal opening in the perineum. It is posterior to the urethra and anterior to the rectum. The vagina receives the penis and its semen during sexual intercourse, provides the exit for menstrual flow, and is the birth canal at the end of pregnancy. The vulva (Fig. 16.3) includes the clitoris, labia majora and minora, and Bartholin glands. The clitoris is erectile tissue that responds to sexual stimulation. The Bartholin glands keep the mucosa of the vagina moist and lubricated during sexual intercourse. Both the labia majora and minora are paired folds of skin on either side of the urethral and vaginal openings that prevent drying of their mucous membranes.

The mammary glands of the breast (Fig. 16.4) produce milk to nourish the infant. After birth, the alveolar glands produce milk that enters the lactiferous ducts on

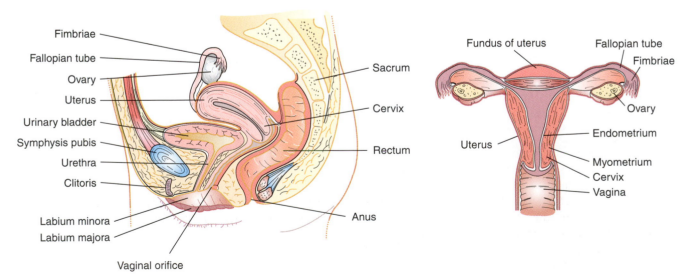

Figure 16.2 Female reproductive system.

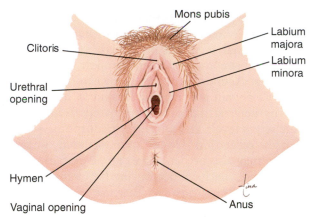

Figure 16.3 Vulva of female external genitals; inferior view of the perineum. *(From Scanlon, VC, and Sanders, T: Essentials of Anatomy and Physiology, ed. 6. Philadelphia: F.A. Davis, 2011, p 497, with permission.)*

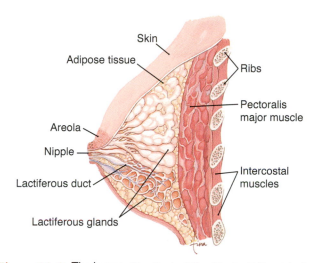

Figure 16.4 The breast. *(From Scanlon, VC, and Sanders, T: Essentials of Anatomy and Physiology, ed. 6. Philadelphia: F.A. Davis, 2011, p 498, with permission.)*

its way to the nipple. Milk formation is dependent on hormone action of prolactin from the anterior pituitary. Also, the infant's sucking at the nipple stimulates the hypothalamus to send impulses to the posterior pituitary gland to secrete oxytocin, causing the release of milk. The pigmented area around the nipple is called the *areola*.

SEXUAL HEALTH

The only mammals known to express caring and loving in the sexual act are human beings. For males and females, the function of sexuality is twofold—reproduction and the enhancement of caring and pleasure.

The World Health Organization identifies *sexual health* as a state of physical, emotional, mental, and social well-being related to sexuality; it is not merely the absence of disease, dysfunction, or infirmity. Sexual health requires a positive and respectful approach to sexuality and sexual relationships, as well as the possibility of having pleasurable and safe sexual experiences, free of coercion, discrimination, and violence. For sexual health to be attained and maintained, the sexual rights of all persons are to be respected, protected, and fulfilled. Refer to Chapter 7 for additional information pertinent to this chapter.

Infertility

MALE INFERTILITY AND FEMALE INFERTILITY

ICD-10: N46.9 (MALE INFERTILITY)
ICD-10: N97.9 (FEMALE INFERTILITY)

Description

Infertility is defined as the failure to become pregnant after 1 year of regular, unprotected intercourse, even after one or more pregnancies. According to the Centers for Disease Control and Prevention (CDC), 2.1 million couples experience infertility or other conditions that impair their ability to have children. Female fertility normally peaks at age 24 and diminishes after age 30, with pregnancy occurring rarely after age 50. Hormonal balances, the ovulation cycle, and vaginal secretions determine female fertility. A female is most fertile within 24 hours of ovulation.

Male fertility usually peaks at age 25 and declines after age 40. Sperm count, semen composition, and bodily hormonal changes affect male fertility. The greatest fertility for a male occurs when he has sexual intercourse four times a week.

Etiology

Causes of infertility in females include hormonal problems, nutritional deficiencies, infections, tumors, and anomalies of the reproductive organs, such as cervical mucous problems, uterine cavity abnormalities, and tubal factors. In males, persistent infertility may be caused by sperm deficiencies, congenital abnormalities, endocrine imbalances, surgical intervention, and infections and chronic inflammation of the testes, epididymis, or vas deferens. In both males and females, advancing age is a factor in fertility. Other causes include heavy alcohol or illegal drug abuse, obesity (especially in women), and radiation exposure. In 10% of the cases, the cause remains unknown.

Signs and Symptoms

Inability to conceive after 1 year of regular, unprotected intercourse is a sign of infertility.

Diagnostic Procedures

In a female, a complete medical, surgical, and gynecologic history and physical examination are essential. The laboratory studies ordered may include urinalysis, complete blood count (CBC), blood hormone levels, and immunologic or antibody testing that detects spermicidal antibodies in the woman's serums. X-rays to visualize the uterus and fallopian tubes, called **hysterosalpingography** (HSG), may be necessary to detect uterine or tubal abnormalities. Endoscopy of the uterus, the endometrium, the fallopian tubes, the ovaries, and the abdominal and pelvic areas may be done. Pelvic ultrasound may be ordered. One test that may be done is an analysis of cervical mucus within 1 hour after coitus to check for motile sperm cells. This test is called the Huhner test. Vaginal smears or an endometrial biopsy may be required. A laparoscopy may be ordered to detect abnormalities of the abdominal and pelvic areas.

In a male, a complete ejaculate following sexual abstinence for 4 days should be examined within 1 to 2 hours of collection. A complete physical examination, including rectal and genital palpation, is essential. The laboratory studies ordered may include a sperm count, CBC, reproductive hormone levels, and urine 17-ketosteroid levels to measure testicular function. Cystoscopy and catheterization of ejaculatory ducts may be ordered to detect any occlusion or stenosis of the tubes. Vasography and seminal vesiculography may be necessary.

Treatment

The treatment of infertility is dependent on the cause. In a female, treatment may include any of the following:

- Salpingostomy
- Lysis of adhesions
- Removal of ovarian abnormalities
- Correction of endocrine imbalance
- Alleviation of **cervicitis** (inflammation of the cervix)
- Hormone therapy
- Microsurgical excision of tubal obstructions

In males, treatment may include any of the following:

- Surgical correction of any abnormality
- Correction of testicular hypofunction secondary to hypothyroidism
- Surgical correction of hydrocele or **varicocele,** which is a dilation of the complex network of veins that comprise part of the spermatic cord to form a palpable swelling within the scrotum
- Hormone therapy

Assisted reproductive technology (ART) may be tried. The technologies include in vitro fertilization (IVF) (the most common method), gamete intrafallopian transfer (GIFT), zygote intrafallopian transfer (ZIFT), and tubal embryo transplant (TET). All of these procedures stimulate the eggs, combine the eggs with sperm, and return the eggs to the female's body. (See the Glossary for definitions of each of the different types of ART.)

Complementary Therapy

Traditional Chinese medicine can work in conjunction with traditional medicine by designing acupuncture treatments that complement and support other medical procedures. Acupuncture treatment can help regulate the body's system and may be helpful to females who have just been artificially inseminated. Acupuncture lowers stress levels and increases endorphins while it enhances relaxation. Meditation, guided imagery, and yoga may also be beneficial. Some practitioners in Eastern medicine have been using herbs for centuries to enhance fertility; however, any use of herbs should be discussed with a primary care provider (PCP).

✈ CLIENT COMMUNICATION

Encourage women to have children during the years when they are most fertile—in their 20s and 30s. Smoking increases the risk of infertility, and as few as five alcoholic drinks a week can impair conception. Being severely overweight or underweight can be a factor in infertility. Female marathon runners and those who exercise excessively are prone to menstrual irregularities and may have problems getting pregnant.

Prognosis

About 60% of the couples treated for infertility achieve pregnancy. Many others undergo fertility treatment using ART; some cases are untreatable. The emotional impact on infertile couples is not to be discounted. Anxiety and depression are often noted.

Prevention

The only prevention of infertility in females and males generally involves avoiding the causative factors leading to acquired infertility, such as infections, drugs and alcohol, trauma, and environmental agents. Infertile couples may suffer loss, and they may experience guilt and anger. Information and support systems can be helpful to some.

Sexually Transmitted Diseases

GONORRHEA

✔ **REPORTABLE DISEASE**

ICD-10: A54.00

Description

Gonorrhea is a contagious bacterial infection of the epithelial surfaces of the genitourinary tract in males and females. In the United States, the gonorrhea rate is 111 cases per 100,000 population. The highest reported cases occur among sexually active teenagers and young adults.

Etiology

Gonorrhea is caused by the bacterium *Neisseria gonorrhoeae*. The disease is transmitted during sexual intercourse with an infected partner or through other forms of intimate sexual contact. The bacterium can grow in the mouth, throat, eyes, and anus. Infants born to infected mothers can contract gonorrhea during vaginal delivery.

Signs and Symptoms

The signs and symptoms of gonorrhea vary according to the site and duration of the infection, the particular characteristics of the infecting strain, and whether the infection remains localized or becomes systemic. It is worth emphasizing, however, that many cases of gonorrhea, especially in females, are asymptomatic or produce symptoms so slight that the infected individual ignores them.

The presenting symptoms of an infected male are typically those of acute urethritis: pus or **purulent** urethral discharge, pain, and urinary frequency. A purulent discharge from the pharynx or rectum with accompanying pain may be the presenting symptom among persons who participate in oral and anal sex.

The symptoms of an infected female are typically those of acute cervicitis: purulent greenish-yellow discharge from the cervix, urinary frequency, and itching and burning pain. Other symptoms may include pelvic pain with muscular rigidity or abdominal tenderness and distention.

In the neonate, gonorrheal ophthalmia neonatorum may result. This is a severe, hyperacute inflammation of the membrane lining the inner surface of the eyelids and covering the white of the eye. Gonorrheal ophthalmia neonatorum may produce a purulent discharge from the eyes 2 to 3 days after birth. Eyelid edema may be evident as well.

Diagnostic Procedures

Bacterial cultures (Gram stain) from the site of infection generally establish the diagnosis. Gonorrhea present in the urethra can be diagnosed by testing a urine sample.

Treatment

Antibiotics are given, but increasing numbers of strains are resistant to penicillin; therefore, a large number of new and very potent antibiotics are necessary, including ceftriaxone (Rocephin), cefixime (Suprax), and ciprofloxacin (Cipro). Many people with gonorrhea also have chlamydia, so testing for other STDs is important. Clients are advised to have a second culture 1 to 2 weeks after the first and an additional culture in about 6 months to ensure that they no longer have the disease.

Complementary Therapy

Emphasize treating the disease and stimulating the immune system. Elimination of fatty foods, sugar, white flour, salt, and caffeine will help to boost the immune system. Vitamins and herbal supplements may be recommended but are not to replace antibiotic therapy.

⊙ CLIENT COMMUNICATION

Practicing safer sex is advised. Remind individuals to take all of their medications and to return for follow-up cultures. Testing of all partners is essential so treatment can begin as necessary.

Prognosis

The prognosis is good with prompt diagnosis and treatment of localized gonorrheal infections. Systemic gonorrheal infections may produce joint destruction or life-threatening complications, such as meningitis or endocarditis. Pelvic inflammatory disease (PID) is a serious complication of gonorrheal infection among women, producing fever, nausea, vomiting, and tachycardia. Men may have epididymitis as a result of gonorrhea.

Prevention

The use of condoms, avoidance of multiple partners, and the tracing of the sexual contacts of an infected individual can prevent the spread of gonorrhea. Instillation of a 1% silver nitrate solution in the eyes of the neonate has reduced the incidence of gonorrheal ophthalmia neonatorum.

GENITAL HERPES

ICD-10: A60.9

Description

Genital, or venereal, herpes is a highly contagious viral infection of the male and female genitalia. Unlike other STDs, genital herpes tends to recur spontaneously. The disease has two stages. During the active stage, characteristic skin lesions and other accompanying symptoms may occur. During the latent stage, the individual is asymptomatic. The incidence of genital herpes is beginning to decline, but at least 45 million individuals over age 12 have it.

Etiology

Genital herpes is caused by the herpes simplex virus (HSV). Two strains of the virus—designated HSV-1 and HSV-2—may produce the disease. Most cases of genital herpes, however, are attributable to HSV-2. The disease is transmitted through direct contact with infected bodily secretions. Infection typically occurs during sexual intercourse, oral-genital sexual activity, kissing, and hand-to-body contact. A particularly life-threatening form of the disease can occur in infants infected by the virus during vaginal birth.

Signs and Symptoms

During the active phase of the disease, males and females may present with characteristic skin lesions on their genitals, mouth, and/or anus (Fig. 16.5). These appear as multiple, shallow ulcerations, pustules, or erythematous vesicles. The diffuse redness of the skin, or erythema, is caused by dilation of the superficial capillaries. The vesicles tend to rupture, causing acute pain and consequent itching. Other generalized symptoms may include fever, headache, malaise, muscle pain, anorexia, and dysuria. Leukorrhea may be a further symptom in females.

Diagnostic Procedures

Physical examination looking for the characteristic lesions is usually sufficient for diagnosis. Scraping and biopsy of the ulceration with evidence of HSV-2 may be required to confirm the diagnosis. Blood tests can detect antibodies to HSV-1 or HSV-2.

Treatment

Acyclovir is an effective treatment for genital herpes. Newer agents include famciclovir and valacyclovir. These drugs will not eradicate the virus, but when taken as soon as an outbreak occurs, they can shut down virus production. Secondary infections need to be prevented or speedily managed. Topical medications may be ordered to reduce edema and pain. Clients are encouraged to keep lesions clean and dry.

Complementary Therapy

Complementary therapy aims to diminish discomfort and hasten recovery. An ice pack applied to sores at the beginning of eruptions can help. Cool compressions or baking soda also soothes lesions. A topical cream made from the *Prunella vulgaris* plant has shown promise in reducing skin lesions.

CLIENT COMMUNICATION

Clients may be embarrassed about their disease; reassure them that they can lead a sexually healthy life so long as they adhere to proper precautions.

Prognosis

Genital herpes cannot be cured. The prognosis varies according to the individual's age, the severity of the infection, the promptness of treatment, and the individual's immunological response. It is estimated that as many as 80% of individuals with primary genital herpes infections will experience a recurrence within 12 months. The virus is also associated with cervical cancer.

Prevention

No proven method of prevention among adults has been established other than avoiding sexual intercourse and other sexually intimate contact with infected individuals when lesions or symptoms of herpes are present and using condoms during all sexual exposure. Transmission of the disease to neonates can be minimized through cesarean delivery when it is known that the mother is infected.

GENITAL HUMAN PAPILLOMAVIRUS (HPV) INFECTION

ICD-10: B97.7

Description

Genital human papillomavirus (HPV) is the most common of the STDs. There are over 40 types that can infect the genital areas of men and women, including the penis; vulva; anus; and the rectal, cervical, and vaginal linings. Genital warts (one type of HPV) are circumscribed, elevated skin lesions, usually seen on the external genitalia or near the anus. Approximately 20 million Americans are currently infected with HPV. Most persons do not realize they are infected or that they are passing the virus to their partner.

Etiology

Genital HPV is typically spread from person to person during intimate sexual contact. A pregnant woman can pass HPV to her neonate during vaginal delivery. Genital warts have a prolonged incubation period of 1 to 6 months and grow rapidly in the presence of heavy perspiration, poor hygiene, or pregnancy.

Signs and Symptoms

Most individuals with HPV do not develop symptoms. However, some types of HPV (usually known

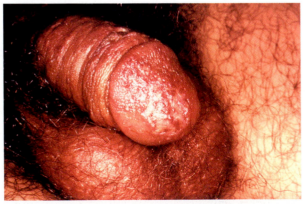
Figure 16.5 Genital herpes on the glans penis and penile shaft.
(Centers for Disease Control and Prevention. Dr. N. J. Flumara and Dr. Gavin Hart, 1976.)

as "low-risk") are the cause of genital warts. Clients may be asymptomatic or may experience tenderness in the area of the wart. Genital warts appear as solitary or clustered lesions. In males, the warts typically occur at the end of the penis or in the perianal area. In females, the warts typically appear near the opening of the vagina, and they commonly spread to the perianal area. Other types of HPV (known as high-risk) can cause cervical cancer.

Diagnostic Procedures

There is no test for HPV. It usually goes away on its own. The characteristic appearance and location of genital warts are usually sufficient for diagnosis. Cervical cell changes that can lead to cervical cancer can be identified on routine Papanicolaou (Pap) tests.

Treatment

There is no cure for the virus; a healthy immune system can usually deter HPV naturally. Genital warts can be removed by topical medication, carbon dioxide laser treatment, cryosurgery, electrocautery, or debridement. Small warts may require no treatment. Cervical cancer is treatable when diagnosed early.

Complementary Therapy

An ointment made of vitamin A and herbs may be topically applied to genital warts.

➤ CLIENT COMMUNICATION

Encourage hand washing after the application of topical treatments. Recommend the use of condoms. Sexually active females are encouraged to have annual Pap tests as identified by their age and risk factors. Encourage clients to know the sexual histories of their partners and to limit their number of sexual partners.

Prognosis

Low-risk HPV infection responds well to treatment. The prognosis is variable for high-risk HPV or cervical cancer. Spontaneous "cures" are rare, and the remainder of cases may be unresponsive to treatment.

Prevention

Girls and women can be protected against many cervical cancers by the HPV vaccine. This vaccine is recommended for all boys and girls between the ages of 11 and 12. Additionally, should the vaccination not be given between those ages, it is now suggested that young men can receive the vaccine until the age of 21 and young women until 24 years of age. The Pap test can identify abnormal changes in the cervix so they can be removed before cancer develops. Some specialists recommend yearly Pap tests for men who participate in

receptive anal intercourse, which places them at greater risk for anal cancer. This diagnostic procedure can catch early detection and guide appropriate interventions.

SYPHILIS

✔ **REPORTABLE DISEASE**

ICD-10: A53.9

Description

Syphilis is a highly infectious, chronic STD characterized by lesions that may involve any organ or tissue. After a brief decline in cases in the late 1990s, cases have again begun to rise.

Etiology

Syphilis is caused by the bacterium *Treponema pallidum*. The bacteria are transmitted via direct contact with infected lesions, typically through vaginal, oral, or anal intercourse or through contact with infected bodily fluids. Syphilis also may be contracted via transfusion with infected blood (a rare occurrence). In pregnant females, *T. pallidum* can cross the placenta and infect the fetus, causing serious fetal damage.

The bacteria rapidly penetrate skin or mucous membranes. From the point of infection, they spread into the lymphatic system and the blood, producing a systemic infection. Typically, the bacteria will have been carried throughout the body long before the first clinical symptoms appear.

Signs and Symptoms

Untreated, syphilis typically progresses through three clinical stages, each with characteristic signs and symptoms. Some infected individuals are asymptomatic or present with symptoms that are not readily evident on casual inspection.

Primary syphilis, which has an incubation period of about 3 weeks, is characterized by the appearance of a distinctive red, ulcerated, painless lesion, called a **chancre,** at the point of infection. In males, the chancre typically appears on the penis; however, lesions also may appear on the anus or within the rectum. Among females, the lesion typically appears on the labia of the vagina or within the vagina or on the cervix. Among both males and females, chancres also may appear on the lips, tongue, fingers, or nipples. The appearance of the chancre may be accompanied by regional lymphadenopathy, a disease of the lymph nodes, usually manifested as swelling of the nodes. It must be emphasized that the chancres are *highly contagious*. During this stage, the chancre usually heals within 3 to 12 weeks without treatment.

Secondary syphilis can produce a host of symptoms, many of which may be mistaken as symptoms of other diseases. Most frequently, however, individuals at this stage of the disease present with a rash characterized by uniform macular, papular, pustular, or nodular lesions. These typically, but not exclusively, appear on the palms or soles. In moist areas of the body, these lesions can erode and become contagious. Various general or systemic manifestations may accompany the rash, including headache, malaise, gastrointestinal (GI) upset, sore throat, fever, patchy hair loss, and brittle nails. This stage generally lasts 3 to 6 months.

After the manifestations of secondary syphilis subside, a latent stage of the disease begins in which the infected individual is generally asymptomatic. The bacteria may remain latent indefinitely. In nearly half of untreated individuals with latent syphilis, manifestations of the final, or tertiary, stage of the disease begin to appear 2 to 7 years after the initial infection. However, some cases may not appear until 20 years after the initial infection. In tertiary syphilis, the *Treponema* bacteria may cause life-threatening damage to the aorta of the heart, the central nervous system, or the musculoskeletal system; no organ system is immune from damage. Consequently, the symptoms of tertiary syphilis mimic the symptoms of other organ system diseases, making diagnosis difficult.

Diagnostic Procedures

The most sensitive test available for detecting syphilis is the fluorescent treponemal antibody-absorption (FTA-ABS) test. A rapid plasma reagin (RPR) test or a Venereal Disease Research Laboratories (VDRL) test also may be performed.

Treatment

Penicillin, given intramuscularly or via IV, is the antibiotic of choice for the treatment of all stages of syphilis. Doxycycline may be used in the event of allergic reaction to penicillin. Any lesions should be kept as dry and clean as possible. An RPR or the VDRL test typically accompanies the drug therapy to ensure the *Treponema* bacteria have been eradicated.

Complementary Therapy

There are no complementary therapies that will kill the bacterium.

 CLIENT COMMUNICATION

The use of condoms is highly recommended. Clients are encouraged to limit and know their sexual partners as well as their partners' sexual history. Regular screening for STDs is recommended for those persons at risk.

Prognosis

The prognosis varies with the age of the affected individual and with the stage at which the disease is detected and treated. The prognosis for complete recovery is very good for adults treated for primary and secondary syphilis. Although tertiary syphilis also can be successfully treated, any organ system damage that has been done is generally irreversible. Untreated, the disease may lead to life-threatening cardiac, central nervous system, or musculoskeletal disorders. Fetuses infected with syphilis have a very poor prognosis, with spontaneous abortion or stillbirth occurring in nearly 20% of cases.

Prevention

The use of condoms during sexual intimacy can reduce the possibility of transmitting or acquiring syphilis, but contact tracing of intimate partners and serological screening remain the most important methods in limiting the spread of this disease. Sexual partners should be evaluated and treated even if they show no symptoms.

TRICHOMONIASIS

ICD-10: A59.00

Description

Trichomoniasis is a protozoal infestation of the vagina, urethra, or prostate. It is a common STD, with about 7.4 million new cases occurring each year in women and men.

Etiology

Trichomonas vaginalis, a motile protozoan, is the cause of trichomoniasis. The disease usually is transmitted via sexual intercourse or vulva to vulva contact with an infected partner. Women may increase their susceptibility to *Trichomonas* infection by using vaginal sprays and over-the-counter douches. These preparations may change the natural flora of the vagina, creating a more hospitable environment for the parasite.

Signs and Symptoms

About 70% of the females with trichomoniasis are asymptomatic. When symptoms occur, they are usually those of acute vaginitis: a strong-smelling, greenish yellow, frothy vaginal discharge, possibly accompanied by itching, swelling, dyspareunia, and dysuria. Symptoms may persist for several months if untreated.

In most males, the disease is asymptomatic. When symptoms are present, they are typically those of urethritis, such as dysuria and urinary frequency.

Diagnostic Procedures

The diagnosis of trichomoniasis is facilitated by wet-mount microscopic examination of vaginal or seminal discharges. The disease also may be detected through urinalysis.

Treatment

The treatment of choice is oral metronidazole (Flagyl). Alcohol should be avoided during treatment and for 24 to 48 hours afterward because of its adverse reaction with Flagyl. Treatment of all partners with antiparasitic drugs usually cures trichomoniasis. After treatment, there should be a follow-up examination.

Complementary Therapy

Following diagnosis and treatment of trichomoniasis by a PCP, many naturopaths recommend the following:

- Increase good bacteria or probiotics found in products like yogurt.
- Herbs, such as garlic, echinacea, goldenseal, and tea tree oil, may be formulated.
- Eliminate all sugar from the diet and take a good multivitamin each day.

 CLIENT COMMUNICATION

Practicing abstinence during treatment periods is recommended.

Prognosis

The prognosis is good with proper treatment, although reinfection may occur.

Prevention

Over-the-counter douches and vaginal sprays should be avoided; abstinence or the use of condoms is recommended. Being in a long-term, mutually monogamous relationship with an uninfected partner is encouraged. Introducing more probiotics into the diet and eliminating all sugar may prove to be quite helpful.

Vaginitis (Yeast Infection)

The most common inflammations of the vagina, or vaginitis, are usually bacterial vaginosis, trichomoniasis, or yeast infection. Yeast infection is caused by an overgrowth of the fungus *Candida*. Burning, itching, swelling of the vulva and vagina, and pain upon urination are common symptoms. There may be a thick, white, cottage cheese–like vaginal discharge with an offensive odor. Antifungal medicines, with or without a prescription, are commonly used in treatment. They come in the form of creams, tablets, ointments, or vaginal suppositories. It is important to obtain a proper diagnosis prior to treatment, as the same symptoms may be due to a more serious infection, such as bacterial vaginosis or trichomoniasis. See http://www.womenshealth.gov/publications/our-publications/fact-sheet/vaginal-yeast-infections.html for additional information.

CHLAMYDIAL INFECTIONS

✔ *REPORTABLE DISEASE*

ICD-10: A74.9

Description

Chlamydial infection is a sexually transmitted infection that is now highly prevalent and is among the most potentially damaging of all the STDs in the United States. In 2014, the CDC reported 1.8 million cases of chlamydia infection and stated that perhaps twice as many cases were undetected.

Etiology

Chlamydial infection is caused by the bacterium *Chlamydia trachomatis*. Transmission is usually through oral, vaginal, or anal sexual contact with an infected person. A neonate exposed to the bacteria in the birth canal during delivery may develop an eye infection called *conjunctivitis*.

Signs and Symptoms

An individual may be asymptomatic or present with mild symptoms; this disease is sometimes called the "silent STD" because symptoms are often absent. Sexual transmission occurs unknowingly. Clinical manifestations in many females may resemble those of gonorrhea and include itching and burning in the genital area, mucopurulent vaginal discharge, and cervicitis. In males, there is discharge from the penis with a burning sensation on urination. The scrotum may be swollen. *C. trachomatis* can also cause rectal inflammation during anal intercourse or infect the throat when oral sex with an infected individual is practiced.

Diagnostic Procedures

Diagnosis can be confirmed by cytological and serological studies, which reveal *C. trachomatis* in infected body fluids. The bacteria also appear in a urine sample. Chlamydia is easily confused with gonorrhea because the symptoms of both diseases are similar and they often occur concurrently.

Treatment

The recommended treatment is an antibiotic such as azithromycin taken for 1 day or doxycycline taken for 7 days. Penicillin, often used to treat other STDs, will not cure chlamydia. All partners should be treated.

Complementary Therapy

See "Trichomoniasis."

 CLIENT COMMUNICATION

Remind clients to refrain from sexual activity until treatment is completed and to take all prescribed medication. Inform sexual partners so they can be tested and treated as necessary.

Prognosis

The prognosis is good if treatment is instituted early. If left untreated, complications include disease of the fallopian tubes, PID, and infertility in females. Males may suffer from epididymitis and become sterile.

Prevention

The use of condoms during sexual activity can reduce the possibility of transmitting or acquiring chlamydial infection. Contact tracing of intimate partners and screening of at-risk individuals remain the most important methods of limiting the spread of this infection.

COMMON SYMPTOMS OF SEXUALLY TRANSMITTED DISEASES (STDs)

Individuals with STDs may present with the following common symptoms, which deserve attention from health-care professionals:

- Dysuria, hematuria, urinary frequency or incontinence, purulent discharge, or burning and itching on urination
- Pelvic or genital pain
- Any skin ulcerations, especially in the genital area
- Fever and malaise
- Dyspareunia

Male Reproductive Diseases and Disorders

BENIGN PROSTATIC HYPERPLASIA

ICD-10: N40.0

Description

Benign prostatic hyperplasia (BPH) is an enlarged prostate. Growth occurs in one of two ways: In the first, the cells multiply and squeeze the urethra; in the second, the cells grow into the urethra and the bladder outlet area. The second type usually requires surgery (Fig. 16.6). The condition is common in males over age 50, and the incidence increases with age. It is only clinically significant if the enlarging, hyperplastic portion of the prostate obstructs urinary flow.

Etiology

The etiology of BPH is not well understood, but it seems to be due to metabolic and hormonal changes associated with aging. In clinically significant BPH, the gland compresses the urethra or the neck of the bladder, obstructing urinary flow.

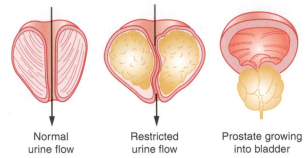

Normal urine flow | Restricted urine flow | Prostate growing into bladder

Figure 16.6 Benign prostatic hyperplasia showing restricted urinary flow and prostate growing into the bladder.

Signs and Symptoms

Individuals may report symptoms of urinary obstruction, such as difficulty in initiating urination or in completely emptying the bladder in the first stage. As the obstruction increases in size, symptoms may include nocturia, dribbling, urinary frequency, hematuria, weak urine stream, and incontinence.

Diagnostic Procedures

Symptomatology of the individual and a digital rectal examination are usually sufficient for diagnosis, but blood tests to determine the level of prostate-specific antigen (PSA) and prostatic acid phosphatase (PAP) are helpful in ruling out prostate cancer. Primary care providers will have clients complete the American Urological Association (AUA) Prostate Symptom Index questionnaire that is designed to evaluate urinary difficulties and to help diagnose BPH. Urodynamic tests can be used to measure the volume and pressure of urine in the bladder as well as its flow. Uroflowmetry records urine flow and how quickly the bladder is emptied. A pressure flow study determines the pressure in the bladder and can detect a blockage. The postvoid residual (PVR) measures the amount of urine remaining in the bladder after urination.

Treatment

Often providers and clients wait for treatment to see how far symptoms progress. This is known as "watchful waiting." Some alpha blocker medications that act to shrink the prostate or relax the muscles in the prostate have shown moderate success. Thermotherapy that includes laser, transurethral microwave therapy (TUMT), or Prostiva RF (radio frequency) therapy may be chosen. These methods heat and destroy the constricting tissue while preserving the urethra and nonprostatic tissues. Various surgical procedures, such as transurethral prostate resection (TURP), holmium laser enucleation of the prostate (HoLEP), transurethral incision of the prostate (TUIP), or transurethral ultrasound-guided laser incision of the prostate (TULIP) may be performed.

Complementary Therapy

Naturopaths recommend eating whole, fresh, unrefined, and unprocessed organic foods as much as possible and increasing water consumption. Clients are advised to avoid such prostatic irritants such as caffeine, alcohol, tobacco, and red pepper; take 30 g of zinc picolinate daily; and increase their intake of amino acids. An herbal remedy made from saw palmetto products may be beneficial. The client should add soy to the diet and increase consumption of tomatoes for their content of lycopene. Symptomatic treatment may include prostatic massage and cool sitz baths.

 CLIENT COMMUNICATION

Remind clients of the importance of regular follow-up examinations and surgical choices while in the "watchful" stage of the disorder. Men are sensitive to their sexuality and will want to discuss their fear of impotence and/or incontinence if surgery is a choice.

Prognosis

Prognosis is good with proper intervention. There is a surgical success rate of 80% to 90%. Impotence or incontinence is usually not a problem. There may be retrograde ejaculation, but this does not affect sexual pleasure. If untreated, infections may ascend to the kidney, or various urinary obstructive disorders may result. Complications include cystitis, dilation of the ureters, hydronephrosis, pyelonephritis, and uremia.

Prevention

No specific prevention is known for BPH, but older males should be encouraged to have a regular prostate examination to detect any enlargement.

PROSTATITIS

ICD-10: N41.X*

Description

Prostatitis is inflammation of the prostate gland. The condition may be acute or chronic, with the chronic type being more common in males over age 50. Acute prostatitis is more common in young and middle-aged men.

Etiology

Prostatitis may be either bacterial or nonbacterial in origin. Bacterial causes of the disease include *Escherichia coli*, *Klebsiella*, *Enterobacter*, *Proteus*, *Staphylococcus*, *Streptococcus*, and *Pseudomonas*. Trauma from horseback or bicycle riding, use of a urinary catheter, and HIV infection can lead to prostatitis also. Routes of infection can be via the urethra or the bloodstream. In nonbacterial prostatitis, no infectious agent is detectable.

Signs and Symptoms

Acute prostatitis clients may describe low back pain, pain in the pelvic region, perineal fullness or pain, fever, dysuria, hematuria, and urinary frequency and urgency. When palpated, the prostate may be enlarged, tender, and boggy. An individual with chronic prostatitis may be asymptomatic or experience sporadic, mild forms of acute symptoms and be prone to urinary tract infections (UTIs).

Diagnostic Procedures

The primary care provider may have clients complete a National Institutes of Health (NIH) Chronic Prostatitis Symptom Index to aid in diagnosis. Rectal examination suggests prostatitis. A firm diagnosis depends on a comparison of urine cultures of specimens obtained by the Meares and Stamey technique. Four specimens are collected: one when the client starts voiding, another midstream, another after the client stops voiding and the physician massages the prostate to produce secretions, and a final voided specimen. A significant increase in colony count in the specimens confirms prostatitis. Cystoscopy may be ordered; any of the urodynamic tests may be run; also see Diagnostic Procedures in "Benign Prostatic Hyperplasia."

Abnormally high urine leukocyte counts in the absence of detectable bacteria are indicative of nonbacterial prostatitis.

Treatment

Antibiotic and/or antimicrobial therapy is initiated, and the client may be advised to rest and increase fluid intake. Alpha blockers may lessen symptoms. Analgesics, antipyretics, and stool softeners also may be ordered. Sitz baths may be recommended. Regular ejaculation may help promote drainage of prostatic secretions.

Complementary Therapy

See "Benign Prostatic Hyperplasia." Both biofeedback and acupuncture have been used to reduce the pain and discomfort that accompanies prostatitis.

 CLIENT COMMUNICATION

Remind clients to eat nutritional meals and have adequate fluid intake. Provide individuals with information about possible complications and treatment choices as necessary.

Prognosis

Acute prostatitis responds well to treatment; however, chronic prostatitis does not. Complications may include

*The X represents the fourth and fifth digits that are often required and supplied once more detailed information about the disease or disorder is made known to the provider.

epididymitis, cystitis, and urethritis. Chronic prostatitis predisposes one to recurrent urinary tract infections, urethral obstruction, acute urinary retention, and abnormalities in semen and infertility.

Prevention

Early treatment of UTIs is the best prevention.

EPIDIDYMITIS

ICD-10:N45.X

Description

Epididymitis is inflammation of the epididymis due to infection. The condition is typically unilateral and is one of the most common infections of the male reproductive system, especially those in the age bracket of 19 to 35 years.

Etiology

Epididymitis can occur as a result of prostatitis, a UTI, tuberculosis, or STDs such as gonorrhea and chlamydia. *Chlamydia trachomatis* and *Neisseria gonorrhoeae* are the most common infectious agents that cause epididymitis in sexually active males.

Signs and Symptoms

The epididymis may become enlarged, hard, and tender, causing pain. Scrotal and groin tenderness, fever, and malaise also may occur. Groin tenderness is the result of enlarged lymph nodes in the groin. Clients may "waddle" as they walk, trying to protect the scrotal area. There may be blood in semen, a discharge from the penis, and enlarged lymph nodes in the groin area.

Diagnostic Procedures

A swab sample from urethral discharge is used to determine the presence of bacteria. Ultrasound may be ordered, especially if the symptoms were sudden and the pain is severe. Urinalysis and urine cultures help in the diagnosis. An increased leukocyte count is common.

Treatment

Antibiotic and/or antimicrobial therapy appropriate for the particular causative agent is initiated. If an STD is found to be the cause, then sexual partners need treatment as well.

Complementary Therapy

Wearing scrotal support and taking analgesics may be helpful. Bed rest may be necessary in the acute phase. Scrotal elevation and cool compresses (30 minutes or less) to relieve pain and reduce swelling may be helpful.

⊖ **CLIENT COMMUNICATION**

Remind clients to take all their medications and analgesics as necessary. When clients are feeling better, encourage walking and the use of an athletic supporter.

Prognosis

The inflammation generally responds well to therapy, but portions of the epididymis may be scarred. Orchitis may occur as a complication to epididymitis; it causes infection of the testes and can lead to sterility. Any pain, swelling, and redness of the testes should be reported immediately to the PCP. Orchitis can be the result of mumps, so young males should receive the mumps vaccine.

Prevention

Early treatment of UTI is the best prevention. The use of a condom during sexual intimacy is recommended, especially if the causative agent was sexually transmitted.

PROSTATIC CANCER

ICD-10: C61

Description

Prostatic cancer is a malignant neoplasm of the prostate tissue. The majority of these neoplasms are classified as adenocarcinomas. Prostatic cancer is the second leading cause of cancer deaths in males (after lung cancer). Prostate cancer tends to metastasize, often spreading to the bones of the spine or pelvis before it is detected. The American Cancer Society reports that an estimated 220,800 new cases will be reported in 2015. The disease is rare before age 50.

Etiology

Four factors are suspected in this cancer:

1. Family or racial predisposition (African Americans have the highest prostate cancer rate in the world).
2. Exposure to environmental or chemical elements (e.g., Vietnam War veterans exposed to Agent Orange have a higher incidence of prostate cancer; therefore, military service information is important in any social and medical history).
3. Coexisting STDs
4. Endogenous hormonal influence

Eating high amounts of fat-containing animal products has also been implicated.

Signs and Symptoms

Most individuals with prostatic cancer are asymptomatic on diagnosis. When symptoms are present, they are typically those of urinary obstruction, such as dysuria, difficulty in voiding, urinary frequency, lower back pain, or urinary retention. Hematuria, bone pain or tenderness, unintentional weight loss, and lethargy may also be symptoms.

Diagnostic Procedures

A digital rectal examination will help in diagnosing the tumor. A biopsy is essential for confirmation of the diagnosis. Computed tomography (CT) or ultrasonography may be useful in localizing and gauging the extent of the tumor.

A PSA blood test is used to differentiate prostate cancer from BPH. This test is advised for all males over age 50 on a yearly basis. The alpha-methylacyl-CoA racemase (AMACR) test is newer and is more sensitive in detecting cancer of the prostate. AMACR is a genetic marker for prostate cancer.

Treatment

The course of treatment selected depends on the stage and grade of the disease and the client's physical condition and age. Surgery may be performed to remove the prostate and adjacent affected tissues. Various hormonal therapies also may be attempted to limit prostatic cell growth, including **orchiectomy** (surgical removal of the testis) and estrogen therapy. Medications may be given to block the production of testosterone, commonly referred to as *chemical castration*. However, unlike orchiectomy, this procedure is reversible. Radiation therapy may be tried in some cases, and this further helps to relieve bone pain. **Cryoablation** of the prostate may be effective in destroying the cancer cells of the prostate by freezing them. Chemotherapy may be used in treating advanced stages of the disease. Many older clients, in discussions with their PCPs, choose a watchful waiting approach.

Complementary Therapy

A component of soy called *genistein* appears to inhibit the growth of prostate cancer. The supplement is available without a prescription and has been a popular therapy for prostate cancer in Asia for many decades. The supplement seems to work best when given before surgery, radiation therapy, or chemotherapy. This is an example of integrative medicine at work.

➤ CLIENT COMMUNICATION

Explain all possible treatments to clients. The PCP can discuss the implications of surgery, any possibilities of impotence, and the potential for curing the disease.

Prognosis

The earlier the cancer is detected, the better is the prognosis. Survival rates for all stages combined have steadily increased and are now approaching 100% when diagnosed early.

Prevention

There is no known method of prevention.

TESTICULAR CANCER

ICD-10: C62.XX

Description

Testicular cancer is a malignant neoplasm of a testis. There are various forms of the disease, classified according to the type of testicular tissue from which the malignancy originates. The disease primarily affects young to middle-aged males and is rare in males over age 40.

Etiology

The cause of cancer of the testes is essentially unknown. Predisposing factors include cryptorchidism, even after this condition has been surgically corrected, and being born to a mother who used diethylstilbestrol during pregnancy. It is rare in nonwhite males.

Signs and Symptoms

The first sign is often a smooth, firm, painless mass of varying size in the testicles. Rarer symptoms may include breast enlargement and nipple tenderness.

Diagnostic Procedures

Diagnosis generally is through regular self-examination and palpation of the testes during a routine physical examination. Further tests such as ultrasound and CT or magnetic resonance imagining (MRI) may be necessary to differentiate the cell type of the mass. Some blood tests can help diagnose testicular cancer when the cancer secretes high levels of certain proteins or tumor markers that show up in the blood.

Treatment

Treatment may include any combination of surgery (orchiectomy or retroperitoneal node dissection), radiation, and chemotherapy, as determined by the tumor cell type and staging.

Complementary Therapy

No significant complementary therapy is indicated.

CLIENT COMMUNICATION

Provide information on the disease and appropriate treatment methods. Reassure clients that sterility and impotence need not follow unilateral orchiectomy and that synthetic hormones can restore hormone imbalance.

Prognosis

The prognosis varies according to cancer type and staging. Cure rates of higher than 96% can be expected following the successful treatment of early-stage testicular cancers.

Prevention

Although no specific prevention is known, early detection is crucial to successful treatment. Young males should be encouraged to perform monthly self-examination of the testes.

COMMON SYMPTOMS OF MALE REPRODUCTIVE DISEASES AND DISORDERS

Males may present with the following common complaints, which deserve attention from health-care professionals:

- Any urinary complaints such as frequency, urgency, incontinence, dysuria, or nocturia
- Pain in any of the reproductive organs or any unusual discharge
- Swelling or enlargement of any of the reproductive organs
- Any sexual disorder or concern

Female Reproductive Diseases and Disorders

PREMENSTRUAL SYNDROME

ICD-10: N94.3

Description

Premenstrual syndrome (PMS) is a distinct cluster of physical and psychological symptoms that regularly recur 3 to 14 days before the onset of menstruation and are relieved by the onset of menses. Surveys show 30% to 40% of women experience mild to severe PMS. PMS appears more frequently in women in their 30s and 40s.

Etiology

The cause of PMS is not clearly understood, although it is thought to be multifactorial. PMS is different for each woman. Some theories suggest that the condition may be attributable to water retention, estrogen-progesterone imbalance, psychological factors, or dietary deficiencies. Some believe there is a relationship between PMS and changes in the endorphin levels.

Signs and Symptoms

The particular assortment of symptoms and their severity vary among women. Symptoms associated with PMS include the following:

- Irritability
- Anxiety or depression
- Sleeplessness
- Fatigue
- Acne
- Appetite changes or food cravings
- Headache or backache
- Syncope
- Lowered resistance to infections
- Nervousness
- Arthralgia
- Abdominal bloating and weight gain
- Heart palpitations
- Swollen and tender breasts
- Easily bruised skin

The signs and symptoms may affect a female's ability to perform normal tasks and can affect relationships.

Diagnostic Procedures

Diagnosis depends on the timing of the symptoms rather than on the appearance of any specific set of symptoms. Consequently, women with PMS should be encouraged to keep a journal recording the onset, duration, and intensity of all symptoms for at least 3 months. Evaluation of estrogen and progesterone levels in the blood to check for imbalances should be performed. Blood tests may be done to rule out other hormonal imbalances or anemia. A history and physical examination will be done to eliminate other diseases and disorders.

Treatment

There is no one effective treatment for PMS. It is helpful to take a multivitamin every day that includes 400 micrograms of folic acid. A calcium supplement with vitamin D may also ease some PMS symptoms. A reduction of salt intake for 2 weeks before menses will minimize water retention. Sometimes diuretics and analgesics are ordered. Avoidance of stimulants (coffee, nicotine, and alcohol) and simple sugars and an increase in lean protein are suggested. Proper diet, exercise, and sufficient amounts of rest are important. Reduction in stress, relaxation techniques, and medication may be ordered to relieve the symptoms.

Complementary Therapy

Continuing a daily exercise and relaxation program can improve emotional and physical symptoms. Some practitioners recommend vitamins B_6 and E, magnesium, zinc, and oil of evening primrose capsules. Herbs and acupuncture have been used as well.

CLIENT COMMUNICATION

Educate clients on keeping a journal of signs and symptoms and dietary intake. Encourage support from family members, and stress the importance of following any prescribed treatment. Clients can become easily discouraged; offer support as needed.

Prognosis

The prognosis is variable. The disorder is considered chronic but will cease at menopause and does not have long-term effects.

Prevention

There is no known prevention for PMS.

Premenstrual Dysphoric Disorder Diagnosis

Premenstrual dysphoric disorder (PMDD; ICD-10: N94.3) is a severe form of PMS related to the brain chemical serotonin. Women who have five or more of the following symptoms or more severe forms of those identified in PMS are diagnosed with PMDD:

- Feelings of despair; possible suicide thoughts
- Panic attacks
- Severe mood swings; crying
- Lasting irritability or anger that affects others
- Disinterest in daily activities
- Feeling out of control
- Physical symptoms as described in PMS

Treatment for PMDD is similar to that for PMS, but antidepressants such as selective serotonin reuptake inhibitors (SSRIs) are often prescribed and can be helpful. Sometimes birth control pills that stop ovulation from occurring are given.

AMENORRHEA

ICD-10: N91.2

Description

Amenorrhea is the absence of **menarche,** the initial menstrual cycle, beyond age 16 (primary amenorrhea) or the absence of menstruation for 6 months in a female who has previously had regular, periodic menses (secondary amenorrhea) and is not menopausal.

Etiology

Medically significant primary or secondary amenorrhea may be caused by a variety of hormonal imbalances capable of preventing ovulation. Primary amenorrhea is influenced by hereditary factors; environment; body build; and physical, mental, and emotional development. Secondary amenorrhea may be caused by pregnancy, stress, or tension. Several forms of congenital anatomic defects, such as the absence of a uterus, may cause amenorrhea. The condition is also associated with endometrial problems, bulimia, anorexia, polycystic ovarian syndrome, ovarian or pituitary tumors, malnutrition, psychological stress, or too much physical exercise.

Signs and Symptoms

A young female reporting delayed menarche by age 16 or a female reporting skipped periods for 3 to 6 months or longer should be carefully assessed for amenorrhea.

Diagnostic Procedures

A thorough physical and pelvic examination will rule out pregnancy and anatomic abnormalities. Analysis of blood and urine samples may reveal hormonal difficulties. A hormonal medication may be given that normally would trigger menstruation and can tell if a lack of estrogen might be the cause of the amenorrhea. Ultrasound, CT scans, and laparoscopy with an endometrial biopsy may be necessary to detect tumors.

Treatment

Treatment is dependent on the cause, if it is known. Hormone therapy usually starts the menstrual cycle, but some cases of this disorder may require more aggressive treatment, such as surgery for anatomic defects or tumor or cyst removal.

Complementary Therapy

Practitioners recommend that females who exercise intensively and tend toward malnourishment eat at least an additional 500 calories a day. Whenever exercising, the client should eat an adequate and well-balanced diet to compensate for the increased metabolism and get ample rest.

CLIENT COMMUNICATION

Encourage clients to seek medical attention for amenorrhea so that any underlying cause may be treated. It should not be ignored. A discussion with the PCP will help to determine what steps to take to restore menstruation to a more regular cycle.

Prognosis

Prognosis is good when the underlying cause can be determined and corrected. It is important that an accurate record of the menstrual cycle be kept to aid in the detection of amenorrhea.

Prevention

Preventive measures include adequate diet and a balanced physical exercise program.

CHAPTER EPISODE—PART II

Allison is now in her mid-20s and her menses continue to be of concern. She has irregular menses, is newly diagnosed with hypothyroidism, and when menses occurs, it is still extremely painful. Allison has decided to go back to her gynecologist for some answers.

- What might her doctor's diagnosis be?
- What diagnostic procedures might be performed to assist in the diagnosis?

DYSMENORRHEA

ICD-10: N94.6

Description

Dysmenorrhea is pain associated with menstruation. It is one of the most frequent gynecologic disorders, affecting more than half of menstruating women. Dysmenorrhea is divided into primary and secondary categories. Primary dysmenorrhea is not associated with any identifiable pelvic pathological disorder, whereas secondary dysmenorrhea accompanies some underlying pelvic pathology or disease condition. Dysmenorrhea is more commonly seen among women who had early onset of menses, have long and/or heavy menstrual periods, and who smoke. Obesity and alcohol consumption may contribute to dysmenorrhea as well.

Etiology

A specific cause of primary dysmenorrhea is difficult to pinpoint. Hormonal imbalances such as increased **prostaglandin** secretions may be the cause. Prostaglandins are a class of chemically related fatty acids present in many body tissues; they have the ability to stimulate smooth muscle contractions or lower blood pressure. The hormone vasopressin is known to be involved in some cases of dysmenorrhea, causing hypersensitivity in the endometrium, reduced uterine blood flow, and pain. Secondary dysmenorrhea arises as a consequence of some other problem, such as endometriosis, cervical stenosis, polycystic ovarian syndrome (PCOS), or PID. Secondary dysmenorrhea is occasionally associated with uterine polyps or benign tumors.

Signs and Symptoms

Aching, spasmodic, colicky, cramping pains in the lower abdominal area are the classic symptoms. The pain may radiate to the thighs, back, and genitalia. Headache, nausea, diarrhea, fatigue, irritability, dizziness, and syncope may result. These symptoms usually start just before or immediately after menses and subside within 18 to 24 hours.

Diagnostic Procedures

A detailed medical history is taken, and pelvic examination is performed to determine the cause. Cervical culture may be obtained to rule out STDs and a white blood cell count (WBC) to exclude infection. Abdominal and transvaginal ultrasound may be ordered. A hysterosalpingogram may be used to exclude endometrial polyps, **leiomyomas** (tumor of smooth muscle tissue), and abnormalities of the uterus.

Treatment

Analgesics and NSAIDs usually are sufficient for relieving the pain of this disorder. Moreover, when taken before menses, aspirin is an inhibitor of prostaglandins. Other analgesics may be ordered. Heat applied to the abdomen can provide comfort. Sometimes oral contraceptives may be prescribed to relieve pain by suppressing ovulation. Uterine leiomyomas may require surgery.

Complementary Therapy

Eating whole grains, legumes, fruit, vegetables, and nuts is recommended. The client should avoid sugars, alcohol, caffeine, dairy products, and salt. Supplements such as vitamin B, calcium, magnesium, and zinc may be ordered. Acupuncture is useful for pain reduction.

 CLIENT COMMUNICATION

Listen to the concern of clients, who best understand their dysmenorrhea. Encourage clients to eat a balanced diet and to exercise.

Prognosis

The prognosis for primary dysmenorrhea is good but can be frustrating. For secondary dysmenorrhea, the prognosis is dependent on the cause. Careful evaluation of the pain is necessary in order to avoid delay in a diagnosis that could be serious or life-threatening—ectopic pregnancy or pelvic neoplasm.

Prevention

Correction of any hormonal imbalance may be helpful in the prevention of dysmenorrhea.

OVARIAN CYSTS AND TUMORS

ICD-10: N83.XX

Description

Benign cysts of the ovary are derived from ovarian follicles that do not break open to release the egg. Corpus luteum cysts—small, yellow structures on the ovary—are formed from the mass of follicle cells left behind after an ovum is released. Cysts may occur any time from puberty to menopause. Nonneoplastic cysts (tumors) usually are small and produce few symptoms. Dermoid or benign cystic tumors, or **teratomas,** also are common in the ovary; they become large and cause pain. Other types of ovarian cysts include endometrioma and polycystic ovarian cysts. Endometrioma is cyst-containing endometrial tissue that is attached to the ovary, causing pain during sexual intercourse or menses. Polycystic ovarian cysts are caused when eggs mature within sacs but are not released. This is known as PCOS (see Chapter 11), a complex endocrine disorder involving mainly females of childbearing age. Cystadenomas form on the outer surface of the ovary and are often filled with a watery fluid or thick gel.

Etiology

The etiology of ovarian cysts and tumors is not known; however, genetics are thought to play a part, especially in PCOS. The cause may be defects in the ovary or the result of hypothalamic-pituitary dysfunction. Irregular menstrual cycles, increased upper body fat, hypothyroidism, and tamoxifen therapy for breast cancer are possible risk factors.

Signs and Symptoms

Some cysts are asymptomatic. Large cysts may produce pelvic pain, low back pain, and dyspareunia. Cysts that are mobile and can twist may produce acute spasmodic abdominal pain. Urinary retention can result if a large fluid-filled cyst presses on the area near the bladder. Any time the pain is accompanied by fever and vomiting, is sudden and severe, or causes faintness or dizziness, medical attention should be sought.

Diagnostic Procedures

Visualization of the ovaries through ultrasonography is most commonly used. CT scans can further assess the extent of the condition. Blood tests to check hormone levels of LH, FSH, estradiol, and testosterone may indicate potential problems.

Treatment

Watchful waiting is the normal course of action when there are no symptoms. Cysts may disappear spontaneously through reabsorption or silent rupture or may require drug-induced ovulation therapy or surgical resection. Surgery may be necessary for diagnosis as well as treatment of most ovarian tumors, especially if any question exists regarding malignancy or if the cysts continue to grow. Laparoscopy or laparotomy are the surgeries of choice. Oral contraception may be useful to regulate periods and encourage ovulation.

Complementary Therapy

A balanced diet and control of weight may be useful in some types of ovarian cysts. Some recommend a vegetarian diet with organic foods. Clients should avoid fried foods, coffee, tobacco, alcohol, and sugar.

⊖ CLIENT COMMUNICATION

It is important to inform clients of this disease process so they understand the treatment plan. Offer support as needed, especially if infertility results.

Prognosis

Prognosis varies according to whether the diagnosis indicates nonneoplastic cysts or a true ovarian neoplasm. Some cysts may cause infertility problems. Chronic **anovulation** predisposes one to endometrial cancer, cardiovascular disease, and hyperinsulinemia.

Prevention

There is no known prevention of ovarian cysts and tumors.

ENDOMETRIOSIS

ICD-10: N80.X

Description

Endometriosis is the appearance and growth of endometrial tissue in areas outside the endometrium, the lining of the uterine cavity. The misplaced endometrial tissue generally is found within the pelvic area, but it can appear anywhere in the body (Fig. 16.7). Despite its location at an ectopic site (outside the uterus), the tissue still responds to the hormonal signals of the female's menstrual cycle, but the "menstruating" tissue cannot be sloughed off through the vagina. This situation gives rise to a variety of symptoms and may lead to scarring of the ectopic site. Endometriosis affects 5.5 million females in the United States during their active reproductive years.

Etiology

The cause of endometriosis remains unknown, although various theories have been proposed, such as a familial susceptibility. One theory is that some menstrual tissue backs up through the fallopian tubes and implants in the abdomen. Another theory is that the endometrial tissue is distributed through the blood or lymph systems. Research by the Endometriosis Association found a significant connection to endometriosis from dioxin, which is a toxic chemical by-product of pesticide manufacturing, bleached pulp and paper products, and medical and municipal waste incineration.

Signs and Symptoms

Dysmenorrhea occurs along with pain in the lower back and the vagina. The severity of the pain does not necessarily indicate the extent of the disease. There is pain at the ectopic site during menses. Clients may report profuse menses, infertility, dyspareunia, dysuria, and even painful defecation.

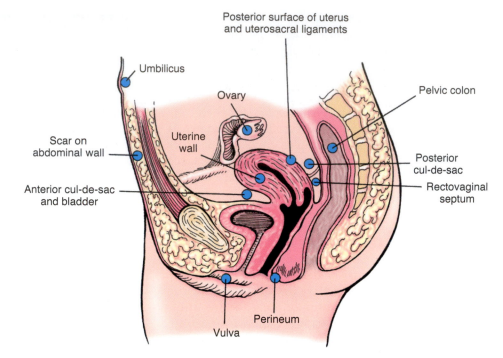

Figure 16.7 Possible sites of endometriosis. *(From Venes, D, and Thomas, CL [eds]:* Taber's Cyclopedic Medical Dictionary, *ed. 21. Philadelphia: F.A. Davis, 2009, p 768, with permission.)*

Diagnostic Procedures

A physical examination and a thorough health history are indicated. Diagnosis is usually made by laparoscopically visualizing the ectopic deposits within the pelvis. Palpation may detect tender nodules or areas of the pelvis. These nodules become more tender during menses. The disease is usually staged from 1 (superficial or minor lesions) to 4 (deep involvement and dense adhesions).

Treatment

Treatment goals include relieving the pain and discomfort, shrinking or slowing endometrial growths, preserving fertility, and preventing recurrence. Pain medications may be prescribed or taken over the counter. Hormone therapy that will completely suppress the menstrual cycle may be recommended. This therapy includes birth control pills, progesterone drugs, a testosterone derivative, and gonadotropin-releasing hormone drugs. Laparoscopy may be used to lyse adhesions. **Panhysterosalpingo-oophorectomy,** which is surgical removal of the entire uterus, including the cervix, ovaries, and fallopian tubes, may be indicated in severe cases.

Complementary Therapy

Clients are advised to increase intake of essential fatty acids found in salmon, seeds, and nuts and to reduce intake of meat, eggs, and dairy products. Refer to "Ovarian Cysts and Tumors" for additional information. Many find pain relief from acupuncture.

⊖ CLIENT COMMUNICATION

It is important to dispel any myths clients may have. If infertility results, ART may be tried. Clients need support and reassurance. Often there are support systems in a community for women with endometriosis or fertility issues.

Prognosis

The prognosis varies according to the location of the ectopic sites and the intensity of symptoms experienced by each individual. A primary complication of endometriosis is infertility. Women who want to have a child may be advised not to postpone pregnancy.

Prevention

There is no known prevention of endometriosis.

UTERINE LEIOMYOMAS

ICD-10: C79.82

Description

Uterine leiomyomas are often mislabeled as fibroids or fibroid tumors, but they are not composed of fibrous tissue. Rather, they are composed of smooth muscle tissue. These benign tumors may vary in size, number, and location within the uterine muscle. They are the most common tumors in females, and they tend to calcify after menopause.

Etiology

The etiology of leiomyomas is not known, but their development is stimulated by estrogen. Therefore, they grow during pregnancy or when using high-dose estrogen birth control pills. Conversely, their growth is lessened after pregnancy or with the use of low-dose estrogen birth control pills.

Signs and Symptoms

Frequently, leiomyomas are asymptomatic. If symptoms do occur, they may include pelvic pressure, pain, stress urinary incontinence or urinary frequency, constipation, and menorrhagia. A palpable mass may be detected during a routine pelvic examination. The growths vary in size and increase during pregnancy or with oral contraceptive use.

Diagnostic Procedures

The client's symptoms and a thorough history and physical examination, including palpation of the tumor, are essential for diagnosis. Additionally, ultrasonography, MRI, hysterosonography, and hysterosalpingography may be also performed.

Treatment

Treatment is dependent on age, the desire to have children, tumor status, and the severity of symptoms. If the tumors are small, no treatment may be necessary other than periodic monitoring of the growth of the leiomyomas, or watchful waiting. A pelvic examination every 6 to 12 months may then be advised. Certain medications may shrink the fibroids. MRI-guided ultrasound surgery may be performed to heat and destroy small tumors. Surgical removal of the tumors may be done (myomectomy), or a hysterectomy may be performed.

Complementary Therapy

There is no known complementary therapy for uterine leiomyomas.

⊙ CLIENT COMMUNICATION

Encourage clients to be watchful of any new signs and symptoms and report them to the PCP.

Prognosis

Only a very small percentage of leiomyomas develop into a malignancy. Some tumors may outgrow their blood supply, become infected, or undergo degenerative changes. The leiomyomas may cause infertility. Additionally, if the client is pregnant, spontaneous abortion or premature labor may occur.

Prevention

No prevention is known for uterine leiomyomas.

PELVIC INFLAMMATORY DISEASE

ICD-10: N70.XX

Description

Pelvic inflammatory disease is an acute, subacute, or recurrent or chronic infection of the uterus, fallopian tubes, or ovaries. There may be inflammation of the cervix (cervicitis), uterus (endometritis), fallopian tubes (salpingitis), and ovaries (oophoritis). More than 1 million women in the United States suffer from PID; more than 100,000 are infertile as a result of PID.

Etiology

The causes of PID include infections from, most commonly, *N. gonorrhoeae* or *C. trachomatis*; (2) infections following **parturition** (the act of giving birth); and (3) iatrogenic causes—for instance, PID may follow **conization** (the excision of cervical tissue for diagnostic testing), cervical cauterization, or insertion of an intrauterine device (IUD) or biopsy curette. PID is most common in young nulliparous females (women who have never produced a viable offspring). However, PID can also occur after childbirth, abortion, or miscarriage.

Signs and Symptoms

Often there are no symptoms at all while serious damage is being done to reproductive organs. This disease may exhibit both acute and chronic symptoms. Acute symptoms include sudden pelvic pain, a purulent and foul-smelling vaginal discharge, fever, sexual dysfunction, **metrorrhea** (abnormal uterine bleeding), and rebound pain. Chronic symptoms, such as cervical dysplasia; alteration in size, shape, and organization of mature cells; and laceration may go undetected for an indefinite period of time.

Diagnostic Procedures

PID is difficult to diagnose because the symptoms are subtle. Diagnosis includes taking a smear of uterine secretions for culture. Laboratory tests may include erythrocyte sedimentation rate, WBC count, and a measurement of C-reactive protein (CRP) in the blood. An elevated CRP level indicates an inflammation. Ultrasonography may be used to identify a uterine mass.

Treatment

Appropriate antibiotics are the best treatment for PID. The quicker antibiotic therapy begins, the less likely there is to be serious damage to reproductive organs. Supplemental therapy may include analgesics and bed rest. Surgery may be necessary if there is an abscess in the fallopian tube or ovary.

Complementary Therapy

Abstinence is recommended during the infectious stage. Clients are urged to know the sexual history of their partners and to limit sexual partners. If there is pain, acupuncture may be used to reduce it. A daily multivitamin and additional vitamin C may help the body fight the infection; eating a balanced diet is recommended. Herbalists may recommend castor oil packs (castor oil poured on a clean folded cloth and warmed) placed on the lower abdomen for up to 20 minutes each day for 7 days.

 CLIENT COMMUNICATION

Remind clients of the importance of taking all their antibiotic medication. Stress the seriousness of PID, and encourage clients to comply with the treatment plan and inform the primary care provider of possible complications. It is necessary that all sexual partners are checked and treated for any infection.

Prognosis

The prognosis of PID is good when treatment is instituted early and few complications occur. If treatment is delayed, scar tissue and adhesions can form. Recurrences are possible.

Prevention

There is no known prevention other than promptly treating any STD, being in a long-term monogamous relationship with a partner who is not infected, and abstaining from sexual intimacy during treatment for PID.

MENOPAUSE

ICD-10: N95.1

I used to have Saturday night fever; now I have Saturday night hot flashes. —Maxine

Description

Menopause is not a disease but rather is the natural cessation of menses and ovarian function, with a resultant decrease in estrogen and progesterone levels.

Etiology

Menopause occurs naturally in women between ages 45 and 55. It also can be surgically induced by oophorectomy, or it can result from malnutrition or from a disease that has an adverse effect on hormone balance. Premature menopause can be idiopathic.

Signs and Symptoms

Menstrual irregularities, a decrease in the amount of menstrual flow, and, finally, cessation of menses are the common symptoms. These symptoms occur over a period of months or years. Ordinarily the hormone levels gradually decrease, allowing the body to adjust to the hormonal changes. However, if the hormone levels suddenly drop, symptoms can be more severe. Changes occur in the body systems, sometimes producing hot flashes, night sweats, syncope, tachycardia, and loss of elasticity in the skin. There is a reduction in size and firmness of breast tissue, some atrophy of the genitalia, and a decrease in secretion from Bartholin glands. Some females experience transient psychological symptoms, such as depression, poor memory, and loss of interest in sexual activity.

Diagnostic Procedures

A careful history usually suggests menopause. Blood serum levels of estradiol, FSH, and LH are screened.

Treatment

Some individuals need no treatment; others may require hormone replacement therapy (HRT), counseling, or both, if symptoms are severe. It is recommended that a woman have a screening mammogram before HRT. A woman who requires HRT should be informed of the possible increased risks. (See the box "Weighing the Risks and Benefits of Hormone Replacement Therapy.") Some medications can lessen the symptoms of menopause. They include low doses of some antidepressants, such as paroxetine, venlafaxine, and fluoxetine. Gabapentin is effective for reducing hot flashes, and clonidine (normally used to control high blood pressure) is also helpful.

Complementary Therapy

Clients are advised to increase calcium intake and exercise in moderation. Caffeine, alcohol, and spicy foods are to be avoided. Kegel exercises are recommended to strengthen the muscles of the vagina and pelvis. Practicing slow, deep breathing at the onset of a hot flash is helpful. Acupuncture, yoga, tai chi, and meditation have been helpful to many. Using a water-based lubricant during sexual intercourse can ease any discomfort.

 CLIENT COMMUNICATION

A good understanding of menopause is essential because the signs and symptoms vary widely among women.

Prognosis

The prognosis is good; women move on to lead healthy and normal lives for many years. Postmenopausal women may suffer bone loss and eventual osteoporosis or changes in cholesterol levels as a result of decreased estrogen levels. Therefore, bone density studies and blood cholesterol levels should be monitored during regular physical examinations.

Prevention

Menopause cannot be prevented, but there are ways to reduce the symptoms. Controlling blood pressure and cholesterol, eating a low-fat diet, not smoking, exercising regularly, taking calcium and vitamin D, and discussing possible bone loss with a PCP are ways clients can reduce symptoms.

Weighing the Risks and Benefits of Hormone Replacement Therapy

HRT was first prescribed in the 1940s for postmenopausal women to treat their symptoms and to prevent postmenopausal conditions such as osteoporosis. However, two recent studies questioned whether the benefit of HRT outweighs its risks. The first study, conducted by the National Institutes of Health, looked at the effect of HRT taken as combination therapy versus a placebo. The study was halted because it found that the overall risks of HRT therapy exceeded the benefits. The risks included more coronary heart disease events, more strokes, serious blood clots, and invasive breast cancers. The benefits the study found were fewer colorectal cancers and fewer hip fractures.

A second study, completed in Britain, suggested that HRT can increase the risk of dying from breast cancer in addition to raising the risk of getting the disease. The researchers also determined that stopping HRT seemed to reduce the risk fairly quickly. It has been found that treatment for osteoporosis with ultralow doses of estrogen appears to be safe and increases bone density in older females.

The research suggests that estrogen-only therapy would cause fewer breast cancer occurrences than the combination HRT. The risk of endometrial cancer with estrogen-only therapy is well documented; therefore, this type of HRT is generally given only to women who have had a hysterectomy. The Food and Drug Administration recommends that women take the lowest dose for the shortest possible duration, less than 5 to 7 years. More research may be needed. However, the decision to use either estrogen-only or combination HRT after menopause must be made between a woman and her PCP, who together can weigh the possible risks and benefits. The NIH recommends that taking hormones should be reevaluated every 6 months. Weighing the possible risks and benefits is also necessary when considering estrogen therapy for the treatment of osteoporosis.

OVARIAN CANCER

ICD-10: C56.9

Description

Ovarian cancer is the sixth most common cancer among females and the fifth leading cause of cancer deaths in the United States. The National Cancer Institute projects an estimated 21,980 new cases of ovarian cancer will be reported in 2015 in the United States and that there will be approximately 14,180 deaths. More women die of ovarian cancer than from cervical and endometrial cancer combined. Women who take oral contraceptives for at least 5 years decrease their risk of ovarian cancer by 60%. Ovarian cancer has been called the silent killer because it usually is not found until it has spread to other organs. New evidence, however, indicates that there are recognizable symptoms in the early stages. Delaying the diagnosis results in a poorer prognosis.

Etiology

The exact cause of ovarian cancer is unknown, but contributing factors include infertility, familial tendency, HRT with estrogen only, obesity, and use of the male hormone androgen to treat endometriosis. Some researchers believe the monthly tissue-repair process that follows the release of the ovum may establish a situation in which genetic errors can occur. There is an increased risk for ovarian cancer in women who carry the *BRCA1* and *BRCA2* breast cancer genes. A new genetic variation identified as basonuclin-2 (*BNC2*) is more common than *BRCA1* and *BRCA2* but also appears to raise a woman's risk of ovarian cancer. Another genetic link comes from an inherited syndrome called hereditary nonpolyposis colorectal cancer (HNPCC) that also puts these women at greater risk for ovarian cancer.

Signs and Symptoms

Clients who consistently experienced urinary urgency; pelvic pain; abdominal pressure, fullness, and bloating; persistent indigestion or nausea; unexplained bowel habits; loss of appetite; increased abdominal girth; dyspareunia; lack of energy; low back pain; and changes in menstruation should report their symptoms to their PCP. An ovarian tumor can grow to considerable size (about the size of an onion) before producing any symptoms. Tumor rupture, infection, or torsion (twisting) may cause pain.

Diagnostic Procedures

Clinical evaluation, complete history, and physical examination are necessary. Transvaginal sonography, abdominal ultrasound, or CT scan may be used. CBC and blood chemistries may be ordered. Surgical exploration is the only way to grade and stage a tumor. Histological studies are done.

An early test for the diagnosis of ovarian cancer uses the HE4 biomarker, which is secreted into the blood by ovarian cancer cells. Another test used to detect ovarian cancer detects the protein CA125 and often is unreliable, so the hope is that the HE4 test will be more reliable in the earlier stages of the disease.

Treatment

Treatment is dependent on the grading and staging of the tumor. In some cases, surgery to remove the tumor and chemotherapy are done and, less frequently, radiation, as it is not considered effective in treating ovarian cancer. Surgical procedures may include a total abdominal hysterectomy and bilateral salpingo-oophorectomy with tumor resection. Surgery is often followed by chemotherapy. A procedure that may be used if the cancer is advanced involves injecting chemotherapy medications directly into the abdomen where higher levels of the drug can reach the cancer cells than is possible through IV chemotherapy. Palliative care is needed for clients undergoing chemotherapy treatment. Immunotherapy to boost the immune system can help combat the cancer. A new option is the drug bevacizumab (Avastin), which works to disrupt the blood supply to the tumor, hopefully causing it to shrink.

Complementary Therapy

Controlled amino acid therapy (CAAT) is achieved by taking certain foods out of the diet for a short time and replacing them with a scientifically supported formula of amino acids. CAAT works with chemotherapy to enhance its benefits and shut down the energy supply to cancer cells. A special diet is prescribed when clients are treated with CAAT and should never be undertaken without the strict supervision of the PCP or oncologist. Green tea and ginger capsules can help reduce nausea. Acupuncture, meditation, and aromatherapy helps some.

⊙ CLIENT COMMUNICATION

Help clients understand the staging and typing of ovarian cancer and subsequent treatment plans. If the client is young and wishes to have children, special attention to treatment is necessary. If chemotherapy is part of treatment, encourage clients to report any side effects so they can be treated. If the ovarian cancer is in the final stages, seek support of others on the health-care team to help the client and the family.

Prognosis

The prognosis is dependent on the type and stage of the cancer when it is diagnosed. If the cancer is detected early, the 5-year survival rate is approximately 95%; if the cancer has progressed, the prognosis drops to 35%.

Prevention

The best prevention of ovarian cancer is a yearly pelvic examination. A Pap test will detect ovarian cancer only in its advanced stages. Genetic testing is available to test whether a female carries mutations of the *BRCA1* and *BRCA2* breast cancer genes. Mutations of these genes put females at higher risk for the development of both ovarian and breast cancer. Factors that can reduce the risk of ovarian cancer include taking oral contraceptive pills, pregnancy followed by breastfeeding, and tubal ligation or hysterectomy.

Diseases and Disorders of the Breasts

FIBROCYSTIC BREASTS

ICD-10: N60.19

Description

Fibrocystic breasts have palpable lumps or cysts that fluctuate in size with the menstrual cycle. The condition is seen more frequently in women aged 30 to 55 and rarely after menopause. Fibrocystic breast tissue exhibits fluid-filled round or oval cysts, fibrosis, and hyperplasia of the cells lining the milk ducts or lobules of the breast (Fig. 16.8). Fibrocystic breasts are fairly common; more than half of women experience fibrocystic breast changes at some point in their lives. Medical professionals stopped using the term *fibrocystic breast disease* because fibrocystic breasts are not considered a disease.

Etiology

The causes of fibrocystic breasts are not well understood, but they are linked to the hormonal changes associated with ovarian activity. There is a tendency for fibrocystic breasts to run in families.

Signs and Symptoms

There may be widespread lumpiness or a localized mass, usually in the upper, outer quadrant of the

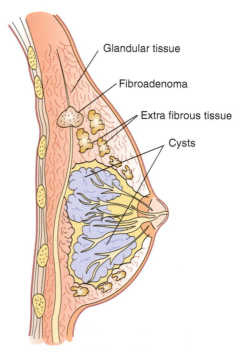

Glandular tissue

Fibroadenoma

Extra fibrous tissue

Cysts

Fibrocystic breast

Figure 16.8 Fibrocystic breast illustrating fibroadenoma.

breast. Pain, tenderness, and feeling of fullness are likely before menstruation. There can be fluctuating size of breast lumps, nonbloody nipple discharge (rare), and changes in both breasts.

Diagnostic Procedures

Monthly breast self-examinations cannot be overemphasized. Palpation is essential. A mammogram is especially useful if there is any suspicious change in the breast. Ultrasound is particularly helpful in distinguishing between fluid-filled breast cysts and any solid masses. When a suspicious area is discovered through these tests, a biopsy is essential to confirm the diagnosis. The clinical picture of pain, fluctuation in size, and lumpiness helps to differentiate fibrocystic breasts from breast cancer.

Treatment

No treatment is usually warranted; however, severe pain or large cysts may need treatment. Treatment is usually fine-needle aspiration to draw the fluid from the cyst or, on rare occasions, surgical excision. Acetaminophen or ibuprofen can reduce pain; oral contraceptives to lower the hormone levels linked to fibrocystic breasts may be prescribed. Breast pain also may be lessened with a good supportive bra. Caffeine intake may be restricted, salt intake reduced, and a low-fat diet advised because some studies indicate that these steps may reduce symptoms.

Complementary Therapy

Many women take one capsule of evening primrose oil up to three times a day to manage symptoms of fibrocystic breasts. It is believed that evening primrose oil may replace linoleic acid in women who are deficient in this essential fatty acid, as it can help to make breast tissue less sensitive to hormonal influences. Removing all forms of caffeine from the diet is suggested.

⊕ CLIENT COMMUNICATION

Teach clients how to perform breast self-examinations. Fibrocystic breasts often feel lumpy, and clients can best assess whether the lumps they feel are normal or abnormal.

Prognosis

The prognosis is good, although exacerbations may continue until menopause, after which they subside. Fibrocystic breasts can make breast examination and mammography more difficult to interpret, possibly causing a few early cancerous lesions to be overlooked.

Prevention

There is no known prevention. Monthly self-examination of the breasts and regular mammography are advised. Reducing caffeine and fat in the diet are other helpful measures.

CHAPTER EPISODE—PART III

After many diagnostic procedures and blood work, the PCP determined that Allison has polycystic ovarian syndrome (PCOS).

- What therapies might be suggested to her?
- What foods should she avoid to help reduce symptoms?
- If Allison's chronic anovulation continues, what is she predisposed for?

BENIGN FIBROADENOMA

ICD-10: D24.1

Description

A fibroadenoma is a benign, well-circumscribed solid tumor of fibrous and glandular breast tissue. It is a common tumor occurring in women under age 30.

Etiology

The cause of a fibroadenoma is unknown.

Signs and Symptoms

The breast mass is typically round, firm, smooth-edged, discrete, and relatively movable. It is nontender and usually discovered by accident.

Diagnostic Procedures

Palpation, followed by a mammogram, is essential for diagnosis. Digital mammography transfers images to a computer, where the radiologist can zoom in, magnify, and view the entire breast at one time. The images can also be stored and transferred for later viewing. The distinctive characteristics of this kind of tumor make it easy to diagnose, but it must be differentiated from a cyst or carcinoma through ultrasound and biopsy (see Fig. 16.8).

Treatment

The mass is excised under local anesthesia.

Complementary Therapy

No significant complementary therapy is indicated.

⊕ CLIENT COMMUNICATION

Teach clients how to perform breast self-examinations (Fig. 16.9). Fibroadenoma masses often feel round and firm and may be movable. Clients are the best indicator of any new growths but often fear the lump is breast cancer.

Prognosis

The prognosis is good after excision of the tumor.

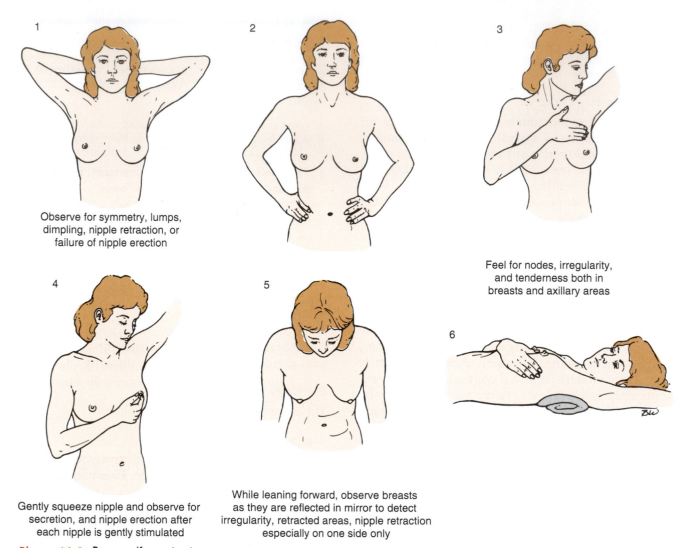

Observe for symmetry, lumps, dimpling, nipple retraction, or failure of nipple erection

Feel for nodes, irregularity, and tenderness both in breasts and axillary areas

Gently squeeze nipple and observe for secretion, and nipple erection after each nipple is gently stimulated

While leaning forward, observe breasts as they are reflected in mirror to detect irregularity, retracted areas, nipple retraction especially on one side only

Figure 16.9 **Breast self-examination.** *(From Venes, D, and Thomas, CL [ed]:* Taber's Cyclopedic Medical Dictionary, *ed. 21. Philadelphia: F.A. Davis, 2009, p 310, with permission.)*

Prevention

There is no known prevention for fibroadenomas.

CARCINOMA OF THE BREAST

ICD-10: C50.XX

Description

Breast cancer encompasses a variety of malignant neoplasms of the breast. It usually begins in the cells of the lobules (milk-producing glands) or the ducts that drain milk from the lobules to the nipple. It is the most common site of cancer in females and until recently was the leading cause of cancer deaths among women in the United States, a position that is now occupied by lung cancer.

Etiology

Breast cancer is caused by a genetic abnormality; however, only 5% to 10% of cancers are due to an abnormality inherited from a mother or father. The largest group of breast cancers is the result of genetic abnormalities related to aging and the "wear and tear" of life in general. The risk of breast cancer is higher in women with biopsy-confirmed atypical hyperplasia, a long menstrual history, and obesity after menopause. Smoking, alcohol consumption, a diet high in fat and red meat, and little or no daily exercise places one at greater risk as well.

Signs and Symptoms

The earliest sign of breast cancer is an abnormality shown on a mammogram. Breast changes, such as a lump, thickening, dimpling, swelling, skin irritation, distortion, retraction or scaliness of the nipple, nipple discharge, pain, and tenderness are the most common signs and symptoms. Advanced symptoms include edema, redness, nodularity or ulceration of the skin, and enlargement or shrinkage of the breast. Some cancers exhibit no symptoms.

Diagnostic Procedures

The best method of early detection continues to be the monthly self-examination of the breast. Mammography and ultrasonography are also frequently used screening methods. CT scan and MRI may be ordered. Diagnosis, however, must be made without delay because of the possibility of metastasis. Biopsy is essential for definitive diagnosis. Diagnosed breast cancer is staged and typed according to its pattern of growth.

Treatment

Treatment depends on the stage of breast cancer and the client's preferences. Curative treatment nearly always involves surgical management of the cancer. Possible surgeries are lumpectomy or mastectomy with accompanying radiation (either external or internal), chemotherapy, or hormone therapy. Whether lymph nodes under the arm are removed depends on the likely spread of the disease. Radiation may be done before surgery to shrink the tumor or postoperatively to destroy any remaining malignancy. If surgery is done, breast reconstruction may follow. Targeted cancer therapy is another treatment that may be used. This therapy targets specific characteristics of cancer cells, such as a protein that allows the cancer cells to grow rapidly and abnormally. Targeted therapy is generally less likely than chemotherapy to harm normal, healthy cells.

The tumor tissue is tested for the presence of hormone receptors to determine whether the tumor is estrogen and/or progesterone dependent. If it is, hormonal therapy may include medications to lower or block hormone production. Also, removal of the ovaries or adrenal glands and administration of testosterone, may be attempted to halt tumor regrowth or to prevent its spread.

Complementary Therapy

Importance is placed on enhancing the immune system and on working with the oncologist to make traditional treatment easier to handle. Treatments that have been effective for some individuals include acupuncture, aromatherapy, chiropractic, guided imagery, hypnosis, massage, meditation, music therapy, Reiki, spirituality and prayer, support systems, tai chi, and yoga.

⊙ CLIENT COMMUNICATION

Information is vital so that clients can make the choices appropriate for treatment. Referral to others who have been successfully treated can be beneficial.

Prognosis

The most reliable indicator of the prognosis is the stage of the breast cancer. In the early stages, the prognosis is good, especially if no metastasis has occurred. According to the American Cancer Society, the 5-year survival rate for localized breast cancer has risen to 97%. If the cancer has spread regionally, however, the survival rate is reduced to 77%. Since 1989, deaths from breast cancer have declined by about 3%. The reasons are believed to be advances in treatment and earlier detection.

Inflammatory Breast Cancer

Inflammatory breast cancer (IBC) is a rare (1% to 5% of all breast cancers) but aggressive form of breast cancer in which the cancer cells block the lymph vessels in the skin of the breast. The breast often looks swollen and red, or "inflamed." It tends to be diagnosed in younger women and occurs more frequently in African Americans than in whites.

Symptoms may include redness, swelling, and breast warmth. The breast may also appear pink, reddish purple, or bruised. The skin may have ridges or appear pitted, like the skin of an orange (called *peau d'orange*). Other symptoms include heaviness, burning, aching, increase in breast size, tenderness, or an inverted nipple. IBC has more likely metastasized at the time of diagnosis than other breast cancers. As a result, the 5-year survival rate for patients with IBC is only between 25% and 50%.

Breast Reconstruction

Breast reconstruction is generally done after mastectomy. The plastic surgeon rebuilds the breast contour, the nipple, and the areola. According to the American Cancer Society, the goals of reconstruction are:

- To provide symmetry of the breasts when the woman is wearing a bra.
- To permanently regain the client's breast contour.
- To prevent the need for an external prosthesis.

Several surgical options are available, including the use of a breast implant, using the client's own tissue flap (section of skin, fat, and muscle, which are removed from the abdomen or other area of the client's body), or a combination of the two. The surgery can be done immediately after a mastectomy or delayed until the client completes radiation.

Two websites to visit for more detailed information are http://www.cancer.org (search for breast reconstruction) or http://www.cancer.gov/cancerinfo (search for breast reconstruction).

Prevention

There is no known prevention of breast cancer. Breast self-examination and regular mammography cannot prevent breast cancer but can detect it early and increase the chance for a favorable prognosis.

COMMON SYMPTOMS OF FEMALE REPRODUCTIVE SYSTEM DISEASES AND DISORDERS

Women may present with the following common symptoms, which deserve attention from health-care professionals:

- Premenstrual and postmenstrual complaints, such as amenorrhea, dysmenorrhea, and metrorrhea; skin changes; and psychological reactions to hormonal changes
- Lower abdominal or pelvic pain
- Consistent bloating or fullness
- Any abnormal vaginal discharge or itching
- Fever
- Dyspareunia or any sexual dysfunction
- Breast changes, such as unusual swelling, lumpiness, mass formation, pain, or nipple abnormalities

Diseases and Disorders of Pregnancy and Delivery

Complementary Therapy

Complementary therapy in pregnancy is aimed at achieving a healthy pregnancy and preventing any difficulties. A well-balanced diet is advised, as is the avoidance of any harmful substances. These substances include caffeine, nicotine, and recreational and prescription drugs (prescription drugs need to be avoided unless specifically advised by the PCP, who will seek medications that are not harmful to the unborn). Adequate rest, "mental breaks," moderate exercise, and a positive outlook are beneficial to both mother and baby.

⟶ CLIENT COMMUNICATION

Pregnancy is most often a happy time in a woman's life. Any problem that causes difficulties during pregnancy requires special consideration. Pay attention to psychological and emotional needs of those affected by the problem. Remind clients to report any signs of spotting or bleeding and cramping immediately. Prompt treatment of any pelvic infection is encouraged. Any occurrence that ends the pregnancy before delivery is traumatic and grieving occurs. Remind clients that a difficult loss in pregnancy one time does not mean that a healthy full-term pregnancy is impossible in the future.

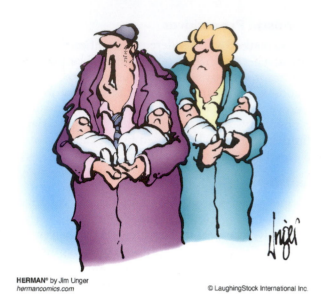

HERMAN® by Jim Unger
hermancomics.com
© LaughingStock International Inc.

"That's the last time we'll use this hospital!"

HERMAN© is reprinted with permission from LaughingStock Licensing Inc., Ottawa, Canada. All rights reserved.

SPONTANEOUS ABORTION

ICD-10: O03.9

Description

Spontaneous abortion, or miscarriage, is the expulsion of the conceptus before the 20th week of pregnancy. As many as 10% to 20% of pregnancies may end in spontaneous abortion; the incidence is higher in first pregnancies, and most occur in the first 7 weeks. The risk is higher in women over age 35 and those who have had a previous spontaneous abortion.

Etiology

Spontaneous abortion may be a result of defective development of the embryo (chromosomal abnormalities), faulty implantation of the fertilized ovum, placental problems, maternal infections or serious chronic disease, hormonal imbalances, trauma, or an unknown cause.

Signs and Symptoms

A pink or brown discharge may precede the onset of cramping and increased vaginal bleeding. The cervix will dilate, and the uterine contents will be expelled. The discharge may appear as a clotty menstrual flow. If the entire contents are expelled, bleeding and cramping stop. If any contents remain, cramping and bleeding continue.

Diagnostic Procedures

Evidence of the expelled uterine contents, pelvic examination, and laboratory studies will confirm the occurrence of a spontaneous abortion.

Treatment

If remnants of the conceptus remain in the uterus, **dilation and curettage (D&C)** should be performed or medication given to expel the remaining contents. A normal menstrual cycle will usually follow in a few weeks.

Prognosis

The prognosis for full recovery is good, barring any complications, such as hemorrhage, anemia, or infections.

Prevention

The progression of a spontaneous abortion usually cannot be prevented. However, it is less likely to occur if early, comprehensive prenatal care is received and environmental hazards (e.g., x-rays, drugs and alcohol, high levels of caffeine, and infectious diseases) are avoided.

ECTOPIC PREGNANCY

ICD-10: O00.X

Description

Ectopic pregnancy occurs when the fertilized ovum implants and grows somewhere other than in the uterine cavity. The most common ectopic site is within one of the fallopian tubes. Less frequently, ectopic implantation occurs in an ovary or in the abdominal cavity (Fig. 16.10). There is no way to save an ectopic pregnancy. It cannot turn into a normal pregnancy.

Etiology

Ectopic pregnancy is often due to scarring or inflammation of the fallopian tubes as a result of infection, such as chlamydia or gonorrhea, or it may be due to congenital malformations of the tubes. Endometriosis, PID, and tumors can cause ectopic pregnancy. In general, any factor that impedes the migration of the fertilized ovum into the uterus before attachment takes place increases the likelihood of an ectopic pregnancy.

Signs and Symptoms

Signs of early pregnancy may be present. There also may be abdominal pain and tenderness and slight vaginal bleeding. A rupture of a fallopian tube due to the development of the conceptus is life-threatening and will cause severe abdominal pain and intra-abdominal bleeding.

Diagnostic Procedures

A pelvic examination and a careful history may suggest ectopic pregnancy. A serum pregnancy test and an ultrasound examination likely will be used in this determination. Laparoscopy and exploratory laparotomy also may help in the diagnosis of this condition.

Treatment

Laparotomy is frequently necessary. A ruptured fallopian tube may require removal. All attempts will be made to save the ovary. Transfusion of whole blood may be necessary in the event of severe intra-abdominal bleeding or hypovolemic shock.

Prognosis

The prognosis is good when emergency treatment is sought quickly. If rupture of the tube occurs, complications may include hemorrhage, shock, and peritonitis.

Prevention

Prompt treatment of any genitourinary infection may help reduce the likelihood of ectopic pregnancy. Having an ectopic pregnancy increases the possibility of a second ectopic pregnancy unless any underlying cause can be corrected.

PREGNANCY-INDUCED HYPERTENSION (PREECLAMPSIA AND ECLAMPSIA)

ICD-10: O014.X, O15.X, O16.X

Description

Pregnancy-induced hypertension (PIH) is a hypertensive disorder that may develop during the third trimester. Most health-care professionals prefer to use the more precise terms *preeclampsia* and *eclampsia* to designate the condition. Preeclampsia, the nonconvulsive form of PIH, is the initial cluster of symptoms characterized by hypertension, edema, and proteinuria. Eclampsia, the convulsive form of PIH, is the subsequent group of symptoms

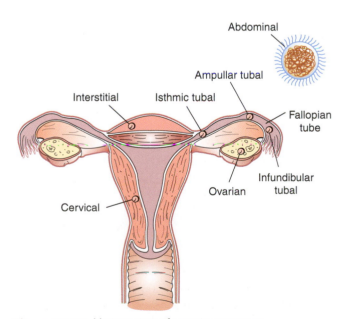

Figure 16.10 Various sites of ectopic pregnancy.

characterized by convulsions and coma. Eclampsia is a medical emergency. The condition is more likely to occur in women in their first pregnancy, or **primigravidas,** who are ages 12 to 18, or in women older than age 35 who have had multiple pregnancies.

Etiology

The cause of preeclampsia and eclampsia is not known, but some evidence suggests it is related to maternal nutrition. Predisposing factors include preexisting vascular and renal disease.

Signs and Symptoms

Hypertension, generalized edema, proteinuria, and sudden weight gain are the classic symptoms of preeclampsia. High sodium ingestion may be a contributing factor. Headache, vertigo, malaise, irritability, epigastric pain, and nausea also may occur. Eclampsia symptoms may include tonic-clonic convulsions, coma, crackling or **rhonchi** (rattling in the throat), rhythmic **nystagmus** (involuntary movement of the eyeball), and oliguria or **anuria.**

Diagnostic Procedures

Elevated—especially steadily rising—blood pressure, proteinuria, and oliguria are suggestive of preeclampsia. If the pregnant woman's urine exhibits low levels of placental growth factor and vascular endothelial growth factor, she is at high risk for PIH. Once PIH is identified, the gynecologist can more closely monitor the pregnancy for indications of PIH. The clinical picture of convulsions confirms a diagnosis of eclampsia.

Treatment

In preeclampsia, the goal of treatment is to prevent eclampsia and to deliver a healthy infant. Bed rest is advised, with sedatives prescribed. Antihypertensives may be necessary. The fetus may be delivered as soon as it is judged viable, possibly via cesarean section. At the onset of eclampsia, the client is hospitalized and intensive treatment is instituted. With careful monitoring, the goal is to manage severe cases until 32 to 34 weeks into the pregnancy and mild cases until 36 to 37 weeks. This helps reduce complications from premature delivery.

Prognosis

The prognosis is good for preeclampsia. In eclampsia, the maternal mortality rate is about 15%. In the United States, however, maternal deaths are rare.

Prevention

Adequate nutrition, good prenatal care, and control of high blood pressure during pregnancy are important. Urinalysis to detect high levels of protein is essential. Early treatment of preeclampsia can prevent eclampsia.

PLACENTA PREVIA

ICD-10: O44.10

Description

In placenta previa, the placenta is implanted abnormally low in the uterus so that it covers all or part of the internal cervical os, or opening (Fig. 16.11). Placenta previa is an obstetric complication that occurs in the second and third trimesters of pregnancy. This condition is dangerous because the placenta may prematurely separate from the uterus, causing maternal hemorrhaging and interrupting oxygen flow to the fetus. Bleeding occurs when the stretching and thinning of the uterus caused by the developing fetus creates a tear in the placenta somewhat at its margins. There are three types of placenta previa: (1) marginal or low implantation in which the placenta approaches the edge of the cervix, (2) partial placenta previa in which the placenta only partly covers the cervix, and (3) total placenta previa in which the placenta completely covers the cervix.

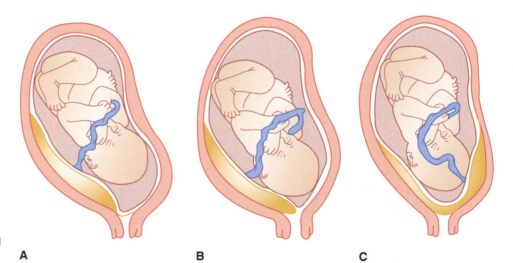

Figure 16.11 Placenta previa.
(A) Low marginal implantation.
(B) Partial placenta previa. (C) Central (total) placenta previa.

A   **B**   **C**

Etiology

The cause is unknown, but predisposing factors include multiparity, scars in the uterine lining, and previous uterine surgery.

Signs and Symptoms

A typical symptom is painless, bright-red bleeding, generally occurring in the third trimester, that may become more severe. The fetus may present in a variety of positions, but the situation is not critical as long as fetal heart tones remain strong. Vital signs may indicate shock.

Diagnostic Procedures

Ultrasonography is the primary diagnosis tool for placenta previa.

Treatment

If bleeding is not severe, bed rest at home is often advised with a decrease in activity. Hospitalization becomes necessary if bleeding is severe or cannot be stopped. Treatment is aimed at controlling and treating blood loss, delivering a healthy infant, and preventing complications. A cesarean section may be necessary.

Prognosis

The maternal prognosis depends on the amount of bleeding; the fetal prognosis depends on gestational age, blood loss, and consequences of possible anoxia. Complications include shock and maternal or fetal death.

Prevention

There is no known prevention for placenta previa.

ABRUPTIO PLACENTAE

ICD-10: O45.XX

Description

Abruptio placentae is the premature separation of a normally implanted placenta from the uterine wall at about the 20th week of gestation. The condition is most common in multigravidas.

Etiology

The cause is unknown, but predisposing factors include trauma, PIH, multiparity, diabetes, advanced maternal age, smoking, heavy use of alcohol during pregnancy, and cocaine abuse.

Signs and Symptoms

Abruptio placentae presents a wide range of symptoms, depending on the separation of the placenta and the amount of blood loss. There may be mild to moderate bleeding; continuous pain; or sudden, severe abdominal pain with boardlike rigidity, tenderness of the uterus, hemorrhage, and the onset of shock.

Diagnostic Procedures

Ultrasonography, pelvic examination, and history will help confirm the diagnosis. A CBC is likely ordered.

Treatment

The goals of treatment are to control the bleeding, deliver a healthy infant, and prevent complications. Hospitalization is required, and a cesarean section is typically performed. IV fluids and blood replacement may be necessary.

Prognosis

The maternal prognosis is good if the bleeding can be controlled. The fetal prognosis depends on gestational age and the amount of blood loss.

Prevention

There is no known prevention, but clients are advised to avoid drinking, smoking, and using recreational drugs during pregnancy and to get early and continuous prenatal care. Early recognition and proper management of conditions, such as diabetes and high blood pressure, in the mother also decrease the risk.

PREMATURE LABOR/PREMATURE RUPTURE OF MEMBRANES

ICD-10: O60.XX (PREMATURE LABOR)
ICD-10: O42.XX (PREMATURE RUPTURE OF MEMBRANES)

Description

Premature rupture of membranes (PROM) is early rupture of the amniotic sac. Premature labor is the early onset of rhythmic uterine contractions after fetal viability but before fetal maturity. Close to 90% of term clients and 50% of preterm clients go into labor within 24 hours after rupture. It is the most common diagnosis with preterm delivery.

Etiology

These conditions may be caused by cervical incompetence, preeclampsia, multiple pregnancy, abruptio placentae, anatomic malformations, infections, or fetal death. A predisposing factor may be poor prenatal care.

Signs and Symptoms

There may be a blood-tinged flow from the vagina, with uterine contractions and cervical dilation or **effacement**. PROM is marked by the flow of amniotic fluid from the vagina.

Diagnostic Procedures

Diagnosis is confirmed by prenatal history and vaginal and physical examination. Ultrasonography also may be used. Electronic fetal monitoring is used to confirm the fetal condition.

REALITY EPISODE

Carmina was expecting her second baby. She was due in 2 weeks. Riding home on a very full subway, she was particularly uncomfortable and had to ask a gentleman to give up his seat. A "grandmotherly type" next to her began a conversation about when the baby was due. Carmina began to relax and feel a little better when she felt the warm gush between her legs. She knew her water had broken, and she felt the first hard labor pain.

What can Carmina do? How can others on the subway help?

Treatment

When pregnancy is 36 weeks and beyond, management of PROM consists of delivery. Clients in active labor should be allowed to progress; those who are not will be induced with oxytocin. Those not yet in active labor and when there is no fetal distress may be discharged until labor begins, usually within 48 hours.

Prior to 36 weeks of pregnancy, delivery is delayed when there is no active labor, no infection, and no fetal distress. Clients are closely monitored for infection. Cultures for gonococci, *Chlamydia,* and group B streptococci are obtained. Symptoms, vital signs, uterine tenderness, odor of the **lochia,** and leukocyte counts are monitored.

Prognosis

The maternal prognosis is good with proper attention and care. The fetal prognosis depends on gestational age.

Prevention

The best prevention is good prenatal care.

Cesarean Birth (C-Section)

A C-section is a surgical procedure that is performed when a vaginal birth is not possible or is unsafe or when the health of the mother or neonate is at risk. The infant is delivered through an incision made in the abdomen and the uterus. C-section decisions may be made before labor and delivery when the neonate's head or body is too large to pass through the mother's pelvis or the mother's pelvis is too small (Fig. 16.12). Multiple births, placenta previa, horizontal or sideways position of the neonate in the uterus, or a breech (buttocks first) presentation also may dictate a C-section. During labor and delivery, C-sections may be necessary when there is failure of the labor to progress, when the cord is compressed or prolapsed, and when there is abruptio placentae or fetal distress. If the C-section is an emergency, the time from incision to delivery can take 10 to 15 minutes, with the delivery of the placenta and suturing of the incision requiring an additional 45 minutes.

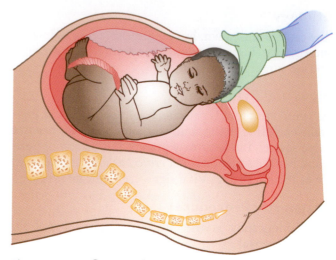

Figure 16.12   Cesarean delivery.

COMMON SYMPTOMS OF DISEASES AND DISORDERS OF PREGNANCY AND DELIVERY

Pregnant women may present with the following common complaints, any of which deserve attention from health-care professionals:

- Abdominal pain, tenderness, or cramping
- Unusual discharge that is pink, red, or brown in color or that is clotted
- Hypertension, rapid weight gain, edema, and malaise

SUMMARY

Human sexuality defines human beings. Some diseases and disorders are unique to either the male or the female reproductive system, yet they share numerous common factors. Because the reproductive system has the purpose of both reproduction and enhancement of caring and pleasure, any dysfunction clearly affects sexuality and self-image.

 DavisPlus | For more resources and to sharpen your skills with interactive exercises, visit *DavisPlus* at http://davisplus.fadavis.com. Keyword *Tamparo.*

ONLINE RESOURCES

Assisted reproductive technology
http://www.cdc.gov/art/artreports.htm

Endometriosis
http://www.endometriosisassn.org

Female reproductive health
http://www.womenshealth.gov

Inflammatory breast cancer
http://www.ibcresearch.org/

Ovarian cancer
http://www.apjohncancerinstitute.org/cancer/ovarian.htm

Prostate cancer
http://www.cancer.gov/cancertopics/types/prostate

http://www.cancer.org/research/cancerfactsstatistics/
cancerfactsfigures2015/

Sexually transmitted diseases
http://www.cdc.gov/STD

CASE STUDIES

Case Study 1

Roberta Hills, a sexually active 15-year-old girl, is informed by her boyfriend that he has gonorrhea. Roberta had noted that she has a slight vaginal discharge and some urinary difficulties, but she thought these were just symptoms of a UTI, because she has had a UTI twice before.

Case Study Questions
1. If Roberta calls the provider's office, what is she likely to be advised to do?
2. Can Roberta's symptoms be those of a UTI? Can they be symptoms of gonorrhea? Explain.
3. Based on the assumption that the symptoms are those of a UTI, what diagnostic tests are ordered? What action will be taken if gonorrhea is suspected?

Case Study 2

Linda Benedict, a 38-year-old woman, visits her PCP because she has been experiencing pain and tenderness in her left breast. The pain appears to be localized. In reply to the provider's question, Linda reports that she has been examining her breasts monthly and has not noted any lumps or abnormalities. Linda is examined, and no abnormalities are found. She is advised to return in 6 months; if the pain is still present, the PCP tells her a mammogram will be ordered.

Case Study Questions
1. What are the recommendations of the American Cancer Society that apply to this situation?
2. Is pain an early symptom of cancer? What might be causing Linda's discomfort?

Case Study 3

Dean Moore is a 67-year-old man diagnosed with benign prostatic hyperplasia. Surgery is suggested, but Dean fears impotence and incontinence.

Case Study Questions
1. How might a medical professional respond to Dean regarding his fears?
2. What other possible treatments might be considered?

REVIEW QUESTIONS

Matching

Match each of the following definitions with its correct term:

Sexually Transmitted Diseases

_____ 1. Caused by various types of papillomavirus

_____ 2. Caused by a motile protozoal infection

_____ 3. Caused by bacterium Treponema pallidum

_____ 4. Caused by the simplex virus

a. Genital herpes

b. HPV infection

c. Gonorrhea

d. Chlamydial infection

e. Syphilis

f. Trichomoniasis

Disorders of the Breast

_____ 5. Breast mass that is well circumscribed and solid

_____ 6. Lumpiness in upper, outer breast quadrant

_____ 7. Breast dimpling, swelling, skin irritation, lump, nipple discharge

a. Fibrocystic breasts

b. Benign fibroadenoma

c. Carcinoma of the breast

Male and Female Reproductive Diseases/Disorders

_____ 8. Most common male reproductive infection

_____ 9. Symptom is painless, smooth, firm mass in testis

_____ 10. Cluster of symptoms 3 to 14 days prior to menses

_____ 11. More than 1 million women have this disease

_____ 12. First prescribed to treat postmenopausal women

a. PMS

b. Testicular cancer

c. HRT

d. Epididymitis

e. PID

Short Answer

1. What are the two functions of sexuality in humans?

   a. _____

   b. _____

2. Can you name two inflammatory diseases of the male reproductive system and distinguish between them?

   a. _____

   b. _____

3. What are two common diagnostic procedures for prostatic cancer?

   a. _____

   b. _____

4. What is the difference between amenorrhea and dysmenorrhea?

5. Spell out the following abbreviations:

   a. BPH _____

   b. PMDD _____

   c. PID _____

   d. VDRL _____

   e. PSA _____

Multiple Choice

Place a checkmark next to the correct answer:

1. What might diseases of the breast include?

   _____ a. Leiomyomas

   _____ b. Fibroadenoma

   _____ c. Trichomoniasis

   _____ d. PCOS

2. What is the most commonly known STD?

   _____ a. Gonorrhea

   _____ b. Genital HPV infection

   _____ c. Genital herpes

   _____ d. Syphilis

3. What are two reproductive diseases that go undetected and are considered silent?

   _____ a. Prostatitis and epididymitis

   _____ b. Syphilis and trichomoniasis

   _____ c. Chlamydia and ovarian cancer

   _____ d. Ovarian cysts and endometriosis

4. What might an effective treatment for PMS be?

   _____ a. Reduction in salt intake

   _____ b. Reduction in caffeine and other stimulants

   _____ c. Proper diet and exercise

   _____ d. All of the above

5. Pregnancy-induced hypertension

_____ a. Causes an implanted ovum outside the uterine cavity

_____ b. Is diagnosed by ultrasonography

_____ c. Results in the premature separation of the placenta from the uterine wall

_____ d. Is also called *preeclampsia* and *eclampsia*

Discussion Questions/Personal Reflection

1. Discuss reasons a couple might choose ART. What are the advantages and disadvantages?

_____

_____

_____

_____

_____

_____

_____

_____

_____

_____

2. Discuss various complications that can occur during pregnancy. Identify any known preventative measures that could be taken.

_____

_____

_____

_____

_____

_____

_____

_____

_____

_____

_____

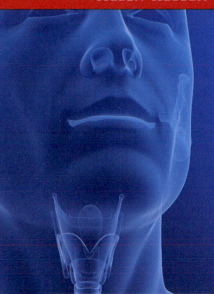

Life is either a daring adventure or nothing at all.
—HELEN KELLER

17

Eye and Ear Diseases and Disorders

● *chapter outline*

● *key words*

Amblyopia (ăm″blē•ō′pē•ă)
Atropine (ăt′rō•pēn)
Cellulitis (sĕl•ū•lī′tĭs)
Conjunctiva (kŏn″jŭnk•tī′vă)
Diplopia (dĭp•lō′pē•ă)
Macula (măk′ū•lă)

Myringotomy (mĭr•ĭn•gŏt′ō•mē)
Phacoemulsification (făk″ō•ē•mŭl′sĭ•fĭ•kā″shŭn)
Photophobia (fō″tō•fō′bē•ă)
Seborrhea (sĕb•ŏr•ē′ă)
Serous (sēr′ŭs)

Stapedectomy (stā″pĕ•dĕk′tō•mē)
Suppurative (sŭp′ū•ră″tĭv)
Tinnitus (tĭn•ī′tŭs)
Tonometer (tŏn•ŏm′ĕ•tĕr)
Tympanoplasty (tĭm″păn•ō•plăs′tē)
Vertigo (vĕr′tĭ•gō)

Upon successful completion of this chapter, you will be able to:

- Interpret key terms.
- Describe eye and ear anatomy and physiology.
- Name four common refractive errors.
- Identify the signs and symptoms of nystagmus.
- Describe the treatment for stye, or hordeolum.
- Discuss the prognosis of corneal abrasions.
- List the various causes of cataracts.
- Restate the prognosis for and prevention of glaucoma.
- Discuss the process that causes retinal detachment.
- List the prevention of age-related macular degeneration.
- Describe the symptoms of strabismus.
- Identify the signs and symptoms of conjunctivitis.

- Describe uveitis.
- Restate the signs and symptoms of blepharitis.
- Describe the etiology of keratitis.
- Identify the treatment for impacted cerumen.
- Describe the etiology of external otitis, or swimmer's ear.
- Compare and contrast serous otitis media with suppurative otitis media.
- Define *otosclerosis*.
- Discuss the treatment for motion sickness.
- Identify the treatment for Ménière disease.
- Recall the client communication for hearing loss.
- List at least three common symptoms for both eye and ear diseases and disorders.

EYE AND EAR ANATOMY AND PHYSIOLOGY REVIEW

CHAPTER EPISODE—PART I

Emory is an 11-month old baby girl who is generally happy and playful. Developmentally she is on track and is enjoying exploring the world around her. Recently Emory has not been acting like her normal happy self. She has had a runny nose and has been fussy for the past two days. This afternoon she spiked a fever of 102°F.

- What could be causing Emory's discomfort?
- What should Emory's parents do?

The most important sensory receptors are our eyes and the ears. The eye is the primary organ for sight, and the ear is the primary organ for sound and equilibrium. Impairment of either of these sensory receptors can be a traumatic experience and can cause serious disability.

Eyes

The eyes contain the receptors for light stimuli and are the organs of vision. Eyes are protected within the orbits by surrounding bones, the eyelids, the eyelashes, the eyebrows, and the **conjunctiva,** or inner mucous membrane surface of the eyelids. The meibomian glands on the inner surface of the upper and lower eyelids produce lipidlike secretions to help keep the eye moist. When the eye blinks, the upper lid presses on the oil, pulling a sheet of oil upward to coat the tear layer and keep it from evaporating. The lacrimal apparatus produces and removes tears. Tears assist in keeping the outer part of the eye and the conjunctiva moist.

The eye is a hollow, spherical organ composed of three layers (Fig. 17.1). The outer layer consists of the sclera (an opaque, white portion of the eye) and the cornea (an anterior window of the eye). The cornea bends the light rays as they pass through its convex curvature.

The middle layer of the eye consists of the choroid coat, the ciliary body, and the iris. The choroid coat contains the blood vessels of the eye and melanin. The melanin absorbs light within the eyeball and prevents glare. The ciliary body contains the ciliary muscles, which contract and relax to change the shape of the lens of the eye and form a ring around it.

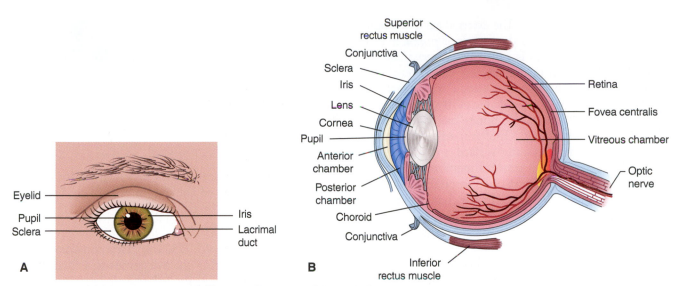

Figure 17.1 (A) The human eye and (B) internal anatomy of the eyeball.

Ligaments hold the lens in place. The lens focuses the light rays precisely on the retina. The colored portion of the eye is the iris, and it controls the amount of light entering the eye by controlling the size of the pupil. The pupil is the opening in the center of the iris through which light passes to the lens.

The inner layer of the eye contains the retina, which lines the interior of the eye. It contains the rods (for light detection) and cones (for color detecting) and neurons. The **macula** is a yellow disk on the retina directly behind the lens. In the center of the macula is a small depression called the *fovea centralis* that contains only densely packed cones. The fovea is the area of the sharpest, bright-light vision. The sight impulses formed by the rods and cones are transmitted to ganglion neurons that converge at the optic disk, forming the optic nerve. Blood vessels nourish the eye. The space between the cornea and the lens is called the *anterior cavity,* which is filled with aqueous humor. The aqueous humor helps to maintain the shape of the cornea and is responsible for the pressure of the eye. Behind the lens is the posterior cavity, which is filled with a clear gel-like substance called *vitreous humor*. The vitreous humor helps to maintain the shape of the eye by pressing firmly against the wall of the eye.

Refraction is the process of bending the light rays and is produced by the cornea and lens. There is further bending by the lens (accommodation) to provide fine adjustments, focusing the image on the retina. Once the light stimulus is on the retina, it must convert into impulses that are sent to the brain via the optic nerve. In the brain, the impulses are interpreted as visual images.

Ears

Ears are the organs of hearing and equilibrium (Fig. 17.2). The ear is divided into three parts: the external, the

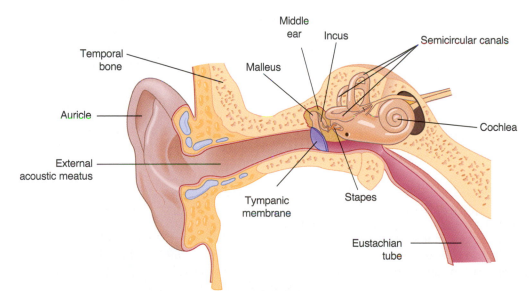

Figure 17.2 Outer, middle, and inner ear structures in a frontal section through the right temporal bone.

middle, and the inner parts. The external ear is the outer, funnel-like structure called the *auricle* or *pinna*, and the external auditory meatus is called the *external auditory canal*. Hearing begins in the external ear, where sound waves are carried through the auricle and canal. The middle ear consists of the tympanic cavity, the tympanic membrane, and three small bones called the *ossicles* (malleus, incus, and stapes). The tympanic membrane is a thin layer of skin on its outer surface, and on the inner surface, it is covered with mucous membrane. Sound is transmitted from the auditory canal through the auditory meatus. The sound is conducted by the change in pressure on the eardrum and then the three ossicles vibrate.

The auditory or eustachian tube connects the middle ear to the throat or nasopharynx and mouth. The tube helps maintain equal air pressure on both sides of the eardrum, which is essential for normal hearing.

The inner ear, embedded in the temporal bone, consists of three semicircular canals and a cochlea. The canals provide a sense of equilibrium, and the cochlea contains the organ of Corti, the hearing receptors. The space between the bony and membranous labyrinths is filled with perilymph, whereas the membranous labyrinth contains endolymph. These fluids are essential in the hearing function of the inner ear. In the inner ear, sound is conducted via the organ of Corti receptor cells and nerves.

Figures 17.1 and 17.2 illustrate the major parts of the eye and ear.

Eye Diseases and Disorders

REFRACTIVE ERRORS

ICD-10: H40.9

Description

Refractive errors are defects in visual acuity resulting from the inability of the eye to effectively focus light on the surface of the retina (Fig. 17.3). Four common refractive errors are:

- *Hyperopia (ICD-10: H52.03):* This condition occurs when light entering the eye comes to a focus behind the retina so that vision is better for distant objects. This condition is commonly called *farsightedness,* which causes difficulties in seeing objects that are close. Hyperopia often results when the globe of the eye is abnormally short in length from front to back.
- *Presbyopia (ICD-10: H52.4):* This refractive error is a form of farsightedness that causes the eye to lose its ability to focus. Unlike hyperopia, however, presbyopia results from a loss of elasticity in the crystalline lens of the eye. When the eye focuses on a distant object, muscles encircling the lens contract, stretch, or flatten it. When the eye focuses on a nearby object, the muscles relax, allowing the lens

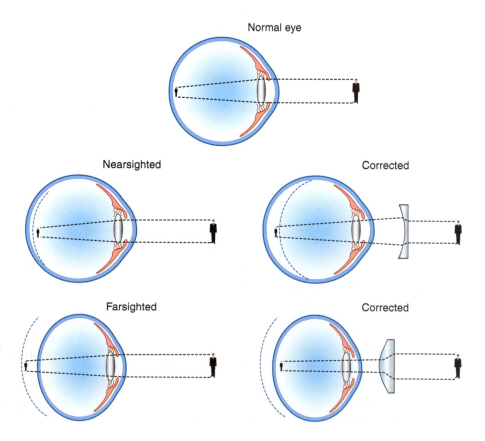

Figure 17.3 Errors of refraction compared with the normal eye. Corrective lenses are shown for nearsightedness and farsightedness. *(Adapted from Scanlon, VC, and Sanders, T: Essentials of Anatomy and Physiology, ed. 6. FA Davis, Philadelphia, 2011, p. 224, with permission.)*

to resume a more spherical shape. In presbyopia, however, the lens remains in a comparatively flattened position after the muscles have relaxed. This condition is a consequence of advancing age.

- *Myopia (ICD-10: H52.1):* This condition occurs when light entering the eye comes to a focus in front of the retina so that vision is better for nearby objects. Consequently, this condition is commonly called *nearsightedness*. With myopia, close objects are seen clearly, but objects farther away appear blurred. Myopia often results when the eyeball is abnormally long from front to back.
- *Astigmatism (ICD-10: H52.20):* This refractive error occurs when light entering the eye is focused unevenly or diffusely across the retina so that some of the visual field appears properly focused while some does not. The condition is caused by variations in the curvature over certain portions of the lens or cornea of the eye, creating out-of-focus vision.

Etiology

Except for presbyopia, which is a consequence of advancing age, it is not known what causes some individuals to develop visual defects, whereas others do not. Some types of refractive errors, however, show a strong familial pattern, suggesting a genetic predisposition to acquiring them. For example, when both parents have astigmatism, their offspring will also have astigmatism.

Signs and Symptoms

In addition to the characteristic visual deficits described, general symptoms of refractive errors may include squinting, headaches, and frequent rubbing of the eyes. Seeing halos around bright lights is also common.

Diagnostic Procedures

The diagnosis of refractive errors usually involves testing for visual acuity using the Snellen eye chart, dilation for ophthalmoscopic examination of the interior of the eye, and tests to detect eye muscle function.

Treatment

Treatment of refractive errors involves the prescription and fitting of corrective lenses in the form of either eyeglasses or contact lenses (see Fig. 17.3). An alternative to corrective lenses is laser eye surgery, which permanently changes the shape of the cornea. Laser-assisted in situ keratomileusis (LASIK) can be performed on individuals with varying degrees of nearsightedness, farsightedness, and astigmatism. In the surgery, a microsurgical knife cuts a hinge flap in the cornea that is then lifted out of the way. A laser reshapes underlying corneal tissue. The flap is then replaced and quickly adheres to the eyeball. Other surgical alternatives include the following:

- Photorefractive keratectomy (PRK): This procedure does not create a corneal flap but uses laser to treat myopia, hyperopia, and astigmatism. PRK involves the use of a cool ultraviolet light-beam laser to ablate or remove very tiny bits of tissue from the surface of the cornea in order to reshape it. When the cornea is reshaped, it works better to focus light into the eye and onto the retina, providing clearer vision than before. Both nearsighted and farsighted people can benefit from PRK.
- Astigmatic keratectomy: This is an incision to reduce certain degrees of astigmatism by smoothing an irregular cornea into a more normal shape.
- Intrastromal corneal rings: In this procedure, clear, thin polymer inlays are used to correct low myopia only. Two ultrathin arcs are surgically implanted in the peripheral area of the cornea. The arcs flatten the cornea to the degree required to correct the myopic condition. The procedure does not cut or remove any tissue, although the segments can later be removed or replaced to correct for possible sight changes as the eye ages.

Complementary Therapy

The American Academy of Ophthalmology identifies a number of studies regarding the effectiveness of complementary therapy for several eye diseases and disorders. Some of the therapies mentioned include visual training for refractive errors and acupuncture for age-related macular degeneration. Visual training for refractive errors can help enhance efficiency and processing of one's vision. While acupuncture for age-related macular degeneration is identified by the American Academy of Ophthalmology, no strong evidence is provided to indicate whether it is truly effective as a treatment. See http://one.aao.org/guidelines-browse?filter=complementarytherapy assessment for details.

➔ CLIENT COMMUNICATION

If multifocal lenses are prescribed, clients may need continued encouragement to get used to them. If contacts, either hard or soft, are prescribed, clients need to be fully informed of their care, use, and safety. In the case of laser surgery, clients must understand good postoperative follow-up and the importance of keeping the eye moist.

Prognosis

With corrective lenses and/or surgery, the prognosis is good for persons with refractive errors.

Prevention

There are no specific preventive measures for any of these refractive errors.

NYSTAGMUS

ICD-10: H55.00

Description

Nystagmus is repetitive, involuntary, and rapid movement of the eye. The eyes may move side to side (horizontal nystagmus), up and down (vertical nystagmus), or in a rotary or turning pattern. One or both eyes may be affected.

Etiology

Nystagmus may be either congenital or acquired. The congenital form is rare and is usually mild when it does occur. Acquired nystagmus results from disease processes that produce lesions in the portions of the brain or the structures within the ears that help govern eye movement. Ménière disease can cause nystagmus. Chronic visual impairment, certain antiseizure medications, or alcohol abuse also may produce this condition by harming the labyrinth. Head injuries from vehicle crashes or cerebrovascular accident or stroke can also cause nystagmus.

Signs and Symptoms

The symptoms of nystagmus are continuous horizontal, vertical, or circular eye movements (or a combination of these). Blurred vision may also be reported.

Diagnostic Procedures

The tests to determine nystagmus include CT or MRI scans of the head, electrooculography that measures eye movements using tiny electrodes, and vestibular testing. Vestibular testing records eye movements and response to caloric stimulation. The caloric test measures responses to warm and cold water circulated through a small, soft tube in the ear canal.

Treatment

Treatment must be directed at the underlying cause of the nystagmus, if possible. In some instances, nystagmus disappears when underlying causes are corrected.

Complementary Therapy

In nystagmus, a cure may not be possible; however, avoidance of sugar, eggs, dairy products, fats, fried foods, alcohol, tobacco, and caffeine has proved helpful to some. Exposure to fluorescent lighting should be minimized when possible.

⊕ CLIENT COMMUNICATION

A careful review of clients' medications may be necessary in acquired nystagmus. Carefully explain the diagnostic procedures and listen to clients' concerns.

Prognosis

The prognosis for nystagmus depends on the underlying cause.

Prevention

There is no specific prevention for nystagmus.

STYE (HORDEOLUM)

ICD-10: H00.019

Description

A stye (hordeolum) is a localized, purulent, inflammatory infection of one or more of the sebaceous glands of the eyelid. Styes commonly occur on the skin surface at the edge of the lid or on the surface of the conjunctiva, the mucous membrane structure that lines the inner surface of the eyelids.

Etiology

Styes usually result from infection by staphylococcal bacteria. An eyelash is often found in the center of the stye. Frequently, it is secondary to blepharitis or immunoglobulin M (IgM) deficiency.

Signs and Symptoms

The chief signs and symptoms are pain and tenderness of an intensity directly related to the amount of swelling. There is redness at the site.

Diagnostic Procedures

Visual examination is all that is necessary in most cases to make a diagnosis; however, a culture may be taken to isolate staphylococci.

Treatment

Most styes disappear on their own in 5 to 7 days, but warm compresses applied to the eyes for up to 10 minutes four times a day may be prescribed to hasten the pointing of the abscess. Removal of an eyelash may be followed by pus drainage. An incision and drainage of the abscess under local anesthesia may be necessary. Antibiotic eyedrops or ointment may be used. In some cases, the infection warrants the use of oral antibiotics.

Complementary Therapy

Once the infection has been treated, the eye may be dry. The eye can be rinsed with a normal saline solution, as some over-the-counter eyedrops may irritate the eye.

⊕ CLIENT COMMUNICATION

It is essential that clients keep the affected eye clean and avoid rubbing or irritating it. Remind clients to return in 2 to 4 weeks for follow-up assessment by the primary care provider or ophthalmologist.

Prognosis

The prognosis is good with treatment, but recurrences are common. A complication of a hordeolum is an inflammation, or **cellulitis,** of the eyelid.

Prevention

Prevention includes cleanliness, proper eye care, and keeping hands away from the eyes.

Dry Eye Syndrome

Millions of Americans suffer from dry eye syndrome, which is caused by a problem with the quality of the tear film that lubricates the eye. There are three layers to the eye's tears: (1) The mucus layer coats the cornea; (2) the aqueous layer provides moisture, oxygen, and other nutrients to the cornea; and (3) the outer lipid layer is an oily film that helps prevent evaporation. Tears are formed in the glands around the eye; with each blink, the eyelids spread tears over the eye. Tears that respond to injury or emotion are known as *reflex tears* and do little to lubricate a dry eye.

Dry eyes are part of the normal aging process, but hot, dry, windy climates and high altitudes can cause dry eye as well. Air-conditioning, cigarette smoke, and reading or working at a computer screen for a long time without a break are also causes of dry eye syndrome. Contact lens wearers have dry eyes, and some medications cause dryness. Symptoms include burning, itching, irritation, redness, and blurred vision that improves with eye blinking. The condition is diagnosed when a primary care provider or ophthalmologist measures the production, evaporation rate, and the quality of the tear film. Using preservative-free artificial tears on a regular basis is the most common treatment for dry eye syndrome. On occasion, closing the tear drain in the eyelid with special inserts may be instituted. These plugs trap the tears on the eye. Drinking at least eight glasses of water each day is helpful. Clients are to be reminded not to rub their eyes and to blink regularly when reading or looking at a computer screen for long periods of time. The recommendation is that after every 20 minutes at the computer screen, look away for 20 seconds.

CORNEAL ABRASION

ICD-10: S05.00XA*

Description

A corneal abrasion is a painful scrape or scratch on the transparent anterior cellular layer of the eye known as the cornea. This transparent window covers the iris, the circular colored portion of the eye.

Etiology

Corneal abrasions may be produced by foreign bodies, such as dirt, dust, or metal particles trapped between the cornea and the eyelid. A scratch also may result from fingernail contact with the cornea or from wearing poorly fitting or scratched contact lenses. A hot cigarette ash flying into the eye may cause a corneal abrasion. A common cause of a corneal abrasion occurs from an accidental poke in the eye by a young child. Corneal abrasions can also occur when the eyes are rubbed excessively when they are irritated.

Signs and Symptoms

Pain, redness, and tearing are common symptoms; there may be the sensation that something is constantly in the eye. Visual acuity may be impaired, depending on the size and location of the abrasion. The eyes quite often tear. Pain is felt when eyes are exposed to bright light. The muscles around the eye may spasm, causing squinting.

Diagnostic Procedures

A medical history and visual examination may be all that are necessary to suggest the diagnosis. Instilling the affected eye with a fluorescein stain will help highlight the presence of any corneal lesion; the injured area will appear green when examined with a flashlight.

Treatment

If a foreign body is indeed present in the eye, irrigation of the corneal surface may be attempted, or a topical anesthetic may be administered and the object removed. Once the eye surface is clear of debris, an antibiotic ophthalmic ointment is often prescribed. The eye may or may not be patched by the ophthalmologist. Recent evidence shows that patching the eye probably does not help and may actually have a negative impact on the healing process. However, clients are advised to rest the eye, keeping it closed as much as possible, and to not read, watch television, or drive.

Complementary Therapy

No significant complementary therapy is indicated.

CLIENT COMMUNICATION

Encourage clients to strictly follow the prescribed treatment because an abrasion may cause loss of vision. Further damage to the eye can be avoided by wearing protective eye gear when in situations where anything might fly into the eye.

*The X represents the fourth digit that is often required and supplied once more detailed information about the disease or disorder is made known to the provider.

Prognosis

The prognosis is good with treatment and usually resolves in 24 to 48 hours. Complications of untreated corneal abrasion include ulceration of the cornea and permanent vision loss.

Prevention

Prevention of corneal abrasions includes wearing protective eyewear when engaging in hazardous occupations or sports and following recommendations for cleaning and wearing contact lenses.

CATARACT

ICD-10: H26.9*

Description

A cataract is an opacity, or clouding, of the crystalline lens of the eye or its surrounding membrane (Fig. 17.4). The condition may be unilateral or bilateral. A cataract develops slowly, affecting visual acuity. It is very common, especially in older persons. Worldwide, half of all individuals have cataracts or have had cataract surgery by the time they are age 80.

Etiology

Cataracts are caused by a change in the chemical composition of the lens, resulting in a loss of lens transparency. These changes can be caused by aging (senile cataracts), eye injuries (traumatic cataracts), certain diseases (secondary cataracts), and genetic diseases such as myotonic dystrophy, neurofibromatosis, or birth defects (congenital cataracts).

Signs and Symptoms

A gradual loss or blurring of vision is the common symptom. Colors appear faded. Some people report seeing halos around lights, and some have problems driving at night because of glare from the lights of oncoming cars. As a cataract matures, the pupil of the eye may appear white to an observer. The condition is painless.

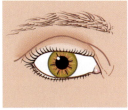 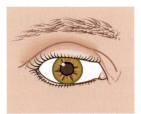

Normal, clear lens   Lens clouded by cataract

Figure 17.4 Cataract.

Diagnostic Procedures

A visual acuity test is performed to check the vision for clarity and sharpness. Ophthalmoscopy, penlight examination, or slit-lamp examination are used to confirm the diagnosis. Pupil dilation is needed to see the retina and look for any other problems. Tonometry is used to measure fluid pressure inside the eye.

Treatment

Treatment varies depending on the degree of visual impairment and on the age, general health, and occupation of the affected individual. Once the cloudy, natural lens of the eye is removed, the person needs a substitute lens to focus the eye. Surgical extraction of the defective lens is followed by refractive correction using eyeglasses, contact lenses, or surgically implanted artificial lenses called *intraocular lenses* (IOLs). The most common surgical methods to remove cataracts are intracapsular and extracapsular extraction and **phacoemulsification.** The latter uses an ultrasonic device that disintegrates cataracts so they can be aspirated and removed. Laser is used less frequently.

Complementary Therapy

Unfortunately, cataracts cannot be prevented by vitamin, mineral, or protein supplements. Protecting eyes from ultraviolet light and wearing sunglasses outside can be very helpful.

⊸ CLIENT COMMUNICATION

Clients may be advised to make accommodations prior to the removal of their cataracts. Using a magnifying glass for reading, increasing the lighting in the home environment, and wearing sunglasses to block ultraviolet B (UVB) rays are recommended.

Prognosis

The prognosis is excellent with surgery, and visual acuity is improved in 97% to 98% of cases.

Prevention

Currently there is no known prevention for most cataracts, but regular eye examinations, especially after age 65, and wearing sunglasses when outside to protect the eye from harmful UVB rays can help clients maintain healthy eyes.

*Unspecified cataract. Codes with a higher degree of specificity can be assigned once more detailed information about the disease or disorder is made known.

GLAUCOMA

ICD-10: H40.9*

Description

Glaucoma is a condition in which accumulating fluid pressure within the eye damages the retina and optic nerve, often causing blindness. The buildup of pressure occurs because more fluid, called *aqueous humor,* is produced than can be drained from the eye. Open-angle glaucoma is the most common form of this condition and results from the obstruction of passages within the eye that form the trabecular meshwork, which drains the aqueous humor into the lymphatic system. In the United States, glaucoma affects 2% of the population older than age 40. The condition may be unilateral or bilateral.

Etiology

Primary forms of the condition, such as open-angle glaucoma, are idiopathic; however, a strong familial tendency toward developing glaucoma suggests that unknown genetic factors may be involved. It also may arise secondary to a wide variety of other diseases, or it may be induced by certain drugs or toxins. Glaucoma most often occurs in adults over age 45, but it can also occur in young adults, children, and even infants. Those of African American, Irish, Russian, Japanese, Hispanic, Inuit, or Scandinavian descent are at an increased risk. Individuals who are over age 45 or have a family history of glaucoma, severe myopia, or diabetes are also at risk. Those who had a previous eye injury may also be at risk.

Signs and Symptoms

The most common forms of glaucoma develop asymptomatically and often are not detected until irreparable damage has already occurred to the retinas or optic nerves. When symptoms appear late in the course of the disease, they may include mild aching in the eyes and visual disturbances, such as seeing halos around lights or a noticeable loss of peripheral vision.

Diagnostic Procedures

A positive family history for the disease should suggest a potential diagnosis of glaucoma. One of the various instruments used to measure intraocular pressure, a **tonometer,** can detect elevations in eye pressure. Ophthalmoscopic inspection of the retinal surface is essential to determine whether retinal damage has occurred. Vision-field testing, done periodically, can help determine the extent of peripheral vision loss, and results are compared over time by the ophthalmologist.

Treatment

Glaucoma treatment may include prescription eyedrops, laser surgery, or microsurgery in order to lower eye pressure. Eyedrops either reduce the formation of fluid in the front of the eye or increase its outflow. Laser surgery slightly increases the outflow of the fluid from the eye in open-angle glaucoma or eliminates fluid blockage in angle-closure glaucoma. Microsurgery for glaucoma is an operation called a *trabeculectomy.* In this procedure, a new channel is created to drain the fluid, thereby reducing the intraocular pressure that causes glaucoma. In the United States, medications are used first, but there is increasing evidence that some individuals may respond better with early laser surgery or microsurgery.

Complementary Therapy

Antioxidant supplements such as carotene, vitamin C, and vitamin E identified as beneficial for cataracts may have the same effect on glaucoma. Keep the client's primary care provider informed of the glaucoma treatment.

➔ CLIENT COMMUNICATION

It is important that clients understand they have to administer their eye medication exactly as prescribed. Regular eye examinations should be scheduled for follow-up.

Prognosis

The prognosis usually is good with early treatment. Drug therapy must be maintained for life.

Prevention

It is important for all persons over age 20 to have ophthalmoscopic examinations that include a test for glaucoma every 3 to 5 years.

RETINAL DETACHMENT

ICD-10: H33.XXX*

Description

Retinal detachment is the complete or partial separation of the retina from the choroid layer of the eye (Fig. 17.5); it leads to the loss of retinal function and blindness. The condition occurs as a result of a hole or break in the retina that allows vitreous humor to accumulate between the two layers.

Etiology

Retinal detachment usually is caused by head trauma. Hemorrhages or tumors of the outer (choroid) layer also

---

*Unspecified glaucoma. Codes with a higher degree of specificity can be assigned once more detailed information about the disease or disorder is made known.

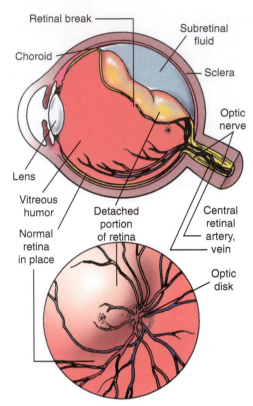

Figure 17.5 **Retinal detachment.** *(From Venes, D, and Thomas, CL [eds]: Taber's Cyclopedic Medical Dictionary, ed. 21. FA Davis, Philadelphia, 2009, p 2025, with permission.)*

may cause the condition. Certain systemic diseases such as diabetes mellitus may predispose one to the condition. Spontaneous retinal detachments also may occur among elderly persons, those who are very nearsighted, or those who have a family history of retinal detachment.

Signs and Symptoms

An individual with retinal detachment may report seeing cobwebs, floating spots, flashes of light, or the sensation of a shade coming across the eye. These signs worsen and are followed by a dark shadow extending from the periphery inward. As more of the retina detaches from the choroid surface, progressive loss of vision occurs. The condition is painless. **Retinal detachment is a medical emergency.**

Diagnostic Procedures

Ophthalmoscopic examination while the pupils are fully dilated reveals the detached portion of the retina suspended in the vitreous humor of the eye.

Treatment

Small holes are treated with laser surgery or a freeze treatment called *cryopexy*. The goal of both procedures is to "weld" the retina back in place. During laser surgery, tiny burns are made around the hole to weld the retina back into place. Cryopexy freezes the area around the hole and helps reattach the retina. Some treatments

for retinal detachments may require a hospital stay. In some cases, a tiny synthetic band is attached to the outside of the eyeball to gently push the wall of the eye against the detached retina. A vitrectomy may also be performed to remove the vitreous, a gel-like substance that fills the center of the eye and helps the eye maintain a round shape. Gas or silicone oil is injected into the eye to replace the vitreous and reattach the retina. During the healing process, the eye makes fluid to replace the gas and fill the eye.

Complementary Therapy

No significant complementary therapy is indicated.

> ⊖ **CLIENT COMMUNICATION**
>
> The diagnostic procedure using an ophthalmoscope with the eye dilated can be a prolonged examination that clients find very uncomfortable. It can feel like looking directly into the sun, so it is important to explain the procedure and its importance for diagnosis and follow-up care. After surgery, return visits for checkups are essential to monitor progress and prevent any complications.

Prognosis

The prognosis is good if surgical repair is successful. The prognosis is worse if the portion of the retina that produces the sharpest vision (the macula lutea) is detached. Even under the best circumstances, after multiple attempts at repair, treatment sometimes fails and vision may eventually be lost. Without treatment, retinal detachment may become total in a few months.

Prevention

There is no specific prevention for retinal detachment other than following safety measures that minimize its risk.

AGE-RELATED MACULAR DEGENERATION

ICD-10: H35.30

Description

Macular degeneration is a slowly progressive disease that produces changes in the pigmented cells of the retina and macula. These pigmented cells are more concentrated in the macula. The result is progressive loss of fine vision in one or both eyes. There are two types of age-related macular degeneration (AMD or ARMD): the dry, or non-neovascular, form and the wet, or neovascular, form. The dry form accounts for about 90% of people with AMD. It is a slowly progressive mild vision loss. The wet form may come on abruptly and begins with proliferation under the retina. The vessels leak, hemorrhage, and form scars that produce significant central vision loss. AMD is the leading cause of new blindness in the United States, and it affects millions of elderly Americans.

Etiology

Macular degeneration usually is a result of the aging process. Risk factors include increasing age (60 years or older), hyperopia, light iris color, positive family history, hypertension, cigarette smoking, and obesity. AMD may be inherited (especially the wet form), or it may result from injury, inflammation, or infection.

Signs and Symptoms

Dry macular degeneration usually starts with the appearance of spots on the retina called *drusen*. Similar to age spots, drusen do not change vision very much; rather, the person will notice relatively mild visual loss with distortion. It is believed these spots are deposits or debris from deteriorating tissue. Gradual central vision loss may occur with dry AMD but usually is not nearly as severe as wet AMD symptoms. Early in macular degeneration, there may be no symptoms; however, as the degeneration continues, the person experiences painless visual loss and/or distortion and should have an immediate eye examination. The individual usually notices that sharp vision is affected and often is unable to read or do close work.

Diagnostic Procedures

Macular degeneration may be detected during a routine eye examination. An Amsler chart or grid is used to detect small changes in vision when they first appear. It looks similar to graph paper, with horizontal and vertical lines. The person with macular degeneration may notice distortion of the grid pattern, such as bent lines and irregular box shapes or a gray shaded area. A fluorescein angiography may be ordered.

Treatment

No U.S. Food and Drug Administration–approved treatments exist yet for dry macular degeneration, although nutritional intervention may help prevent its progression to the wet form. Laser therapy may be used and may delay or prevent the onset of blindness. If scarring or atrophy has occurred, the condition cannot be reversed.

Complementary Therapy

Clients are advised to eat a low-fat, low-cholesterol diet and eat foods high in vitamins E and C and lutein, which are found in spinach, kale, and other dark green, leafy vegetables. Advise clients to wear sunglasses with UV protection, not to smoke, and to avoid secondhand smoke. Weight reduction can be helpful in reducing hypertension (a risk factor).

 CLIENT COMMUNICATION

As the loss of sight continues, suggest magnifiers and special devices to read fine print such as in newspapers. Audiobooks can be especially beneficial to an avid reader. Encourage clients to join a macular degeneration support system to learn how others cope. Help may be needed from family members in the preparation and administration of daily medication and meals. Be aware of safety measures for the blind.

Prognosis

The disease slowly progresses, especially without treatment, and can eventually lead to blindness. Early diagnosis and treatment are helpful.

Prevention

As noted under "Complementary Therapy," many researchers believe that the nutrients zinc, lutein, zeaxanthin, and vitamins A, C, and E help lower the risk of AMD or slow the progression of dry AMD.

 REALITY EPISODE

It has been a few months since Jeri's work allowed her time to visit her parents, who live 1,000 miles away. Jeri knows there have been changes. Dad recommended she rent a car to drive the 20 miles from the airport. In the past, they always came to pick her up. Dad drives when they go out to dinner. He seems confident, but Jeri is concerned when he asks her mother to read the street signs. (This is especially alarming because her mother is in the early stages of Alzheimer disease and is not always accurate in her assessment.) When ordering from the menu, her father jokes about having to put on his "cheaters," but then he always needed his glasses to read. When the bill comes for dinner, he is unable to see the figures; the lights are dim and there is votive candlelight at the table. He picks up the votive to take a closer look. When Jeri asks if she can help, he hands her the bill to have her check the order and give him the total. Jeri offers to drive home, but Dad says, "Thanks, but I am okay." Jeri knows, however, that he is not. The next morning, she and Dad have some alone time. He tells Jeri that in the last few weeks his vision has changed. Everything is blurry except around the edges. The ophthalmologist says it is macular degeneration. Nothing can be done for him, and it will get worse. He worries about his wife of 60 years and her mental deterioration. Jeri now has grave concerns about both of them—Dad is losing his eyesight; Mom has Alzheimer disease.

Put yourself in Jeri's place. What steps need to be taken to try to keep her parents as safe as possible?

Benefits of high levels of antioxidants and zinc for halting or slowing development of macular degeneration have been widely reported based on results released in 2001 from the Age-Related Eye Disease Study (AREDS) conducted by the National Eye Institute. Periodic vision testing is advisable for everyone, but especially for those who have a family history of retinal problems.

STRABISMUS

ICD-10: H50.9*

Description

Strabismus is a disorder in which the eyes cannot be directed to focus on the same object. The condition may affect one or both eyes. The eye may turn inward—convergent strabismus (esotropia), or cross-eye; or it may turn outward—divergent strabismus (exotropia), or walleye (Fig. 17.6).

Etiology

Causes of strabismus include genetics, inappropriate development of the "fusion center" of the brain, problems with the control center of the brain, and injuries or other problems to muscles and nerves. Up to 5% of all children have some type or degree of strabismus; about half of these children have a positive family history for the defect. There has been the belief that the most common cause of strabismus is lazy eye or **amblyopia,** but amblyopia and strabismus are not the same condition. Strabismus can cause amblyopia, however.

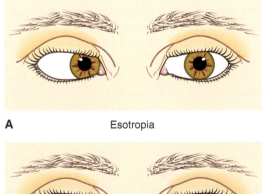

A   Esotropia

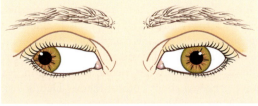

B   Exotropia

Figure 17.6 Strabismus: esotropia; exotropia

Unspecified strabismus

Signs and Symptoms

There may be double vision (**diplopia**) and blurred vision. The affected eye will appear to wander. If both eyes are involved, they may appear crossed or give the child a "walleyed" appearance. The child may stumble and appear to be clumsy. He or she may squint in an effort to see better.

Diagnostic Procedures

The most important diagnostic tool is the history that indicates the age of onset, duration of turning of the eye, and family history of strabismus. The ophthalmologist attempts to rule out amblyopia and uncorrected refractive error and measures the amount of deviation. A complete ophthalmologic examination is necessary. A neurological examination may be indicated as well.

Treatment

The aim of treatment is to attain the best possible vision while trying to obtain binocular vision. Treatment depends on the cause. Eye exercises and corrective lenses may be ordered. Some miotics (drugs that act on the ciliary muscles) may be prescribed to make accommodation better. Botulinum toxin may be injected into the eye muscle to temporarily paralyze the eye muscle. In about 2 months, the medication wears off, and permanent correction occurs in about half the cases. Surgical correction may be necessary. If amblyopia is a problem, treatment often consists of covering the normal eye, forcing the child to use the deviating one.

Complementary Therapy

No significant complementary therapy is indicated; however, children can be encouraged to play with objects that encourage hand-eye coordination.

⊕ CLIENT COMMUNICATION

Family members must be taught the importance of helping the child follow the treatment plan because it can be difficult on the child. Patience is needed, especially if an eye patch is warranted.

Prognosis

In general, the earlier treatment is begun, the more rapid is the improvement and the more effective is the treatment. By age 6, the vision in the deviating eye usually has become so suppressed that treatment is not effective and vision loss is permanent.

Prevention

There is no known prevention.

Eye Inflammations

CONJUNCTIVITIS

ICD-10: H10.9

Description

Conjunctivitis is inflammation of the conjunctiva, the mucous membrane that lines the inner surface of the eyelids and the anterior portion of the eyeball. Inflammation causes small blood vessels in the conjunctiva to become more prominent, giving a pink cast to the whites of the eyes, hence the term *pinkeye*. The condition may be unilateral or bilateral. It is the most common ocular disease worldwide.

Etiology

Acute, sometimes epidemic, outbreaks of conjunctivitis are caused by infection from certain viruses or bacteria. Commonly, the infection is transmitted by the person's own hand or by contaminated washcloths or towels. The infection usually lasts about 2 weeks. Conjunctivitis also may be caused by irritation from heat, cold, chemicals, allergies, or exposure to UV light.

Signs and Symptoms

Conjunctivitis is marked by red, swollen conjunctivae, which may itch, burn, or cause pain, especially when blinking. There may be a discharge in one or both eyes that forms a crust during the night. The eyes may tear excessively and may be overly sensitive to light, although conjunctivitis rarely affects vision.

Diagnostic Procedures

Physical examination reveals inflammation of the conjunctivae. Stained smears of conjunctival scrapings may reveal monocytes, polymorphonuclear leukocytes, and macrophages. Culture and sensitivity tests identify the specific causative organism and indicate appropriate treatment.

Treatment

Treatment varies depending on the causative agent, but antibiotic therapy for bacterial conjunctivitis may involve eyedrops or systemic medication. For the viral form of conjunctivitis, antibiotics are not prescribed, and the inflammation has to run its course. Often, warm compresses applied to the eye three or four times a day for 10 to 15 minutes are recommended.

Complementary Therapy

Using a boric acid compress may offer some relief. Boil 1 teaspoon of boric acid in 1 cup water and let cool. Soak sterile cotton balls or gauze pads in solution, and apply over closed eyes for 10 minutes three to four times daily. Vitamin A (10,000 IU per day), vitamin C (250 to 500 mg twice daily), and zinc (30 to 50 mg per day) can strengthen the adult immune system and encourage healing.

⟳ CLIENT COMMUNICATION

Educate clients to keep objects and hands away from the infected eye. Advise clients that any solution or compress put on or in the eye must be sterile. If children are infected, it is best they stay at home and not share towels or toys; girls are advised not to share makeup. Advise clients to wear dark glasses, if the sun is bothersome.

Prognosis

The prognosis is good if degeneration of the conjunctiva or corneal damage does not occur. The disease normally is benign and self-limiting.

Prevention

Prevention involves careful hygiene, proper hand washing, and the use of clean washcloths and towels to prevent infection.

UVEITIS

ICD-10: H20.00

Description

Uveitis is inflammation of the uveal tract, which is the principal vascular connective tissue component of the eye (iris, ciliary body, choroid). The iris, ciliary body, or choroid may be affected separately or in combination. It may occur in the anterior or posterior portion of the tract. This condition is usually unilateral.

Etiology

Uveitis may be associated with autoimmune disorders, or it may be idiopathic. Uveitis may be caused by microbial infections or debilitating diseases, such as AIDS, tuberculosis, herpes zoster infection, and histoplasmosis, or it may result from improperly healed corneal abrasions. Allergies, chemicals, trauma, or surgery may also be the cause.

Signs and Symptoms

Symptoms include pain; intense, unusual intolerance of light (**photophobia**); blurred vision; redness; and dark, floating spots in the vision. The primary care provider may note severe ciliary congestion, tearing, and a pupil that is nonreactive when exposed to light.

Diagnostic Procedures

An ophthalmic examination that includes a slit-lamp inspection is necessary for diagnosis. A complete medical history likely reveals any underlying medical issues that relate to the diagnosis.

Treatment

Treatment is specific to the particular type of uveitis and should be prompt and vigorous. Treatment may involve wearing dark glasses, using eyedrops to dilate the pupil and relieve pain, or using steroid eyedrops or ointment as prescribed. **Atropine,** an anticholinergic agent that counteracts the effects of parasympathetic stimulation, is used so that the pupil remains dilated to reduce the likelihood of adhesions. If the uveitis is caused by a body-wide infection, treatment may involve antibiotics and powerful anti-inflammatory medicines called *corticosteroids*. Analgesics may be prescribed, and intraocular pressure must be monitored.

Complementary Therapy

See "Complementary Therapy" for conjunctivitis.

 CLIENT COMMUNICATION

Clients should wear dark green eyeglasses both inside and outside. If uveitis recurs, encourage a good medical workup to determine the underlying cause.

Prognosis

Most uveitis subsides in a few weeks with treatment. It may persist despite treatment. Adhesions may develop that can cause glaucoma, cataracts, or even retinal detachment. Uveitis can recur.

Prevention

There is no known prevention other than prompt treatment of the infections and debilitating diseases mentioned previously.

BLEPHARITIS

 ICD-10: H01.009

Description

Blepharitis is an inflammation of the edges of the eyelids that is commonly ulcerative or nonulcerative, involving hair follicles and glands that open onto the surface. It is classified into two types: Anterior blepharitis appears on the outside front edge of the eyelid where eyelashes attach. Posterior blepharitis appears at the inner edge of the eyelid that is in contact with the eye. It affects people of all ages, is not contagious, and generally does not cause any permanent damage to eyesight.

Etiology

Ulcerative forms of blepharitis usually result from infection by staphylococcal bacteria. Nonulcerative forms may be due to allergy or exposure to dust, smoke, or chemical irritants. The condition also may arise secondary to an increase in the sebaceous secretion (**seborrhea**) of the eyelids or pediculosis of the eyelashes or eyebrows.

Signs and Symptoms

The affected individual may experience burning and itching and the feeling of a foreign body in the eye. The eyes usually appear red-rimmed. Both dry and oily scales may be present on the eyelid margins. For some, blepharitis causes only minor irritation and itching. However, it can lead to more severe signs and symptoms such as blurring of vision, missing eyelashes, and inflammation of other eye tissue, particularly the cornea.

Diagnostic Procedures

Blepharitis is diagnosed through a comprehensive eye examination. A medical history may reveal the presence of any general health problems that may contribute to the eye problem. External examination of the eye, including lid structure and margins, skin texture, and eyelash appearance, is important. Evaluation of the lid margins, base of the eyelashes, and meibomian gland openings using bright light and magnification helps to determine the type of blepharitis. Staphylococcal blepharitis frequently exhibits mild sticking together of the lids, thickened lid margins, and missing eyelashes. Seborrheic blepharitis appears as greasy flakes or scales at the base of eyelashes and some eyelid redness. Ulcerative blepharitis is characterized by matted, hard crusts around the eyelashes that, when removed, leave small sores that ooze and bleed. In severe cases, the cornea may also become inflamed.

Treatment

The key to treating most types of blepharitis is keeping the lids clean and free from crusts. Warm compresses can be applied to loosen the crusts, followed by gentle washing of the eyes. Stopping the use of eye makeup may be necessary for a period of time. Staphylococcal blepharitis requires antibiotic treatment. Artificial tear solutions or lubricating ointments may be prescribed. Contact lens wearers may have to temporarily discontinue wearing them during treatment.

Complementary Therapy

See "Complementary Therapy" for conjunctivitis.

 CLIENT COMMUNICATION

Cleanliness in and around the eyes cannot be overstressed. Show clients how to clean the eyelid margins and keep them free from exudate. Remind clients to always wash their hands thoroughly prior to any procedure performed on their eyes.

Prognosis

The prognosis is good with proper treatment and care, but some forms of the disease tend to recur and become chronic, especially the seborrheic type. Blepharitis may lead to keratitis.

Prevention

Cleanliness and proper eye care are the best preventive measures for blepharitis.

KERATITIS

ICD-10: H16.9*

Description

Keratitis is inflammation of the cornea that usually occurs unilaterally. Trevor John Mills, MD, MPH, Chief of Emergency Medicine, Veterans Affairs Northern California Health Care System, reports that approximately 25,000 Americans develop infectious keratitis annually.

Etiology

Keratitis is most frequently due to infection of the cornea by herpes simplex virus (HSV); by certain bacteria, such as *Staphylococcus pneumoniae* and *Pseudomonas aeruginosa;* or by fungi. The condition also may arise secondary to syphilis. Noninfectious keratitis may be caused by prolonged exposure to dry air or intense light, or it may result from corneal trauma.

Signs and Symptoms

Symptoms of keratitis include irritation, tearing, and photophobia. There may be redness of the eyelid and conjunctiva or mucopurulent discharge from the eye. When the cause is HSV-1, an upper respiratory infection (URI) with facial cold sores may be the precursor. When prolonged exposure to dry air or intense light is the cause of keratitis, the symptoms are exhibited about 12 hours later. The person experiences severe photophobia.

Diagnostic Procedures

Slit-lamp examination of the corneal surface confirms the diagnosis. Fluorescein staining may reveal the characteristic dendritic ulcer of HSV infection. Vision testing may indicate decreased visual acuity, and the medical history may reveal a recent URI.

Treatment

Topical treatment with eyedrops and ointment is likely to be prescribed. Depending on the specific cause, antibiotic, antifungal, or antiviral medication may be necessary. An eye patch may be recommended for a period of time.

Complementary Therapy

No significant complementary therapy is indicated.

*Unspecified keratitis

⊕ CLIENT COMMUNICATION

See the Client Communication section in "Blepharitis."

Prognosis

The prognosis is good when the condition is properly treated, but untreated keratitis may lead to corneal ulcerations (a medical emergency) and blindness.

Prevention

The best prevention for keratitis is proper eye care, proper contact lens usage, and avoidance of offending infections.

COMMON SYMPTOMS OF EYE DISEASES AND DISORDERS

Individuals may present with the following common symptoms, which deserve attention from health-care professionals:

- Any visual disturbance or change in vision
- Pain or burning in the eye and any of its structures
- Eye redness
- Photophobia

CHAPTER EPISODE—PART II

Emory's parents offer her Tylenol to ease the discomfort and help reduce the fever. Although this seems to reduce the symptoms, Emory's fever returns every 4 hours, just prior to when her next Tylenol dose would be given. Her mother notices that Emory occasionally pulls on her right ear.

- What should Emory's mother do now?
- Should Emory be taken to her pediatrician's office at this time? Justify your response.

Ear Diseases and Disorders

Impacted Cerumen

ICD-10: H61.23

Cerumen is the soft, brown, waxy secretion found in the external canal of the ear. The ear makes cerumen in order to clean itself. Cerumen protects the ear and should not be

Continued

Impacted Cerumen—cont'd

routinely removed unless impacted. Abnormal accumulation and eventual impaction of cerumen within the ear canal can cause temporary hearing loss. Cerumen may accumulate because of dryness and scaling of the skin or excessive hair in the ear canal. Individuals with narrow or tortuous ear canals may be predisposed to the condition. Common symptoms are gradual loss of hearing, **tinnitus,** or a feeling of fullness in the ear. When cerumen adheres to the wall of the canal, it can be softened by repeated instillation of oil eardrops or hydrogen peroxide and then irrigated with water. Suction may also be used to remove wax, especially with clients who have narrow ear canals, eardrum perforation or tube in their ears, or an immune deficiency. Under no circumstances should cotton-tipped swabs or hairpins be pushed into the ears to try to remove the wax. Oral jet irrigators and ear candling are not recommended.

EXTERNAL OTITIS (SWIMMER'S EAR)

ICD-10: H60.XXX*

Description

External otitis (swimmer's ear) is inflammation of the external ear canal. The ear canal becomes inflamed if it has been scratched or if a skin condition such as eczema is present. If it is the result of a fungal infection from swimming, it is commonly called *swimmer's ear.*

Etiology

The inflammation may be caused by a bacterial or fungal infection or by a dermatologic condition such as seborrhea or psoriasis. Predisposing factors include swimming or bathing in contaminated water or trauma to the ear canal from attempts to clean or scratch the ear. The frequent use of earphones, earplugs, or earmuffs may create a favorable environment within the ear canal in which bacteria and fungi may propagate. The most common bacterial infections are caused by *Staphylococcus aureus* and *Pseudomonas* species. *Aspergillus* is the most common fungus to cause external otitis.

Signs and Symptoms

Pain, pruritus, and a red, swollen ear canal are common presenting symptoms. Drainage from the ear may be either purulent or watery and may be foul-smelling.

Diagnostic Procedures

An otologic examination confirms the diagnosis. White blood cell count may be normal or elevated.

A bacterial culture of ear canal scrapings, as well as sensitivity tests, may be carried out if an infection is suspected.

Treatment

Antibiotics and analgesics may be prescribed. The ear must be kept dry and clean, and it should be protected from trauma. Eardrops or ointments may be instilled. Heat compresses may reduce the pain to the area.

Complementary Therapy

A known remedy for swimmer's ear involves making a solution of a large pinch of powdered boric acid dropped into 1 pint of ethyl alcohol (not methyl alcohol). After shaking well, fill an eyedropper with the mixture and fill the ear with it. Let it sit for a minute, then turn the head to drain. Do this one more time and wipe any excess liquid off. Repeat three times a day for 5 days.

 CLIENT COMMUNICATION

If clients are swimmers, suggest the use of earplugs. If symptoms reappear or persist, instruct clients to see their primary care provider for prompt treatment.

Prognosis

External otitis tends to recur and become chronic. When untreated, it can cause hearing loss.

Prevention

Prevention includes wearing earplugs when swimming, bathing, or showering. To minimize the risk of trauma to the ear canal, clients should not clean the ear with any foreign objects.

OTITIS MEDIA

ICD-10: H66.90

Description

Otitis media is an accumulation of fluid within the middle ear. The condition is subclassified into either **serous** or **suppurative,** according to the composition of the accumulating fluid. In serous otitis media, the fluid is comparatively clear and sterile, secreted from the membranes lining the inner ear. In suppurative otitis media, the fluid is the product of pus-producing bacteria. The pressure from the accumulating fluid, in either form of the condition, may be sufficient to occasion temporary hearing loss. Both serous and suppurative forms of the disease may occur as acute or chronic conditions. Otitis media is most common among children.

Etiology

Acute serous otitis media may occur spontaneously or following an upper respiratory tract infection. It also may be occasioned by rapid changes in atmospheric pressure, such as when flying or diving, or by allergic reactions. The chronic form of serous otitis media may develop from the acute condition, or it may result from the overgrowth of adenoidal tissue or chronic sinus infections. Suppurative otitis media is caused by the introduction of pyogenic microorganisms into the middle ear, usually *Haemophilus influenzae, S. pneumoniae,* or *Moraxella catarrhalis.* The condition often follows the flu or a cold and may be induced by overly forceful nose blowing. Swimming in contaminated water also may result in a middle ear infection.

Variations in the structure or function of the eustachian tubes may strongly predispose an individual to the development of otitis media. Narrowing or constriction of the eustachian tubes may interfere with the normal drainage of secretions from the middle ear. Individuals with eustachian tubes that are shorter, wider, or more horizontally placed than normal may be more prone to infectious forms of otitis media.

Signs and Symptoms

The symptoms vary with the severity of the infection. A person with serous otitis media usually experiences only a sensation of fullness or pressure in the affected ear, along with varying degrees of hearing impairment. Suppurative otitis media, on the other hand, is usually manifested by pain in the affected ear and is often accompanied by general symptoms of infection such as fever and chills. Both conditions may cause dizziness.

Diagnostic Procedures

Examination of the affected ear with an otoscope reveals bulging of the eardrum. Often the eardrum has a cherry-red discoloration. Fluid bubbles may be discernible behind the eardrum. The individual's WBC count is usually elevated in cases of suppurative otitis media.

Treatment

Antibiotics are ordered to control suppurative otitis media, and analgesics may be prescribed to relieve pain and discomfort of either form. Recently, many primary care providers have been opting not to use antibiotics except in the most severe cases. Decongestants may be ordered to promote drainage. In severe cases, drainage may be accomplished by needle aspiration; by surgical incision of the tympanic membrane, a procedure called **myringotomy;** or by surgery to correct the eardrum, called **tympanoplasty.** For chronic forms of otitis media, the acute attacks must be treated as previously described, but surgery, such as myringoplasty and tympanoplasty, may

also be necessary. In some cases, especially in children, tubes are surgically inserted into the tympanic membrane to equalize pressure between the atmosphere and the middle ear. In most cases, the tubes are removed after 6 to 18 months, or they may fall out on their own.

Complementary Therapy

Stollery Children's Hospital at the University of Alberta published research data from studies indicating that complementary therapy may help children with ear infections. Most of the studies, however, had significant limitations that made it difficult to offer advice based on their conclusions, whether positive or negative.

 CLIENT COMMUNICATION

It must be stressed that clients should finish their course of antibiotics even when they are feeling well. Follow-up care is needed especially in cases when the infection recurs. Instruct in any preoperative and postoperative care that may be necessary. Children especially need to understand procedures and special care. Many infections are becoming difficult to treat because of their increasing resistance to antibiotics, due to an unnecessary overprescribing of antibiotics. (See Chapter 4 section on antimicrobial resistance).

Prognosis

The prognosis for an individual with either form of acute otitis media usually is good if he or she receives prompt treatment. Chronic otitis media, however, may lead to scarring, adhesions, and severe ear damage with hearing loss.

Prevention

Prompt treatment of any URI infection and otitis media is recommended.

CHAPTER EPISODE—PART III

Despite continuing to give Emory Tylenol every 4 hours, Emory's parents have decided to take her to the pediatrician's office to be evaluated. Emory's fever has now persisted for nearly 4 days. Emory is pulling on her right ear often and is extremely fussy.

- What equipment do you think Emory's pediatrician will use to examine her?
- What might the pediatrician find upon examination of Emory?
- What kind of medication might be prescribed to Emory to treat the findings?

Perforated Eardrums

Perforated eardrums can be caused by serious infections or injury and trauma. Most will heal spontaneously within about 3 months. However, if a dirty item such as a stick caused the injury, antibiotics are likely necessary. If healing fails, a tympanoplasty to repair the eardrum may be required. The perforated eardrum can also be treated with a myringoplasty, where a tissue graft is used to seal the hole.

OTOSCLEROSIS

ICD-10: H80.23

Description

Otosclerosis is a metabolic imbalance that causes new bone to grow over the end of the stapes, especially around the oval window, with resulting immobilization of the stapes. Eventually the bone becomes fixed and no vibration occurs, eliminating the transfer of sound to the inner ear and causing permanent hearing loss. The disease occurs primarily among women, usually appearing between ages 15 and 40 and affects about 3 million Americans.

Etiology

Otosclerosis is an idiopathic condition, but because the disease shows a familial pattern, genetic factors are suspected. This condition is often aggravated by pregnancy.

Signs and Symptoms

A gradual bilateral hearing loss of low tones and/or soft sounds is the first sign. Tinnitus may accompany the condition. Affected clients may turn their head to hear better or may notice they cannot use the telephone on the affected ear.

Diagnostic Procedures

Basic hearing tests are conducted with a tuning fork. Clients demonstrate a conductive hearing loss, and a Rinne test determines if the bone conduction is better than the air conduction. A Weber test identifies the ear with the greater conductive hearing loss.

Treatment

In the early or mild stages of otosclerosis, the only treatment may be hearing aids. However, as the calcium buildup on the stapes progresses, hearing loss becomes more severe. Sodium fluoride tablets may help prevent the progression of otosclerosis, but only if the condition has also affected the inner ear. There is hope that continued bone-remodeling research may be able to identify potential new therapies. At some point, surgery is indicated. The ear that is most affected may undergo excision of the stapes, or **stapedectomy,** and a prosthesis will be inserted. The other ear may need the same surgery later. About 85% of clients report a good improvement in hearing following surgery.

Complementary Therapy

No significant complementary therapy is indicated.

⊙ CLIENT COMMUNICATION

Clients may need help adjusting to the hearing loss. If surgery is needed, prepare clients for possible balance disturbances and the sensation of spinning around in space (**vertigo**) for a short time following surgery.

Prognosis

The prognosis improves following surgery, although some degree of lasting hearing impairment is characteristic of the disease.

Prevention

There is no known prevention for otosclerosis.

MOTION SICKNESS

ICD-10: T75.3XXA*

Description

Motion sickness consists of nausea, vomiting, and vertigo induced by irregular or rhythmic movements, such as may occur during airplane, boat, or automobile travel.

Etiology

This disorder is caused by any motion capable of disturbing the equilibrium of the organs of balance in the inner ear (the semicircular canals). Strong emotions, such as fear and grief, and digestive upset or offensive odors may exacerbate the problem.

Signs and Symptoms

An individual affected by motion sickness may experience loss of equilibrium, nausea, vomiting, dizziness, diaphoresis, pallor, headache, and anorexia. Symptoms may disappear almost immediately after the inciting motion has ceased, or they may persist for hours or days.

Diagnostic Procedures

Diagnosis is made by history and complaints made by the client.

Treatment

Ongoing attacks of motion sickness usually are successfully treated with antihistamines, antiemetics, or sedatives. A transdermal medicated patch may be suggested.

Complementary Therapy

While results are mixed, ginger may prevent or ease the symptoms of motion sickness. It can be taken as fresh ginger tea, slices of candied ginger, ginger candy, ginger gum, or powdered ginger in capsules. Relaxation breathing exercises have been known to assist as well.

➔ CLIENT COMMUNICATION

Clients should avoid exposure to the offending motion whenever possible. They should keep the following in mind when traveling:

- On a ship, seek a cabin in the front, the middle, or the upper deck.
- On a plane, seek a seat over the front edge of the wing; let the air vent flow to the face.
- On a train, sit near the front and next to a window; face forward.
- In an automobile, drive or sit in the front passenger's seat.
- Focus on the horizon or a distant object; do not read.
- Keep the head still or rested against the seat back.
- Do not smoke or sit near smokers.
- Avoid greasy, spicy foods and alcohol.
- Take an over-the-counter antihistamine 30 to 60 minutes before travel.
- Consider the transdermal patch.
- Dry soda crackers and a carbonated beverage may help settle the stomach.

Prognosis

Although the condition may be severe enough to be debilitating for some, the symptoms of motion sickness usually disappear with the restoration of equilibrium.

Prevention

For more information than provided here, the Centers for Disease Control and Prevention produces the *CDC Health Information for International Travel* (commonly called the "Yellow Book") with detailed information about medications that might be prescribed for the prevention of motion sickness.

MÉNIÈRE DISEASE

ICD-10: H81.0

Description

Ménière disease is a chronic inner ear syndrome marked by attacks of vertigo, progressive deafness, tinnitus, and a sensation of fullness in the ears. The condition usually appears in persons between ages 40 and 50.

Etiology

The cause of Ménière disease is not known, but the disease process appears to destroy the hair cells within the cochlea. Experts on Ménière disease think that a rupture of the membranous labyrinth allows the endolymph to mix with perilymph, causing the symptoms of Ménière disease. Scientists are investigating several possible causes, such as noise pollution and viral infections, as well as biological factors.

Signs and Symptoms

The classic symptoms are severe vertigo, tinnitus, and sensorineural hearing loss. An acute attack of vertigo may cause nausea, vomiting, sweating, and loss of balance. These attacks may occur several times a year, but remissions also can last several years.

Diagnostic Procedures

When all three classic symptoms are present, the diagnosis is not difficult. Further testing using audiometry and radiographs of the internal meatus of the ear may be necessary. The primary care provider may request an MRI to rule out brain involvement. Accurate measurement and characterization of hearing loss are of critical importance in the diagnosis of Ménière disease.

Treatment

There is no cure for Ménière disease. A salt-free diet, diuretics, antihistamines, and mild sedatives are helpful in long-term care. Changes in medications that either control allergies or improve blood circulation in the inner ear may help. Eliminating tobacco use and reducing stress levels are more ways some people can lessen the severity of their symptoms. If the disease persists and causes debilitating vertigo, surgical intervention may be necessary. Labyrinthectomy (removal of the inner ear sense organ) can effectively control vertigo but sacrifices hearing. Vestibular neurectomy, selectively severing a nerve from the affected inner ear organ, usually controls the vertigo and preserves hearing but carries surgical risks. Recently, the administration of the ototoxic antibiotic gentamicin directly into the middle ear space has gained popularity worldwide for the control of the vertigo of Ménière disease.

Complementary Therapy

No significant complementary therapy is indicated.

➤ CLIENT COMMUNICATION

Instruct clients on what foods are low in sodium, with a dietary goal of fewer than 2,000 mg per day. Be sure clients are aware of side effects of any prescribed medication.

Prognosis

The prognosis varies, but usually recurrent attacks over several years lead to residual tinnitus and hearing loss.

Prevention

There is no known prevention for Ménière disease.

HEARING LOSS AND DEAFNESS

ICD-10: H91.90

Description

Hearing loss can involve one or both ears and can be mild, moderate, or severe. Approximately 17% (36 million) of American adults report some degree of hearing loss. Hearing loss more commonly affects elderly people and is part of the aging process. Currently, 50% of people over age 75 have hearing difficulties. It is estimated that by 2050, about one-fifth of the population will be age 55 or older.

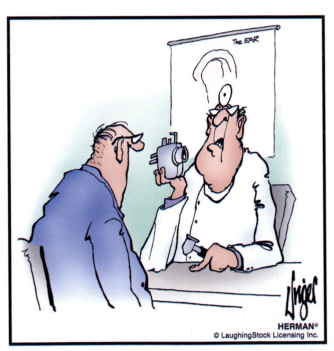

"We implant this behind your left ear and you won't even know it's there."

(HERMAN© is reprinted with permission from LaughingStock Licensing Inc., Ottawa, Canada. All rights reserved.)

Etiology

Deafness can occur at any age. In children, deafness may be congenital and may be transmitted as a dominant, autosomal-recessive, or sex-linked recessive trait. It may also be due to trauma, toxicity, or infection during pregnancy or delivery. The most common cause of deafness in children is otitis media, meningitis, and Down syndrome. Deafness in children can contribute to difficulties in the development of language skills.

In adults, the cause of the hearing loss may be idiopathic. It tends to be familial. The many causes include infection, ototoxic drugs, exposure to noise, tumors, trauma, and the aging process. It can result from otosclerosis, Ménière disease, or a sensorineural loss with damage to the cochlear or vestibulocochlear nerve. A mixed hearing loss (conductive and sensorineural loss) and a functional loss (psychogenic) may occur. A functional loss is usually the result of an emotional disturbance.

Signs and Symptoms

Early symptoms usually include difficulty in hearing in a large group, tinnitus, and having to turn up the television volume. If the hearing impairment is moderate to severe, there may be personality and attitude changes. Sometimes a hearing loss affects the person's safety when a fire alarm or someone uninvited entering the home cannot be heard. Most individuals with a hearing loss do not notice the loss; family members and friends usually bring it to their attention.

Diagnostic Procedures

The goals in evaluating the hearing loss are to determine the nature of the hearing impairment (conductive and/or sensorineural), its severity, the anatomy of the impairment (external ear, middle ear, inner ear, or central nerve pathway), and the etiology. A history and physical examination will assist in the diagnosis. The Weber and Rinne tuning fork tests help to differentiate the diagnosis. An audiological examination is ordered. A CT or MRI scan may be prescribed to rule out tumors or other abnormalities.

Treatment

In general, conductive hearing losses can be treated surgically, whereas the sensorineural hearing losses are permanent. Surgery may be tympanoplasty or stapedectomy. Hearing aids may be ordered. Technology has greatly improved all types of hearing aids. Assistive devices are available for lectures and theater. Cochlear implants might be performed if the hearing loss is severe and hearing aids are not helping. These prostheses convert sound energy to electrical energy and can be used to stimulate the eighth nerve directly. Usually within 3 months of implantation, the person understands speech without visual cues.

Complementary Therapy

No significant complementary therapy is indicated.

➔ CLIENT COMMUNICATION

When talking to someone with a hearing loss, face the person and get his or her attention before speaking. When someone is wearing a hearing aid, there usually is no need to speak louder, but speaking more clearly and slowly is helpful. Many hard-of-hearing people lip-read. If asked to repeat what is said, rephrase the statement. Remember, a hearing aid makes the sounds louder but does not improve a person's ability to discriminate words or understand speech.

Prognosis

The prognosis is dependent on the cause of the hearing loss or deafness. If the loss is conductive, the hearing generally returns to normal once it is treated, whereas if the loss is sensorineural, no treatment is curative. Hearing aids are required.

Prevention

Exposure to loud noises, especially via headsets or heavy machinery, should be avoided. Ear protection should be worn as a preventative measure. Good ear hygiene is essential. Yearly auditory examinations are recommended. Prompt treatment of ear infections is good prevention.

COMMON SYMPTOMS OF EAR DISEASES AND DISORDERS

Individuals may present with the following common symptoms, which deserve attention from health-care professionals:

- Hearing loss
- Tinnitus
- Ear pressure
- Loss of balance
- Pain
- Dizziness

SUMMARY

The senses, specifically sight and sound, provide essential information about the environment. With decreased or lost sight or hearing, activities of daily living can be affected drastically. Many assistive devices exist to help. Health-care professionals must be aware of the challenges clients face without sight and hearing because teaching is an essential aspect of treatment. Many diseases and disorders of the eye and ear are preventable and treatable. Again, education is necessary.

 DavisPlus | For more resources and to sharpen your skills with interactive exercises, visit DavisPlus at http://davisplus.fadavis.com. Keyword *Tamparo*.

ONLINE RESOURCES

Complementary and Alternative Research and Education Program

http://www.care.ualberta.ca/en/~/media/care/Resources/OtitisMedia2011.pdf

Motion sickness medications

http://wwwnc.cdc.gov/travel/yellowbook/2010/chapter-2/motion-sickness.aspx

Strabismus

http://www.strabismus.org

CASE STUDIES

Case Study 1

During a general physical examination, Marmie Smith, a 60-year-old woman, complains of what appears to be a painless, gradual loss of sight. In response to questions, Marmie reports that she perceives halos around most light sources, such as lamps and headlights. The primary care provider notes that her eyes have a white cast to them.

Case Study Questions

1. What condition is likely indicated by these signs and symptoms?

2. What treatment options and/or recommendations will the primary care provider have to consider?

Case Study 2

A mother notices that her preschooler, Darlene, doesn't always respond when called. It also seems that Darlene sits very close to the television and turns the volume up quite high. The mother suspects a hearing problem.

Case Study Questions

1. What ear diseases or disorders might cause hearing loss in a young child?

2. What treatments might be ordered for the various possible diseases?
3. Discuss the prognosis for each possible ear disease.

Case Study 3

Eileen McCannes, a 35-year-old woman, slowly begins losing her hearing. Three years later, she visits an otologist, who performs an examination, including an audiogram. The results are clear; Eileen has a moderate hearing loss. The otologist prescribes in-the-ear hearing aids. With some effort, Eileen learns to hear with the aids. Eileen is now 55 years old, her hearing continues to worsen, and she has a severe hearing loss with behind-the-ear hearing aids. She reads lips.

Case Study Questions

1. What can Eileen expect as she ages?
2. What can be done to facilitate Eileen hearing when she goes to her medical clinic?
3. Where will Eileen have more trouble hearing?

REVIEW QUESTIONS

Matching

Match each of the following definitions with its correct term:

_____ 1. Cerumen

_____ 2. External otitis

_____ 3. Otitis media

_____ 4. Otosclerosis

_____ 5. Tinnitus

_____ 6. Ménière disease

_____ 7. Uveitis

_____ 8. Hyperopia

_____ 9. Blepharitis

_____ 10. Cataract

a. Earache or inflammation of middle ear

b. Noise or ringing in ear

c. Opacity of crystalline lens of the eye

d. Causes severe vertigo

e. Swimmer's ear

f. Farsightedness

g. Hearing loss due to aging

h. Ear wax

i. Spongy bone in labyrinth's capsule

j. Inflammation of the uveal tract

k. Inflammation of the cornea

l. Inflammation of edges of the eyelids

Short Answer

1. What is the name of the most common bacteria or fungus that causes swimmer's ear?

_____

2. Can you identify the common treatments for otitis media?

_____

3. What is one important teaching tip for a client with a hearing loss or deafness?

_____

4. In macular degeneration, what are client communications for the health-care professional?

_____

5. When a client has an eye infection, what are some of the preventive measures a health-care professional can suggest?

_____

Multiple Choice

Place a checkmark next to the correct answer:

1. What is another name for a stye?

_____ a. Abrasion

_____ b. Macula

_____ c. Drusen

_____ d. Hordeolum

2. For which eye disease is an intraocular lens likely to be implanted or fitted?

_____ a. Corneal abrasion

_____ b. Macular degeneration

_____ c. Cataract

_____ d. Retinal detachment

3. A tonometer, ophthalmoscopic inspection, and periodic vision-field testing will be ordered in which of the following eye diseases?

_____ a. Macular degeneration

_____ b. Glaucoma

_____ c. Cataract

_____ d. Uveitis

4. You use the term *swimmer's ear* with your client; what term do you put in the medical chart?

_____ a. External otitis

_____ b. Otitis media

_____ c. Otosclerosis

_____ d. Ménière disease

5. How is deafness best described?

_____ a. Occurs only with old age

_____ b. Generally caused by injury to the ear

_____ c. Refers only to a sensorineural problem

_____ d. Is always genetic

Discussion Questions/Personal Reflection

1. Identify what a primary care provider looks for in a physical examination of both the eye and the ear.

_____

_____

_____

_____

_____

_____

_____

_____

2. Describe the prognosis for strabismus.

_____

_____

_____

_____

_____

_____

_____

_____

_____

Appendix 1

Diagnostic Procedures

A

acid perfusion test: One test used to measure esophageal function. This test reproduces the pain of heartburn by placing a nasogastric tube into one nostril down into the esophagus. A dilute solution of hydrochloric acid is sent down the tube, followed by a saline solution.

alanine aminotransferase (ALT): Test used to check for liver damage; it measures the amount of ALT enzyme in a blood sample taken via venipuncture.

allergy testing: Skin test for identifying allergens to confirm allergic contact sensitization. Types include:

intradermal test: A small amount of allergen is injected into the skin; more sensitive than the skin prick test.

skin patch test: The suspected substance is applied to an adhesive patch that is placed on the skin for 24 to 72 hours.

skin prick test: A drop of solution containing a possible allergen is place on the skin where a series of scratches or needle pricks have been made.

amniocentesis: Surgical puncture of the amniotic sac, which surrounds the fetus in utero, to remove amniotic fluid; can detect genetic disorders and evaluate an adverse uterine environment.

Amsler chart: Grid that looks similar to graph paper with horizontal and vertical lines. The person with macular degeneration may notice distortion of the grid pattern, such as bent lines and irregular box shapes, or a gray-shaded area.

angiography: Radiographic visualization of blood vessels, with or without the injection of a radiopaque material. Common types include cerebral, coronary, renal, pulmonary, and abdominal angiography.

ankle-brachial index (ABI): Used to check for peripheral arterial disease of the legs; it predicts the severity of the disease.

anorectal function test: Evaluates bowel muscle function.

anorectal manometry: Test to measure anal sphincter muscles, rectal sensation, and neural reflexes necessary for normal bowel movement.

antibody titers: Measures the amount of antibody against a particular antigen in the blood taken via venipuncture.

anti-DNA antibodies: Measures antinative DNA antibody levels in a serum sample obtained by venipuncture.

antinuclear antibody (ANA): Diagnostic test to help screen for autoimmune disorders, especially of systemic lupus erythematosus (SLE) for which peripheral blood smears are taken and a fluorescein-tagged antihuman gamma globulin is used. If the LE factor is present, the specimen will fluoresce.

antistreptolysin O (ASO) titer: Blood test to measure antibodies against antistreptolysin O that is produced by group A *Streptococcus*.

arterial blood gases (ABGs): Percutaneous arterial puncture is made to assess the gas exchanges of oxygen and carbon dioxide in the lungs by measuring the partial pressures of oxygen and carbon dioxide.

aspartate aminotransferase (AST): Venipuncture is performed to measure this cardiac enzyme. Aspartate aminotransferase is essential to energy production; used to detect recent myocardial infarction, to differentiate acute hepatic disease, and to monitor clients with cardiac and hepatic disease. May be performed at the same time as ALT.

audiogram: Record made by a delicate instrument, the audiometer, of the threshold of hearing; identifies a person's hearing ability.

auscultation and percussion (A & P): Auscultation is listening to the sounds within the body, usually using a stethoscope. Percussion is using the fingertips to tap the body lightly to determine size, position, and consistency of body structures and fluids.

B

barium (contrast) enema: (Also called a *lower GI.*) Radiograph of the lower gastrointestinal tract; barium, given as an enema, is the contrast medium.

barium (contrast) swallow: (Also called an *upper GI.*) Radiograph of the upper gastrointestinal tract; barium, given by mouth, is the contrast medium.

bilirubin levels: Blood test to determine the level of bilirubin in the circulating blood; venipuncture is used to obtain the blood sample.

biopsy: Test that removes cells or tissues for examination to determine presence or extent of disease.

blood glucose testing: Measures the amount of glucose in the blood; common for detecting diabetes or prediabetes. Types of tests include:

fasting glucose (FBS): Done when the client has not eaten for 8 hours.

oral glucose tolerance test: Measures blood glucose after a person fasts for at least 8 hours and 2 hours after drinking a liquid containing 75 grams of glucose dissolved in water.

random blood sugar (RBS): A number of random blood glucose tests are taken throughout the day, regardless of when a meal was consumed.

2-hour postprandial blood sugar: Measures blood glucose 2 hours after a meal.

blood pressure: Measures cardiac function; records the blood force on peripheral arteries during the cardiac cycle; stethoscope and sphygmomanometer are used.

blood serum for hormones: Radioimmunoassay (see *radioimmunoassay*) and competitive protein binding are two testing methods commonly used to measure serum hormone levels; blood samples are carefully drawn so as to correspond with or avoid times of peak secretions for the particular hormones being tested.

blood smear: A drop of blood is placed on a slide and examined microscopically; examination of blood cells is helpful in diagnosing many diseases.

blood urea nitrogen (BUN): Measures nitrogen in the blood coming from urea; performed to determine how well kidneys are functioning.

body mass index (BMI): Measures body fat based on height and weight as applied to adults.

bone marrow biopsy: Bone marrow fluid and cells can be removed through aspiration or needle biopsy of bone tissue; examination gives important data about blood disorders.

bone mineral density (BMD): Test that measures bone mineral density to diagnose osteoporosis. BMD determines the amount of mineralized tissue in grams per square centimeter in the area of bone scanned. (See *dual-energy x-ray absorptiometry [DEXA]*).

bone scintiscan: Nuclear imaging test (using radioactive materials injected into a vein) to help diagnose bone disease or detect bone cancer.

bronchial washings: A procedure in which saline is instilled through a bronchoscope as cells and microorganisms from the upper airways are aspirated into a trap; material is then centrifuged, stained, and examined by microscopy or cultured if infection is suspected.

bronchoscopy: Visualization of the larynx, trachea, and bronchi through a metal or fiber-optic scope with a light; also used for bronchial washings, removal of foreign bodies, and biopsy.

C

caloric test: This test uses water temperature differences to diagnose acoustic nerve damage.

carbon 13 (^{13}C) urea breath test: Breath test for detecting bacteria in persons with dyspepsia and ulcer-like symptoms.

carcinoembryonic antigen (CEA): Blood test used to monitor the effectiveness of cancer therapy; also helps determine how widespread the cancer (especially colon and rectal cancer) is.

cardiac catheterization: Catheter is passed into the right (veins to inferior vena cava) or left (arteries to the aorta) side of the heart; can determine blood pressure and blood flow in the heart.

cardiac enzymes: See *creatinine phosphokinase (CPK)* and *aspartate aminotransferase*.

cardiac stress test: Evaluates the heart and vascular system during physical exercise; helpful in identifying partial blockage to coronary arteries.

catheterization of ejaculatory ducts: Catheter is passed into the ejaculatory ducts to determine blockage or disease.

cerebral angiography: (See *angiography*.) Radiographic visualization of blood vessels of the brain after injection of radiopaque material into the arterial bloodstream. CT scan is a less hazardous procedure and is more commonly used.

cerebrospinal fluid (CSF) analysis: Lumbar puncture between the third and fifth lumbar vertebrae is commonly used to measure CSF pressure and to obtain CSF to diagnose viral or bacterial meningitis, brain tumor and hemorrhages, and chronic central nervous system infections.

chemistry screens: Tests performed on blood to determine values of any number of factors, such as calcium, phosphorus, creatinine, uric acid, cholesterol, total protein, alkaline phosphatase, glucose, blood urea nitrogen, and sodium.

cholecystogram: Used to detect biliary tract disease. A series of radiographs of the gallbladder is taken after the ingestion of contrast medium.

chorionic villus sampling (CVS): Prenatal test of chorionic villi sample removed from the placenta to provide information about the genetic makeup of the fetus.

colonoscopy: Visual examination of the lower bowel with a colonoscope. Biopsy and surgical excision can be accomplished through the scope.

colorectal transit study: A test to evaluate colon function and motility; helps in diagnosis of pathological constipation.

complement-fixation test: Common blood assay used to determine if antigen-antibody reactions have occurred; it can measure the severity of an infection.

complete blood cell count (CBC): Venipuncture usually is performed to give a complete picture of all the blood's formed elements. A CBC usually includes hemoglobin, hematocrit, red and white blood cell counts, and a differential white blood cell count.

complete neurological examination: Series of tests and procedures to assess functioning of cranial nerves, motor and sensory systems, and superficial and deep tendon reflexes.

computed tomography (CT) scan: Noninvasive radiographic technique more sensitive than conventional radiography; a scanner and detector circle the client while sending an array of focused x-rays through the body; allows a specialist to distinguish tumors, abscesses, hemorrhages, and white and gray brain tissue.

computed tomography angiogram (coronary): A technique that noninvasively determines if fatty deposits or calcium deposits have built up in the coronary arteries.

creatinine phosphokinase (CPK): Venipuncture is performed to measure CPK, an enzyme that speeds up the creatine-to-creatinine transformation in muscle cells and brain tissue. Its purpose is to detect acute myocardial infarction or reinfarction and evaluate chest pain and skeletal muscle disorders.

cryoablation: Destruction of tissue.

culture and sensitivity: Withdrawing of tissue or fluid, placing it on a suitable culture media, and determining whether or not bacteria grow. If bacteria do grow, they are identified by bacteriologic methods. Tests are then done to determine the susceptibility of the client's bacterial infection to antibiotics. A viral culture will detect viral growth in a sample.

cystoscopy: Urinary bladder is distended with water or air while the client is sedated. Examination of the bladder with a fiber-optic scope is done to obtain biopsy samples and to remove polyps. (See *voiding cystoscopy*.)

cystourethrography: Radiographic examination of the bladder and urethra by use of contrast media cytology during urination.

D

DNA testing: This test allows determination of heritage through the examination of deoxyribonucleic acid in a person's cells.

Doppler ultrasonography: Noninvasive test evaluating blood flow in the major veins and arteries of arms, legs, and extracranial cerebrovascular system. A handheld transducer directs high-frequency sound waves to the area being tested. Transcranial Doppler (TCD) is a test to measure the velocity of blood flow through blood vessels in the brain.

dual-energy x-ray absorptiometry (DEXA): Test to measure bone mineral density at sites especially susceptible to fracture to diagnose osteoporosis before any fractures occur. (See *bone mineral density* test.)

dynamic infusion cavernosometry and cavernosography (DICC): Test that pumps fluid into the penis at a known rate and pressure. It measures the vascular pressure in the corpus cavernosum during an erection. Cavernosography injects a contrast material prior to x-ray to visualize any leakage.

E

echocardiography: Noninvasive diagnostic test using ultrasound to visualize internal cardiac structures. A special transducer is placed on the client's chest, and it directs ultra-high-frequency sound waves toward cardiac structures, which reflect these waves. The echoes are converted to electrical impulses and displayed on an oscilloscope.

ejaculatory or semen analysis: Uses semen specimen to evaluate the volume of seminal fluid, sperm count, and sperm motility; also used to detect semen on a person who has been raped, identifying the blood group of an alleged rapist, or to prove sterility in a paternity suit.

electrocardiography (ECG): Recording of electric currents emanating from the heart muscle. Electrodes are placed on the client to obtain the reading.

electroencephalography (EEG): Recording of electric currents developed in the brain by placing electrodes on the skull.

electrolyte analysis: Analysis of electrolytes (sodium, potassium, chloride, and bicarbonate) to evaluate fluid and acid-base status.

electrooculography (EOG): Electrodes placed on the skin next to the eyes to measure changes between the front and back of the eyeball as the eye moves; can detect retinal pigment epithelium dysfunction.

electromyography (EMG): The process of creating a graphic recording of muscle contraction as a result of electrical stimulation.

ELISA (enzyme-linked immunosorbent assay): Rapid enzyme immunochemical assay method in which either an antibody or antigen can be coupled to an enzyme. Used to detect certain bacterial antigens and antibodies as well as hormones. One of the primary diagnostic tests for many infectious diseases, including HIV.

endomysium antibody (EMA): This test helps to determine how effective a gluten-free diet is for an individual with celiac disease.

endoscopic retrograde cholangiopancreatography (ERCP): Radiographic examination of the pancreatic ducts and hepatobiliary tree after injection of a contrast medium into the duodenal papilla. It is used to diagnose pancreatic disease.

endoscopy: Visual inspection of any cavity of the body by means of an endoscope.

Epworth sleepiness scale (ESS): Measures daytime sleepiness by use of a short questionnaire. (See *multiple sleep latency test [MSLT]*.)

erythrocyte sedimentation rate (ESR): Blood specimen is obtained by venipuncture to measure the time required for erythrocytes in whole blood to settle to the bottom of a vertical tube; may be one of the earliest disease indicators.

esophageal acid testing: A test to determine the amount of acid in reflux. The 24-hour esophageal pH test is performed by passing a catheter through the nose into the esophagus. A sensor on the tip of the catheter senses acid and records over a 24-hour period; recorder is attached to the other end of the catheter, which is wrapped around the ear and attached to the recorder at the waist. (See *acid perfusion test*.)

esophageal manometry: A test to measure the pressure inside the lower part of the esophagus. A thin, pressure-sensitive tube or esophageal probe is passed through the mouth or nose into the stomach. The tube is pulled slowly back into the esophagus and measures the muscle contractions along the way.

esophagogastroduodenoscopy: Upper barium swallow.

exfoliative cytology: Microscopic examination of cells that have shredded or scaled off the surface epithelium. The cells are obtained from sputum, lesions, secretions, urine, aspirations, smears, or washings.

F

fluorescein angiography: This eye test uses special dye and a camera to visualize blood flow in the retina and choroid.

fluorescent treponema antibody-absorption test (FTA-ABS): Serum or CSF test that provides the most sensitive treponemal antibodies in all stages of syphilis.

G

gastric analysis: Evaluates gastric function by measuring the contents of a fasting client's stomach for acidity, appearance, and volume.

gastroscopy: Inspection of the stomach interior using a gastroscope.

Glasgow coma scale: The test provides a score in the range 3 to 15; the sum of the scores obtained from three categories measures consciousness.

glucose tolerance test: Checks to determine how the body metabolizes glucose. Blood is drawn before and after a glucose-containing liquid is swallowed.

glycated hemoglobin test (A1c): Measures the amount of sugar attached to the hemoglobin in red blood cells; results are given as a percentage. This test gives an indication of how well diabetes is controlled.

Gram stain: Staining procedure in which microorganisms are stained with crystal violet, followed by iodine solution; decolorized with alcohol; and counterstained with safranin. The retention of either the violet or pink color is a means to identify and classify bacteria. Gram-positive bacteria retain the violet color; gram-negative bacteria lose the violet color and are counterstained red.

H

heart catheterization: Percutaneous intravascular insertion of a catheter into any chamber of the heart or great vessels for diagnosis, assessment of abnormalities, interventional treatment, and evaluation of the effects of pathology on the heart and great vessels.

hematocrit: Used to measure the percentage of packed red cells in a whole blood sample obtained by finger stick or venipuncture.

hemoglobin: Venipuncture or finger stick is done to measure the amount of hemoglobin found in whole blood; used to measure the severity of anemia or polycythemia.

hemoglobin electrophoresis: Evaluates different types of hemoglobin in the blood.

hepatobiliary iminodiacetic acid (HIDA) scan: A scan to track production and flow of bile through the small intestine to show any blockage.

histoplasmin skin test: Form of delayed hypersensitivity skin testing to detect a systemic fungal respiratory disease due to *Histoplasma capsulatum*.

Holter monitor: A machine to record the heart's rhythms over a period of 24 to 48 hours during normal activity.

Huhner test: Postcoital examination of cervical mucus to assess characteristics of the mucus as correlated with the phase of the woman's menstrual cycle and number, motility, and ability of the sperm to cross the cervical mucus.

hysterosalpingography: Radiography of the uterus and uterine tubes after the introduction of an opaque material through the cervix.

hysterosonography: A transvaginal ultrasound to capture inside the uterus; evaluate uterine abnormalities.

I

immunofluorescence microscopy: This test labels antigens or antibodies with a fluorescent dye.

immunoglobulin E (IgE): Test using either serum or urine that provides a detailed separation of the individual immunoglobulin (IgG, IgA, IgD, IgM, IgE) to identify the presence of monoclonal protein and its type.

immunohistochemical test: Test performed on a serum sample to detect the presence of an antibody directed against antigens in cells or tissue sections that are mounted on glass slides.

interferon-gamma release assays (IGRAs): Blood tests to identify individuals at increased risk for developing tuberculosis.

intravenous cholangiogram: Radioisotope is injected intravenously, and radiographs are taken of the bile ducts.

intravenous pyelogram (IVP): Contrast medium is injected intravenously, and radiographs are taken as the medium is cleared from the blood by glomerular filtration. The renal calyces, renal pelves, ureters, and urinary bladder are all visible on film.

in vitro lymphocyte transformation test: An in vitro test to detect lymphocyte function.

isotope scanning: A small amount of radioactivity is injected into the body's vein in order to obtain a series of pictures of different organs.

K

kidneys ureters bladder (KUB): Radiographs taken of the kidneys, ureters, and bladder.

L

laparoscopy: Small incision is made in the abdominal wall to visualize the interior of the abdomen using a laparoscope. It is used to examine the ovaries or fallopian tubes and as a gynecologic sterilization technique.

laryngoscopy: Visual examination of the interior of the larynx using a laryngoscope.

low-dose dexamethasone suppression test: This test may be performed whenever there is unexplained excessive glucocorticoid secretion. Dexamethasone is given orally every 6 hours for 2 days, and adrenocorticotropic hormone (ACTH) stimulation is monitored to determine pathology.

low-dose helical CT scan: This spiral CT scan continually rotates to take several 3-dimensional x-rays of the lungs.

lumbar puncture: Also called a *spinal tap*. (See *cerebrospinal fluid [CSF] analysis*.)

lupus erythematosus (LE) test: Blood sample is mixed with laboratory-treated antigens. If the sample contains antinuclear antibody, the LE factor will react with the antigen, causing swelling and rupture of the nuclear material. Phagocytes from the serum engulf the foreign particles and form LE cells, which are then detected by microscopic examination.

lymph node biopsy: Lymph node tissue is removed and examined under a microscope for signs of infection or a disease.

lymphoscintigraphy: A special type of nuclear medicine imaging that provides pictures called *scintigrams* of the lymphatic system; used to identify the first node to receive lymph drainage from a tumor, to detect blockage in the lymph system, and to assess the stage of cancer.

M

magnetic resonance angiogram (MRA): Type of MRI using a magnetic field and pulses of radio wave energy to provide pictures of blood vessels inside the body.

magnetic resonance cholangiopancreatography (MRCP): MRI using a magnetic field and pulses of radio wave energy to visualize the biliary and pancreatic ducts; can be used to determine if gallstones are lodged in any of the ducts surrounding the gallbladder.

magnetic resonance imaging (MRI): A radiological technique using magnetism, radio waves, and a computer to produce images of body structures. An individual is surrounded by a magnetic field, which causes hydrogen atoms to line up in a certain fashion. A signal is released when the atoms move back to their original places and is processed by the computer. Ionizing radiation is not required.

mammogram: Radiograph of the mammary gland or breast.

Mantoux test: A skin test to determine if there has been exposure to *Mycobacterium tuberculosis* that causes tuberculosis.

mental status examination (MSE): Observations a mental health specialist uses to understand a client's presentation to help in a diagnosis.

microscopic urine: Urine sample is centrifuged; then the cells, casts, and crystals are viewed to detect infection, obstruction, inflammation, trauma, or tumors.

multiple sleep latency test (MSLT): A nap study to see how quickly a client falls asleep in quiet situations during the day; the MSLT is a standard way to measure the level of daytime sleepiness.

myelography: Radiograph of the spinal cord after the injection of a contrast medium; used to identify and study spinal lesions caused by trauma and disease. It has been largely replaced by CT scan or MRI.

N

National Institutes of Health (NIH) Chronic Prostatitis Symptom Index: Using a questionnaire, provides a method of evaluating symptoms and quality of life in men with chronic prostatitis.

neurological assessment: Several examinations, tests, and procedures are performed to help make a diagnosis of nervous system diseases. Tests likely include CT and MRI scans, cerebral angiogram, electroencephalogram, electromyogram, and a nerve conduction study.

nocturnal polysomnography: Test of sleep cycles and stages using continuous EEG recordings of brain waves, electrical activity of muscles, eye movement (electrooculogram), breathing rate, blood pressure, blood oxygen level, heart rhythm, and direct observation of a person during sleep.

noncontrast spiral CT: (Also called *helical CT*.) X-rays are used to scan an entire area while the person lies still on a table. The table passes through the donut-shaped CT scanner. The scanner rotates around the client while a computer creates images from the scan and assembles them into a three-dimensional model.

O

ophthalmologic examination: (Also called a *refraction examination*.) An examination that includes a series of tests to check vision and eye health.

ophthalmoscopy: Allows magnified examination of inner structures of the eye; the ophthalmoscope has a light source and a special viewing device.

Ortolani sign: Procedure to evaluate the stability of the hip joints in newborns and infants. With the infant on his or her back, the joints are manipulated, and if a clicking or popping sensation (Ortolani sign) is felt or heard, the joint is unstable.

otologic examination: Ear examination; may include the use of an otoscope, a tuning fork, and an audiometer.

P

palpation: The health-care provider touches and feels the client's body to examine the size, consistency, texture, location, and tenderness of an organ or body part.

Papanicolaou (Pap) test: Diagnostic test for early detection of cancer cells by a simple smear method. The sample is usually taken from the cervix through a vaginal speculum.

patch test: See *allergy testing*.

pelvic examination: Includes both an inspection of the vulva, vagina, and cervix for abnormalities and a bimanual palpation of the uterus, fallopian tubes, and ovaries. A Pap smear often is done at the same time.

penlight examination: Performed with a lighted instrument to check pupil reactivity.

perfusion lung scan: Client receives IV injection with radioactive particles that pass through the larger blood vessels but are temporarily trapped in small blood vessels. The images show blood perfusion in the lungs.

phenylketonuria (PKU) test: (Also called the *Guthrie screening test*.) Heel stick on an infant is done to collect three drops of blood for screening to check for elevation of serum phenylalanine; performed about 4 days after milk feeding has begun.

pH studies: Determines the acidity or alkalinity level of gastrointestinal secretions. The pH electrode to be used is swallowed by the client. Studies also can be done on blood and urine.

phlebography: Radiography of the veins after the injection of a radiopaque contrast medium.

polymerase chain-reaction test: Process that permits making, in a laboratory, unlimited numbers of copies of genes, beginning with a single molecule of DNA to investigate and diagnose numerous bacterial diseases, viruses associated with cancer, and genetic diseases.

portable cardiorespiratory monitoring: A compact, portable monitor to acquire, classify, record, and display cardiorespiratory data in an online manner; detects apnea, blood oxygen saturation, and heart rate.

positron emission tomography (PET): Indirect visualization using an intravenous injection of a radionuclide contrast substance, which becomes concentrated in the organ being studied. Then the scanning transmits the findings to the computer, where analysis can take place. It is used to diagnose and evaluate certain disease conditions and tumors.

postvoid residual (PVR): Measures urine volume in women with overactive bladder.

potassium hydroxide (KOH) examination: Most sensitive test for superficial fungal infections; involves placing the hair or scales of the lesion on a microscopic slide with a few drops of KOH solution. The KOH dissolves the keratinous material for better visualization.

PPD tuberculin test: Intradermal injection of a purified protein derivative (PPD) tuberculin antigen. A delayed reaction occurs in clients infected with tubercle bacillus, whether or not there are clinical manifestations of disease.

proctoscopy: Visual examination of the rectum using a proctoscope.

prostate-specific antigen (PSA): Serology test to detect, classify, and stage prostatic cancer.

prostatic acid phosphatase (PAP): Formally a major tumor marker for prostate cancer that has been replaced with the PSA; can be used to predict recurrence in men undergoing radical prostatectomy for localized prostate cancer.

pulmonary angiography: A procedure using contrast media and x-rays to show blood flow through the lungs.

pulmonary artery catheterization (PAC): Permits evaluation of ventilation function through spirometer measurements; performed on clients with pulmonary dysfunction.

pulmonary function studies: Number of different tests to determine the ability of the lungs to exchange oxygen and carbon dioxide.

pulse oximetry: Widely used procedure to measure oxygen saturation of arterial blood during breathing.

R

radiography: Process of obtaining an image for diagnosing a radiologic modality.

radioimmunoassay: Technique in radiology used to determine the concentration of an antigen, antibody, or other protein in the serum. (See *blood serum for hormones*.)

random blood glucose test: See *blood glucose testing*.

rapid blood test for methicillin-resistant *Staphylococcus aureus*: This test can detect MRSA and less dangerous strains of the staph bacterium in just 2 hours.

rapid diagnostic tests (RDT): Developed to make accurate malaria diagnoses in locations where microscopy services are not available; finger-stick or venous blood is used, and the result is known in 10 to 15 minutes; a laboratory is not required.

rapid HIV antibody test: A number of tests are available to offer faster and easier response to determine if the virus is present. The following website provides a detail of the four tests currently approved by the FDA http://www.cdc.gov/hiv/basics/testing.html

rapid plasma reagin (RPR) test: Substitute for the venereal disease research laboratory (VDRL) test to detect syphilis. It uses a cardiolipin antigen to detect reagin, which is the antibody relatively specific to the causative agent for syphilis.

real-time RT-PCR (reverse transcription-polymerase chain reaction): The most sensitive test available to detect RNA in a single cell; quantitates gene expression.

rectal examination: Digital examination to detect polyps, early cancer, lesions, inflammatory conditions, and hemorrhoids. It also can show how far the uterus is displaced in the female and reveals the texture and size of the male prostate.

rectal manometry: Measures rectal sphincter function and peristaltic contractions.

red blood cell (erythrocyte) count: Usually performed with a CBC; measures the number of red blood cells in a liter of blood.

Reed-Sternberg cells: These giant multinucleated cells seen under light microscopy are an indication of Hodgkin lymphoma.

refraction test: Defines any vision or refractive error and determines any correction necessary.

reticulocyte count: Venipuncture is performed and the number of immature erythrocytes in the blood is determined; important in diagnosing certain blood disorders, especially anemia.

rheumatoid factor blood test: Blood test to detect rheumatoid arthritis; present in about 80% of adults with rheumatoid arthritis.

Rinne test: Hearing test to evaluate air and bone conduction. A tuning fork is placed on the mastoid process.

S

scan: Image obtained from a system that compiles information in a sequence pattern, such as CT, ultrasound, or MRI; scintiscan.

scintiscan: Produces a map of scintillations observed when a radioactive substance is introduced into the body. The intensity of the record indicates the differential accumulation of the substance in the various body parts.

sensitivity test: See *allergy testing*.

serum B$_{12}$: Venipuncture is done for a quantitative analysis of serum vitamin B$_{12}$ levels. Usually done concurrently with a serum folic acid because deficiencies of the two are common causes of megaloblastic anemia.

serum bilirubin: Measures serum levels of bilirubin; helps evaluate liver function, jaundice, biliary obstruction, and hemolytic anemia.

serum calcium, phosphorus, total protein, or serum electrolytes: This series of tests performed on a blood sample determines levels of calcium, phosphorus, and protein in the blood. (See *chemistry screens*.)

serum creatinine (serum creatinine kinase): Creatinine in blood serum provides a sensitive measure of tissue damage, especially renal damage. Creatinine levels are directly related to the glomerular filtration rate. (See *chemistry screens*.)

serum ferritin: Serum ferritin levels are related to the amount of available iron stored in the body. This test screens for iron deficiency and overload, measures iron storage, and can distinguish between iron deficiency and chronic inflammation.

serum folate: See *serum folic acid*.

serum folic acid: This test on a blood sample measures the levels of folic acid; helps to diagnose megaloblastic anemia and to determine folate stores in pregnancy.

serum gonadotropin: See *serum human chorionic gonadotropin (hCG)*.

serum human chorionic gonadotropin (hCG): Production of hCG begins very quickly after the fertilized ovum is implanted into the uterine wall; the blood test reveals the presence of hCG if pregnancy has occurred.

serum protein electrophoresis: Measures serum albumin and globulins in an electric field by separating the proteins on the basis of size, shape, and electric charge at pH 8.6; helps to diagnose hepatic disease, protein deficiency, blood and renal disorders, and gastrointestinal and neoplastic diseases.

sigmoidoscopy: Visual inspection of the sigmoid flexure of the large intestine using a sigmoidoscope.

skin (intradermal or scratch) test: See *allergy testing*.

slit-lamp examination: Allows an ophthalmologist to visualize the anterior portion of the eye. The slit lamp is an instrument with a special lighting system and a binocular microscope.

Snellen chart: Visual screening using a standardized chart with block letters arranged in rows of decreasing size. A large E chart or one with animals and familiar objects may be used for children.

sputum culture: Examination of the material raised from the lungs and bronchi during deep coughing to determine pathogens.

StaphSR assay: Rapid blood test to detect *Staphylococcus aureus* (SA) and *methicillin-resistant Staphylococcus aureus (MRSA)*.

stool culture: Feces will be examined to determine pathogens that cause gastrointestinal disease; a chemical test may also be done on the stool specimen to detect occult blood.

stool occult blood: Chemical test performed on a stool specimen to detect occult or hidden blood.

straight-leg raising test: The leg is raised with the knee straight to determine low back and leg pain. If pain radiates down the back of the leg below the knee, the test is positive, indicating that one or more nerve roots leading to the sciatic nerve may be compressed or irritated.

sweat test: Measures sodium and chloride in sweat to diagnose cystic fibrosis; people with cystic fibrosis have 2 to 5 times the normal amount of sodium and chloride in their sweat.

synovial fluid analysis: Sterile needle is inserted into a joint space to obtain a fluid specimen; aids in diagnosing arthritis, relieving pain and distention, and administering local drug therapy.

T

thoracentesis: Surgical puncture of the pleural space to remove fluid for analysis or treatment.

thyroid function tests: Tests of thyroid function, including physical examination; some tests include determination of thyroid hormone levels.

Tinel sign: Cutaneous tingling sensation produced by pressing on or tapping the nerve trunk that has been damaged or is regenerating following trauma.

tissue transglutaminase (tTG) antibody: This antibody is important in diagnosing celiac disease; the value of this antibody in long-term follow-up is controversial.

tonometry: Measurement of tension or pressure, especially of the eye for detection of glaucoma.

toxicology screen: Tests used on blood or urine to detect toxic substances.

transesophageal echocardiogram (TEE): An ultrasound transducer that uses high-frequency sound waves to produce a graphic outline of the heart's movement. It is positioned on an endoscope, inserted down the throat into the esophagus; it provides a close look at the heart's valves and chambers without interference from the ribs or lungs.

transillumination test: Uses a light shining through a body area or organ to check for abnormalities; often used on the head, scrotum, or chest of newborn or breast of adult female.

transthoracic echocardiogram (TTE): The echocardiogram probe is placed on the chest wall to get heart images through the chest wall.

transvaginal sonography (transvaginal ultrasound, or TVS): Test that examines the vagina, uterus, fallopian tubes, ovaries, and bladder through an instrument that is inserted into the vagina and causes sound waves to bounce off pelvic organs. The echoes created are sent to a computer to produce a sonogram.

"triple screen" blood test—alpha-fetoprotein (AFP), human chorionic gonadotropin (hCG), and estriol: Tests maternal blood for three specific substances—AFP, hCG, and estriol; often helps in estimating a person's chances of having an abnormality.

tumor markers in blood (CEA, PSA): See *carcinoembryonic antigen (CEA)* and *prostate-specific antigen (PSA)*.

U

ultrasonography: Use of ultrasound to produce an image or photograph of an organ or tissue. Ultrasound echoes are recorded as the sound waves strike tissues of different densities.

upper gastrointestinal endoscopy: Allows visualization of the upper gastrointestinal tract to diagnose inflammatory, ulcerative, and infectious disease, neoplasms, and other lesions.

ureteroscopy: Process of examining the inside of the urinary tract (specifically the urethra and bladder) with an endoscope.

urinalysis: Voided specimen in a clean container is obtained to test for color, appearance, formed elements, casts, odor, transparency, and specific gravity.

urinary antigen test: This test is an immunochromatographic membrane assay that detects cell wall C-polysaccharide common to all types of pneumonia.

urine calcium and phosphates: Measures the urine levels of calcium and phosphates, which are essential for formation and resorption of bone; requires a 24-hour urine specimen.

urine catch, 24-hour: Urine is collected over a 24-hour period to measure quantity as well as physical and chemical characteristics.

urine creatinine: Measures the levels of creatinine in urine; used to help assess glomerular filtration and to check the accuracy of 24-hour urine collection based on relative contrast levels of creatinine excretion.

urine culture: Clean-voided midstream sample is collected for evaluation of urinary tract infections; the specimen is studied under a microscope, and a colony count is made to determine the presence of infection.

urine flowmetry (uroflowmetry): Test to measure the volume of urine excreted, the speed it is excreted, and how long excretion takes; helps in evaluating urinary tract function.

urodynamic tests: Measures bladder function and efficiency.

V

vaginal smear: With a cotton-tipped applicator or wooden spatula, vaginal secretions are collected for microscopic examination.

vasography: Used when ultrasound is uncertain; radioactive dye is injected into the vas deferens and ejaculatory ducts; the X-ray is taken as the dye flows through the ducts to detect blockage.

Venereal Disease Research Laboratory (VDRL) test: This test is used to screen for primary and secondary syphilis. A serum sample usually is used, but a specimen of cerebrospinal fluid may be used as well.

venography: Test performed to view the veins (usually in leg); dye is used, and x-rays are viewed as the dye flows through the veins.

vesiculography: X-ray of the seminal vesicles following injection of radiopaque medium.

vestibular testing: A number of tests to help determine problems with the vestibular portion of the inner ear; helps isolate dizziness symptoms to a specific cause that can often be treated.

videoplethysmography: A relatively new method to detect atrial fibrillation via facial feature recordings that illustrate a subtle change in skin color and uneven blood flow.

vision-field test: Eye test to detect dysfunction in central and peripheral vision.

voiding cystoscopy: Examination of the bladder to determine urine excretion. (See *urine flowmetry*.)

W

Weber test: Test for unilateral deafness. A vibrating tuning fork held against the midline of the top of the head. In those with equal hearing ability in the ears, the sound is perceived as being located at the top of the head; to a person with unilateral conductive deafness, the sound is perceived as being more pronounced on the diseased side; in persons with unilateral nerve deafness, the sound is perceived as being louder in the good ear.

Western blot test, ELISA/Western blot: A set of blood tests to diagnose chronic HIV infection.

West Nile virus (WNV) IgM capture ELISA: Diagnostic test detects the levels of a particular type of antibody, IgM, in a client's serum. IgM antibodies can be detected within the first few days of the onset of illness and can assist in diagnosis of WNV.

white blood cell count (WBC): Test made on whole blood to report the number of leukocytes in a cubic millimeter. The WBC may rise or fall in disease and is diagnostically useful only when interpreted in light of the client's clinical status.

X

x-ray of kidneys, ureters, and bladder (KUB): Provides radiographs of the kidneys, ureters, and bladder to evaluate the urinary tract and kidney structure, size, and position.

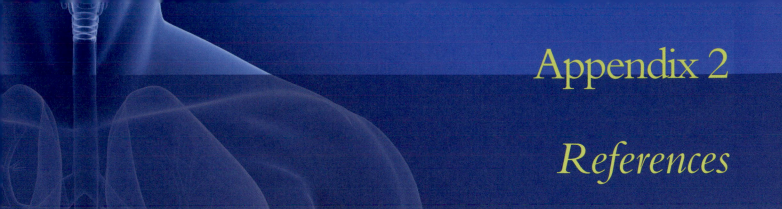

BOOKS

American Psychiatric Association: *Diagnostic and Statistical Manual of Mental Disorders*, ed. 4. Text Revision. Washington, DC: American Psychiatric Association, 2000.

Barankin, B, and Freiman, A: *Derm Notes Pocket Guide*. Philadelphia: FA Davis, 2006.

Deglin, JH, and Vallerand, AH: *Davis's Drug Guide for Nurses*, ed. 11. Philadelphia: FA Davis, 2009.

Diamond, J: *The Life Energy in Music* (Vols. 1 and 2). Valley Cottage, NY: Archaeus Press, 1983.

Frisch, NC, and Frisch, LE: *Psychiatric Mental Health Nursing*, ed. 4. Clifton Park, NY: Thomson Delmar Learning, 2010.

Gorman, LM, and Sultan, DF: *Psychosocial Nursing for General Patient Care*, ed. 3. Philadelphia: FA Davis, 2008.

The Institute of Medicine: *Relieving Pain in America. A Blueprint to Transforming Prevention, Care, Education, and Research*. Washington, DC: National Academies Press, 2011: http://www.ncbi.nlm.nih.gov/books/NBK92525/.

Kligler, B, and Lee, R: *Integrative Medicine Principles for Practice*. New York: McGraw-Hill, 2004.

Lake, JH: *Textbook of Integrative Mental Health Care*. New York: Thieme Medical Publishers, 2007.

Lake, JH, and Spiegel, D (eds): *Complementary and Alternative Treatments in Mental Health Care*. Arlington, VA: American Psychiatric Publishing, 2007.

Laurence, P, and Dana, B: *The Laughter Prescription*. New York: Ballantine Books, 1982.

Leeuwen, AM, and Poelhuis-Leth, DJ: *Davis's Comprehensive Handbook of Laboratory Tests with Nursing Implications*, ed. 3. Philadelphia: FA Davis, 2009.

Lindh, WQ, Pooler, MS, Tamparo, CD, and Dahl, BM: *Delmar's Comprehensive Medical Assisting Administrative and Clinical Competencies*, ed. 5. Clifton Park, NY: Delmar Cengage Learning, 2010.

Mumber, MP: *Integrative Oncology: Principles and Practice*. London: Taylor and Francis, 2006.

Nurse's 5-Minute Clinical Consult Diseases. Ambler, PA: Lippincott Williams & Wilkins, 2007.

Nurse's 5-Minute Clinical Consult Diagnostic Tests. Ambler, PA: Lippincott Williams & Wilkins, 2008.

Rakel, D: *Integrative Medicine*, ed. 3. Philadelphia: Saunders Elsevier, 2012.

Scanlon, VC, and Sanders, T: *Essentials of Anatomy and Physiology*, ed. 6. Philadelphia: FA Davis, 2011.

Sommers, MS, Johnson, SA, and Beery, TA: *Diseases and Disorders: A Nursing Therapeutics Manual*, ed. 3. Philadelphia: FA Davis, 2007.

Stuart, GW: *Principles and Practice of Psychiatric Nursing*, ed. 109. St. Louis, MO: Elsevier Mosby, 2013.

Taber's Cyclopedic Medical Dictionary, ed. 22. Philadelphia: FA Davis, 2013.

U.S. Department of Health and Human Services, National Institutes of Health. *What You Need to Know About Cancer of the Colon and Rectum*. NIH Publication No. 06-1552, May 2006.

ARTICLES

Complementary and alternative medicine use among adults and children; United States, 2012. U.S. Department of Health and Human Services, Centers for Disease Control and Prevention, National Health Statistics Reports, No. 79, February 10, 2015.

Complementary and alternative medicine: Healthy Lifestyle Consumer health: http://www.mayoclinic.com Accessed October 18, 2014.

Greenwald, JL, Burstein, GR, Pincus, J, and Branson, B: A rapid review of rapid HIV antibody tests. Boston Medical Center, Hospital Medicine Unit. Current Science Inc., Boston, MA, 2006.

Guidance for industry: Final rule declaring dietary supplements containing ephedrine alkaloids adulterated because they present an unreasonable risk; Small Entity Compliance Guide. U.S. Department of Health and Human Services, Food and Drug Administration, Center for Food Safety and Applied Nutrition, July 17, 2008.

Preventing emerging infectious diseases: A strategy for the 21st century. U.S. Department of Health and Human Services, Centers for Disease Control and Prevention (CDC), Atlanta, GA, 1998.

Whalen, J: Atrial-fibrillation patients have increasing options for treatment. *Wall Street Journal*, Personal Journal, July 14, 2009.

Whitlock, G: Obesity takes years off your life. *Lancet* (online edition), March 18, 2009.

Winslow, R: How ice can save your life: Therapeutic hypothermia. *Wall Street Journal*, Personal Journal, October 6, 2009.

CHAPTER 1 URL REFERENCES

Body mass index calculator: http://www.nhlbi.nih.gov/health/educational/lose_wt/BMI/bmicalc.htm

Burns: http://www.ncbi.nlm.nih.gov/pmc/articles/PMC449823/

Huntington disease: http://www.ncbi.nlm.nih.gov/pubmedhealth/PMH0001775/

Immunodeficiency disorders: http://www.nlm.nih.gov/medlineplus/ency/article/000818.htmSpider bites: http://www.medicinenet.com/spider_bites_black_widow_and_brown_recluse/article.htm

CHAPTER 2 URL REFERENCES

Complementary and alternative medicine: Evaluate treatment claims: http://www.mayoclinic.org/healthy-living/consumer-health/in-depth/alternative-medicine/art-20046087

Complementary and alternative medicine in the United States, National Center for Complementary and Integrative Health (NCCIH): http://nccihnih.gov/

Food and Drug Administration: http://www.fda.gov

The Healing Art of Laughter: http://www.mondaymag.com/news/146909085.html

http://www.laughteryoga.org/english

CHAPTER 3 URL REFERENCES

American Pain Society: http://www.ampainsoc.org

Association for Applied Psychophysiology and Biofeedback: http://www.aapb.org

International Association for the Study of Pain: http://www.iasp-pain.org

CHAPTER 4 URL REFERENCES

Antimicrobial resistance: http://www.who.int/mediacentre/factsheets/fs194/en/

DEET (*N,N*-diethyl-3-methylbenzamide): http://www.deet.com/faqs.html

Emergency preparedness and response/bioterrorism: http://emergency.cdc.gov

Emerging and re-emerging infectious diseases: NIH Curriculum Series [Internet], www.ncbi.nlm.nih.gov/books/NKB20370/

HIV infection/AIDS: http://www.avert.org/worldstats.htm

MERS: http://www.cdc.gov/features/novelcoronavirus/

Morbidity and Mortality Weekly Report: http://www.cdc.gov/mmwr

National Center for Health Statistics: http://www.cdc.gov/nchs

Reportable diseases. Find greater detail on reportable infections, diseases, or conditions: http://www.in.gov/isdh/files/ReportableDiseaseList.pdf

West Nile Virus: Chicagotribune.com. 2014 West Nile Virus Season Update and Safety Tips: http://www.chicagotribune.com/suburbs/batavia-geneva-st-charles/community/chi-ugc-article-2014-west-nile-virus-season-update-and-safety-2014-05-05-story.html

CHAPTER 5 URL REFERENCES

American Cancer Society: http://www.acs.org

http://www.cancer.org/cancer/cancerbasics/signs-and-symptoms-of-cancer

Cancer facts and figures: http://www.cancer.org/acs/groups/content/@research/documents/webcontent/acspc-042151.pdf

National Cancer Institute: http://www.cancer.gov

Measles vaccine for cancer treatment: http://www.mayoclinic.org/medical-professionals/clinical-updates/neurosciences/update-measles-virus-novel-therapy-glioblastoma

U.S. Department of Health and Human Services: http://www.hhs.gov

CHAPTER 6 URL REFERENCES

American Heart Association: http://www.heart.org

Cleft Palate Foundation: http://www.cleftline.org

Cystic Fibrosis Foundation: http://www.cff.org

Muscular Dystrophy Association: http://www.mda.org/disease/DMD.html

National Down Syndrome Society: http://www.ndss.org

National Organization on Fetal Alcohol Syndrome: http://www.nofas.org

Spina Bifida Association: http://www.spinabifidaassociation.org

United Cerebral Palsy: http://www.ucp.org

CHAPTER 7 URL REFERENCES

Anxiety and Depression Association of America: http://www.adaa.org

Autism Society: http://www.autism-society.org

Autism Speaks: http://www.autismspeaks.org/index.php

Centers for Disease Control and Prevention: http://www.cdc.gov/

Children and Adults with Attention-Deficit/Hyperactivity Disorder: http://www.chadd.org

National Alliance on Mental Illness: http://www.nami.org

National Institute of Mental Health: http://www.nimh.nih.gov/index.shtml

PTSD: National Center for PTSD: http://www.ptsd.va.gov/index.asp

Substance Abuse and Mental Health Services Administration (SAMHSA): http://www.samhsa.gov

CHAPTER 8 URL REFERENCES

Warts: http://www.nlm.nih.gov/medlineplus

CHAPTER 9 URL REFERENCES

Arthritis: http://www.arthritis.org

Fibromyalgia: http://www.fmaware.org
https://www.rheumatology.org/Practice/Clinical/Patients/Diseases_And_Conditions/Fibromyalgia/

Myasthenia gravis: http://www.myasthenia.org

Osteomyelitis: http://www.nlm.nih.gov/medlineplus/ency/article/000437.htm

Systemic lupus erythematosus: http://www.lupus.org

CHAPTER 10 URL REFERENCES

ALS Association: http://www.alsa.org

Alzheimer's Association: http://www.alz.org/index.asp

American Brain Tumor Association: http://www.abta.org

Cerebral aneurysm: http://www.brainaneurysm.com

Epilepsy Foundation: http://www.epilepsyfoundation.org

Hemiplegia: http://www.nlm.nih.gov/medlineplus/paralysis.html

Meningitis: http://www.cdc.gov/meningitis/about/faq.html

Neuropathy Association: http://www.neuropathy.org

Paralysis: http://www.nlm.nih.gov/medlineplus/paralysis.html

Transient ischemic attack: http://www.americanheart.org/presenter.jhtml?identifier=4781

Traumatic brain injury: http://www.ninds.nih.gov/disorders/tbi/tbi.htm
http://www.aans.org/Patient%20Information.aspx

CHAPTER 11 URL REFERENCES

Diabetes mellitus: http://www.diabetes.org

Hormone Health Network: www.hormone.org

Hypopituitarism: http://www.pituitary.org/disorders/hypopituitarism.aspx

National Endocrine and Metabolic Diseases Information Service: http://endocrine.niddk.nih.gov/pubs/addison/addison.htm

Polycystic Ovarian Syndrome Association: http://www.pcosupport.org

CHAPTER 12 URL REFERENCES

American Heart Association: http://www.americanheart.org

Aplastic anemia, folic acid deficiency anemia, pernicious anemia: http://www.nhlbi.nih.gov/health/dci/Diseases

Coronary artery disease: http://www.nhlbi.nih.gov/health/dci/Diseases/Cad/CAD_WhatIs.html

Endocarditis: http://www.endocarditis.org/index.html

Hodgkin lymphoma: http://www.cancer.gov/cancertopics/types/hodgkin

Lymphedema: http://www.lymphnet.org

Medical Daily: http://www.medicaldaily.com/facetime-your-heart-your-face-can-help-diagnose-atrial-fibrillation-300470

Myocarditis Foundation: http://www.myocarditisfoundation.org

National Cancer Institute (cancer staging): http://www.cancer.gov

CHAPTER 13 URL REFERENCES

American Academy of Allergy, Asthma, & Immunology/Sinusitis: http://www.aaaai.org

American Association of Sleep Apnea: http://www.sleepapnea.org

COPD International: http://www.copd-international.com

Lung cancer: http://www.cancer.gov/cancertopics/types/lung

Pneumothorax (collapsed lung): http://www.pneumothorax.org

Pulmonary hypertension: http://www.americanheart.org

CHAPTER 14 URL REFERENCES

Celiac disease: http://www.CeliacCentral.org

Crohn disease, IBS, and ulcerative colitis: http://www.ccfa.org

Viral hepatitis: http://www.medicinenet.com

CHAPTER 15 URL REFERENCES

Bladder cancer: http://www.cancer.gov/cancertopics/pdq/treatment/bladder/Patient

Cystitis and urethritis: http://www.onlinemedicare.org/diseases/cystitis-and-urethritis.html

Eating hints for cancer patients: http://www.cancer.gov/cancertopics/eatinghints

National Kidney Foundation: http://www.kidney.org

CHAPTER 16 URL REFERENCES

Assisted reproductive technology: http://www.cdc.gov/art/artreports.htm

Endometriosis: http://www.endometriosisassn.org

Female reproductive health: http://www.womenshealth.gov

Inflammatory breast cancer: http://www.ibcresearch.org/

Ovarian cancer: http://www.apjohncancerinstitute.org/cancer/ovarian.htm

Prostate cancer: http://www.cancer.gov/cancertopics/types/prostate

http://www/cancer.org/cancer/prostatecancer/

Sexually transmitted diseases: http://www.cdc.gov/STD

CHAPTER 17 URL REFERENCES

Complementary and alternative medicine for pediatric otitis media: www.ncbi.nlm.nih.gov/pubmed/23562352

Motion sickness medications: http://wwwnc.cdc.gov/travel/yellowbook/2010/chapter-2/motion-sickness.aspx

Strabismus: http://www.strabismus.org

5-ASA	5-aminosalicylic acid
^{13}C	carbon 13

A

A_{1C}	glycated hemoglobin
AAA	abdominal aortic aneurysm
AAFP	American Academy of Family Physicians
AAP	American Academy of Pediatrics
ACE	angiotensin-converting enzyme
ACIP	Advisory Committee on Immunization Practices
ACS	American Cancer Society
ACTH	adrenocorticotropic hormone
ADA	American Diabetes Association
ADH	antidiuretic hormone
ADHD	attention deficit-hyperactivity disorder
AED	automated external defibrillator
AFP	alpha-fetoprotein
AHRQ	Agency for Research Health and Quality
AIDS	acquired immune deficiency syndrome
ALL	acute lymphocytic leukemia
ALS	amyotrophic lateral sclerosis
ALT	alanine aminotransferase
AMACR	alpha-methylacyl-CoA racemase (a genetic marker)
AMD	age-related macular degeneration (also ARMD)
AML	acute myeloblastic leukemia
ANS	autonomic nervous system
APA	American Psychiatric Association
APS	American Pain Society
APSGN	acute poststreptococcal glomerulonephritis
ARBD	alcohol-related birth defects
ARDS	acute respiratory distress syndrome
AREDS	Age-Related Eye Disease Study
ARMD	age-related macular degeneration (also AMD)
ARND	alcohol-related neurodevelopmental disorder
ART	assisted reproductive technology
ARV	antiretroviral drug
ASD	atrial septal defect

ASD	autism spectrum disorders
AST	aspartate aminotransferase
AUA	American Urological Association

B

bCG	bacille Calmette-Guérin
BMI	body mass index
BMT	bone marrow transplant
BNC2	basonuclin-2 gene
BPH	benign prostatic hyperplasia
BRCA1	breast cancer susceptibility gene 1
BRCA2	breast cancer susceptibility gene 2
BRM	biological response modifier
BUN	blood urea nitrogen

C

CAAT	controlled amino acid therapy
CAD	coronary artery disease
CAM	complementary and alternative medicine
CBC	complete blood count
CBT	cognitive behavioral therapy
CDC	Centers for Disease Control and Prevention
CEA	carcinoembryonic antigen
CF	cystic fibrosis
CFS	chronic fatigue syndrome
CFTR	cystic fibrosis transmembrane conductance regulator
CHD	coronary heart disease
CHF	congestive heart failure
CK	creatine kinase
CLL	chronic lymphocytic leukemia
CML	chronic myelocytic leukemia
CNS	central nervous system
CO_2	carbon dioxide
COPD	chronic obstructive pulmonary disease
CP	cerebral palsy
CP	cleft palate
CPAP	continuous positive airway pressure
CPK	creatine phosphokinase
CPK-MB	creatine phosphokinase myocardial band
CPR	cardiopulmonary resuscitation
CRP	C-reactive protein
CRRT	continuous renal replacement therapy
CSF	cerebrospinal fluid

CT	computed tomography
CTA	computed tomography angiogram
CVA	cerebrovascular accident
CVS	chorionic villus sampling

D

DBT	dialectical behavior therapy
D&C	dilation and curettage
DDH	developmental dysplasia of the hip
DEET	*N,N*-diethyl-3-methylbenzamide
DEXA	dual-energy x-ray absorptiometry
DFA	direct fluorescent antibody
DHEA	Dehydroepiandrosterone
DICC	dynamic infusion cavernosometry and cavernosography
DMARD	disease-modifying antirheumatic drug
DNA	deoxyribonucleic acid
DRE	digital rectal examination
DSM-V	*Diagnostic and Statistical Manual of Mental Disorders*, Fifth Edition
DTaP	diphtheria and tetanus toxoids and pertussis vaccine—pediatrics
DVT	deep venous thrombosis

E

EAP	employee assistance programs
EBV	Epstein-Barr virus
ECG	electrocardiogram
ECM	erythema chronicum migrans
ECT	electrical convulsive therapy
EDS	excessive daytime sleepiness
EEG	electroencephalogram
EFT	emotional freedom technique
EGD	esophagogastroduodenoscopy
ELISA	enzyme-linked immunosorbent assay
EMA	endomysium antibody
EMDR	eye-movement desensitization and reprocessing
ERCP	endoscopic retrograde cholangiopancreatography
ESBL	extended-spectrum beta-lactamase
ESR	erythrocyte sedimentation rate
ESRD	end-stage renal disease
ESSR	enlarge, stimulate, swallow, rest

F

FAS	fetal alcohol syndrome
FASD	fetal alcohol spectrum disorders
FDA	U.S. Food and Drug Administration
FSA	flexible spending account
FSH	follicle-stimulating hormone
FTA-ABS	fluorescent treponemal antibody-absorption

G

GAD	generalized anxiety disorder
GDM	gestational diabetes mellitus

GERD	gastroesophageal reflux disease
GH	growth hormone
GHB	gamma hydroxyl butyrate
GI	gastrointestinal
GIFT	gamete intrafallopian transfer
GRP	gastrin-releasing peptide

H

HAART	highly active antiretroviral therapy
HAV	hepatitis A virus
HBV	hepatitis B virus
hCG	human chorionic gonadotropin
HCV	hepatitis C virus
HDL	high-density lipoprotein
HDV	hepatitis D virus
HEV	hepatitis E virus
hGH	human growth hormone
HGV	hepatitis G virus
Hib	*Haemophilus* influenza type b vaccine
HIDA	hepatobiliary iminodiacetic acid
HIV	human immunodeficiency virus
HNPCC	hereditary nonpolyposis colorectal cancer
HoLEP	holmium laser enucleation of the prostate
HPV	human papillomavirus; genital human papillomavirus
HRT	hormone replacement therapy
HSA	health savings account
HSG	hysterosalpingography
HSV	herpes simplex virus
HSV-1	herpes simplex virus type 1
HSV-2	herpes simplex virus type 2
HTLV-1	human T-cell leukemia virus-1

I

IASP	International Association for the Study of Pain
IBC	inflammatory breast cancer
IBD	inflammatory bowel disease
IBS	irritable bowel syndrome
ICD	implantable cardioverter-defibrillator
IF	intrinsic factor
IgA	immunoglobulin A
IgE	immunoglobulin E
IgG	immunoglobulin
IgM	immunoglobulin M
IOL	intraocular lens
IUD	intrauterine device
IV	intravenous
IVF	in vitro fertilization
IVP	intravenous pyelogram

K

KOH	formula for potassium hydroxide
KUB	x-ray studies of the kidney, ureter, and bladder

L

LASIK	laser-assisted in situ keratomileusis
LDH	lactate dehydrogenase
LDL	low-density lipoprotein
LE	lupus erythematosus
LES	lower esophageal sphincter
LH	luteinizing hormone
LRG	leucine-rich alpha-2 glycoprotein
LSD	lysergic acid diethylamide
LTH	luteotropic hormone

M

MAOI	monoamine oxidase inhibitor
MERS	Middle East Respiratory syndrome
MHPA	Mental Health Parity Act
MI	myocardial infarction
MMR	measles/mumps/rubella immunization
MMRV	measles/mumps/rubella/varicella immunization
MRA	magnetic resonance angiography
MRCP	magnetic resonance cholangiopancreatography
MRI	magnetic resonance imaging
MRSA	methicillin-resistant *Staphylococcus aureus*
MRT	moral recognition therapy
MS	multiple sclerosis
MSA	medical savings account
MSAFP	maternal serum alpha-fetoprotein
MSE	mental status examination
MSLT	multiple sleep latency test

N

NAMI	National Alliance on Mental Illness
NCCIH	National Center for Complementary and Integrative Health
NCCLS	National Committee for Clinical Laboratory Standards
NCHS	National Center for Health Statistics
NCI	National Cancer Institute
NDRI	norepinephrine and dopamine reuptake inhibitors
NIDA	National Institute on Drug Abuse
NIH	National Institutes of Health
NIMH	National Institute of Mental Health
NSAID	nonsteroidal anti-inflammatory drug
NSCLC	non–small-cell lung cancer
NTD	neural tube defect

O

OCD	obsessive-compulsive disorder
OTC	over-the-counter

P

PAA	peripheral artery aneurysm
$PaCO_2$	partial pressure of carbon dioxide
PAP	prostatic acid phosphatase or Papanicolaou
PBSCT	peripheral blood stem cell transplantation
PCA	patient-controlled analgesia
PCI	percutaneous coronary intervention
PCOS	polycystic ovary syndrome
PCP	primary care provider
PCR	polymerase chain reaction
PDA	patent ductus arteriosus
PDT	photodynamic therapy
PET	positron emission tomography
PID	pelvic inflammatory disease
PIH	pregnancy-induced hypertension
PKU	phenylketonuria
PLMD	periodic limb movement disorder
PMDD	premenstrual dysphoric disorder
PMS	premenstrual syndrome
PNS	peripheral nervous system
PPD	purified protein derivative (for tuberculin test)
PPH	primary pulmonary hypertension
PPI	proton pump inhibitor
PPND	postpartum or paternal postnatal depression
PRK	photorefractive keratectomy
PROM	premature rupture of membranes
PRSP	penicillin-resistant *Streptococcus pneumoniae*
PSA	prostate-specific antigen
PT	physical therapy/therapist
PTH	parathyroid hormone
PTSD	post-traumatic stress disorder
PUVA	psoralen and ultraviolet A therapy
PVR	postvoid residual

R

RA	rheumatoid arthritis
RBC	red blood cell
RCC	renal cell carcinoma
RDT	rapid diagnostic test
REM	rapid eye movement
RLS	restless leg syndrome
RPR	rapid plasma reagin

S

SAD	seasonal affective disorder
SAMHSA	Substance Abuse and Mental Health Services Administration
SARS	severe acute respiratory syndrome
SBS	shaken baby syndrome
SCLC	small-cell lung cancer
SEER	National Cancer Institute's Surveillance and Epidemiology and End Results
SG	substantia gelatinosa

SIDS	sudden infant death syndrome
SLE	systemic lupus erythematosus
SNRI	serotonin and norepinephrine reuptake inhibitors
SSRI	selective serotonin reuptake inhibitors
STD	sexually transmitted disease

T

T_3	triiodothyronine
T_4	thyroxine
TAA	thoracic aortic aneurysm
TB	tuberculosis
TBI	traumatic brain injury
TCA	tricyclic antidepressant
TCD	transcranial Doppler
TCM	traditional Chinese medicine
TEE	transesophageal echocardiogram
TEF	transesophageal fistula
TENS	transcutaneous electrical nerve stimulation
TET	tubal embryo transplant
TGA	transposition of great arteries
THC	tetrahydrocannabinol
TIA	transient ischemic attack
TIG	tetanus immune globulin (human)
TMS	transcranial magnetic stimulation
TSH	thyroid-stimulating hormone
tTG	tissue transglutaminase
TUIP	transurethral incision of the prostate

TULIP	transurethral ultrasound-guided laser incision of the prostate
TUMT	transurethral microwave therapy
TURP	transurethral prostate resection

U

UPPP	uvulopalatopharyngoplasty
URI	upper respiratory infection
UTI	urinary tract infection
UV	ultraviolet
UVB	ultraviolet B

V

VA	Veteran's Administration
VDRL	Venereal Disease Research Laboratories
VEGF	vascular endothelial growth factor
VHF	viral hemorrhagic fever
VRE	vancomycin-resistant enterococcus
VSD	ventricular septal defect
VZIG	varicella zoster immune globulin
VZV	varicella-zoster virus

W

WBC	white blood cell
WHO	World Health Organization
WNV	West Nile virus

Z

ZIFT	zygote intrafallopian transfer

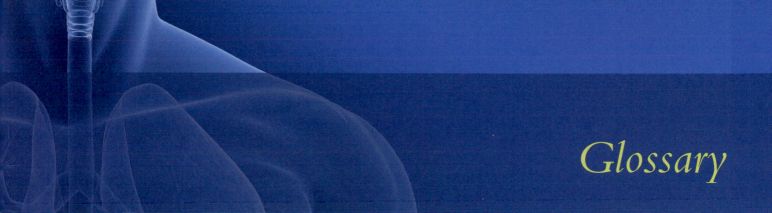

Glossary

A

abrade: To chafe; to roughen or remove by friction.

acetabulum: Rounded cavity on the outer surface of the hip bone that receives the head of the femur.

adenoma: Tumor of a gland or cancerous growth in glandular epithelial tissue.

adjuvant analgesic: Any drug whose primary purpose is not generally used or prescribed for pain but can also serve as an analgesic for some pain conditions.

agnosia: Loss of ability to understand or interpret auditory, visual, or other forms of sensory information even though the respective sensory organs are functioning properly.

agraphia: Loss of ability to convert thought into writing.

albumin: One of a group of simple plasma proteins in humans that can act as a source for rapid replacement of tissue proteins.

alexia: Loss of ability to understand the written language.

allogeneic: Belonging to the same species but having a different genetic constitution.

alogia: Inability to speak owing to a mental condition or a symptom of dementia.

alopecia: Absence or loss of hair, especially on the head.

alveoli (pulmonary): The microscopic air sacs in the lungs where the exchange of carbon dioxide and oxygen occurs.

amblyopia: Unilateral reduction in visual acuity in which there is no apparent pathological condition of the eye.

amino acid: Any one of a large group of organic compounds constituting the primary building blocks of proteins.

amygdala: Almond-shaped section of the brain used to form emotional reactions.

analgesic: Drug or other agent used to relieve pain.

anaphylaxis: Allergic reaction of the body to a foreign body or other substance. Sometimes used to refer exclusively to a sudden, unusually severe, and possibly life-threatening allergic reaction.

anaplasia: Loss of structural differentiation, as seen in malignant neoplasms.

anastomosis: Surgical, traumatic, or pathological formation of a connection between two normally separate tubular structures or organs in the body.

aneurysm: Abnormal, saclike bulge in the wall of an artery, a vein, or the heart.

ankylosis: Immobility of a joint.

anorexia: Loss of appetite for foods.

anoxia: Absence of oxygen.

antibody: Protein substance produced by the body's immune system in response to and interacting with a specific antigen.

anticholinergic (drug): Drug or agent that inhibits the action of the neurotransmitter chemical acetylcholine, blocking parasympathetic nerve impulses, with consequent reduction of smooth-muscle contractions and various bodily secretions.

antiemetic: Drug or other agent used to prevent or stop vomiting.

antigen: Any substance that, when introduced into the body, causes the production of a specific antibody by the immune system.

antipruritic: Agent that prevents or relieves itching.

antipyretic: Drug or agent that reduces fever.

anuria: Absence of urine formation.

aphasia: Loss or impairment of the ability to communicate through speech, writing, or signs due to dysfunction of brain centers.

apnea: Temporary cessation in breathing.

arrhythmia (cardiac): Irregularities in the force or rhythm of heart action caused by disturbances in the discharge of cardiac impulses from the heart's sinoatrial node or their transmission through the heart's conductile tissue.

arthralgia: Pain in a joint.

ascites: Abnormal accumulation of fluid in the peritoneal cavity.

atelectasis: In a neonate, the failure of the lung to completely expand at birth; generally, a collapsed lung. The collapse may be complete or partial.

atropine: Anticholinergic agent that counteracts effects of parasympathetic stimulation.

auscultation: Listening to sounds produced by the internal organs or other body parts for diagnostic purposes.

autologous: Originating within an individual, especially a factor present in tissues or fluids.

avolition: Lack of motivation for work or other goal-oriented activity.

azotemia: Presence of urea in the blood.

B

bacteremia: Bacteria in the blood.

bacteriuria: The presence of bacteria in the urine.

bilirubin: Orange- to yellow-colored compound in the blood plasma, produced by the breakdown of hemoglobin following the normal or pathological destruction of red blood cells. It is collected by the liver to produce bile.

bilirubinuria: Presence of bilirubin in the urine. May be indicative of a liver or blood disorder.

biotin: Component of the vitamin B complex essential for the metabolism of fat and carbohydrates.

blast: Precursor of the final, mature form of a cell.

blastomycosis: Infection caused by the fungus *Blastomyces dermatitidis;* the infection can be cutaneous but usually affects the lungs.

bleb: Irregularly shaped elevation of the epidermis. A blister.

blepharoptosis: Drooping of the upper eyelid.

bradycardia: Abnormally slow heartbeat, generally characterized by a pulse rate below 60 beats per minute.

bradykinesia: Extreme slowness of movement.

bronchiole: One of the many smaller passages conveying air to the lung.

bruit: Abnormal noise of venous or arterial origin heard during auscultation.

bulla (pl. bullae): Large (generally greater than 0.5 cm) fluid-filled blister.

C

cachexia: Marked wasting away of the body, usually as a consequence of chronic disease.

calyx (pl. calyces): Cuplike extension of the renal pelvis that encloses the papilla of a renal pyramid; urine from the papillary duct empties into it.

carcinoembryonic antigen (CEA): A tumor marker indicating malignancies of the colon, stomach, pancreas, lungs, and breasts.

carcinogen: Any substance or agent that can produce cancer.

carcinoma in situ: Malignant cell changes in the epithelial tissue that do not extend beyond the basement membrane; "cancer in place."

cardiac tamponade: A life-threatening condition in which elevated pressures within the pericardium impair the filling of the heart during diastole.

cardiomegaly: Increase in the volume of the heart or the size of the heart muscle tissue.

cardioversion: Restoration of normal sinus rhythm by chemical or electrical means.

catatonia: Abnormality of movement and behavior arising from a disturbed mental state.

cellulitis: Inflammation of cellular or connective tissue.

cerebrospinal fluid: Clear fluid that bathes the ventricles of the brain and the central cavity of the spinal cord.

cervicitis: Inflammation of the cervix.

chancre: Firm, red, ulcerated sore. A chancre is the primary indication of syphilis; it occurs at the point of entry of the infection.

Cheyne-Stokes respiration: Breathing pattern disturbance characterized by a period of deep, rapid respirations followed by a period of shallow respirations or no respirations at all. The cycle rhythmically repeats every 45 seconds to 3 minutes.

Chiari malformation: A condition in which the inferior poles of the cerebellar hemispheres and the medulla protrude through the foramen magnum into the spinal canal. It is one of the causes of hydrocephalus and is usually accompanied by spina bifida cystica and meningomyelocele. Also called *Arnold-Chiari deformity*.

chromosome: In human cells, a linear structure in the nucleus composed of DNA and proteins and bearing part of the genetic information of the cell. Each human cell (except for egg or sperm cells) has 46 chromosomes, occurring in 23 pairs.

chyme: Nearly liquid mixture, composed of partially digested food and gastric secretions, that is found in the stomach and duodenum during digestion of a meal.

claudication: Lameness; limping.

clubbing: Condition characterized by bulbous swelling of the tips of the fingers and toes.

coccidioidomycosis: Also called *San Joaquin Valley fever*, it is caused by *Coccidioides immitis,* a fungus common in the dry desert soils of California, New Mexico, Nevada, and Arizona.

colectomy: Surgical removal of all or a portion of the colon.

comedo: Plug of dried, discolored fatty matter clogging a pore of the skin; commonly called a *blackhead*.

conization: Surgical removal of a cone of tissue, such as excision of cervical tissue for microscopic examination.

conjunctiva: Mucous membrane lining the eyelids.

contracture: Permanent shortening or contraction of a muscle, often producing physical distortion or deformity.

cordotomy: Surgical division of one or more of the lateral nerve pathways emerging from the spinal cord to relieve pain.

coryza: Common cold. An acute inflammation of the nasal mucous membrane accompanied by profuse nasal discharge.

craniotomy: Surgical incision through the cranium.

creatinine: Nitrogen-based compound formed in muscle tissue, passed into the bloodstream, and excreted in the urine. Elevated levels of creatinine in the blood may indicate a kidney disorder.

crepitation: Crackling sound, such as that produced by the grating ends of a broken bone.

cryoablation: A procedure to remove tissue through the use of extreme cold.

cyanosis: Bluish discoloration of the skin and mucous membranes due to an increased proportion of unoxygenated hemoglobin in the blood.

cystectomy: Removal of a cyst. Excision of the cystic duct and the gallbladder. Excision of all or part of the urinary bladder.

D

debridement: Removal of dead or damaged tissue or other matter, especially from a wound.

decompensate: Inability to maintain defense mechanisms in response to stress, resulting in personality disturbance or psychological imbalance.

delusion: A false belief brought about without appropriate external stimulation and inconsistent with one's own knowledge and experience.

deoxyribonucleic acid (DNA): An acid containing the genetic instructions used in the development and functioning of all living organisms.

diaphoresis: Sweating, especially when profuse or medically induced.

diastole: Period of cardiac muscle relaxation alternating with systole or contraction.

digoxin: The most frequently prescribed digitalis glycoside to treat clients with congestive heart failure, atrial fibrillation, atrial flutter, and supraventricular tachycardia.

dilatation: Expansion or enlargement of an organ or vessel.

dilation and curettage (D&C): The uterine cervical canal is expanded (dilated) to allow scraping (curettage) of the surface lining of the uterus.

diplopia: Double vision.

diuretic: Drug or agent that promotes the secretion of urine.

ductus arteriosus: Connection between the aorta and the pulmonary artery in the fetus; it allows most of the blood pumped by the left ventricle to bypass the lungs (which do not function in the fetus) and enter the systemic circulation. In some infants, the connection persists after birth; the condition is known as *patent ductus arteriosus.*

dysphagia: Difficulty in swallowing or inability to swallow.

dysphasia: Impairment of speech resulting from a brain lesion.

dysplasia: Alteration in size, shape, and organization of mature cells.

dyspnea: Labored or difficult breathing, generally indicating an insufficient amount of oxygen in the blood.

dystonia: Prolonged muscular contractions that may cause twisting (torsion) of body parts, repetitive movements, and increased muscular tone.

dysuria: Difficult or painful urination, symptomatic of numerous conditions.

E

echolalia: Involuntarily repeating words spoken by others.

edema: Excessive accumulation of fluid in bodily tissues. May be localized or general.

effacement: Dilation of the cervix.

effusion: Seeping of fluid into a body cavity or part.

electrodesiccation: Method of electrosurgery in which tissue is destroyed by dehydration with a probe generating a series of short, high-frequency electric sparks.

electrolytes: Ionized salts present in blood and tissue fluids and within cells. They are involved in all metabolic processes and are essential to the normal functioning of all cells.

embolism: Obstruction of a blood vessel by foreign substances or a blood clot.

embolus: Clot or undissolved mass carried through the circulatory vessels by the blood or lymph flow. An embolus may be a blood clot, piece of tissue, fat globule, or air bubble. (Compare with *thrombus.*)

empyema: An abscess caused by infected pleural fluid.

enanthems: Mucous membrane eruption.

en bloc: To remove as one piece (in surgery).

endophthalmitis: A bacterial or fungal infection inside the eye causing inflammation of the vitreous and/or aqueous humors.

endoplasmic reticulum: A network of sacs that manufactures, processes, and transports chemical compounds for use inside and outside the cell; responsible for the production of the protein and lipid components of most of the cell's organelles.

endorphin: One of a group of naturally occurring substances, produced by the central nervous system, that reduce the perception of pain. (See *enkephalin.*)

enkephalin: Substance produced in the brain that acts opiate-like and produces analgesia. (See *endorphin.*)

enteropathy: Any disease of the intestine.

epididymis (pl. epididymides): A small, oblong organ resting on and beside the posterior surface of a testis, consisting of a convoluted tube 13 to 20 feet long, enveloped in the tunica vaginalis, ending in the ductus deferens.

epigastric: Pertaining to the epigastrium, the region of the abdomen over the pit of the stomach.

epistaxis: Hemorrhage from the nose; a nosebleed.

epithelial: Pertaining to the layer of cells forming the outer surface of the body, the lining of the body cavities, and principal tubes and passageways.

erythema (erythematous): Diffused redness of the skin due to dilation of the superficial capillaries.

exanthems: Any eruption or rash of the skin (not the mucous membrane). Term often used to describe childhood or infectious rashes.

excoriation: Abrasion of the skin or the surface of any organ by trauma, chemical agents, burns, or other causes.

exfoliative cytology: Microscopic examination of cells that have been shed from or scaled off the surface epithelium. Performed for diagnostic purposes.

exophthalmos: Abnormal protrusion of the eyeball.

exudate: Fluid discharged through vessel walls and collected in adjacent tissue. It has a high content of protein and cellular debris. (Compare with *transudate*.)

F

fecalith: Hard, solid, intestinal mass formed around a core of fecal material.

fibrillation (ventricular): Cardiac arrhythmia characterized by the rapid, incomplete, and uncoordinated contractions of the muscle fibers of the heart ventricles. Can lead to cardiac arrest. (See *arrhythmia*.)

fibrinogen: A protein synthesized by the liver and present in blood plasma that is converted into fibrin through the action of thrombin in the presence of calcium ions.

fissure: Groove, natural division, cleft, slit, or deep furrow in organs; an ulcer or cracklike sore.

fistula: Abnormal tubelike passage from a normal cavity or tube to a free surface or cavity.

folate: Salt or ester of folic acid.

fontanel: Incompletely ossified space or soft spot between the cranial bones of the skull of a fetus or infant.

foramen magnum: Opening in the occipital bone through which the spinal cord passes from the brain.

G

ganglion: Mass of nervelike cell bodies lying outside the brain and spinal cord.

genotype: Description of the combination of genes of an individual, either with respect to a single trait or with respect to a larger set of traits. (Contrast with *phenotype*.)

gliadin: Water-soluble protein present in the gluten of wheat. The sticky mass that results when wheat flour and water are mixed is due to gliadin.

globulin: One of the plasma proteins to control osmotic pressure within capillaries.

glycogen: Molecule that is the principal storage form of glucose in human cells.

glycosuria: Presence of sugar, particularly glucose, in the urine.

goitrogens: Substances that cause goiters. These occur in nature in certain foods, including turnips, rutabagas, and cabbage.

gustatory: Associated with the sense of taste or eating.

H

hallucination: False perception having no relation to reality and not accounted for by exterior stimulus.

hematemesis: Vomiting blood.

hematochezia: Passage of bright red blood in the stool.

hematopoietic: Related to the formation of red blood cells.

hematuria: Blood in the urine.

hemiparesis: Paralysis affecting only one side of the body.

hemoglobin: Oxygen-carrying pigment in red blood cells.

hemolysis: Rupturing of red blood cells with the resulting release of hemoglobin into the plasma.

hemoptysis: Coughing and spitting up blood due to bleeding in any portion of the respiratory tract.

hemostasis: An arrest of bleeding or of circulation.

hepatomegaly: Enlargement of the liver.

heritability: Genetic or inheritable trait(s).

heterozygous: Possessing different genes from each parent for a particular trait.

hirsutism: Condition marked by excessive growth of hair in unusual places, especially in women.

histoplasmosis: Also called *Darling disease*, it is caused by *Histoplasma capsulatum*.

homeostasis: Tendency of the body systems to maintain stability even though they are exposed to continually changing outside forces.

homozygous: Possessing identical genes from each parent for a particular trait.

hydronephrosis: Swelling of the renal pelvis of the kidney with urine due to obstructed outflow.

hydroureter: Distention of the ureter with fluid due to obstructed outflow.

hyperchlorhydria: Excessive amount of hydrochloric acid in the stomach.

hyperglycemia: Abnormally high levels of glucose in the blood.

hyperkalemia: Excessive amount of potassium in the blood, usually caused by inadequate excretion of potassium or the shift of potassium from tissues.

hyperlipemia: Excess levels of fatlike substances called *lipids* in the blood.

hyperparathyroidism: Oversecretion of parathyroid hormone by the parathyroid glands.

hyperplasia: Overproliferation of normal cells within a normal tissue structure.

hypersomnia: Excessive daytime sleepiness.

hypertrophy: Increase in size or volume of an organ or other body structure that is produced entirely by an increase in the size of existing cells, not by an increase in the number of cells.

hypoalbuminemia: Abnormally low levels of a protein called *albumin* in the blood plasma.

hypoglycemia: Abnormally low levels of glucose in the blood.

hypophysectomy: Removal of the pituitary gland.

hypovolemic shock: Condition of severe physiologic distress caused by such a large decrease in the circulating blood volume that the body's metabolic needs cannot be met.

hypoxemia: Decreased oxygen in arterial blood.

hypoxia: Decreased concentration of oxygen in the inspired air and body tissues.

hysterosalpingography: Use of x-rays to visualize the uterus and fallopian tubes.

I

iatrogenic: Caused by treatment; for instance, an infection caused by a failure of surgical antiseptic precautions.

idiopathic: Of unknown cause.

ileostomy: Surgically created opening in the abdominal wall so the end of the lower small intestine (ileum) can be brought to the surface forming a stoma to evacuate feces. May be temporary or permanent.

incontinence: Inability to control the passage of urine, semen, or feces due to one or more physiological or psychological conditions.

induration: Area of hardened tissue; the process of hardening.

in situ: In place. (See *carcinoma in situ*.)

intoxication: Recent ingestion of a substance with significant behavioral or psychological changes.

intrathecal: Within the spinal canal or a sheath.

intromission: Insertion of the penis into the vagina.

ischemia: Temporary deficiency of blood in a body part due to a constriction or obstruction of a blood vessel.

J

jaundice: Condition characterized by a yellowish discoloration of the skin, whites of the eyes, and bodily fluids resulting from the accumulation of bilirubin in the blood. Caused by any of several disease processes in which the normal production and secretion of bile are disrupted.

K

keratin: Hard, fibrous protein that is the primary constituent of hair and nails.

keratolytic: Agent used to loosen and remove the outer layer of the epidermis.

ketoacidosis: Abnormally high concentrations in the blood or tissues of organic compounds called *ketone bodies*: beta-hydroxybutyric acid, acetoacetic acid, and acetone. It is sometimes called *ketosis*. The condition is frequently associated with diabetes mellitus.

ketone: A substance containing the carbonyl group attached to two carbon atoms. Acetone is an example of a simple ketone.

kyphoscoliosis: Abnormal backward and lateral curvature of the spine.

L

lacteals: Lymphatic capillaries in a villus of the small intestine that absorb fatty acids and other fat-soluble products of digestion.

leiomyoma: Tumor of smooth-muscle tissue.

leukopenia: Abnormal decrease in the number of circulating white blood cells.

lipiduria: Lipids in the urine.

lochia: Postpartum discharge of blood, mucus, and tissue from the uterus.

lumbar: Pertaining to the part of the back between the thorax and pelvis.

lumen: Space within an artery, vein, intestine, or other tubular structure.

luxation: Displacement of organs or articular surfaces; complete dislocation of a joint.

lymphadenopathy: Disease of the lymph nodes, usually manifested as swelling of the nodes.

lymphangitis: Inflammation of lymph vessels.

lymphocytopenia: Presence of abnormally small numbers of lymphocytes in the circulating blood.

M

macrophage: Any of the class of cells within the body tissues having the ability to engulf particular substances and microorganisms.

macula: Small, colored spot or thickening.

malaise: Generalized feeling of illness, discomfort, or depression indicative of some underlying disease or disorder.

maxillomandibular advancement: Surgical treatment for obstructive sleep apnea; both the upper jaw (maxilla) and lower jaw (mandible) are moved forward to enlarge the airway.

McBurney point: Point of special abdominal tenderness indicating acute appendicitis. It lies over and corresponds with the normal position of the appendix.

meconium: First feces of a newborn infant, made of salts, amniotic fluid, mucus, bile, and epithelial cells. The substance is greenish black, almost odorless, and tarry.

megakaryocyte: Large bone marrow cell with large or multiple nuclei. It gives rise to blood platelets.

meiosis: Process of two successive cell divisions, producing cells, egg, or sperm that contain half the number of chromosomes in somatic cells. When fertilization occurs, the nuclei of the sperm and ovum fuse and produce a zygote with the full chromosome complement.

melanin: Dark pigment that gives color to skin and hair.

menarche: Initial menstrual cycle, marking the onset of fertility.

meninges: Three membranes covering the brain and spinal cord.

menorrhagia: Excessive menstrual flow in duration or quantity, or both.

mesothelioma: A malignant tumor derived from the mesothelial cells of the pleura, peritoneum, or pericardium. It is found most often in smokers or persons with a history of exposure to asbestos.

metastasis (metastasize): Movement of bacteria or body cells, especially cancer cells, from one part of the body to the other, typically by way of the circulatory system.

metrorrhea: Abnormal uterine discharge.

microbiome: Consists of all the microorganisms that reside in the human body and how they react in a particular environment.

microcephaly: Abnormally small head.

micturition: Urination.

mitochondria: Microscopic cell organelle that contains enzymes for cell respiration.

Mohs micrographic surgery: A method of excising skin tumors a layer at a time until entire tumor is removed. Developed by Frederic Edward Mohs, U.S. surgeon.

mutism: Persistent inhibition of speech seen in some severe forms of mental illness.

myalgia: Muscle pain or tenderness.

myringotomy: Surgical incision of the tympanic membrane (eardrum).

N

nephrectomy: Removal of a kidney.

neuromodulator: Alteration in function or status in response to a stimulus of the nerve.

neuropathic pain: Discomfort that originates in peripheral nerves or the central nervous system rather than from damage in organs or tissues.

neuropeptides: Brain messengers responsible for mood, energy levels, pain and pleasure reception, body weight, and ability to solve problems; they also form memories and regulate the immune system.

neurotomy: Division or dissection of a nerve.

neurotransmitter: Substance produced and released by one neuron that travels across a synapse, exciting or inhibiting the next neuron in the neural pathway.

nevus (pl. nevi): Birthmark or mole; congenital discoloration of the skin due to abnormal pigmentation or vascular tumor.

nociceptive pain: Pain from tissue damage; may be sharp, dull, or aching but does not follow a nerve distribution.

nocturia: Excessive urination at night.

nonopioids: Nonopium drugs, formerly referred to as *nonnarcotic;* includes such drugs as acetaminophen and NSAIDs.

nosocomial: Occurring in a health-care setting.

nuchal rigidity: Stiff neck.

nystagmus: Rhythmic, involuntary movement of the eyeball.

O

occult blood: Minute quantities of blood in feces, urine, and gastric fluid, detectable only by microscopic examination or chemical test.

oliguria: Reduced urine secretion.

oogenesis: The creation of the mature human ovum.

opioids: Any synthetic or natural narcotic that relieves pain, with morphinelike activity.

orchiectomy: Surgical removal of a testis.

orchitis: Inflammation of the testes.

orthopnea: Respiratory condition in which there is discomfort breathing in any but erect standing or sitting positions.

Ortolani sign: The "clunk" felt when an examiner abducts (draws away from the body) and lifts the femurs of a supine infant. The clunk indicates a partial or an incomplete displacement of the hip.

osteomalacia: Disease caused by vitamin D deficiency in adults that causes soft, flexible, brittle, deformed bones.

P

palliative: Treatment provided to relieve the symptoms of a disease rather than to effect a cure.

pallor: Lack of color; paleness, as of the skin.

panhysterosalpingo-oophorectomy: Surgical removal of the entire uterus, including the cervix, ovaries, and fallopian tubes.

Papanicolaou test (smear): Diagnostic test for the early detection of cancer cells. Commonly called *Pap test* or *Pap smear*.

papule: Red, raised area of the skin, generally small and solid.

parasympathetic: Referring to a portion of the automatic (involuntary) nervous system. Activity of the parasympathetic nerves produces effects such as constriction of the pupil of the eye and slowed heart rate.

paresthesia: Sensation of numbness, prickling, or tingling.

parturition: Act of giving birth.

pathogenic: Capable of causing disease.

percussion: Diagnostic technique in which various body surfaces are tapped; the resulting sounds indicate the size, position, and general condition of underlying organs or structures.

pericardiocentesis: Surgical puncture of the membranous sac surrounding the heart to draw out fluid.

peristalsis: Involuntary wavelike contraction occurring along the walls of the hollow tubes of the body, especially the esophagus, stomach, and intestines.

petechia (pl. petechiae): A small, reddish or purplish pinpoint spot on a body surface, such as the skin or mucous membranes, caused by a minute hemorrhage.

pH: Degree of acidity or alkalinity of a solution, expressed in numbers from 0 to 14. Maximum acidity is pH 0 and maximum alkalinity is pH 14. A pH of 7 is neutral.

phacoemulsification: Ultrasonic device that disintegrates cataracts so they can be aspirated and removed.

phagocytosis: Ingestion and digestion of bacteria, other cells, and particles by a class of cells called *phagocytes.*

phenotype: Observable physical characteristics of an individual, determined by the combined influences of the individual's genetic makeup and the effects of environmental factors. (Contrast with *genotype.*)

photophobia: Unusual intolerance of light.

pleurectomy: Surgical excision of a portion of the pleura.

polycythemia vera: Chronic, life-shortening disorder of the bone marrow, involving the tissue producing blood cells. It is primarily characterized by abnormally high numbers of circulating red blood cells.

polydipsia: Excessive thirst.

polymorphonuclear leukocyte: White blood cell that possesses a nucleus composed of 200 or more lobes or parts.

polyphagia: Eating abnormally large amounts of food.

polyposis: Formation of numerous small growths or masses on a mucous membrane surface.

polyuria: Excessive formation and discharge of urine.

postural drainage: Therapeutic technique in which a client is directed to assume a variety of positions that facilitate the drainage of secretions in the lobes of the lungs or the bronchial passages.

prebiotics: A nutrient that stimulates the growth of bacteria living in the large intestine.

primigravida: Woman during her first pregnancy.

probiotics: Substance that has a health-promoting effect on living cells.

prostaglandins: Class of chemically related fatty acids present in many body tissues and having the ability to stimulate smooth-muscle contractions, lower blood pressure, and regulate or influence many other body functions.

prostate-specific antigen (PSA): A tumor marker widely used to detect and monitor prostatic cancer.

proteinuria: An excess of serum proteins in the urine.

prothrombin: A plasma protein coagulation factor synthesized by the liver that is converted to thrombin by prothrombinase and thrombokinase in the presence of calcium ions; sometimes referred to as *coagulation factor.*

pruritus: Severe itching.

pulmonary infarction: Death of a localized area of lung tissue resulting from an interruption of blood flow to that area. Generally caused by a pulmonary embolism.

purulent (discharge): Containing pus.

pustule: Small, raised area of the skin filled with pus or lymph.

pylorus (pyloric sphincter): Lower opening of the stomach leading into the duodenum. The pylorus is closed most of the time by the pyloric sphincter, a ring of muscles that opens at intervals to allow the flow of chyme into the duodenum.

pyoderma: Any acute, pus-causing, inflammatory skin disease.

pyuria: Pus in the urine.

R

radiofrequency catheter ablation: Destruction of electrical conduction pathways in the heart with an intracardiac catheter that removes the abnormal conducting tissue.

radioisotope: Radioactive form of an element. Some are commonly used for diagnostic or therapeutic purposes.

Raynaud phenomenon: Intermittent interruptions of blood supply to the fingers, toes, and sometimes the ears, marked by severe pallor of these parts and accompanied by numbness, tingling, or extreme pain.

Reed-Sternberg cells: Giant connective tissue cells with one or two large nuclei that are characteristic of Hodgkin disease.

reflux: Flowing back or return flow of fluid or other matter.

resection: Excision.

reticulocyte: Immature form of red blood cell, normally comprising about 1% of circulating red blood cells.

retinopathy: Any disease of the retina of the eye.

rhinitis: Inflammation of the nasal mucous membranes.

rhinophyma: Nodular swelling and congestion of the nose associated with acne rosacea.

rhonchus (pl. rhonchi): Rale or rattling in the throat, especially when it resembles snoring.

ribosomes: Microscopic cell organelles that produce proteins for cells.

S

sarcomas: A cancer arising from mesenchymal tissue, such as muscle or bone, which may affect the bones, bladder, kidneys, liver, lungs, parotids, and spleen.

sclerotherapy: Injecting irritating chemicals into vascular spaces or body cavities to harden, fill, or destroy them.

scotomata: Temporary, islandlike, blind gaps in the visual field.

seborrhea: Functional disease of the sebaceous glands marked by an increase in the amount, and often an alteration of the quality, of the sebaceous secretion.

sepsis: Microorganisms released into the bloodstream trigger inflammation throughout the body.

septic: Pertaining to disease-causing organisms or their toxins.

septum: Any wall between two cavities; for example, the atrial septum divides the right and left atria of the heart.

sequela: Condition that is the result of a disease.

serotonin: A chemical found in platelets, gastrointestinal mucosa, mast cells, and the central nervous system; its action on cellular receptors plays a role in intestinal motility, nausea and vomiting, sleep-wake cycles, obsessive-compulsive disorder, depression, and eating.

serous: Pertaining to serum.

somatic: Pertaining to sensation perceived as originating from superficial or muscular structures of the body rather than sensations seeming to come from the internal organs.

spermatogenesis: Process of creating a mature human sperm cell.

spirochete: Member of an order of microorganisms that have a slender, spiral shape.

sputum: Substance expelled by coughing or clearing the throat.

stapedectomy: Excision of the stapes in the ear in order to improve hearing, especially in cases of otosclerosis. The stapes is replaced by a prosthesis.

stratum corneum: Outermost or horny layer of the epidermis.

stridor: Harsh, high-pitched sound during respiration due to obstruction of air passages.

stupor: Condition of unconsciousness or lethargy.

suppurative: Pus producing.

syncope: Transient loss of consciousness due to inadequate blood flow to the brain.

syndrome: A group of symptoms or signs linked by a common pathological history.

syngeneic: Descriptive of individuals or cells without detectable tissue incompatibility.

systole: Contraction of the chambers of the heart; the myocardial fibers shorten, making the chamber smaller and forcing out blood.

T

tachycardia: Abnormally rapid heart beat, generally defined as exceeding 100 beats per minute.

tachypnea: Abnormal, very rapid breathing.

teratogen: Anything that adversely affects normal cellular development in the embryo or fetus. It may be certain chemicals, some therapeutic and illicit drugs, radiation, and intrauterine viral infections.

teratoma: Tumor composed of several different tissue types, none of which are normally found in the area of occurrence. Teratomas usually occur in the testes or ovaries.

tetany: Nervous condition characterized by sharp, painful, periodic muscle contractions, particularly those of the extremities.

thoracentesis: Surgical puncture of the chest wall to remove fluid from either of the pleural cavities.

thoracotomy: Surgical incision in the wall of the chest.

thrombocytosis: A condition pertaining to high platelet count in the blood.

thrombus: Blood clot formed along the wall of a blood vessel or in a cavity of the heart. It may be of sufficient size to obstruct blood flow; or all, or a portion, of it may break off to become an embolus. (*See embolus.*)

thyrotoxicosis: The overproduction of thyroid hormone.

Tinel sign: A cutaneous tingling sensation produced by pressing the nerve trunk that has been damaged or is regenerating following trauma; named for Jules Tinel, French neurologist.

tinnitus: Ringing, buzzing, tinkling, or hissing sound in the ear.

tolerance: Acquired resistance to the effects of a drug.

tonometer: Instrument to measure intraocular pressure.

tophus (pl. tophi): Calculus (stone) or mineral deposit in bone or tissue.

toxemia: Condition in which poisonous products of body cells at a local source of infection or derived from the growth of microorganisms are spread throughout the body in the blood.

transillumination: Visual inspection of a body structure or organ by passing a light through its walls.

transsphenoidal: Through or across the sphenoid bone.

transudate: Fluid discharged through a membrane or vessel wall. In contrast to an exudate, a transudate has a low content of protein or cellular debris.

transurethral resection: (Usually of prostate.) Visualizing the prostate through the urethra; removing tissue by electrocautery or sharp dissection.

tympanoplasty: Surgery to reconstruct or repair the eardrum.

U

urea: Chief nitrogenous constituent of urine.

uremia: Toxic condition associated with chronic renal failure and produced by excess levels of urea, creatinine, and other nitrogen-based compounds in the blood.

urolith: Concretion, or stone, within the urinary tract.

urticaria: Vascular reaction of the skin characterized by the temporary eruption of wheals; hives.

uvulopalatopharyngoplasty: A procedure that removes excess tissue in the throat to make the airway wider; often used to treat obstructive sleep apnea.

V

varices: Abnormally dilated and twisted veins, arteries, or lymph nodes.

varicocele: Dilation of the complex network of veins that comprise part of the spermatic cord to form a palpable swelling within the scrotum.

vasodilator: Drug or agent causing relaxation and expansion of the blood vessels.

vasopressin: Hormone secreted by the hypothalamus that raises blood pressure, increases peristalsis, and promotes resorption of water by the kidney. Synthetic or prepared extracts are administered as antidiuretics. Also known as *antidiuretic hormone* (ADH).

vertigo: Sensation of spinning around in space or of having objects spin around oneself.

villi (intestinal): Tiny fingerlike projections lining the interior of the small intestine that absorb fluid and nutrients.

virulence: Strength of a disease, its capacity to overcome the resistance of the organism.

visceral: Pertaining to the cavity containing internal organs.

W

wheal: Generally round, transient elevation of the skin, which is white in the center, with pale red edges; often accompanied by itching.

withdrawal: Negative physical symptoms that occur after periods of abstinence

Index

Page numbers followed by "f" denote figures, "t" denote tables, and "b" denote boxes.

Index of Diseases and Disorders

Page numbers followed by "f" denote figures, "t" denote tables, and "b" denote boxes.